Master the™
Nursing School
&
Allied Health
Entrance
Exams

20th Edition

PETERSON'S®

About Peterson's

Peterson's® has been your trusted educational publisher for over 50 years. It's a milestone we're quite proud of, as we continue to offer the most accurate, dependable, high-quality educational content in the field, providing you with everything you need to succeed. No matter where you are on your academic or professional path, you can rely on Peterson's for its books, online information, expert test-prep tools, the most up-to-date education exploration data, and the highest quality career success resources—everything you need to achieve your education goals. For our complete line of products, **visit www.petersons.com**.

For more information about Peterson's range of educational products, contact Peterson's, 8740 Lucent Blvd., Suite 400, Highlands Ranch, CO 80129, or find us online at **www.petersons.com**.

Peterson's Updates

Check out our website at **www.petersonspublishing.com/publishingupdates** to see if there is any new information regarding the test and any revisions or corrections to the content of this book. We've made sure the information in this book is accurate and up-to-date; however, the test format or content may have changed since the time of publication.

Table of Contents

PART I: INTRODUCTION

PART II: DIAGNOSING STRENGTHS AND WEAKNESSES

PART III: PRACTICE FOR REGISTERED NURSING SCHOOL ENTRANCE EXAMINATIONS

Contents

Contents

Before You Begin

Now that you've decided on a career in nursing or in one of the allied healthcare fields, you'll need to take an entrance exam for the coursework and degree or certificate that you want. Peterson's *Master the™ Nursing School & Allied Health Entrance Exams* can help you prepare for your test. This book provides review and practice in a variety of subjects so that you can develop the essential skills to do well on whichever test you are required to take.

HOW THIS BOOK IS ORGANIZED

Peterson's *Master the™ Nursing School & Allied Health Entrance Exams* is divided into five parts to facilitate your study and review.

- **Part I** provides an overview of starting your career in the nursing or allied health fields, selecting an educational program, and obtaining financial aid. You'll find an overview of the tests, including how they are organized, the topics they cover, the types and numbers of questions, how to apply to take them, and how they are administered, in addition to techniques on how to reduce text anxiety.

- **Part II** offers diagnostic tests to help you identify your strengths and those areas where you will need to spend more time preparing. This part is divided into three units, each containing a separate diagnostic test: one for those planning to test for registered nursing school, one for those planning to test for allied healthcare, and one for those planning to test for practical/vocational nursing school. New to this edition are English grammar and usage, spelling, and non-verbal ability questions, which appear in each of the three diagnostic tests. Also new to the diagnostic test for practical/vocational nursing school is a section on judgment and comprehension in practical nursing. In the verbal ability, mathematics, and science sections of each diagnostic test, the specific topic of the question is provided at the end of each answer explanation to aid in identifying the areas that you will need to spend more time on while preparing for your test.

- **Part III** focuses on the types of information and questions typically found on registered nursing school entrance exams. Review and practice exercises will help prepare you to answer questions testing your verbal and nonverbal abilities as well as your mathematics, science, and reading comprehension skills.

  - **New:** Unit 4 contains review and test questions on English grammar and usage, spelling, and nonverbal ability, to better reflect the types of questions that are included on the nursing and allied health entrance exams of the Psychological Services Bureau (PSB).

  - **New and Updated:** Unit 6 contains new and updated science content and practice tests pertaining to general biology, chemistry, and physics. Emphasis is on the description of the activities and characteristics of life with respect to humans.

- ○ **New:** Unit 8 introduces the Vocational Adjustment concept and provides sample questions similar the ones included on the PSB nursing and allied health school entrance exams.

- **Part IV** offers practice for allied health school entrance exams. Questions are provided in the areas of verbal and nonverbal ability, mathematics, science, and reading comprehension. The content review for verbal and nonverbal ability, mathematics, and reading comprehension provided in Part III is appropriate for Part IV as well.

  - ○ **New:** Unit 9 contains additional review and test questions on English grammar and usage, spelling, and nonverbal ability.

  - ○ **New and Updated:** Unit 11 contains new and updated science content and test questions pertaining to humans and their environment, astronomy, and environmental science.

- **Part V** tackles review and practice for the practical nursing and vocational nursing school entrance exams. The content review for verbal and nonverbal ability, mathematics, and reading comprehension provided in Part III is appropriate for Part V as well.

  - ○ **New:** Unit 13 contains new practice questions for English grammar and usage, spelling, and nonverbal ability.

  - ○ **New and Updated:** Unit 15 contains new and updated science content and practice tests pertaining to human anatomy and physiology, health, nutrition, and factors affecting your health and the environment.

  - ○ **New:** Unit 17 introduces the concept of Judgment and Comprehension in practical nursing and provides sample questions that pertain to using professional judgment in the nursing profession.

SPECIAL STUDY FEATURES

Peterson's *Master the™ Nursing School & Allied Health Entrance Exams* has several features that will help you get the most from your study time.

Overview

Review units begin with a listing of the major topics in each chapter followed by an introduction that explains what you will be reviewing in the chapter.

Bonus Information

You will find three types of notes in the margin of the book to alert you to important information about the test.

Note

Margin notes marked "Note" highlight information about the test structure itself.

Tip

A note marked "Tip" points out valuable advice for taking nursing and allied health school entrance exams.

Alert

An "Alert" identifies pitfalls in the testing format or question types that can cause mistakes in selecting answers.

HOW TO GET THE MOST OUT OF YOUR REVIEW

Plan to set aside time to study so that you can get the most out of your exam review. Begin by reading the "Top Ten Strategies to Raise Your Score," and then organize your schedule accordingly so that you can dedicate time to your review.

TOP 10 STRATEGIES TO RAISE YOUR SCORE

It's common to feel anxious about taking a test, especially a standardized test or a computer-based test. To help you deal with your anxiety, first, realize that anxiety can be productive. Anxiety can be energizing if you direct the energy toward your goals and away from negative thinking such as "I hate tests. I never do well on tests." Remember that admissions tests are only one thing that committees look at in determining to whom to offer admission. One way to lower your anxiety level is to prepare for the test you will be taking. Practicing ahead of time will boost your confidence. The following are 10 strategies to help you feel confident and do well on your entrance exam.

1. **Use one of the diagnostic tests as a tool.** Taking the diagnostic test that corresponds to your desired career field and studying the answers will help you identify the content that you need to spend the most time reviewing. The answer explanations include the topics and specific content for the verbal ability, math, and science questions, so you will have a quick-and-easy way to decide which topics to spend more time on.

2. **Schedule your study time.** Between now and the time you take your exam, set aside time each day at least six days per week to study. Try to give the same amount of time each day. Find a place that is conducive to studying.

3. **Budget your time on the topics.** Don't move too quickly through the material, but don't get bogged down and spend too much time on one or two topics. Be sure that you are comfortable with each topic before you move on to the next one, but avoid spending too much time early in your schedule on just a couple of topics and then having to rush through the end of your review.

4. **Memorize basic math rules.** Be sure that you know the basic math rules so that you have a firm grasp of what the basic rules are and how to apply them. This will help reduce your stress level.

5. **PRACTICE, PRACTICE, PRACTICE.** Practice may not get you a perfect score, but it will help you score better. Take the diagnostic test and complete each set of exercises in each unit.

6. **Establish a pacing schedule for taking each subtest.** Before you take a diagnostic test, work out what you think will be a reasonable pacing plan so that you can answer every question. Then set the timer and take the test. After you finish the test, see if your plan allowed you to answer all the questions without having to rush at the end. Make adjustments as needed and time yourself as you work through each set of practice tests.

Before the Test

7. **Find the location of the test center.** If you aren't familiar with the location of the test site, take a trial run to find it and find out how long it takes to get there. If you're driving, locate a parking lot or garage. This may seem like overkill, but who wants to arrive at the testing site with 5 minutes to spare and out of breath because you got lost on the way or spent 20 minutes trying to find a parking lot that turned out to be eight blocks away?

8. **Organize what you need for the test.** The night before the test, gather the forms of identification you need to bring with you, your admission ticket, and anything else you may need. The confirmation you received reserving your seat will tell you what you need and what you may not bring. If it doesn't, check the website for the test. Place the items you will bring in a spot where you will see them, such as on your bureau, the table by the door, or on the kitchen counter. Organizing ahead of time may seem unnecessary, but you don't want to waste time the day of the test searching for a photo ID to prove you are who you say you are.

During the Test

9. **Use the features that are given to you.** If you are taking a computer-based test, follow the onscreen instructions as the program explains the functions that are available for your use. Take any tutorial that is offered and be sure that you understand the program before you begin the test.

10. **Use the following general strategies as you work through the test.**

    *   Use your pacing plan.
    *   Skip and return to questions that you aren't sure about.
    *   Eliminate answer choices that you know are incorrect.
    *   Use educated guessing to rule out answers you aren't sure about.

YOU ARE WELL ON YOUR WAY TO SUCCESS

You have made the decision to apply to nursing school and have taken a very important step in that process. Peterson's *Master the™ Nursing School & Allied Health Entrance Exams* will help prepare you for everything you'll need to know on the day of your exam and help you score high on the exam. Good luck!

CHECK OUT OUR WEBSITE OR FIND US ON FACEBOOK, TWITTER, LINKEDIN, AND INSTAGRAM

Want additional test prep tips and advice? Check out **petersons.com** for our complete line of products as well as our insightful blog on the latest news and trends. Or you can join the conversation by liking us on Facebook (**facebook.com/petersons**) or tweeting **@Petersons** on Twitter. Have a LinkedIn profile? Link to Peterson's at **linkedin.com/company/peterson's** or check our library of photos and videos on Instagram **@petersons_com**.

GIVE US YOUR FEEDBACK

Peterson's publishes a full line of books—test prep, education exploration, financial aid, and career preparation. Peterson's publications can be found in high school guidance offices, college libraries and career centers, and your local bookstore or library. You can also find Peterson's books online at **petersons.com**.

We welcome any comments or suggestions you may have about this publication. Please call our customer service department at 800-338-3282 Ext. 54229 or send an email to custsvc@petersons.com. Your feedback will help us make educational dreams possible for you—and others like you.

PART I
INTRODUCTION

About Nursing and Allied Health Programs
and Examinations

About Nursing and Allied Health Programs and Examinations

OVERVIEW

- Getting on the Path to a Career in the Nursing and Allied Health Professions
- Selecting a Nursing Program
- Selecting an Allied Health Program
- Financial Aid Resources
- About the Examinations
- How to Apply to Take an Entrance Examination
- Administration of the Examinations
- Answering Test Questions
- Reducing Test Anxiety
- References

Nursing and allied healthcare professionals are in demand as the large baby boomer generation ages. In 2016, there were nearly 3 million registered nurses (RNs) employed, and the Bureau of Labor Statistics (2018a) projects that employment of RNs will grow by 15% from 2016 to 2026, which is much faster than average. The demand for licensed practical nurses (LPNs) and licensed vocational nurses (LVNs) is also projected to be high. In 2016, there were 724,500 LPNs and LVNs, and the projected growth for this career is 12% from 2016 to 2026, which is also faster than average (Bureau of Labor Statistics, 2018b). Generally, allied health professionals are either technicians (i.e., assistants) or therapists or technologists. In all, there are some 200 different allied health careers, including cardiovascular technologist, radiologic technician, chemotherapy technician, and respiratory therapist. Job openings for allied healthcare professionals are also expected to grow at rates faster than average.

GETTING ON THE PATH TO A CAREER IN THE NURSING AND ALLIED HEALTH PROFESSIONS

As you can see, the nursing and allied health fields offer many opportunities. The path to a fulfilling career in allied health is less defined than that for nursing because of the multiplicity

3

of choices available. According to **explorehealthcareers.org**, "there are five million allied health care providers in the United States, who work in more than 80 different professions and represent approximately 60% of all health care providers."

The type of training and degree or certificate required for an allied health career vary by career. The best strategy to determine the program you will need to realize your career ambitions is to talk to a career counselor, attend career fairs, and search the internet for information about potential careers in your area of interest. Look particularly for professional organizations and associations for healthcare providers. Check whether your specialty requires licensing. Once you have narrowed your choice down to a particular type of job or jobs, begin to search college, community college, and vocational school websites, depending on your potential career choice, for information on career preparation and coursework.

For those interested in a career in nursing, there are four kinds of programs that provide preparation for a nursing career:

1. LPN and LVN programs are usually offered in vocational schools, hospitals, and community colleges. The programs vary in length from 9 to 18 months. The courses include the basic sciences and medical-surgical, pediatric, and obstetrical nursing. Some mental health concepts are included. The major focus is on technical skills. An LPN or LVN works under the supervision of an RN.

2. Associate-degree RN programs are two-year college programs that balance clinical nursing courses (medical, surgical, psychiatric, obstetrical, and pediatric nursing) with general education courses (biological and physical sciences, behavioral sciences, humanities, and electives) to prepare students to make important judgments about patient care. The graduate is technically prepared to assess, plan, and deliver direct patient care in the hospital setting.

3. Hospital-based diploma RN programs prepare students in the same manner as the associate-degree RN programs to function on the nursing team. Most diploma programs are 24 to 30 months long, and the non-nursing courses may be offered through a college.

4. Baccalaureate RN programs are four years long and are offered in colleges and universities. The required courses in the biological, physical, and behavioral sciences are both basic and advanced. These general education requirements, along with courses that provide a broad liberal arts education, are taken during the first two years. The major clinical courses are offered in the third and fourth years and include the five clinical areas previously identified, with an emphasis on community health nursing and the role of the professional nurse as manager. Most nursing programs offering the professional baccalaureate degree admit graduates from the diploma and associate-degree programs with varying degrees of advanced standing.

The graduates of all four programs take a licensing examination. At the current time, there are two kinds of licenses: the practical nurse license and the RN license for graduates of the diploma, associate-degree, and baccalaureate-degree programs.

A nurse may continue studies to receive a master's degree or a doctorate with a major in clinical specialties, teaching, administration, or research, depending on their career choice. There is a great demand for nurses in hospitals, schools, clinics, public health agencies, and many other settings throughout the world. Nurses may enter the military or become anesthetists, writers, consultants, or private practitioners. Nursing provides a foundation for many career opportunities and, more important, a personally and financially satisfying vocation.

Regardless of which kind of nursing program you choose to enter, you will have opportunities to provide an important service. You may enter nursing at one level and expand your skills through practice and additional education. Advancement within the nursing profession comes about in several ways. A practical nurse may decide to become an RN, an upward move. An RN may decide to move from the hospital setting into community-based care, a lateral move that expands the types of services a nurse can provide. An RN who does not have a baccalaureate degree may decide to earn one to step up to a management position.

SELECTING A NURSING PROGRAM

The first factor you should consider when selecting a nursing program is your career goal. Do you plan to work in a hospital or as a member of the health team? Is your ultimate goal to function as a manager or an administrator? Are you primarily interested in teaching? Do you want to specialize in a specific clinical area? Are you planning to work in a community setting, providing services to families? Is your ultimate goal to become an entrepreneur?

The trend today is to license two levels of nursing for entry into the professional services. The assistant level is represented by graduates of the associate-degree nursing programs; the professional level, by graduates of the baccalaureate nursing programs. Baccalaureate education in nursing forms the foundation for graduate education in nursing, where specialization as a clinical practitioner, administrator, or teacher occurs. Other types of graduates (practical nurse and diploma) may achieve these credentials through career mobility programs.

A second factor to consider is cost. The demands of full-time study and the length of the program may necessitate resigning from your current job.

A third factor is your qualification for admission. As the levels of performance increase, so do the academic requirements.

Once you have matched your career goals with a program, you should answer the following questions to help finalize your program choice.

- Is the program approved by the state regulating body?
- Is the program accredited by a voluntary agency?
- What is the program's reputation in terms of graduate performance?
- How do the social and academic environments meet your needs?

SELECTING AN ALLIED HEALTH PROGRAM

Occupations related to allied health are rapidly expanding. The criteria for selecting a program are similar to those for nursing:

- If a license is required to practice, be certain that the program is approved by the regulating body.

- Check to see whether the program is accredited by the appropriate voluntary agency.
- Find out how well the graduates are performing on the licensing examination.
- Consider how well the program meets your short- and long-term career goals.

FINANCIAL AID RESOURCES

Federal financial aid has not kept pace with the increasing cost of postsecondary education. Therefore, it is important to be familiar with sources of funding, eligibility requirements, and application procedures. It is also important to apply as early as possible to a variety of programs.

To apply, complete the Free Application for Federal Student Aid (FAFSA) form online at **https:// fafsa.ed.gov/**. Alternatively, you may obtain a paper copy of the FAFSA from your local high school counseling office, the school to which you are seeking admission, or online from the Department of Education. In a few days (if you applied online) or in approximately six weeks (if you applied using the paper copy), a report is sent back indicating whether you are eligible for financial aid. The schools you identified when filling out the FAFSA receive similar reports so that the amount of aid for which you are eligible and the amount you will have to pay out-of-pocket can be determined.

The amount of money you can receive depends on the need analysis derived from the financial aid form and the financial aid program in which the school, college, or university is participating. The school usually prepares a financial aid package that includes a combination of financial sources to make up the difference between the amount you and your family can contribute and the total costs of the program.

Some financial aid funding sources are loans, which must be paid back at a low interest rate over a prolonged period of time. Other funding sources are grants and scholarships, which do not have to be paid back. The obligation for debt payment requires serious thought, because a default on a loan can affect your credit rating.

When shopping for financial aid, check the accreditation status of the nursing or allied health program and the institution's eligibility for aid. Most accredited nursing or allied health programs are eligible for federal funding, but some institutions have limited federal sources due to high default rates.

Federal Pell Grants

Pell Grants are awarded to students with financial need who have not received their first bachelor's degree or who are enrolled in certain postbaccalaureate programs that lead to teacher certification or licensure. The grant does not have to be repaid and may be supplemented by other funds. Eligibility is based on need, which is calculated by a formula. The amounts of the awards vary yearly and depend on program funding. The maximum award for the 2018–2019 award year was $6,095 per year. You do not have to be a full-time student; however, the amount you receive as a part-time student will be proportionate to your attendance.

Stafford Loans

Stafford loans are offered in two types of loans: Direct Subsidized Loans and Direct Unsubsidized Loans. Direct Subsidized Loans are awarded based on need and do not accrue interest before the repayment period begins as long as you are at least a half-time student or during periods of deferment.

Direct Unsubsidized Loans are not based on need and accrue interest from the time of disbursement. Dependent undergraduate students may borrow $5,500 for the first year, $6,500 for the second year, and $7,500 for the third year and beyond. Independent students and dependent students whose parents are unable to obtain PLUS loans may borrow $9,500, $10,500, and $12,500 for years 1, 2, 3, and beyond, respectively.

PLUS Loans

PLUS loans enable parents with stable credit histories to borrow for the education expenses of each dependent child who is an undergraduate student enrolled at least half-time. The annual maximum is equal to the cost of attendance minus any additional financial aid the student receives.

Consolidation Loans

These loans are designed to help students and parents simplify loan repayment by consolidating several types of federal loans into one loan with one repayment schedule. Student loans cannot be consolidated until they enter repayment.

Campus-Based Programs (Administered by the Financial Aid Office)

Federal Supplemental Educational Opportunity Grants are for undergraduates with exceptional financial need; students who received Federal Pell Grants are given priority in awarding these grants. Students can receive from $100 to $4,000 per year, depending on financial need, the funding at the school, and the school's financial aid policies.

Federal Work Study provides a work-study program for undergraduate and graduate students in financial need. Students are able to earn money through community service and work related to their course of study.

For additional information on federal loans and other aid, visit **https://studentaid.ed.gov/sa/**.

Other Sources of Financial Aid

Peterson's *Scholarships, Grants & Prizes* is a helpful source for information on foundations, religious organizations, fraternities and sororities, and civic groups that provide scholarships and/or loans for educational purposes. In addition, the military offers scholarships through its Reserve Officers' Training Corps (ROTC) Program and through the G.I. Bill for former members of the Armed Services. You should also seek out resources from the organizations related to your field of interest.

ABOUT THE EXAMINATIONS

Each nursing or allied health program selects the entrance examination it requires its applicants to take. Entrance exams aid programs in evaluating the level of preparedness and aptitude of applicants so that they can admit the most qualified applicants. Many different entrance exams are available. Several of the most common of these are covered in this book. These exams are listed according to program type here and then discussed below in greater detail. Moreover, a representative mix of test question types from all of these exams is included in the diagnostic test and all practice tests throughout the book, to ensure that you are well prepared to take any of these exams.

RN program entrance exams:

- Pre-Admission Exam (PAX)
- Psychological Services Bureau (PSB) Registered Nursing School Aptitude Examination (PSB-RN)
- Test of Essential Academic Skills (TEAS)

Allied health program entrance exams:

- PSB Health Occupations Aptitude Examination (PSB-HO)
- TEAS

LPN/LVN program entrance exams:

- PAX
- PSB Aptitude for Practical Nursing Examination (PSB-PN)
- TEAS

PAX

The PAX, developed by the National League for Nursing (NLN), is an entrance exam for applicants to both RN and LPN/LVN programs. Revised in 2016, it now combines in one test what had been previously two separate tests, one for admission to RN programs (NLN-RN) and one for admission to LPN/LVN programs (NLN-PN).

Below are some key points about this exam:

- Computer-based administration
- Four-option multiple-choice question format throughout
- Divided into three main sections
- A total of 160 questions, duration of 2 hours
- Use of calculators determined by each school

The sections of the PAX, as well as the topics, number of questions, and time limit per section, are shown in the table below.

| Section | Subsection | Topics | Items | | Time Limit (min) |
			No.	% of Total	
Verbal	Reading (*Note:* Each passage is 300–450 words.)	Passage 1: 8th–9th grade level	6	N/A	N/A
		Passage 2: 9th–10th grade level	6		
		Passage 3: 10th–11th grade level	6		
		Passage 4: 11th–12th grade level	6		
		Passage 5: 13th–14th grade level	6		
	Subsection Total:		30	19	
	Word knowledge	8th grade level	4	N/A	
		9th grade level	6		
		10th grade level	6		
		11th grade level	5		
		12th grade level	4		
		13th grade level	3		
		14th grade level	2		
	Subsection Total:		30	19	
Section Total:			60	38	45
Mathematics (*Note:* Questions are divided evenly between computation and word problems.)	N/A	Integers	3	N/A	
		Decimals	5		
		Fractions	5		
		Percentages	6		
		Ratio conversion	4		
		Measurement conversion	5		
		Algebra	5		
		Geometry	3		
		Mathematical concepts	4		
Section Total:			40	25	35
Science (*Note:* Cognitive skills are integrated into the general questions, so there are 60 *total* questions in this section.)	General	Biology	20	N/A	
		Human anatomy	7		
		Human physiology	7		
		Physics	5		
		Chemistry	13		
		Health	8		
	Subsection Total:		60		
	Cognitive skills (*Note:* Derived from Bloom's taxonomy.)	Identify facts & terms	18		
		Recognize process & principle	12		
		Apply principle to situation	12		
		Apply research & measurement	9		
		Interpret chart, graph, diagram	9		
	Cognitive Skills Total (integrated into Science questions):		60		
Section Total:			60	37	45
Exam Total:			**160**	**100**	**125**

For more information about the PAX, contact:

>NLN Testing Services
>2408A Lebanon Ave.
>Shiloh, IL 62221
>800-732-8656
>customerhelp@nln.org
>**www.nln.org/testing-services**

PSB Exams

The PSB has developed three different entrance exams: one for admission to RN programs (PSB-RN), one for admission to health occupations programs (PSB-HO), and one for admission to LPN/LVN programs (PSB-PN). Although each is geared to evaluate the readiness of applicants to enter and succeed in its specific program type, all share a common format and therefore are presented together in this section, with differences among them clearly indicated.

Below are some key points about these exams:

- Computer-based or paper-based administration, depending on each school's preference
- Different question formats for different sections, including the following:
  - Three-option multiple-choice (Spelling section)
  - Four-option multiple-choice (Reading Comprehension and Judgment & Comprehension in Practical Nursing Situations sections)
  - Five-option multiple-choice (Academic Aptitude and Information in the Natural Sciences sections)
  - Agree/disagree (Vocational Adjustment Index section)
- Divided into five main sections and three subsections
- PSB-RN and PSB-HO (each): A total of 360 questions, duration of 2 hours and 45 minutes
- PSB-PN: A total of 370 questions, duration of 3 hours
- Use of calculators not permitted, but scratch paper available

The sections of the PBS exams, as well as the topics, number of questions, and time limit per section, are shown in the table below.

Exam	Section	Subsection	Topics	Items		Time Limit (min)
				No.	% of Total	
PSB-RN	Academic aptitude	Verbal	Vocabulary	30	N/A	30
		Arithmetic	Skill & computational speed	30		30
		Nonverbal	Form relationships, shapes, reasoning	30		30
	Section Total:			90	25	90
	Spelling	N/A	Written expression, communication skills	50	14	15
	Reading comp.		Interpretation; comprehension; inferring ideas, purposes, intent	40	11	15
	Natural sciences		Biology, chemistry, health, safety	90	25	30
	Vocational adjustment		Lifestyle, educational & occupational adjustment	90	25	15
Exam Total:				**360**	**100**	**165**
PSB-HO	Academic aptitude	Verbal	Vocabulary	30	N/A	30
		Arithmetic	Skill & computational speed	30		30
		Nonverbal	Form relationships, shapes, reasoning	30		30
	Section Total:			90	25	90
	Spelling	N/A	Written expression, communication skills	50	14	15
	Reading comp.		Interpretation; comprehension; inferring ideas, purposes, intent	40	11	15
	Natural sciences		Biology, chemistry, health, safety	90	25	30
	Vocational adjustment		Lifestyle, educational & occupational adjustment	90	25	15
Exam Total:				**360**	**100**	**165**
PSB-PN	Academic aptitude	Verbal	Vocabulary	30	N/A	30
		Arithmetic	Skill & computational speed	30		30
		Nonverbal	Form relationships, shapes, reasoning	30		30
	Section Total:			90	24	90
	Spelling	N/A	Written expression, communication skills	50	14	15
	Natural sciences		Biology, chemistry, health, safety	90	24	30
	Judgment & comp. in PN situations		Judgment in working situations	50	14	30
	Vocational adjustment		Lifestyle, educational & occupational adjustment	90	24	15
Exam Total:				**370**	**100**	**180**

For more information about the PSB exams, contact:

> PSB, Inc.
> 977 Seminole Trail #317
> Charlottesville, VA 22901
> 434-293-5865
> support@psbtests.com
> **www.psbtests.com**

TEAS

The TEAS, developed by Assessment Technologies Institute (ATI), is an entrance exam for applicants to RN, LPN/LVN, and allied health programs and is normed for each program type separately. The TEAS was revised in 2016 to better align its content with current education standards. The new version, known as "ATI TEAS," replaces the TEAS V.

Below are some key points about this exam:

- Computer-based or paper-based administration, depending on each school's preference
- Four-option multiple-choice question format throughout
- Divided into four main sections
- A total of 170 questions, duration of 3 hours and 29 minutes
- Use of four-function calculators permitted, provided by the testing center

The sections of the TEAS, as well as the topics, number of questions, and time limit per section, are shown in the table below.

Section	Topics	Items		Time Limit (min)
		No.	% of Total	
Reading	Key ideas & details	22	N/A	
	Craft & structure	14		
	Integration of knowledge & ideas	11		
	Pre-test questions	6		
Section Total:		53	31	64
Mathematics	Number & algebra	23	N/A	
	Measurement & data	9		
	Pre-test questions	4		
Section Total:		36	22	54
Science	Human anatomy & physiology	32	N/A	
	Life & physical sciences	8		
	Scientific reasoning	7		
	Pre-test questions	6		
Section Total:		53	31	63
English & language usage	Conventions of standard English	9	N/A	
	Knowledge of language	9		
	Vocabulary acquisition	6		
	Pre-test questions	4		
Section Total:		28	16	28
Exam Total:		**170**	**100**	**209**

For more information about the TEAS, contact:

ATI, LLC
11161 Overbrook Road
Leawood, KS 66211
800-667-7531
www.atitesting.com

HOW TO APPLY TO TAKE AN ENTRANCE EXAMINATION

Different institutions have different requirements and arrangements for testing. Admissions information provided by schools typically lists the exam that you need to take and contact information for the test maker or test administrator, if the latter is different. Typically, you must register online to take the entrance exam. Once at the test provider's website, you should be able to find testing center locations and testing schedules. Register as soon as possible, because testing centers fill up on a first-come, first-served basis. Follow the registration instructions carefully and be sure to download the confirmation email and admission ticket.

The website should also provide specific information about the format and makeup of the exam. Be sure to download this information, as well.

ADMINISTRATION OF THE EXAMINATIONS

The entrance exams are administered by qualified persons at a testing center. Pay careful attention to the information on the testing center's website or in your confirmation email about what you may bring to the test site and what you may have in the exam room with you. Different tests and different testing centers, for example, vary on whether they allow the use of calculators during the exam.

The proctor overseeing the exam administration gives specific instructions for taking the exam. If there is a tutorial for a computer-based test, take it so that you become familiar with the functions that the program has available to you. All tests are timed. Depending on the length of the test, you may or may not have a break. The proctor should tell you when to begin and when to stop.

Some computer-based exams provide a score report immediately on completion. Others send a report within 24–48 hours after completing the exam. Information available from the test maker should describe the process of reporting scores to the institutions you are applying to.

ANSWERING TEST QUESTIONS

Studying the more than 2,200 test questions in this book, which are similar to the questions included in the entrance examinations, enables you to review material you already know, gain new knowledge, and become familiar with the format of timed tests.

After completing the overview of a section, answer the sample test questions. Like the ones on the real exams, the questions in this book are multiple-choice. You are not penalized for incorrect answers in these exams, so use educated guessing if you do not know the answer or aren't sure. A good strategy is to go through the entire test, answering the questions you know, and then go back and make educated guesses for the questions you don't know. Here's how to make an educated guess:

- Carefully read the question (the stem). Look for the clues or the main ideas in the stem that will lead you to the correct answer.

- Go through the entire examination, answering all the questions that you feel sure about. This will give you an overall idea of what the test is about and lessen the time pressure. You may even run across related information that will help you to answer the questions you don't know.

- Now go back to those items you didn't answer and use the test-taking techniques. First, look for the key word(s) or clue(s) in the stem. Keeping that in mind, try to eliminate the choices that do not relate to the clue. Look at the remaining choices to identify similarities to and differences from the stem or clue. Compare the differences with the clue to see if you can eliminate another choice. Select the remaining choice.

Example:

Which of the following observations may be an indication of high blood pressure?
A. Flushed skin
B. Pale skin
C. Cold skin
D. Weak pulse

What is the clue?

Answer: high pressure

Can I eliminate any choices?

Answer: Yes. There is a direct relationship between pressure and force; therefore, choice D cannot be the correct answer.

What are the similarities and differences among choices A, B, and C?

Answer: They all relate to changes in skin characteristics. However, choices B and C are similar. As a matter of fact, if choice B were correct, choice C would also be correct.

The correct answer, then, is choice A.

Now, let's assume that the following question is also on the test.

Why do some people with high blood pressure have flushed skin?
A. The pulse weakens, and blood pools in the skin.
B. The skin temperature lowers, and the skin blood vessels dilate.
C. The increased pressure increases the volume of blood to the arteries.
D. The increased pressure forces the arteries to dilate.

Based on your experience with the previous item, you would immediately eliminate choices A and B. Looking at choices C and D, you might think that both would cause reddened skin. However, you would either eliminate choice D because it contradicts the relationship between pressure and volume, or you would select choice C because it supports the relationship between pressure and volume.

PLEASE PRACTICE THIS TECHNIQUE WITH THE SAMPLE ITEMS!

A summary of the seven steps for preparing to take a nursing school or allied health school entrance examination follows:

1. Study the concepts and principles presented in each section so that you will have a good base of knowledge.

2. Study one section at a time over a period of time—whatever is reasonable for your learning style. Do not cram!

3. Take the tests related to each section immediately after studying the explanatory materials.

4. Follow all directions for each test carefully.

5. Use the guidelines for test taking as presented in this section.

6. Check your answers to diagnose your strengths and weaknesses.

7. Seek additional information from reliable resources in the areas in which you are weak.

REDUCING TEST ANXIETY

Anxiety results from a threat to our well-being that might be real or perceived. This threat makes us uncomfortable and affects our feelings of self-esteem. We then change our behavior in an attempt to seek relief.

Many people become anxious about taking a test because they anticipate that someone is going to make a judgment about them based on their test performance. Is your self-esteem strong enough for you to think, "I can pass this test!"? Or do you lack confidence in yourself and assume, "I am going to fail?"

What can you do to prevent this kind of negative thinking? First, you must realize that anxiety can be both productive and destructive. Anxiety can be energizing if you direct the energy toward your goals and away from the imagined threats. For example, you may have the idea that the admission test will determine your entire future. If you don't pass the test, you imagine that you won't be admitted to the program of your choice. The fact is that admission tests are used along with many other kinds of information to determine your eligibility for entering a program. Therefore, this is not a real threat. On the other hand, if you have made no effort to prepare for this test, then your chances for admission might be threatened.

The secret to success is confidence. You can gain that confidence by completing the practice tests in this book and achieving a score of 80% or above in all areas. This should assure you that you can perform well on the admission test.

Below are a few suggestions on how to reduce test anxiety.

- Set up a time-frame for studying this book. Schedule a few pages per day to avoid a last-minute rush.

- Sharing your anxiety helps to reduce it. Talk to a friend. Explore the "what if" situations and the related options for achieving your career goals.

- Provide an outlet for yourself—perhaps exercise or engage in some other physical activity that you enjoy.

- Think back to how you have handled stress and anxiety in your past experiences. Draw on those experiences.

- Positive thinking is a must. Imagine yourself receiving the results of your test enclosed in a letter of congratulations that you share with your family and friends. Make plans for the next step toward achieving your career goals. Imagine the pleasurable feeling and comfort that comes from a job well done. You'll do just fine!

REFERENCES

Bureau of Labor Statistics, U.S. Department of Labor. (2018a). *Occupational Outlook Handbook: Registered Nurses.* Retrieved from **www.bls.gov/ooh/healthcare/registered-nurses.htm**.

Bureau of Labor Statistics, U.S. Department of Labor. (2018b). *Occupational Outlook Handbook: Licensed Practical and Licensed Vocational Nurses.* Retrieved from **www.bls.gov/ooh/healthcare/registered-nurses.htm**.

U.S. Department of Education, Office of Federal Student Aid. (n.d.a). Subsidized and unsubsidized loans. Retrieved from **https://studentaid.ed.gov/sa/types/loans/subsidized-unsubsidized**.

U.S. Department of Education, Office of Federal Student Aid. (n.d.b). FSEOG (Grants). Retrieved from **https://studentaid.ed.gov/sa/types/grants-scholarships/fseog**.

U.S. Department of Education, Office of Federal Student Aid. (n.d.c). Perkins Loans. Retrieved from **https://studentaid.ed.gov/sa/types/loans/perkins**.

U.S. Department of Education. (2015). Federal Pell Grant Program. Retrieved from **https://www2.ed.gov/programs/fpg/index.html**.

PART II
DIAGNOSING STRENGTHS AND WEAKNESSES

Diagnostic Test for Registered Nursing School

Part II is divided into the following three units:

- Unit 1—Diagnostic Test for Registered Nursing School
- Unit 2—Diagnostic Test for Allied Health School
- Unit 3—Diagnostic Test for Practical/Vocational Nursing School

Each diagnostic test is divided further into six sections: Verbal Ability, Mathematics, Spelling, Nonverbal Ability, Science, and Reading Comprehension. Unit 3 contains a unique seventh section for Judgment and Comprehension in Practical Nursing. The question types are similar to what you will find on each exam.

At the end of each unit, you will find Answer Keys and Explanations. At the end of each explanation in the verbal ability, math, and science sections, you will find the topic or theme assessed in that question. This information will help you identify areas that you should spend more time on as you study and prepare for your exam.

Each section of each diagnostic test begins with directions and a time limit. Set a timer for that amount of time and see how you do answering all the questions in the specific time limit. Knowing how long it takes you will help you determine a pacing plan for each section of the actual exam.

Choose the diagnostic test that matches the career that you are pursuing and complete it to see your strengths and those areas that you need to improve on.

UNIT 1 DIAGNOSTIC TEST FOR REGISTERED NURSING SCHOOL ANSWER SHEET

Verbal Ability

1. Ⓐ Ⓑ Ⓒ Ⓓ   3. Ⓐ Ⓑ Ⓒ Ⓓ Ⓔ   5. Ⓐ Ⓑ Ⓒ Ⓓ   7. Ⓐ Ⓑ Ⓒ Ⓓ   9. Ⓐ Ⓑ Ⓒ Ⓓ

2. Ⓐ Ⓑ Ⓒ Ⓓ   4. Ⓐ Ⓑ Ⓒ Ⓓ Ⓔ   6. Ⓐ Ⓑ Ⓒ Ⓓ   8. Ⓐ Ⓑ Ⓒ Ⓓ   10. Ⓐ Ⓑ Ⓒ Ⓓ

Mathematics

1. Ⓐ Ⓑ Ⓒ Ⓓ   3. Ⓐ Ⓑ Ⓒ Ⓓ   5. Ⓐ Ⓑ Ⓒ Ⓓ   7. Ⓐ Ⓑ Ⓒ Ⓓ   9. Ⓐ Ⓑ Ⓒ Ⓓ

2. Ⓐ Ⓑ Ⓒ Ⓓ   4. Ⓐ Ⓑ Ⓒ Ⓓ   6. Ⓐ Ⓑ Ⓒ Ⓓ   8. Ⓐ Ⓑ Ⓒ Ⓓ   10. Ⓐ Ⓑ Ⓒ Ⓓ

Spelling

1. Ⓐ Ⓑ Ⓒ   3. Ⓐ Ⓑ Ⓒ   5. Ⓐ Ⓑ Ⓒ   7. Ⓐ Ⓑ Ⓒ   9. Ⓐ Ⓑ Ⓒ

2. Ⓐ Ⓑ Ⓒ   4. Ⓐ Ⓑ Ⓒ   6. Ⓐ Ⓑ Ⓒ   8. Ⓐ Ⓑ Ⓒ   10. Ⓐ Ⓑ Ⓒ

Nonverbal Ability

1. Ⓐ Ⓑ Ⓒ Ⓓ Ⓔ   3. Ⓐ Ⓑ Ⓒ Ⓓ Ⓔ   5. Ⓐ Ⓑ Ⓒ Ⓓ Ⓔ   7. Ⓐ Ⓑ Ⓒ Ⓓ Ⓔ   9. Ⓐ Ⓑ Ⓒ Ⓓ Ⓔ

2. Ⓐ Ⓑ Ⓒ Ⓓ Ⓔ   4. Ⓐ Ⓑ Ⓒ Ⓓ Ⓔ   6. Ⓐ Ⓑ Ⓒ Ⓓ Ⓔ   8. Ⓐ Ⓑ Ⓒ Ⓓ Ⓔ   10. Ⓐ Ⓑ Ⓒ Ⓓ Ⓔ

Science

1. Ⓐ Ⓑ Ⓒ Ⓓ   3. Ⓐ Ⓑ Ⓒ Ⓓ   5. Ⓐ Ⓑ Ⓒ Ⓓ   7. Ⓐ Ⓑ Ⓒ Ⓓ   9. Ⓐ Ⓑ Ⓒ Ⓓ

2. Ⓐ Ⓑ Ⓒ Ⓓ   4. Ⓐ Ⓑ Ⓒ Ⓓ   6. Ⓐ Ⓑ Ⓒ Ⓓ   8. Ⓐ Ⓑ Ⓒ Ⓓ   10. Ⓐ Ⓑ Ⓒ Ⓓ

Reading Comprehension

1. Ⓐ Ⓑ Ⓒ Ⓓ   3. Ⓐ Ⓑ Ⓒ Ⓓ   5. Ⓐ Ⓑ Ⓒ Ⓓ   7. Ⓐ Ⓑ Ⓒ Ⓓ   9. Ⓐ Ⓑ Ⓒ Ⓓ

2. Ⓐ Ⓑ Ⓒ Ⓓ   4. Ⓐ Ⓑ Ⓒ Ⓓ   6. Ⓐ Ⓑ Ⓒ Ⓓ   8. Ⓐ Ⓑ Ⓒ Ⓓ   10. Ⓐ Ⓑ Ⓒ Ⓓ

answer sheet

Verbal Ability

10 Questions • 5 Minutes

Directions: For questions 1 and 2, one word is italicized in the sentence shown. Following each sentence are four words or phrases. For each sentence, choose the word or phrase that most nearly corresponds in meaning with the italicized word.

1. The hungry crowd regarded the arrival of the food truck as *auspicious*.
   - A. miraculous
   - B. surprising
   - C. favorable
   - D. ominous

2. The old man had faced many dramatic *vicissitudes* of fortune in his life and thus had learned to adapt to his circumstances, whether good or bad.
   - A. downfalls
   - B. improvements
   - C. repetitions
   - D. changes

Directions: For questions 3 and 4, choose the word that is most different in meaning from the others.

3. A. agitated
   - B. halcyon
   - C. peaceful
   - D. harmonious
   - E. serene

4. A. deleterious
   - B. salubrious
   - C. noxious
   - D. detrimental
   - E. harmful

Directions: For questions 5–7, determine the relationship between the first pair of capitalized words and then decide which of the answer choices shares a similar relationship with the third capitalized word.

5. STEADFAST : WAVERING :: ADAMANTINE :
   - A. pliable
   - B. unreliable
   - C. unyielding
   - D. faithful

6. FISHERMAN : DOCK :: HUNTER :
   - A. gun
   - B. deer
   - C. forest
   - D. tree stand

7. SMOKING : CANCER :: EXERCISE :
   - A. exhaustion
   - B. fitness
   - C. running
   - D. sitting

Directions: For questions 8–10, select the answer that completes the sentence in a grammatically correct manner or that represents the most grammatically correct of all the options.

8. If you study diligently, you are likely to perform _____ on your exam.
   A. well
   B. good
   C. success
   D. goodly

9. _____ a good thing that the dog has _____ own bed, because _____ definitely not sleeping in mine.
   A. Its; it's; its
   B. Its; its; its
   C. It's; it's; it's
   D. It's; its; it's

10. Which of the following sentences is grammatically correct?
   A. She said "How many times does I have to tell you? Stay away from the Smiths' house!"
   B. "She said, How many times do I have to tell you? Stay away from the Smith's house!"
   C. She said, "How many times do I have to tell you? Stay away from the Smiths' house!"
   D. She said, "How many times do I have to tell you stay away from the Smith's house"!

STOP

IF YOU FINISH BEFORE TIME IS CALLED, YOU MAY CHECK YOUR WORK ON THIS SECTION ONLY. DO NOT TURN TO ANY OTHER SECTION IN THE TEST.

Mathematics

10 Questions • 10 Minutes

Directions: Questions 1–10 require logical reasoning and thinking in addition to simple computations to find the solution. Read each question carefully and choose the correct answer from the four choices that follow.

1. Draper Hospital receives a 6% discount on all the pharmaceuticals it purchases. In the month of March, the hospital bought pharmaceuticals worth $82,500 at standard prices. What did the hospital pay after the discount?

   A. $4,950

   B. $33,000

   C. $49,500

   D. $77,550

2. $6 + 4(0.7 - 0.2)(3)^2 =$

   A. 17

   B. 21

   C. 24

   D. 27

3. 14 is what percent of 35?

   A. 75%

   B. 40%

   C. 20%

   D. 4%

4. Willis Medical Supply packages syringes in boxes that are 2 inches wide by 2 inches long by 4 inches tall. If these boxes are shipped in cartons with an interior volume of 16 inches by 24 inches by 8 inches tall, then how many syringes can Willis ship in 5 cartons?

   A. 192

   B. 960

   C. 1,920

   D. 15,360

SHOW YOUR WORK HERE

5. Sequoia Averill recently financed the purchase of a new car priced at $32,000. The finance company required a down payment of 15% of the purchase price. What is the amount of Sequoia's down payment?

A. $2,133

B. $4,200

C. $4,800

D. $27,200

6. Which of the following is true about two parallel lines?

A. They lie in the same plane.

B. The angles created by their crossing are acute.

C. The angles created by their crossing are obtuse.

D. The angles created by their crossing are right angles.

7. A triangle has a height of length 12 and a base of length 9. What is the area of the triangle?

A. 15

B. 54

C. 72

D. 108

8. Rubber gloves cost $11.55 per hundred. What will 160 rubber gloves cost?

A. $6.93

B. $11.71

C. $13.85

D. $18.48

SHOW YOUR WORK HERE

9. Twice the sum of 3 and a number N is 1 less than 3 times the number N. Which equation can you use to find the value of N?

   A. $2(3 + N) - 1 = 3N$

   B. $6 - 2N = 3N - 1$

   C. $2(3 + N) = 1 - 3N$

   D. $6 + 2N = 3N - 1$

10. Herman is covering 20 square tiles with cloth. In order to calculate how much cloth he needs, he must square the length in centimeters, c, of each side of a tile and then add x extra centimeters to account for error. Which equation should Herman use to calculate how much total cloth he will need to cover the 20 tiles?

    A. $20c^2 + x$

    B. $20c^2 + 20x$

    C. $20 + c^2 \times x$

    D. $20c^2 + x^2$

SHOW YOUR WORK HERE

STOP

IF YOU FINISH BEFORE TIME IS CALLED, YOU MAY CHECK YOUR WORK ON THIS SECTION ONLY. DO NOT TURN TO ANY OTHER SECTION IN THE TEST.

Spelling

10 Questions • 5 Minutes

Directions: For questions 1–10, choose the word that is spelled correctly.

1. **A.** recieve
   B. receive
   C. reiceve

2. **A.** respiratory
   B. resperatory
   C. respiritory

3. **A.** dyagnosis
   B. diagnosus
   C. diagnosis

4. **A.** inflammation
   B. inflamation
   C. imflammation

5. **A.** assesment
   B. asessment
   C. assessment

6. **A.** cartiovascular
   B. cardiovascular
   C. cardiovasscular

7. **A.** hemastasis
   B. hemostasis
   C. hemmostasis

8. **A.** farmacology
   B. pharmocology
   C. pharmacology

9. **A.** radiography
   B. radiographie
   C. radioggraphy

10. **A.** viralent
    B. virulent
    C. verulent

STOP

IF YOU FINISH BEFORE TIME IS CALLED, YOU MAY CHECK YOUR WORK ON THIS SECTION ONLY. DO NOT TURN TO ANY OTHER SECTION IN THE TEST.

Nonverbal Ability

10 Questions • 10 Minutes

Directions: For questions 1–10, determine the relationship between the first pair of shapes and then decide which of the answer choices shares a similar relationship with the third shape.

1. ○ is to ● as △ is to?
   A. ○
   B. □
   C. ■
   D. △
   E. ▲

2. △ is to ▷ as ▯ is to?
   A. ▫
   B. ▯
   C. ▮
   D. ▭
   E. ▬

3. ◇ is to ◈ as ○ is to?
   A. ◉
   B. ◎
   C. ●
   D. ▣
   E. ◻

4. ⊂ is to ⊃ as ⊏ is to?
   A. ⊓
   B. ⊔
   C. ⊐
   D. ∩
   E. ∪

5. ○ is to ⌐ as □ is to?
   A. ⌐
   B. ¬
   C. ∟
   D. ⌟
   E. ⊔

6. ⊖ is to ⊘ as ⊕ is to?
   A. ⊘
   B. ⊞
   C. ⊟
   D. ⊗
   E. ◎

7. ○ is to ⌣ as ◙ is to?
   A. ◻
   B. ◗
   C. ◖
   D. ◗
   E. ◒

8. ■ is to ◢ as ▭ is to?
   A. ▫
   B. ▯
   C. ◇
   D. ◇
   E. ▱

9. ▲ is to ■ as ⬠ is to?

    A. ⬣
    B. ⬡
    C. ●
    D. ◆
    E. ▲

10. ○ is to ◉ as ● is to?

    A. ◉
    B. ◻
    C. ☐
    D. ◎
    E. ▣

STOP

> IF YOU FINISH BEFORE TIME IS CALLED, YOU MAY CHECK YOUR WORK ON THIS SECTION ONLY. DO NOT TURN TO ANY OTHER SECTION IN THE TEST.

Science

10 Questions • 10 Minutes

Directions: For questions 1–10, read each question carefully and consider all possible answers. There is only one best answer for each question.

1. The cellular organelle that synthesizes proteins from messenger RNA templates is the
   A. ribosome.
   B. endoplasmic reticulum.
   C. mitochondrion.
   D. Golgi apparatus.

2. A mechanism of sexual reproduction that involves the temporary union of cells to allow for the exchange or transmission of genetic information is called
   A. isogamy.
   B. anisogamy.
   C. conjugation.
   D. oogamy.

3. Which process of human cellular metabolism breaks down glucose into pyruvic acid during the reaction?
   A. Krebs cycle
   B. Glycolysis
   C. Oxidative phosphorylation
   D. Photosynthesis

4. Which type of nucleic acid contains genetic information but is NOT directly involved in protein synthesis?
   A. mRNA
   B. rRNA
   C. tRNA
   D. DNA

5. Which two ions are exchanged as part of a pump mechanism that is necessary for normal transmission of impulses by nerve cells?
   A. Na^+ and Ca^{2+}
   B. H^+ and K^+
   C. K^+ and Ca^{2+}
   D. Na^+ and K^+

6. Which structure of the respiratory system is known as the windpipe?
   A. Bronchiole
   B. Pharynx
   C. Trachea
   D. Diaphragm

7. Which component of blood is involved in clotting?
   A. Erythrocytes
   B. Platelets
   C. Plasma
   D. Leukocytes

8. The structure that is known as the master gland because it regulates the functions of other glands is the
   A. pituitary gland.
   B. pineal gland.
   C. thyroid gland.
   D. adrenal glands.

9. During muscle contraction, the chemical released from axon terminals that diffuses across the synaptic cleft to bind to receptors is a
   A. neurotransmitter.
   B. sodium ion.
   C. potassium ion.
   D. actin filament.

10. In a simple food chain, fungi are classified as
   A. parasites.
   B. producers.
   C. consumers.
   D. decomposers.

STOP

IF YOU FINISH BEFORE TIME IS CALLED, YOU MAY CHECK YOUR WORK ON THIS SECTION ONLY. DO NOT TURN TO ANY OTHER SECTION IN THE TEST.

Reading Comprehension

10 Questions • 20 Minutes

Directions: For questions 1–10, carefully read the passage paragraphs and then answer the accompanying questions, basing your answer on what is stated in the paragraphs. There is only one best answer for each question.

Some Therapies for Asthma Sufferers

A

There are a number of treatments available for asthma sufferers, but some are more effective for certain types of use than others. For example, short-acting beta-2 agonists (bronchodilators) and oral and intravenous corticosteroids are best for rapid relief. They are not for long-term use. However, they can be beneficial for those who have exercise-induced asthma if used before commencing exercise.

B

Inhaled corticosteroids provide long-term control of asthma symptoms. Sometimes, combining a beta-2 agonist with an inhaled steroid is useful for long-term control. Those who have allergy-induced asthma may be prescribed a course of shots for desensitization, that is, a course of specific immunotherapy related to the allergen.

C

Controversial therapies include the use of leukotriene modifiers. These prevent symptoms for up to 24 hours. However, there are a number of recorded side effects. Patients taking this class of drugs have experienced hallucinations, agitations, aggressive behavior, and even thoughts of suicide. Among unproven methods for relief of asthma are breathing techniques, including so-called "yoga breathing," and the ingestion of herbal remedies such as gingko.

1. Which type of treatment is best for rapid relief of asthma symptoms?
   A. Inhaled corticosteroids
   B. Oral and intravenous corticosteroids
   C. Immunotherapy
   D. Yoga breathing

2. Which statement is supported by paragraph C?
   A. Patients who take leukotriene modifiers are likely to have suicidal thoughts.
   B. Yoga breathing is not likely to be an effective treatment for relief of asthma.
   C. Ginko can cause hallucinations.
   D. The main problem with leukotriene modifiers is that they don't work.

Obesity in Children

A

Obesity is a problem that affects children as well as adults. Since the 1970s, childhood obesity has been on the rise among U.S. children. Like their adult counterparts, obese children face a series of health problems. These include hypertension, high cholesterol, and type 2 diabetes, as well as bullying by peers. Being bullied can lead to depression and poor self-esteem. Some obese children may be able to achieve a healthy weight as adults, but the evidence belies this for most obese children. An obese child has a 70% chance of being obese as an adult.

B

It's never too late to help children eat healthful meals and snacks. But parents need to be willing to eat healthfully themselves, which means following the U.S. Department of Agriculture's MyPlate nutrition guide to ensure that they and their children have the right amount of fruits, vegetables, grains, protein, and dairy while reducing the amount of oils, sugar, and fats in their diet. Cooking oils are major ingredients in foods such as cookies, cakes, chips, and donuts. Other foods have what dieticians call empty calories because they have few or no nutrients. These foods include sodas and energy, sports, and fruit drinks; cheese; pizza; ice cream; sausage; hot dogs; bacon; and ribs. Cheese, pizza, ice cream, and ribs may seem less appetizing when you think of them as solid fat. The added sugar in ice cream also adds to it being unhealthful.

C

One way to get around the problem with some of these foods is to buy low-fat or sugar-free versions. For example, you can buy low-fat hot dogs and low-fat cheese as well as plain water and sugar-free sodas. Other foods to look for are unsweetened applesauce, cereals, and gelatin; extra-lean ground meat; and fat-free milk. Drinking plain water is also a good antidote to the empty calories in sodas, flavored waters, and sports drinks.

D

But it's not just parents who need to help children maintain a healthy weight. Schools have to be willing to forego some of their revenue from allowing companies to stock school vending machines with candy bars and sugary drinks, including flavored waters high in sugar content. Owners of stores near schools that sell snacks to students need to be willing to substitute healthful snacks for bags of potato chips, candy bars, and popsicles.

E

Schools have another responsibility, but ultimately it can come down to taxpayers. It's important that children and adolescents get at least 60 minutes or more of physical activity daily according to the FDA. This moderate-to-vigorous activity should include muscle strengthening and bone strengthening. Much of this is done, or could be done, outside of school, but an active physical education program in schools is also an important component. However, when faced with budget deficits and increased pressure to pass state academic tests, districts choose to cut physical education programs to the detriment of their students, especially urban students with no place to play after school.

3. Which of the following would be a better title for this passage?
   A. Parents Need Education on How to Fight Obesity
   B. Schools Have a Responsibility in the Childhood Obesity Trend
   C. Stores That Sell Snacks Need to Change
   D. How to Help Children Achieve and Maintain a Healthy Weight

4. The word *antidote* in paragraph C means
   A. addition.
   B. complement.
   C. remedy.
   D. catalyst.

5. According to the passage, what makes ice cream unhealthful?
   A. Fat content
   B. Sugar content
   C. Lack of nutrients
   D. All of the above

6. Empty-calorie foods are foods that

A. do not offer sufficient nutritional benefit for the number of calories they contain.

B. taste great and have almost no calories.

C. don't have many calories but also lack substance, leaving you feeling empty.

D. foods that are okay to eat in large volumes because they have few calories.

7. What type of activity does the FDA recommend that children engage in daily?

A. Intellectual games

B. Physical activity

C. Nutritional counseling

D. Homework

Making the Decision to Move

A

Are you going to be the caregiver for your parents or for other older relatives, such as a beloved aunt? Where do they live now? How old are they? Have they or you given any thought to having them move close to you? How feasible will it be to take time off and fly or even drive several hours if the person falls and breaks a hip or has a heart attack? How long can you take off from work to be with the person? Will you need to come home and then go back when the person is ready to come home from the hospital or from rehab? These are questions facing many adult children today whose family member or members they will be caring for in later years.

B

And "later" for some of these adult children is right around the corner—or even now. According to the 2010 Census, there were more than 40 million Americans 65 years and older. This is 13% of the total population. By 2050, the percentage is expected to grow to 21%. Of the more than 40 million people 65 years and older, fewer than half—43% or 17 million—are men. The trend line for the percentage, as well as the real number, of Americans 65 years and older has moved steadily upward since 1900. The other notable fact between 2000 and 2010 is that the population of those 65 years and older grew at a faster rate than the total population. Although women over 65 years old still outnumber men in that age group, the number of males over 65 years old increased faster than the number of women.

C

All of this increase in population also means more people needing care. There are various solutions to the problem. One is for the family member or members to move close to the potential caregiver while still young enough to do it on their own, ambulatory, and still able to make new friends as well as experience what their new locales offer in the way of entertainment, hobbies, and lifelong learning. Another option is to allow the older person to remain in the area where they currently live, but have them move into a community with step-up care, that is, a community that provides a continuum of care from totally independent housing to assisted living to nursing facilities. In this way, the potential caregiver is relieved of worry about the person while also being relieved of day-to-day direct-care responsibilities.

8. What does the word *ambulatory* mean in paragraph C?

A. Able to think clearly

B. Able to walk

C. Able to drive a car

D. Able to live independently

9. By 2050, the percentage of the total U.S. population 65 years and older is expected to grow to

A. 21%.

B. 43%.

C. 13%.

D. 40%.

10. What is step-up care?
    A. Aerobics and other fitness classes geared for older adults
    B. An intense level of nursing care required by those with severe dementia
    C. A continuum of care from independent housing to assisted living to nursing facilities
    D. Home health care

STOP

IF YOU FINISH BEFORE TIME IS CALLED, YOU MAY CHECK YOUR WORK ON THIS SECTION ONLY. DO NOT TURN TO ANY OTHER SECTION IN THE TEST.

ANSWER KEYS AND EXPLANATIONS

Verbal Ability

1. C	3. A	5. A	7. B	9. D
2. D	4. B	6. D	8. A	10. C

1. **The correct answer is C.** *Auspicious* means "favorable." Choice A is incorrect because *miraculous* means "occurring through divine intervention," and although this term might be used ironically in this context, it is unlikely the crowd would actually think the arrival of the food truck was by divine intervention. Choice B is incorrect because the crowd may have found the arrival *surprising*, but the word has no relation to *auspicious*. Choice D is incorrect because *ominous*, meaning "foreboding," is an antonym of *auspicious*. (SYNONYMS)

2. **The correct answer is D.** *Vicissitudes* means "*changes* or alterations," for better or worse, often caused by chance, that are life-changing. A clue to this word's meaning is the phrase "whether good or bad" at the end of the sentence. Choice A is incorrect because *downfalls* refers only to bad changes. Choice B is incorrect because *improvements* refers only to good changes. Choice C is incorrect because *repetitions* is nearly opposite in meaning to *vicissitudes* and because repetitions are not dramatic. (SYNONYMS)

3. **The correct answer is A.** *Agitated* means "disturbed, bothered, ill at ease." The words *halcyon, peaceful, harmonious,* and *serene* (choices B through E) are synonyms that relate to states of calmness and peacefulness, which are the opposite of being agitated. (ANTONYMS)

4. **The correct answer is B.** *Salubrious* means "healthful." The words *deleterious, noxious,* *detrimental,* and *harmful* (choices A and C through E) are incorrect because they are synonyms related to causing harm. (ANTONYMS)

5. **The correct answer is A.** This is an antonym analogy. *Wavering* is the opposite of *steadfast*, so you need an answer that is the opposite of *adamantine*, meaning "rocklike, hard." The opposite of this is *pliable* (choice A). Choice B is incorrect because *unreliable* is the opposite of *steadfast* in the first pair of words. Choice C is incorrect because *unyielding* is a synonym of *adamantine*. Choice D is incorrect because *faithful* is a synonym of *steadfast*. (ANTONYM ANALOGY)

6. **The correct answer is D.** This is a person/worker-to-place analogy. A *fisherman* sits or stands on a *dock* to catch fish and a *hunter* sits or stands on a *tree stand* to hunt. Choice A is incorrect because a *hunter* hunts *with* a gun, not *on* a gun. Choice B is incorrect because a *hunter* hunts *for* deer, not *on* a deer. Choice C is incorrect because *forest* is the broader setting where the *hunter* hunts, not the structure the *hunter* sits or stands on while hunting. (PERSON/WORKER-TO-PLACE ANALOGY)

7. **The correct answer is B.** This is a cause-and-effect analogy. *Smoking* causes the condition of *cancer* in the long term, and *exercise* causes the condition of *fitness* in the long term. Choice A is incorrect because *exhaustion* is a short-term, not long-term, effect of *exercise*. Choice C is incorrect

because *running* is a type, not an effect, of *exercise*. Choice D is incorrect because *sitting* is an antonym, not effect, of *exercise*. (CAUSE-AND-EFFECT ANALOGY)

8. **The correct answer is A.** *Well* is an adverb, and thus is an appropriate modifier for the verb *perform*. *Goodly* (choice D) is an archaic form of the adjective *good* (choice B) that is no longer used. In addition, *good* is not an adverb, so choices B and D are incorrect. *Success* (choice C) is a noun and cannot modify *perform*. (GRAMMAR)

9. **The correct answer is D.** The first and third blanks require the meaning "it is," which may be replaced with the contraction *it's*. The second blank requires the possessive pronoun *its* to show that the bed belongs to the dog. Only choice D has the correct forms in all three blanks. Choices A, B, and C are incorrect because they mix up these two concepts in one or all of the three blanks. (GRAMMAR)

10. **The correct answer is C.** Choice A is incorrect because a comma is missing after "said" (a comma should be used to set off a direct quote from the rest of the sentence) and "does" should be "do" (if you convert the question to a statement, this becomes clear: "I *do* have to tell you how many times."). Choice B is incorrect because the opening quotation mark should appear just before "How" and the apostrophe should come after the final "s" in the plural family name to show possession (Smiths' house). Choice D is incorrect because the quotation contains a run-on sentence and Smith's house should be Smiths' house. (GRAMMAR)

Mathematics

1. D	**3.** B	**5.** C	**7.** B	**9.** D
2. C	**4.** B	**6.** A	**8.** D	**10.** B

1. **The correct answer is D.**
    Disc. price = (100% − 6%) × Std. price

    = 94% × Std. price

    = 0.94 × $82,500

    = $77,550

    (PERCENTAGES)

2. **The correct answer is C.**

    $$6 + 4(0.7 - 0.2)(3)^2 = 6 + 4(0.5)(3)^2$$
    $$= 6 + 4(0.5)(9)$$
    $$= 6 + 18$$
    $$= 24$$

    (ORDER OF OPERATIONS, DECIMALS)

3. **The correct answer is B.**

    $$\frac{14}{35} = 0.40, \text{ or } 40\%$$

    (PERCENTAGES)

4. **The correct answer is B.**
    Since the bottom of the carton is 16" × 24", and the syringe boxes are 2" wide × 2" long, one layer of 8 boxes × 12 boxes = 96 boxes fills the bottom of a carton. Cartons are 8" tall and syringe boxes are 4" tall, so two layers of boxes stacked one above another fill a carton.

    $$2 \text{ layers} \times \frac{96 \text{ boxes}}{1 \text{ layer}} = 192 \text{ boxes per carton}$$

    $$5 \text{ cartons} \times \frac{192 \text{ boxes}}{1 \text{ carton}} = 960 \text{ boxes in 5 cartons}$$

    (ORDER OF OPERATIONS; PROBLEM SOLVING)

5. **The correct answer is C.**
    15%($32,000) = 0.15($32,000)

    = $4,800

    (PERCENTAGES)

6. **The correct answer is A.** Parallel lines by definition are lines in the same plane that do not intersect.
    (GEOMETRY DEFINITIONS)

7. **The correct answer is B.**

    $$\text{area of a triangle} = \frac{1}{2}(\text{base})(\text{height})$$
    $$x = \frac{1}{2}(9)(12)$$
    $$x = 54$$

    (AREA)

8. **The correct answer is D.**
    $11.55 ÷ 100 = $0.1155

    $0.1155(160) = $18.48

    (MULTIPLICATION, DIVISION, DECIMALS; PROBLEM SOLVING)

9. **The correct answer is D.** Twice the sum of 3 and the number N is written as $2(3 + N)$, or $6 + 2N$. The phrase "1 less than 3 times the number N" is written as $3N - 1$. Equating these two quantities yields the desired equation. For choice A, the 1 should be subtracted from the right side, not the left side. For choice B, the $2N$ should be added, not subtracted, on the left side. For choice C, the order of the terms on the right side should be switched.
    (ONE VARIABLE)

10. **The correct answer is B.** For each tile, Herman needs $c^2 + x$ centimeters of cloth. He needs this much cloth for each of 20 tiles, so he must multiply this expression by 20. $20(c^2 + x) = 20c^2 + 20x$. Choice A is incorrect because the x should be multiplied by 20 as well (by the distributive property). Choice C has the addition and multiplication signs interchanged.
    (TWO VARIABLES)

Spelling

| 1. B | 3. C | 5. C | 7. B | 9. A |
| 2. A | 4. A | 6. B | 8. C | 10. B |

1. **The correct answer is B.** The correct spelling is *receive*.

2. **The correct answer is A.** The correct spelling is *respiratory*.

3. **The correct answer is C.** The correct spelling is *diagnosis*.

4. **The correct answer is A.** The correct spelling is *inflammation*.

5. **The correct answer is C.** The correct spelling is *assessment*.

6. **The correct answer is B.** The correct spelling is *cardiovascular*.

7. **The correct answer is B.** The correct spelling is *hemostasis*.

8. **The correct answer is C.** The correct spelling is *pharmacology*.

9. **The correct answer is A.** The correct spelling is *radiography*.

10. **The correct answer is B.** The correct spelling is *virulent*.

Nonverbal Ability

1. E	3. A	5. B	7. C	9. A
2. D	4. C	6. D	8. E	10. B

1. **The correct answer is E.** The relationship between the first two shapes is that they are both circles but the first is white whereas the second is black. So, in the second pair, we begin with a white triangle and are looking for a black triangle. Therefore, white circle is to black circle as white triangle is to black triangle.

2. **The correct answer is D.** The relationship between the first two shapes is that they are both triangles but the second is rotated 90 degrees to the right in relation to the first. So, in the second pair, we begin with a vertical rectangle and are looking for a rectangle rotated 90 degrees to the right. Therefore, triangle pointing up is to triangle pointing right as vertical rectangle is to horizontal rectangle.

3. **The correct answer is A.** The relationship between the first two shapes is that they are both white diamonds but the second has a smaller black diamond embedded within it. So, in the second pair, we begin with a white circle and are looking for a white circle with a smaller black circle embedded within it. Therefore, white diamond is to white diamond with a smaller black diamond embedded within it as white circle is to white circle with a smaller black circle embedded within it.

4. **The correct answer is C.** The relationship between the first two shapes is that the second is the mirror image of the first. So, in the second pair, we begin with an open black rectangle pointing right and are looking for its mirror image, which is an open black rectangle pointing left. Therefore, black U pointing right is to black U pointing left as open black rectangle pointing right is to open black rectangle pointing left.

5. **The correct answer is B.** The relationship between the first two shapes is that the second is the upper right portion of the first. So, in the second pair, we begin with a square and are looking for its upper right portion, which is an upper right corner. Therefore, circle is to upper right quadrant circular arc as square is to upper right square corner.

6. **The correct answer is D.** The relationship between the first two shapes is that they are both circles bisected by line segments but the second is rotated 45 degrees to the left in relation to the first. So, in the second pair, we begin with a circle bisected by horizontal and vertical line segments and are looking for a circle similarly bisected but rotated 45 degrees to the left in relation to the first. Therefore, circle bisected by a horizontal line segment is to circle bisected by a diagonal line segment as circle bisected by horizontal and vertical line segments is to circle bisected by two diagonal line segments perpendicular to one another.

7. **The correct answer is C.** The relationship between the first two shapes is the second is the lower half of the first. So, in the second pair, we begin with a black square with a circumscribed white ring and are looking for its lower half. Therefore, white circle is to lower quadrant circular arc as black square with circumscribed white ring is to lower half of black square with circumscribed white ring.

8. **The correct answer is E.** The relationship between the first two shapes is that they are both black parallelograms (quadrilaterals with two pairs of parallel sides), but the first is a rectangle (a parallelogram with four right angles) with unequal adjacent sides, and the second is a rhomboid (a parallelogram with unequal adjacent sides and without right angles). So, in the second pair, we begin with a white rectangle and are looking for a white rhomboid. Therefore, black rectangle is to black rhomboid as white rectangle is to white rhomboid.

9. **The correct answer is A.** The relationship between the first two shapes is that the second has one more side than the first. So, in the second pair, we begin with a pentagon, which has five sides, and are looking for a shape with one more side, or six sides, which is a hexagon. Therefore, triangle is to square as pentagon is to hexagon.

10. **The correct answer is B.** The relationship between the first two shapes is that the second is the negative image, or total inversion, of the first. So, in the second pair, we begin with a black circle and are looking for its negative image. Therefore, white circle is to negative image of white circle as black circle is to negative image of black circle.

Science

1. A	**3.** B	**5.** D	**7.** B	**9.** A
2. C	**4.** D	**6.** C	**8.** A	**10.** D

1. **The correct answer is A.** Ribosomes are the organelles that synthesize proteins from messenger RNA templates. Choice B is incorrect because the endoplasmic reticulum is active in the transport of proteins. Choice C is incorrect because mitochondria are involved in cellular respiration. Macromolecules such as carbohydrates, fats, and proteins are oxidized resulting in the release of ATP, a form of usable energy that all cells require. Choice D is incorrect because the Golgi apparatus functions in the synthesis, modification, sorting, and secretion of cell products. Products of the endoplasmic reticulum are modified and stored in the Golgi apparatus and then sent to other destinations. (THE CELL)

2. **The correct answer is C.** Conjugation is a mechanism of sexual reproduction that involves the temporary union of cells to allow for the exchange or transmission of genetic information. Choice A is incorrect because isogamy is a mechanism of sexual reproduction involving the fusion of gametes of identical size and structure. Choice B is incorrect because anisogamy is a type of heterogamy that involves motile gametes that differ only in size. Choice D is incorrect because heterogamy is a mechanism of sexual reproduction involving the fusion of gametes that differ in size and/or structure, and oogamy is a type of heterogamy that involves gametes that differ in size and structure. (REPRODUCTION)

3. **The correct answer is B.** The glycolysis reaction that takes place in the cytosol in the absence of oxygen breaks down glucose into pyruvic acid. Choice A is incorrect because the Krebs cycle, or citric acid cycle, breaks down pyruvic acid to produce CO_2. Choice C is incorrect because the process of oxidative phosphorylation produces much ATP and releases H_2O. Choice D is incorrect because photosynthesis releases O_2 and takes place only in green plants, not humans. (METABOLISM)

4. **The correct answer is D.** DNA contains genetic information but is not directly involved in protein synthesis. Choice A is incorrect because messenger RNA, or mRNA, is the template for amino acid synthesis and contains the codon sequences. Choice B is incorrect because ribosomal RNA, or rRNA, is the key component of ribosomes, which synthesize proteins. Choice C is incorrect because transfer RNA, or tRNA, matches each specific amino acid to its codon on an mRNA strand. The codon is a three-nucleotide sequence that is specific for only one of the 26 amino acids. Thus, tRNA molecules are able to pick up a specific amino acid and deliver it to a specific amino acid codon. (NUCLEIC ACIDS)

5. **The correct answer is D.** The sodium-potassium pump moves sodium ions (Na+) out of and potassium ions (K+) into the cell during transmission of nerve impulses. The other ions listed are not involved in this pump mechanism. (NERVOUS SYSTEM)

6. **The correct answer is C.** The trachea, or windpipe, is encircled by rings of cartilage so that it always remains open. Choice A is incorrect because the bronchioles are smaller, narrower tubes through which air

is distributed around the lungs. Choice B is incorrect because the pharynx is known as the throat. Choice D is incorrect because the diaphragm is a muscle that aids in breathing. (RESPIRATORY SYSTEM)

7. **The correct answer is B.** Platelets are small fragments in the blood that are important for clotting. Choice A is incorrect because erythrocytes, or red blood cells, are involved in transport of oxygen to the body but not clotting. Choice C is incorrect because plasma is the fluid portion of blood; it is not involved in clotting. Choice D is incorrect because leukocytes, or white blood cells, are involved in immune defense but not clotting. (CIRCULATORY SYSTEM)

8. **The correct answer is A.** The pituitary gland is sometimes called the master gland because it regulates the functions of other endocrine glands. Choice B is incorrect because the pineal gland is a pea-sized gland near the center of the brain that synthesizes and secretes melatonin. Melatonin links biorhythms with environmental light (daily and seasonal). However, this gland does not regulate other glands. Choice C is incorrect because the thyroid gland produces thyroxine (T4) and triiodothyronine (T3) that stimulate and maintain metabolic processes. However, this gland does not regulate other glands. Choice D is incorrect because the adrenal glands are located above the kidneys and secrete hormones in response to stress on the body. However, this gland does not regulate other glands. (ENDOCRINE SYSTEM)

9. **The correct answer is A.** Neurons release neurotransmitters from axon terminals; these neurotransmitters diffuse across the synaptic cleft and bind to receptors. Choice B is incorrect because sodium ions rush into the muscle cell after the neurotransmitter binds with the receptor. Choice C is incorrect because potassium ions rush out of the muscle cell after the neurotransmitter binds with the receptor. Choice D is incorrect because the actin filaments act in muscle contraction by sliding past the myosin filaments, but they are not released from axon terminals. (MUSCULOSKELETAL SYSTEM)

10. **The correct answer is D.** Decomposers are organisms that rely upon nonliving organic matter as a source of energy and material for growth. Fungi are examples of decomposers. Choice A is incorrect because parasites are organisms that live on a host organism and obtain nourishment while harming the health of the host. Choice B is incorrect because producers are organisms that are able to use energy from the sun to make complex organic molecules from simple inorganic substances, such as nitrogen and phosphorous, in their environment. Plants are producers that carry out the process of photosynthesis. Choice C is incorrect because consumers are organisms in a food chain, or food web, that either eat producers or other consumers to obtain energy. Humans are classified as consumers. In particular, humans are omnivores because they eat both producers (plants) and consumers (animals). (ENERGY IN ECOSYSTEMS)

Reading Comprehension

1. B	3. D	5. D	7. B	9. A
2. B	4. C	6. A	8. B	10. C

1. **The correct answer is B.** The answer is stated in paragraph A, sentence 2.

2. **The correct answer is B.** This answer requires an inference. The author describes this technique as "so-called," puts quotes around "yoga breathing," and identifies it as an "unproven method." From this, it is reasonable to infer that the author does not think yoga breathing is likely to be an effective treatment for asthma.

3. **The correct answer is D.** The title of a piece of writing typically reflects the main idea or theme of the piece. Only choice D expresses the general idea, which is about ways to help children achieve and maintain a healthy weight. Choice A is incorrect because the need for parental education is not addressed as such in the passage, only that parents need to eat healthfully also. Choices B and C are too specific; each addresses only one factor discussed in the passage.

4. **The correct answer is C.** *Antidote* means "a remedy." Choices A and B are incorrect because *addition* and *complement* refer to adding consumption of water to the consumption of unhealthy drinks, whereas *antidote* refers to something that competes with and is a substitute for them. Choice D

is incorrect because *catalyst*, which is something that promotes the action of something else, is the opposite of *antidote*, which is something that works against the action of something else.

5. **The correct answer is D.** The answer is stated in paragraph B, sentences 4 to 7.

6. **The correct answer is A.** The answer is stated in paragraph B, sentence 4. Choices B and D simply aren't true, as "empty-calorie foods" are typically high in calories. Choice C may be true in that eating these foods high in fat and sugar may leave a person hungry, but that's not why they are called empty calories, so eliminate choice C. In addition, this information is not stated in the passage and you should base your answers on only what is in the passage.

7. **The correct answer is B.** The answer is stated in paragraph E, sentence 2. The FDA recommends 60 minutes or more of physical activity daily.

8. **The correct answer is B.** *Ambulatory* means "able to walk."

9. **The correct answer is A.** The answer is stated in paragraph B, sentence 4.

10. **The correct answer is C.** The answer is stated in paragraph C, sentence 4.

Diagnostic Test for
Allied Health School

UNIT 2 DIAGNOSTIC TEST FOR ALLIED HEALTH SCHOOL ANSWER SHEET

Verbal Ability

1. Ⓐ Ⓑ Ⓒ Ⓓ   3. Ⓐ Ⓑ Ⓒ Ⓓ Ⓔ   5. Ⓐ Ⓑ Ⓒ Ⓓ   7. Ⓐ Ⓑ Ⓒ Ⓓ   9. Ⓐ Ⓑ Ⓒ Ⓓ

2. Ⓐ Ⓑ Ⓒ Ⓓ   4. Ⓐ Ⓑ Ⓒ Ⓓ Ⓔ   6. Ⓐ Ⓑ Ⓒ Ⓓ   8. Ⓐ Ⓑ Ⓒ Ⓓ   10. Ⓐ Ⓑ Ⓒ Ⓓ

Mathematics

1. Ⓐ Ⓑ Ⓒ Ⓓ   3. Ⓐ Ⓑ Ⓒ Ⓓ   5. Ⓐ Ⓑ Ⓒ Ⓓ   7. Ⓐ Ⓑ Ⓒ Ⓓ   9. Ⓐ Ⓑ Ⓒ Ⓓ

2. Ⓐ Ⓑ Ⓒ Ⓓ   4. Ⓐ Ⓑ Ⓒ Ⓓ   6. Ⓐ Ⓑ Ⓒ Ⓓ   8. Ⓐ Ⓑ Ⓒ Ⓓ   10. Ⓐ Ⓑ Ⓒ Ⓓ

Spelling

1. Ⓐ Ⓑ Ⓒ   3. Ⓐ Ⓑ Ⓒ   5. Ⓐ Ⓑ Ⓒ   7. Ⓐ Ⓑ Ⓒ   9. Ⓐ Ⓑ Ⓒ

2. Ⓐ Ⓑ Ⓒ   4. Ⓐ Ⓑ Ⓒ   6. Ⓐ Ⓑ Ⓒ   8. Ⓐ Ⓑ Ⓒ   10. Ⓐ Ⓑ Ⓒ

Nonverbal Ability

1. Ⓐ Ⓑ Ⓒ Ⓓ Ⓔ   3. Ⓐ Ⓑ Ⓒ Ⓓ Ⓔ   5. Ⓐ Ⓑ Ⓒ Ⓓ Ⓔ   7. Ⓐ Ⓑ Ⓒ Ⓓ Ⓔ   9. Ⓐ Ⓑ Ⓒ Ⓓ Ⓔ

2. Ⓐ Ⓑ Ⓒ Ⓓ Ⓔ   4. Ⓐ Ⓑ Ⓒ Ⓓ Ⓔ   6. Ⓐ Ⓑ Ⓒ Ⓓ Ⓔ   8. Ⓐ Ⓑ Ⓒ Ⓓ Ⓔ   10. Ⓐ Ⓑ Ⓒ Ⓓ Ⓔ

Science

1. Ⓐ Ⓑ Ⓒ Ⓓ   3. Ⓐ Ⓑ Ⓒ Ⓓ   5. Ⓐ Ⓑ Ⓒ Ⓓ   7. Ⓐ Ⓑ Ⓒ Ⓓ   9. Ⓐ Ⓑ Ⓒ Ⓓ

2. Ⓐ Ⓑ Ⓒ Ⓓ   4. Ⓐ Ⓑ Ⓒ Ⓓ   6. Ⓐ Ⓑ Ⓒ Ⓓ   8. Ⓐ Ⓑ Ⓒ Ⓓ   10. Ⓐ Ⓑ Ⓒ Ⓓ

Reading Comprehension

1. Ⓐ Ⓑ Ⓒ Ⓓ   3. Ⓐ Ⓑ Ⓒ Ⓓ   5. Ⓐ Ⓑ Ⓒ Ⓓ   7. Ⓐ Ⓑ Ⓒ Ⓓ   9. Ⓐ Ⓑ Ⓒ Ⓓ

2. Ⓐ Ⓑ Ⓒ Ⓓ   4. Ⓐ Ⓑ Ⓒ Ⓓ   6. Ⓐ Ⓑ Ⓒ Ⓓ   8. Ⓐ Ⓑ Ⓒ Ⓓ   10. Ⓐ Ⓑ Ⓒ Ⓓ

answer sheet

Verbal Ability

10 Questions • 5 Minutes

Directions: For questions 1 and 2, one word is italicized in the sentence shown. Following each sentence are four words or phrases. For each sentence, choose the word or phrase that most nearly corresponds in meaning with the italicized word.

1. The patient's signs and symptoms did not *correlate* with those of influenza, so the physician ruled this diagnosis out.
   A. differ
   B. correspond
   C. combine
   D. contradict

2. The child complained of *intermittent* coughing.
   A. sporadic
   B. severe
   C. regular
   D. chronic

Directions: For questions 3 and 4, choose the word that is most different in meaning from the others.

3. A. tacit
   B. explicit
   C. implicit
   D. implied
   E. understood

4. A. metamorphosis
   B. stasis
   C. conversion
   D. transformation
   E. evolution

Directions: For questions 5–7, determine the relationship between the first pair of capitalized words and then decide which of the answer choices shares a similar relationship with the third capitalized word.

5. SCALPEL : CUT :: NEEDLE :
   A. syringe
   B. pain
   C. inject
   D. medicine

6. DOG : MAMMAL :: CAKE :
   A. dessert
   B. pie
   C. oven
   D. bake

7. FRIDAY : SATURDAY :: APRIL :
   A. March
   B. May
   C. spring
   D. summer

Directions: For questions 8–10, select the answer that completes the sentence in a grammatically correct manner or that represents the most grammatically correct of all options.

8. I've read every book that author has written _____ she's an amazing writer.
   A. ,
   B. ?
   C. "
   D. ;

9. You don't look well; you should _____ down for a while and rest.
   A. lie
   B. lay
   C. laid
   D. layed

10. Which of the following sentences is grammatically correct?
   A. The cat that is black and has white paws belongs to my neighbor.
   B. The cat, that is black and has white paws, belongs to my neighbor.
   C. The cat, that is black and has white paws belongs to my neighbor.
   D. The cat that is black and has white paws, belongs to my neighbor.

STOP

IF YOU FINISH BEFORE TIME IS CALLED, YOU MAY CHECK YOUR WORK ON THIS SECTION ONLY. DO NOT TURN TO ANY OTHER SECTION IN THE TEST.

Mathematics

10 Questions • 20 Minutes

> **Directions:** For questions 1–10, read each question carefully and consider all possible answers. There is only one best answer for each question.

1. $\frac{2}{3} + 3\frac{5}{6} + \frac{4}{9} =$

    A. $3\frac{11}{8}$

    B. $4\frac{17}{18}$

    C. $5\frac{7}{9}$

    D. $10\frac{17}{18}$

    SHOW YOUR WORK HERE

2. If it takes 1.69 ounces of liquid to fill one 50 milliliter cup, how many ounces are needed to fill twelve 50 mL cups?

    A. 1.408

    B. 2.028

    C. 20.28

    D. 35.5

3. A shipment of shoes weighs 3,600 pounds. If the shipment has 2,880 individual shoes, then how many pounds does one *pair* of shoes weigh?

    A. 0.8

    B. 1.6

    C. 1.25

    D. 2.5

4. When you multiply $2\frac{4}{7}$ by $5\frac{1}{5}$, the answer is

    A. $\frac{6}{7}$

    B. $\frac{354}{35}$

    C. $\frac{468}{35}$

    D. 468

5. If $8(x + 3) = 58$, then $x = ?$

    A. 10.25

    B. 6.875

    C. 4.25

    D. 4.0

SHOW YOUR WORK HERE

6. Yang Li operates a fleet of delivery trucks. If he spends an average of $156 per month on oil and $9,821 per month on gasoline, how much does Yang Li pay for oil annually?

    A. $1,872

    B. $8,112

    C. $117,852

    D. $119,724

7. What is the solution to $\frac{3}{4} \div \frac{1}{3}$?

    A. $\frac{9}{4}$

    B. $\frac{3}{2}$

    C. $\frac{2}{3}$

    D. $\frac{3}{12}$

8. Compute: 4.0804 ÷ 0.04   **SHOW YOUR WORK HERE**

   A. 0.010201

   B. 1.0201

   C. 10.201

   D. 102.01

9. Consider the following diagram, where it is assumed that *AB* is parallel to *CD*:

What is the value of *x*?

   A. 4

   B. 6

   C. 8

   D. 10

10. Which of the following is NOT an accurate description of the following quadrilateral?

5 in.

5 in.   5 in.

5 in.

A. Trapezoid

B. Square

C. Parallelogram

D. Rectangle

STOP

IF YOU FINISH BEFORE TIME IS CALLED, YOU MAY CHECK YOUR WORK ON THIS SECTION ONLY. DO NOT TURN TO ANY OTHER SECTION IN THE TEST.

Spelling

10 Questions • 5 Minutes

Directions: For questions 1–10, choose the word that is spelled correctly.

1. A. anadomy
    B. anatomie
    C. anatomy

2. A. ediology
    B. etialogy
    C. etiology

3. A. urinealysis
    B. urinalysis
    C. urinalasis

4. A. newtrition
    B. nutrition
    C. nutrision

5. A. achievement
    B. acheivement
    C. achievment

6. A. innfection
    B. infection
    C. infecksion

7. A. vacsination
    B. vacination
    C. vaccination

8. A. diabetes
    B. dyabetes
    C. diabetus

9. A. sistolic
    B. systtolic
    C. systolic

10. A. elektrocardiography
     B. electrocardiography
     C. electracardiography

STOP

IF YOU FINISH BEFORE TIME IS CALLED, YOU MAY CHECK YOUR WORK ON THIS SECTION ONLY. DO NOT TURN TO ANY OTHER SECTION IN THE TEST.

Nonverbal Ability

10 Questions • 10 Minutes

> **Directions:** For questions 1–10, determine the relationship between the first pair of shapes and then decide which of the answer choices shares a similar relationship with the third shape.

1. ▲ is to ▲ as △ is to?
   - A. □
   - B. △
   - C. ○
   - D. ■
   - E. ●

2. □ is to ▥ as ○ is to?
   - A. ▤
   - B. ◉
   - C. ◎
   - D. ◍
   - E. ▨

3. o━●━o is to ●━o━● as ⋈⋈ is to?
   - A. ⋈⋈
   - B. ⋈⋈
   - C. ✕
   - D. ⋈⋈
   - E. ⋈⋈

4. ⊎ is to +⊂ as ＜ is to?
   - A. •∧
   - B. •＜
   - C. •∨
   - D. ＜•
   - E. ＞

5. ▦ is to ⁚ as ※ is to?
   - A. ✕
   - B. ＋
   - C. ∴
   - D. ⁞
   - E. ⊹

6. △ is to 3 as □ is to?
   - A. 6
   - B. 9
   - C. 12
   - D. 8
   - E. 4

7. ◑ is to ◖ as ◐ is to?
   - A. ○
   - B. ◓
   - C. ◒
   - D. ◴
   - E. ◗

8. ⟨ is to ⟪ as ⟩ is to?
   - A. ⟮
   - B. ⟨
   - C. ⟪
   - D. ⟫
   - E. ⟯

9. ⌈ is to ⌉ as ⋐ is to?

A. ⋒

B. ⋑

C. ⋓

D. ⌊

E. ⌋

10. ⚡ is to ⚡ as φ is to?

A. φ̄

B. ✝

C. ⌊↓⌋

D. ✝̇

E. ⊥

STOP

IF YOU FINISH BEFORE TIME IS CALLED, YOU MAY CHECK YOUR WORK ON THIS SECTION ONLY. DO NOT TURN TO ANY OTHER SECTION IN THE TEST.

Science

10 Questions • 8 Minutes

> **Directions:** For questions 1–10, read each question carefully and consider all possible answers. There is only one best answer for each question.

1. Which cellular organelle is considered the control center of the cell because it contains the genetic information of the cell?
   A. Nucleus
   B. Golgi apparatus
   C. Mitochondria
   D. Ribosome

2. White blood cells, which help to fight infection, are part of which body system?
   A. Musculoskeletal system
   B. Immune system
   C. Integumentary system
   D. Endocrine system

3. Which ABO blood type is known as the "universal donor" type because people of all blood types can safely receive it in a red blood cell transfusion?
   A. Type A
   B. Type B
   C. Type AB
   D. Type O

4. Cells that release chemicals that respond to inflammation at the site of an infection are called
   A. cytotoxic T-cells.
   B. natural killer cells.
   C. interferons.
   D. basophils.

5. Which organ of the digestive system produces bile, which breaks down fats?
   A. Small intestine
   B. Large intestine
   C. Liver
   D. Stomach

6. Which type of muscle tissue is found in the lining of the stomach, intestines, and bladder?
   A. Striated
   B. Cardiac
   C. Skeletal
   D. Smooth

7. Nerve cells that receive signals sent by the brain and deliver them to muscle cells to produce a movement in response to a stimulus are called
   A. sensory neurons.
   B. motor neurons.
   C. brain cells.
   D. interneurons.

8. Which of the following hormones triggers ovulation in females and secretion of testosterone in males?
   A. Luteinizing hormone
   B. Follicle-stimulating hormone
   C. Estrogen
   D. Testosterone

9. Which of the following is a fat-soluble vitamin that is essential for forming clots and thus preventing excessive bleeding when injury occurs?

    A. Vitamin A

    B. Vitamin D

    C. Vitamin E

    D. Vitamin K

10. Which hormone acts to increase the body's basal metabolic rate (metabolism)?

    A. Estrogen

    B. Testosterone

    C. Cortisol

    D. Thyroxine

STOP

IF YOU FINISH BEFORE TIME IS CALLED, YOU MAY CHECK YOUR WORK ON THIS SECTION ONLY. DO NOT TURN TO ANY OTHER SECTION IN THE TEST.

Reading Comprehension

10 Questions • 20 Minutes

Directions: For questions 1–10, carefully read the passage paragraphs and then answer the accompanying questions, basing your answer on what is stated in the paragraphs. There is only one best answer for each question.

At the conclusion of World War II, Japan became an occupied nation. The occupation lasted from 1945 until 1952. Most occupying forces were from the United States. During the occupation, the U.S. military government achieved its two main goals. It brought democracy to Japan and also helped lay the foundation for Japan's economic recovery.

The occupation government helped Japan draft a new constitution. The document removed political power from the emperor, a parliamentary system was put into place, and basic rights were guaranteed for all. Women for the first time were given the right to vote. The constitution also stated that the Japanese army would be limited to a size only large enough for national defense.

In addition to political changes, economic changes were introduced. The right of workers to unionize was written into the constitution. Land reforms were introduced. The chief beneficiaries were tenant farmers. They were allowed to buy land, leading to a new class of independent farmers. The Americans tried to disband the large business corporations that existed in Japan, called zaibatsu. This was unsuccessful because Japan believed it needed the corporations to compete with other nations. Although a small number of companies were dismantled, the system remained. The business experience that existed because of the zaibatsu became a positive factor in Japan's economic growth.

After the occupation ended, Japan experienced extraordinary economic growth. A number of factors contributed to this success. During World War II, many Japanese cities and factories had been destroyed. However, this destruction turned out to be beneficial. The Japanese had to build new factories, which were more productive, efficient, and state-of-the-art than were older factories in other manufacturing centers. This included the United States.

In addition to new manufacturing facilities, Japan was able to take advantage of cheap oil prices in the 1950s and 1960s. Japan also had a large workforce, providing cheap labor for factories. The Japanese had a long tradition of saving money, so banks had money to lend to new businesses. Because Japan had few natural resources, it turned to manufacturing products for export. By the 1970s, Japan was a leader in electronics and began producing high-quality automobiles for export. Japan's economic growth was not just due to its technological and manufacturing advances. The Japanese government's protectionist trade policies also helped Japan become an economic superpower.

1. What were the U.S. military's main goals for Japan during the occupation?

   A. Removing the emperor from power and establishing a parliamentary system

   B. Ensuring the right of workers to unionize and encouraging land reform

   C. Disbanding large business corporations and building modern manufacturing facilities

   D. Bringing democracy and helping establish economic recovery

2. What was the primary way that the occupation government helped bring about political reform in Japan?

   A. It established the right of women to vote.

   B. It helped Japan draft a new constitution.

   C. It disbanded large business corporations.

   D. It built modern factories.

3. Under the political reforms, which group was allowed to buy land?

   A. Tenant farmers

   B. Women

   C. Zaibatsu

   D. Factory workers

4. *Protectionist* refers to policies that

   A. favor a country's own domestic products.

   B. encourage competition from other countries in trade.

   C. call for defensive actions by a country's military.

   D. seek to reduce violent crime in a country's population.

5. Which of the following would be a good title for this passage?

   A. The Successes of Japan's Occupation Government

   B. Life in Occupied Japan

   C. Japan's Unlikely Journey from Occupied Nation to Economic Powerhouse

   D. The Secret to Japan's Manufacturing Success

Proteins and You

Proteins are the most complex and diverse macromolecules in any living organism. They are polymers composed of linear chains of monomers called amino acids. A protein macromolecule typically contains between 200 and 300 amino acids. However, the largest can contain nearly 27,000 amino acids on a single chain. These chains are typically found in the skeletal system and cardiac muscle.

Proteins are responsible for an amazing variety of processes within your body. Enzymes are proteins in your body that make chemical reactions occur up to a million times faster. Without enzymes, these chemical reactions either would not occur or would happen too slowly for bodily functions to take place.

Proteins also keep your body safe. Antibodies are proteins that function within your immune system to help you fight disease. Other proteins help your blood form clots so you don't bleed to death when you get a cut. If you ever find yourself needing to flee from a scary situation, you can thank the proteins in your muscles that help you move. Much of the muscle mass in your body is made of proteins.

Transportation is another important job for proteins. Proteins transport materials in fluids throughout your body. For example, hemoglobin is a protein in your blood that carries oxygen from your lungs to your cells.

The most abundant protein in all the animal kingdom is collagen. The body uses it for strength and support. Collagen surrounds and contains all of your body's cells and organs, and it is in your teeth and bones. Another protein, keratin, provides strength for your hair and fingernails.

The same proteins that help your body function are also at work in animals. Like your hair and fingernails, feathers, fur, wool, and cashmere are all made of keratin. So are animal hooves. Leather, which is derived from animal skin, contains collagen and keratin. Silk, a fiber produced by special caterpillars, is also made of protein.

6. Protein is made up of
   A. rings of collagen.
   B. polymers of keratin.
   C. linear chains of amino acids.
   D. networks of antibodies.

7. From paragraph 5, you can assume that
   A. all proteins in humans are a type of collagen.
   B. collagen is the most abundant substance in the human body.
   C. collagen and keratin serve the same functions in the human body.
   D. proteins in general lend strength to substances they form.

8. Silk is made of
   A. keratin.
   B. protein.
   C. collagen.
   D. enzymes.

Mutations

Suppose you pick what you think is a juicy Red Delicious apple to eat. Then you notice that half the apple is yellow. This is an example of a mutation. It is the result of a change in an organism's DNA. Mutations in nature are random; that is, they are not related to how useful they will be to an organism. Most mutations are neutral or harmless. But some mutations can be helpful to organisms. Still others can be dangerous or even fatal.

When a cell divides normally, it makes a perfect copy of its DNA. However, sometimes a cell does not copy perfectly. There may be an addition or subtraction of nucleotides. There could also be a substitution of nucleotides. All of these changes result in a mutation.

Mutations can be inherited or acquired. There are two ways that a mutation is acquired. A cell's DNA may make a mistake when copying itself. Most often, cells can repair themselves, but not always. The result is a mutation. Mutations can also happen when an organism is exposed to certain chemicals or to radiation. This can cause the DNA to break down.

The addition or subtraction of a nucleotide can cause different proteins to be made. Both can also cause a cell to stop protein production. In either case, the result is usually a harmful mutation. The substitution of one nucleotide for another may not lead to a harmful effect. However, it could alter a protein so that it cannot function normally.

Mutations that are harmful include diseases such as phenylketonuria, which is due to a single mutation on chromosome 12 in both parents. If left untreated, this disease can lead to brain damage and intellectual disabilities. Doctors now regularly test newborns for the mutant gene.

Other mutations can be beneficial and help species evolve. An example is the panda's wrist bone, which has evolved into a thumb. This mutation enables pandas to get a better grip on bamboo, which is a major part of their diet.

Sickle cell is a mutation that is both harmful and beneficial. People with one sickle cell gene are resistant to malaria, a dangerous disease. But if a person inherits the gene for sickle cell from both parents, the mutation may result in sickle cell anemia, a chronic and life-threatening disease.

9. Which of the following is an example of an acquired mutation?

   A. Sickle cell anemia

   B. Phenylketonuria

   C. Cancer resulting from exposure to radiation

   D. A panda's thumb evolving from its wrist bone

10. All genetic mutations result from

   A. a mistake made when a cell is copying its DNA.

   B. a change in an organism's DNA.

   C. exposure to chemicals or radiation.

   D. a substitution of nucleotides.

STOP

IF YOU FINISH BEFORE TIME IS CALLED, YOU MAY CHECK YOUR WORK ON THIS SECTION ONLY. DO NOT TURN TO ANY OTHER SECTION IN THE TEST.

ANSWER KEYS AND EXPLANATIONS

Verbal Ability

1. B	**3.** B	**5.** C	**7.** B	**9.** A
2. A	**4.** B	**6.** A	**8.** D	**10.** A

1. **The correct answer is B.** To *correlate* with is "to *correspond* with" or "to bear a mutual relationship with." Choices A and D are incorrect because *differ* and *contradict* mean the opposite of *correspond*. Choice C is incorrect because the physician is comparing the patient's signs and symptoms with those of influenza, not combining. (SYNONYMS)

2. **The correct answer is A.** *Intermittent* and *sporadic* are synonyms. Choice B is incorrect because *severe* refers to degree or strength whereas *intermittent* refers to irregularity. Choice C is incorrect because *regular* means the opposite of *intermittent*. *Chronic* (choice D) is incorrect because it refers to duration, not to irregularity. (SYNONYMS)

3. **The correct answer is B.** *Explicit* means "clear, obvious, unambiguous." The words *tacit, implicit, implied*, and *understood* are incorrect because they all relate to an unspoken understanding or agreement, which is the opposite of *explicit*. (ANTONYMS)

4. **The correct answer is B.** *Stasis* means "a state of stagnation or little change." The words *metamorphosis, conversion, transformation*, and *evolution* are incorrect because they all relate to radical change, which is the opposite of *stasis*. (ANTONYMS)

5. **The correct answer is C.** This is an object to action analogy. A *scalpel* is used to *cut*, and a *needle* is used to *inject*. Choice A is incorrect because a *syringe* is a device to

which a needle can be attached, not an action of the needle. Choice B is incorrect because *pain* is an effect of being injected with a needle, not the action of the needle. Choice D is incorrect because *medicine* is the object of *inject*, not the action of the *needle*. (OBJECT : ACTION ANALOGY)

6. **The correct answer is A.** This is a part to whole analogy. A *dog* is a part of the class of animals known as *mammals*, and a *cake* is a part of the class of food known as *desserts*. Choice B is incorrect because *pie* is another part of the class of *desserts*. Choice C is incorrect because an *oven* is the place where a *cake* is made, not the class to which it belongs. Choice D is incorrect because *bake* is the action associated with the object *cake*, not the class to which it belongs. (PART : WHOLE ANALOGY)

7. **The correct answer is B.** This is a sequence analogy. *Friday* is immediately followed by *Saturday* as *April* is immediately followed by *May*. Choice A is incorrect because *March* precedes, not follows, *April*. Choices C and D are incorrect because *spring* and *summer* are seasons, not months, and thus are not parallel with *April* the same way that *Saturday* is with *Friday*. In addition, April falls within the season of spring and thus is not in sequence with it. (SEQUENCE ANALOGY)

8. **The correct answer is D.** Two independent clauses such as these may be properly joined by a semicolon. Choice A is incorrect because a comma may only join

two independent clauses if followed by a coordinating conjunction, such as *and* or *but*. Choice B is incorrect because the first independent clause does not make sense as a question. Choice C is incorrect because a quotation mark does not serve as coordinating punctuation. (GRAMMAR)

9. **The correct answer is A.** The infinitive of the verb *lie*, which is intransitive (does not take a direct object) and means "to rest in a horizontal position," is correct in this sentence. Choice B is incorrect because the verb *lay* is transitive (requires a direct object) and means "to set something down," which does not make sense in this sentence. Choice C is incorrect because *laid* is the past tense of the verb *lay*; neither the past tense nor the verb *lay* is correct in this sentence. Choice D is incorrect because it is a misspelling of the past tense of the verb *lay*. (GRAMMAR)

10. **The correct answer is A.** The clause "that is black and has white paws" is necessary for identifying the cat; without it, "the cat" could refer to any cat. Therefore, this clause is essential to the meaning of the sentence and should not be set off by commas. Choices B through D are incorrect because essential clauses should not be set off by commas, as just explained. (GRAMMAR)

Mathematics

1. B	3. D	5. C	7. A	9. C
2. C	4. C	6. A	8. D	10. A

1. **The correct answer is B.**

$$\frac{2}{3} + 3\frac{5}{6} + \frac{4}{9} = \left(\frac{6}{6}\right)\left(\frac{2}{3}\right) + \left(\frac{3}{3}\right)\left(\frac{23}{6}\right) + \left(\frac{2}{2}\right)\left(\frac{4}{9}\right)$$
$$= \frac{12}{18} + \frac{69}{18} + \frac{8}{18}$$
$$= \frac{89}{18}$$
$$= 4\frac{17}{18}$$

(ADDITION OF FRACTIONS)

2. **The correct answer is C.** $1.69(12) = 20.28$
(MULTIPLICATION)

3. **The correct answer is D.**

$$\frac{3,600}{2,880}(2) = 2.5$$

(PROBLEM SOLVING: MULTIPLICATION, DIVISION)

4. **The correct answer is C.**

$$2\frac{4}{7} \times 5\frac{1}{5} = \frac{18}{7} \times \frac{26}{5}$$
$$= \frac{468}{35}$$

(MULTIPLICATION OF COMPLEX FRACTIONS)

5. **The correct answer is C.**

$$8(x + 3) = 58$$
$$8x + 24 = 58$$
$$8x = 34$$
$$x = 4.25$$

(SOLVING EQUATIONS)

6. **The correct answer is A.** $\$156 \times 12 = \$1,872$ (PROBLEM SOLVING: MULTIPLICATION)

7. **The correct answer is A.**

$$\frac{3}{4} \div \frac{1}{3} = \frac{3}{4} \times \frac{3}{1}$$
$$= \frac{9}{4}$$

(DIVISION OF FRACTIONS)

8. **The correct answer is D.**
$4.0804 \div 0.04 = 408.04 \div 4 = 102.01$. The other choices are the result of not moving the decimal point correctly. (MULTIPLICATION OF DECIMALS)

9. **The correct answer is C.**
Since AB is parallel to CD, we know that $\angle A$ is congruent to $\angle C$ since they are corresponding angles. For the same reason, we know that $\angle B$ and $\angle D$ are both right angles. Therefore, $\triangle ABE$ is similar to $\triangle CDE$. As such, corresponding sides are in the same proportion. Applying this yields the equation $\frac{AB}{CD} = \frac{BE}{DE}$, which is equivalent to $\frac{10}{5} = \frac{x+8}{8}$. To solve for x, we cross-multiply to get $80 = 5x + 40$, so that $5x = 40$ and $x = 8$. (GEOMETRY: RIGHT TRIANGLE; ALGEBRA: SOLVING EQUATIONS)

10. **The correct answer is A.** A trapezoid has one pair of parallel sides, whereas the illustrated quadrilateral has two. (GEOMETRY RELATIONSHIPS)

Spelling

1. C	3. B	5. A	7. C	9. C
2. C	4. B	6. B	8. A	10. B

1. **The correct answer is C.** The correct spelling is *anatomy*.

2. **The correct answer is C.** The correct spelling is *etiology*.

3. **The correct answer is B.** The correct spelling is *urinalysis*.

4. **The correct answer is B.** The correct spelling is *nutrition*.

5. **The correct answer is A.** The correct spelling is *achievement*.

6. **The correct answer is B.** The correct spelling is *infection*.

7. **The correct answer is C.** The correct spelling is *vaccination*.

8. **The correct answer is A.** The correct spelling is *diabetes*.

9. **The correct answer is C.** The correct spelling is *systolic*.

10. **The correct answer is B.** The correct spelling is *electrocardiography*.

Nonverbal Ability

1. B	3. D	5. C	7. E	9. B
2. D	4. A	6. E	8. D	10. A

1. **The correct answer is B.** The relationship between the first two shapes is that they are both black triangles but the second is larger than the first. So in the second pair, we begin with a small white triangle and are looking for a large white triangle. Therefore, small black triangle is to large black triangle as small white triangle is to large white triangle.

2. **The correct answer is D.** The relationship between the first two shapes is that the second is the same as the first except that it has vertical stripes whereas the first doesn't. So in the second pair, we begin with a circle and are looking for a circle with vertical stripes. Therefore, square is to square with vertical stripes as circle is to circle with vertical stripes.

3. **The correct answer is D.** The first pair of shapes includes a line segment connecting a white circle to a black circle and a line segment connecting a black circle to a white circle. The relationship between the first two pairs of shapes is that both contain an object and its mirror image, but in the second pair, the objects from the first pair have each been rotated 180 degrees. So in the second set of shapes, we begin with an open hourglass pointing right and open hourglass pointing left and are looking for an open hourglass pointing left and open hourglass pointing right.

4. **The correct answer is A.** The relationship between the first two images is that both contain a U and a plus sign, but in the second image, the plus sign has moved out of and to the left of the U and has grown larger. In addition, the U has rotated 90 degrees to the right. So in the second pair, we begin with a V pointed right with a small circle embedded within it and are looking for a larger circle to the left of a V that has rotated 90 degrees to the right. Therefore, U pointed up with small plus sign embedded within it is to large plus sign and U pointed right as V pointed right with small circle embedded within it is to large circle and V pointed down. You might be tempted to choose B because it resembles the second image in the first pair, but this would mean that the V had not rotated, as the U had rotated in the first pair. Remember that it is the *relationships* you are attempting to match, not necessarily the appearance of the images.

5. **The correct answer is C.** The relationship between the first two images is that the second is the same as the first except it has no plus sign. So in the second pair, we begin with a multiplication sign surrounded by four dots that form a diamond and are looking for the same image except without the multiplication sign, which is four dots that form a diamond. Therefore, plus sign surrounded by four dots that form a square is to four dots that form a square as multiplication sign surrounded by four dots that form a diamond is to four dots that form a diamond.

6. **The correct answer is E.** The relationship between the first two items is that the second represents the number of sides of the shape in the first. So in the second pair, we begin with a square and are looking for the number that represents the number of sides of the square, which is 4. Therefore, triangle is to 3 as square is to 4.

7. **The correct answer is E.** The relationship between the first two shapes is that the second is only the black half of the first. So in the second pair, we begin with a circle with a white left half and black right half and are looking for a right-oriented black semicircle. Therefore, circle with left half black and right half white is to left-oriented black semicircle as circle with left half white and right half black is to right-oriented black semicircle. Another way this analogy could have worked is that the relationship could have centered on the second shape in the first pair being the left half of the first, rather than focusing on it being the black half. However, as a white semicircle is not included among the answer choices, this relationship is clearly not the focus.

8. **The correct answer is D.** The relationship between the first two shapes is that the second is double the first. So in the second pair, we begin with a right single angle bracket and are looking for a right double angle bracket. Therefore, left single angle bracket is to left double angle bracket as right single angle bracket is to right double angle bracket.

9. **The correct answer is B.** The relationship between the first two shapes is that the second is the mirror image the first. So in the second pair, we begin with a doubled U pointed right and are looking for its mirror image, which is a doubled U pointed left. Therefore, inverted L pointed right is to inverted L pointed left as doubled U pointed right is to doubled U pointed left.

10. **The correct answer is A.** The relationship between the first two shapes is that the second is an inversion of the first. So in the second pair, we begin with an up-pointing perpendicular line segment bisecting a circle and are looking for its inversion, which is a down-pointing perpendicular line segment bisecting a circle. Therefore, up-pointing triangle bisected by a line segment is to down-pointing triangle bisected by a line segment as up-pointing perpendicular line segment bisecting a circle is to down-pointing perpendicular line segment bisecting a circle.

Science

1. A	3. D	5. C	7. B	9. D
2. B	4. D	6. D	8. A	10. D

1. **The correct answer is A.** The nucleus is the organelle that is considered the control center of the cell because it contains the genetic information of the cell. The Golgi apparatus, or Golgi body (choice B), plays a role in protein synthesis by making modifications to proteins, processing and sorting them, and then packaging the final protein product in a small sac called a vesicle. The vesicle leaves the Golgi body and transports the protein to the cell membrane where it can leave the cell to carry out its function in the body. The mitochondria (choice C) are the organelles in which energy from organic molecules is converted to ATP. Ribosomes (choice D) are the site of protein synthesis in the cell. (THE CELL)

2. **The correct answer is B.** The immune system is composed of cells that help to fight infection. In particular, these are white blood cells. Choice A is incorrect because the musculoskeletal system is only composed of muscles, bones, joints, ligaments, cartilage, and tendons. Choice C is incorrect because the integumentary system is composed of skin, hair, nails, and sweat and sebaceous glands. It functions to protect the body from injury and dehydration, to maintain a constant temperature in the body, to produce vitamin D, to excrete waste materials and toxins, and to react to microorganisms and chemicals. Choice D is incorrect because the endocrine system is made up of organs that produce and secrete hormones and steroids. (IMMUNE SYSTEM)

3. **The correct answer is D.** Type O red blood cells have neither the A nor the B antigen and so can be safely transfused to individuals of any ABO blood type, because any ABO antibodies (A or B) the person has will not be activated. Choice A is incorrect because type A red blood cells have the A antigen and therefore can only be given to those with type A or AB blood. Choice B is incorrect because type B red blood cells have the B antigen and therefore can only be given to those with type B or AB blood. Choice C is incorrect because type AB red blood cells have both the A and B antigens and therefore can only be given to those with type AB blood. (CARDIOVASCULAR SYSTEM)

4. **The correct answer is D.** Basophils are cells that release chemicals that respond to inflammation at the site of an infection. Choice A is incorrect because cytotoxic T-cells act to recognize and kill infected cells. Choice B is incorrect because natural killer cells are released to attack foreign antigens in the body. Choice C is incorrect because interferons and cytokines are chemicals in the immune system that are released to block viruses from replicating and to activate surrounding cells that have antiviral functions. (IMMUNE SYSTEM)

5. **The correct answer is C.** The liver functions in the digestive system to produce bile, which breaks down fats. Choice A is incorrect because the small intestine, which is a long, muscular tube of narrow diameter where most chemical digestion takes place and most nutrients are absorbed, receives bile from the liver but does not produce it. Choice B is incorrect because the large intestine, where water and vitamins are

absorbed, does not produce bile. Choice D is incorrect because in the stomach, acids and enzymes act to break down proteins and to kill bacteria, but no bile is produced. (DIGESTIVE SYSTEM)

6. **The correct answer is D.** Smooth muscle is found in the lining of the organs such as the stomach, intestines, and bladder, as well as the lining of the blood vessels. Smooth muscle functions to help move materials, such as blood and food, through the body. Smooth muscle is involuntary. Choice A is incorrect because only cardiac and skeletal muscle tissues are striated and they do not line the stomach, intestines, and bladder. Choice B is incorrect because cardiac muscle is the tissue that makes up the heart, not the stomach, intestines, and bladder. Choice C is incorrect because skeletal muscle tissue is attached to bones and moves parts of the skeleton. (MUSCULOSKELETAL SYSTEM)

7. **The correct answer is B.** Motor neurons receive an output signal from interneurons leaving the brain and translate that signal into a motor response, such as causing the muscles in the arm to contract and jerk the hand back in response to the hand touching a hot stove. Choice A is incorrect because sensory neurons receive sensory information from a stimulus; the signal is sent to interneurons before it reaches the brain. Choice C is incorrect because brain cells do not directly deliver a signal to muscle cells. The signal passes through interneurons and then on to motor neurons. Choice D is incorrect because interneurons, or association neurons, are neurons that link sensory neurons to motor neurons. They are found in the brain and the spinal cord. They receive information from the sensory neurons of the peripheral nervous system and transport this signal to the brain and then to motor neurons for the output signal. (NERVOUS SYSTEM)

8. **The correct answer is A.** The function of luteinizing hormone is to release an ovum in females (ovulation) and produce testosterone in males. Choice B is incorrect because follicle-stimulating hormone (FSH) initiates the development of follicles in the ovaries in females but does not trigger the release of the ovum from the follicle. In males, FSH stimulates sperm but not testosterone production in the testes. Choice C is incorrect because the main function of estrogen is to promote female secondary sex characteristics, thicken the endometrial lining, and promote oogenesis. Choice D is incorrect because the main function of testosterone is to promote male secondary sex characteristics and spermatogenesis. (REPRODUCTIVE SYSTEM)

9. **The correct answer is D.** Vitamin K is a fat-soluble vitamin that is essential for the synthesis of clotting factors, which are involved in coagulation following an injury. Choice A is incorrect because vitamin A, although a fat-soluble vitamin, is important for maintaining healthy skin and allowing night vision. Choice B is incorrect because vitamin D, although a fat-soluble vitamin, is essential for absorption of calcium and phosphorus and aids in the growth of bones and teeth. Choice C is incorrect because vitamin E, although a fat-soluble vitamin, is involved in helping form cell structures, DNA, RNA, and red blood cells and may help promote wound healing. (NUTRITION)

10. **The correct answer is D.** Thyroxine is a hormone released by the thyroid gland to stimulate the metabolism. Choice A is incorrect because estrogen is a sex hormone and does not act on the metabolism. Choice

B is incorrect because testosterone is a male sex hormone and does not act on the metabolism. Choice C is incorrect because cortisol is a hormone that is released in response to stress and does not act on the metabolism. (ENDOCRINE SYSTEM)

Reading Comprehension

1. D	3. A	5. C	7. D	9. C
2. B	4. A	6. C	8. B	10. B

1. **The correct answer is D.** The answer is stated in the last sentence of paragraph 1. Choices A through C are all too specific, referring only to certain aspects of the main goals.

2. **The correct answer is B.** The answer is stated in paragraph 2, sentence 1. Choice A is incorrect because it is too specific, as it is included in the new constitution that the occupation government helped Japan draft, and thus is not the *primary* way the occupation government helped bring political reform. Choice C is incorrect because the occupation government did not succeed in disbanding the large business corporations; also, this relates more to economic reform than political. Choice D is incorrect because the building of modern factories is something Japan did itself after the occupation; the occupation government had nothing to do with it.

3. **The correct answer is A.** The answer is stated in paragraph 3, sentences 4 and 5.

4. **The correct answer is A.** Protectionist policies favor a country's own domestic products over those of other countries by imposing high tariffs on imports.

5. **The correct answer is C.** A title should reflect the main idea, or theme, of a piece of writing. It needs to be general enough to touch on all the main points in the passage. Choice A is incorrect because it describes just the first part of the passage and doesn't include the idea that Japan became an economic power after the occupation. Choice B is incorrect for the same reason. It doesn't include what happened to Japan after the occupation. Choice D is incorrect because it focuses too narrowly on only one aspect of Japan's recovery, that is, its success in manufacturing. Only choice C represents the full scope of Japan's recovery.

6. **The correct answer is C.** The answer is stated in paragraph 1, sentence 2.

7. **The correct answer is D.** Paragraph 5 mentions that both collagen and keratin provide strength to the substances they compose; therefore, it seems reasonable to assume that protein, in general, lends strength to the substances it composes. The other answer choices are either false statements or unreasonable assumptions.

8. **The correct answer is B.** The answer is stated in the final paragraph, sentence 5.

9. **The correct answer is C.** The answer is stated in paragraph 3, sentence 6. Choices A, B, and D are all examples of inherited, not acquired, mutations.

10. **The correct answer is B.** The answer is stated in paragraph 1, sentence 4.

Diagnostic Test for Practical/Vocational Nursing School

UNIT 3 DIAGNOSTIC TEST FOR PRACTICAL/ VOCATIONAL NURSING SCHOOL ANSWER SHEET

Verbal Ability

1. Ⓐ Ⓑ Ⓒ Ⓓ   3. Ⓐ Ⓑ Ⓒ Ⓓ Ⓔ   5. Ⓐ Ⓑ Ⓒ Ⓓ   7. Ⓐ Ⓑ Ⓒ Ⓓ   9. Ⓐ Ⓑ Ⓒ Ⓓ
2. Ⓐ Ⓑ Ⓒ Ⓓ   4. Ⓐ Ⓑ Ⓒ Ⓓ Ⓔ   6. Ⓐ Ⓑ Ⓒ Ⓓ   8. Ⓐ Ⓑ Ⓒ Ⓓ   10. Ⓐ Ⓑ Ⓒ Ⓓ

Mathematics

1. Ⓐ Ⓑ Ⓒ Ⓓ   3. Ⓐ Ⓑ Ⓒ Ⓓ   5. Ⓐ Ⓑ Ⓒ Ⓓ   7. Ⓐ Ⓑ Ⓒ Ⓓ   9. Ⓐ Ⓑ Ⓒ Ⓓ
2. Ⓐ Ⓑ Ⓒ Ⓓ   4. Ⓐ Ⓑ Ⓒ Ⓓ   6. Ⓐ Ⓑ Ⓒ Ⓓ   8. Ⓐ Ⓑ Ⓒ Ⓓ   10. Ⓐ Ⓑ Ⓒ Ⓓ

Spelling

1. Ⓐ Ⓑ Ⓒ   3. Ⓐ Ⓑ Ⓒ   5. Ⓐ Ⓑ Ⓒ   7. Ⓐ Ⓑ Ⓒ   9. Ⓐ Ⓑ Ⓒ
2. Ⓐ Ⓑ Ⓒ   4. Ⓐ Ⓑ Ⓒ   6. Ⓐ Ⓑ Ⓒ   8. Ⓐ Ⓑ Ⓒ   10. Ⓐ Ⓑ Ⓒ

Nonverbal Ability

1. Ⓐ Ⓑ Ⓒ Ⓓ Ⓔ   3. Ⓐ Ⓑ Ⓒ Ⓓ Ⓔ   5. Ⓐ Ⓑ Ⓒ Ⓓ Ⓔ   7. Ⓐ Ⓑ Ⓒ Ⓓ Ⓔ   9. Ⓐ Ⓑ Ⓒ Ⓓ Ⓔ
2. Ⓐ Ⓑ Ⓒ Ⓓ Ⓔ   4. Ⓐ Ⓑ Ⓒ Ⓓ Ⓔ   6. Ⓐ Ⓑ Ⓒ Ⓓ Ⓔ   8. Ⓐ Ⓑ Ⓒ Ⓓ Ⓔ   10. Ⓐ Ⓑ Ⓒ Ⓓ Ⓔ

Science

1. Ⓐ Ⓑ Ⓒ Ⓓ   3. Ⓐ Ⓑ Ⓒ Ⓓ   5. Ⓐ Ⓑ Ⓒ Ⓓ   7. Ⓐ Ⓑ Ⓒ Ⓓ   9. Ⓐ Ⓑ Ⓒ Ⓓ
2. Ⓐ Ⓑ Ⓒ Ⓓ   4. Ⓐ Ⓑ Ⓒ Ⓓ   6. Ⓐ Ⓑ Ⓒ Ⓓ   8. Ⓐ Ⓑ Ⓒ Ⓓ   10. Ⓐ Ⓑ Ⓒ Ⓓ

Reading Comprehension

1. Ⓐ Ⓑ Ⓒ Ⓓ   3. Ⓐ Ⓑ Ⓒ Ⓓ   5. Ⓐ Ⓑ Ⓒ Ⓓ   7. Ⓐ Ⓑ Ⓒ Ⓓ   9. Ⓐ Ⓑ Ⓒ Ⓓ
2. Ⓐ Ⓑ Ⓒ Ⓓ   4. Ⓐ Ⓑ Ⓒ Ⓓ   6. Ⓐ Ⓑ Ⓒ Ⓓ   8. Ⓐ Ⓑ Ⓒ Ⓓ   10. Ⓐ Ⓑ Ⓒ Ⓓ

Judgment and Comprehension

1. Ⓐ Ⓑ Ⓒ Ⓓ   3. Ⓐ Ⓑ Ⓒ Ⓓ   5. Ⓐ Ⓑ Ⓒ Ⓓ   7. Ⓐ Ⓑ Ⓒ Ⓓ   9. Ⓐ Ⓑ Ⓒ Ⓓ
2. Ⓐ Ⓑ Ⓒ Ⓓ   4. Ⓐ Ⓑ Ⓒ Ⓓ   6. Ⓐ Ⓑ Ⓒ Ⓓ   8. Ⓐ Ⓑ Ⓒ Ⓓ   10. Ⓐ Ⓑ Ⓒ Ⓓ

answer sheet

Verbal Ability

10 Questions • 5 Minutes

Directions: For questions 1 and 2, one word is italicized. Following each sentence are four words or phrases. For each sentence, choose the word or phrase that most nearly corresponds in meaning with the italicized word.

1. The young woman wanted to undergo bariatric surgery, but her healthcare provider informed her that this treatment was *contraindicated*.
   A. ineffective
   B. warranted
   C. unavailable
   D. inadvisable

2. The student's favorite part of biology class was learning about the *taxonomy* of all living things.
   A. classification
   B. origin
   C. adaptability
   D. similarity

Directions: For questions 3 and 4, choose the word that is most different in meaning from the others.

3. A. presume
   B. guess
   C. conjecture
   D. perceive
   E. suppose

4. A. subjective
   B. biased
   C. intuitive
   D. instinctive
   E. detached

Directions: For questions 5–7, determine the relationship between the first pair of capitalized words and then decide which of the answer choices shares a similar relationship with the third capitalized word.

5. CHICAGO : NORTH AMERICA :: BEIJING :
   A. China
   B. Eastern hemisphere
   C. Hebei Province
   D. Asia

6. RISKY : LIFE-THREATENING :: PROFICIENT :
   A. competent
   B. bungling
   C. amateurish
   D. masterful

7. INTELLIGENCE : PROFESSOR ::
   AGILITY :
   A. nimbleness
   B. training
   C. acrobat
   D. accountant

Directions: For questions 8–10, select the answer that completes the sentence in a grammatically correct manner or that represents the most grammatically correct of all options.

---

8. Between _____, I hated that movie.
   A. you and I
   B. you and me
   C. we two
   D. I and you

9. The exam was much _____ than I thought it would be.
   A. easy
   B. more easier
   C. easier
   D. easiest

10. Which of the following sentences is grammatically correct?
    A. Because you are my friend; I'm telling you the truth.
    B. Because you are my friend I'm telling you the truth.
    C. Because you are my friend, I'm telling you the truth.
    D. Because you are my friend. I'm telling you the truth.

STOP

IF YOU FINISH BEFORE TIME IS CALLED, YOU MAY CHECK YOUR WORK ON THIS SECTION ONLY. DO NOT TURN TO ANY OTHER SECTION IN THE TEST.

Mathematics

10 Questions • 10 Minutes

Directions: For questions 1–10, read each question carefully and decide which option is the best answer.

1. What is the answer when the following fractions are added together:

   $\frac{1}{2}, \frac{3}{5}$, and $\frac{7}{10}$?

   A. $\frac{11}{7}$

   B. $1\frac{4}{5}$

   C. $2\frac{2}{5}$

   D. $3\frac{3}{5}$

   SHOW YOUR WORK HERE

2. What is the product of 7.19 and 3.68?

   A. 1.9538

   B. 10.87

   C. 25.4692

   D. 26.4592

3. What is the difference when you subtract 72.3047 from 743.22

   A. 20.173

   B. 102.790

   C. 670.9153

   D. 735.9895

4. When 31.187 is divided by 0.05, the answer is

   A. 0.62374

   B. 6.2374

   C. 62.374

   D. 623.74

5. Express 48% as a fraction and reduce it to its lowest terms.

A. $\dfrac{1.2}{50}$

B. $\dfrac{12}{25}$

C. $\dfrac{5}{12}$

D. $\dfrac{48}{100}$

SHOW YOUR WORK HERE

6. Write the ratio 6 to 11 as a fraction.

A. 6.11

B. 11:6

C. $\dfrac{11}{6}$

D. $\dfrac{6}{11}$

7. What is the difference between
$\dfrac{5}{7}$ and $\dfrac{6}{21}$?

A. $\dfrac{1}{14}$

B. $\dfrac{2}{7}$

C. $\dfrac{3}{7}$

D. $\dfrac{11}{21}$

8. A patient receives medicine at the pre-scribed constant rate of 33 ml every 2 hours. How many ml of medicine does the patient receive in 12.8 hours?

A. 185.4

B. 211.2

C. 212.3

D. 221.1

9. A baker needs $2\frac{1}{4}$ cups of flour, $2\frac{3}{8}$ cups of milk, and $\frac{1}{3}$ cup of sugar to make a dozen popovers. How many total cups of these ingredients are needed to make the popovers?

SHOW YOUR WORK HERE

A. $4\frac{23}{24}$

B. $4\frac{8}{15}$

C. $4\frac{5}{8}$

D. $4\frac{1}{3}$

10. If there are 63 patients in the emergency room at Metro Medical Center, and $\frac{1}{9}$ of these patients are critical, how many non-critical patients are in the ER?

A. 7

B. 54

C. 55.99

D. 56

STOP

IF YOU FINISH BEFORE TIME IS CALLED, YOU MAY CHECK YOUR WORK ON THIS SECTION ONLY. DO NOT TURN TO ANY OTHER SECTION IN THE TEST.

Spelling

10 Questions • 5 Minutes

Directions: For questions 1–10, choose the word that is spelled correctly.

1. A. microorganism
   B. microrganism
   C. mycroorganism

2. A. hemorrage
   B. hemerrhage
   C. hemorrhage

3. A. obstetrics
   B. obstretics
   C. obstetricks

4. A. introvenous
   B. intravenous
   C. innervenous

5. A. carbohydrate
   B. carbahydrate
   C. carbohidrate

6. A. labrotory
   B. laboratory
   C. laborotory

7. A. flebotomy
   B. phlebotomy
   C. phlebodomy

8. A. esofagus
   B. esophogus
   C. esophagus

9. A. ventricole
   B. ventrical
   C. ventricle

10. A. integumentary
    B. entegumentary
    C. integomentary

STOP

IF YOU FINISH BEFORE TIME IS CALLED, YOU MAY CHECK YOUR WORK ON THIS SECTION ONLY. DO NOT TURN TO ANY OTHER SECTION IN THE TEST.

Nonverbal Ability

10 Questions • 10 Minutes

Directions: For questions 1–10, determine the relationship between the first pair of shapes and then decide which of the answer choices shares a similar relationship with the third shape.

1. ◤ is to ◣ as ⋏ is to?

   A. ⊤

   B. ⊥

   C. ⊢

   D. ⋋

   E. ⊣

2. ⊕ is to ✚ as ⊗ is to?

   A. ✕

   B. ◯

   C. ◁✕

   D. ⋈

   E. ⋈

3. ╋ is to ✚ as ✕ is to?

   A. ✕

   B. ☒

   C. ◁☒

   D. ✖

   E. ☒▷

4. ⋏ is to ✦ as ▲ is to?

   A. ●

   B. ■

   C. ▼

   D. ▶

   E. ⬟

5. ▲ is to ▼ as ■ is to?

   A. ◆

   B. ◆

   C. ▪

   D. ◆

   E. ■

6. ▷ is to ◀ as ▶ is to?

   A. ◀

   B. ▷

   C. ◁

   D. △

   E. ▽

7. • is to ◯ as ■ is to?

   A. ⊙

   B. □

   C. ■

   D. ⊡

   E. ◼

8. ⌒ is to ⌓ as ◗ is to?

   A. ●

   B. ◗

   C. ▶

   D. ◆

   E. ◎

9. ◖ is to ● as ◀ is to?

   A. ◆

   B. ■

   C. ◀

   D. ▶

   E. ▲

10. ╬ is to ∟ as ◆ is to?

   A. ◆

   B. ◣

   C. ◤

   D. ◥

   E. ◢

STOP

IF YOU FINISH BEFORE TIME IS CALLED, YOU MAY CHECK YOUR WORK ON THIS SECTION ONLY. DO NOT TURN TO ANY OTHER SECTION IN THE TEST.

Science

10 Questions • 10 Minutes

Directions: For questions 1–10, read each question carefully and consider all possible answers. There is only one best answer for each question.

1. The blood vessels that carry blood from all over the body back to the heart are the
   A. arteries.
   B. bronchioles.
   C. capillaries.
   D. veins.

2. The lower chambers of the heart are called
   A. atria.
   B. ventricles.
   C. arteries.
   D. valves.

3. The organ that is the largest single mass of lymphatic tissue in the body and that contains lymphocytes and macrophages involved in immune response is the
   A. thymus.
   B. lymph node.
   C. liver.
   D. spleen.

4. Bile stored in the gallbladder aids in the process of emulsification, which is the breakdown of
   A. proteins.
   B. carbohydrates.
   C. fats.
   D. sugars.

5. The functional unit of the kidneys, which is involved in filtering blood of wastes, is known as the
   A. neuron.
   B. nephron.
   C. hepatocyte.
   D. osteocyte.

6. Cords of dense regular connective tissue that attach muscles to bone are
   A. tendons.
   B. ligaments.
   C. joints.
   D. cartilages.

7. In a developing embryo, which of the following occurs during weeks 1 to 4 of gestation?
   A. The heart forms and begins to beat.
   B. Limbs become more distinct and digits appear.
   C. Gender is distinguishable on the basis of external genitalia.
   D. Fetal movements are commonly felt by the mother.

8. Which nutrient is the body's primary source for energy?
   A. Vitamins
   B. Protein
   C. Lipids
   D. Carbohydrates

9. Which of the following is an essential mineral?
   A. Tocopherol
   B. Phosphorous
   C. Biotin
   D. Omega-3

10. Which of the following is known as "bad" cholesterol because of its association with the accumulation of fatty plaques in the arteries that increases the risk of heart disease?

 A. High-density lipoproteins (HDLs)

 B. Low-density lipoproteins (LDLs)

 C. Very low-density lipoproteins (VLDLs)

 D. Amino acids

STOP

IF YOU FINISH BEFORE TIME IS CALLED, YOU MAY CHECK YOUR WORK ON THIS SECTION ONLY. DO NOT TURN TO ANY OTHER SECTION IN THE TEST.

Reading Comprehension

10 Questions • 20 Minutes

Directions: For questions 1–10, carefully read the passage paragraphs and then answer the accompanying questions, basing your answer on what is stated in the paragraphs. There is only one best answer for each question.

Listening to Music Through the Years

When listening to music today, you are most likely listening to it on a digital device. However, the first audiences for music were in the streets, music halls, theaters, and clubs. By the late 1800s and early 1900s, musicians had begun to record their music in recording studios. Fans bought the music on discs known as records that were played on phonograph machines, one disc at a time. By the 1920s, the records were made of vinyl, a type of plastic. Over the years, companies produced them in different sizes and speeds: 78s, 45s, and 33 1/3s. The larger records held several songs. Companies soon figured out how to build phonograph machines that could stack several records at a time.

Phonograph machines were large, and many were actually built into pieces of furniture. Even smaller phonographs sat on tables or cabinets. There was nothing portable about phonographs until around the 1940s, when companies began making them in little suitcases.

During the 1970s and 1980s, audiotape cassettes gradually replaced vinyl records. Each cassette tape could hold ten or so songs. Fans listened to these tapes in cassette players. Some players were large and known as "boom boxes"; they could be carried around by a handle or on the shoulder. Others were personal tape players, such as the Sony Walkman®. In the late 1980s, compact discs (CDs) began replacing cassette tapes, and CD players began to replace tape players. Instead of walking around with earphones connected to tape players, people were plugged into personal CD players.

The first digital audio players, popularly known as MP3 players (after the name of the popular file format for digital music), were produced in the late 1990s. In the early 2000s, Apple® launched the iPod®, which would go on to become one of the most popular digital audio players of all time. Soon people were walking around with digital audio players with earbuds in their ears. These new music players were so small they could fit into a pocket or hook onto a belt. Around the same time that digital audio players were gaining popularity, smartphones emerged, many of which had built-in digital audio players. Now people could download their music to dedicated digital audio players, such as the iPod®, and smartphones, as well as to their desktops, laptops, and tablets. Instead of buying music in a "record store," people began buying digital copies online from sites such as Apple® Inc.'s iTunes®. In recent years, many people have begun to dispense with purchasing and downloading digital music files and are turning to streaming music directly from the internet on their digital devices.

Today, musicians still record in studios, but how we listen to their music has greatly changed.

1. Before phonographs, people mostly listened to music
   A. on vinyl record players.
   B. on 8-track tapes.
   C. as audiences at live performances.
   D. in their homes.

2. CDs began replacing cassette tapes in the late
   - **A.** 1960s.
   - **B.** 1970s.
   - **C.** 1980s.
   - **D.** 1990s.

3. A popular personal cassette tape player was known as the
   - **A.** Walkman®.
   - **B.** Boom box.
   - **C.** MP3 player.
   - **D.** iPod®.

Green Jobs for a New Economy

In the not too distant past, if you were looking for a job, you'd read the "Help Wanted" ads in the newspaper, or you would check trade and association publications for open positions within a specific industry. Today, most job listings have migrated to the internet, where you will find hundreds of job websites. How do you decide which ones to search and what to look for? Here are a few ideas to help you concentrate your search in the best places.

Remember that job boards are not just for searching when you are looking for a job. They can be indispensable when you are deciding on a career to pursue. They contain valuable information that can help direct your career choice, including job titles related to your interests; the regions of the country where particular jobs are most common (e.g., the Southwest and Southeast, where many people are retiring); types of employers (e.g., public or private, nonprofit, small companies, or large corporations); and salary ranges.

Examples of major internet sites to search for jobs include Monster.com, CareerBuilder, LinkedIn, Indeed, and ZipRecruiter. Choose one of the websites and type in your job area, such as "licensed practical nurse," and see what job opportunities come up. You can search for jobs in a specific city or nationwide and for specific industries such as hospitals, correctional institutions, and community clinics. You can also search for full-time, part-time, *per diem*, and temporary employment.

You can also look at the websites of professional organizations and unions that represent licensed practical nurses. Many of these organizations have job boards, and their postings are the most closely aligned with the group's specialties. Don't overlook your school's career counseling and job placement offices either.

4. The word *indispensable* means
   - **A.** handy.
   - **B.** essential.
   - **C.** frustrating.
   - **D.** confusing.

5. If searching on a popular job website for a position as an RN, which of the following pieces of information would you be *least* likely to find on the site?
   - **A.** Average salaries for different regions of the country
   - **B.** Listings for positions in public facilities
   - **C.** Regions of the country with most job openings
   - **D.** Code of ethics employer expects you to adopt

6. A good title for this article is
   - **A.** Using Job Boards to Find Your Next Job
   - **B.** Tips for Finding Job Listings and Career Information
   - **C.** Deciding on Your Career Path
   - **D.** How Technology Has Changed the Job Search

7. *Per diem* in this context most likely refers to employment that is
   A. without pay.
   B. on an as-needed basis.
   C. compensated according to an hourly rate.
   D. salaried.

Potential Relief for Patients with Alzheimer's Disease

There is an ongoing debate about the effectiveness of the drugs used to treat Alzheimer's disease. At this time, there are no drugs available that can cure or even stop the disease's progression. However, available drugs can lessen symptoms. But should a particular patient be prescribed one of these drugs? If so, when? For how long? Does the patient actually have Alzheimer's disease, or is the patient suffering from dementia? Complicating decisions about treatment is the difficulty in diagnosing Alzheimer's disease because a definitive diagnosis cannot be made until a patient is dead and an autopsy is performed. Patients may be assumed to have the disease because of the symptoms they present. Some patients may actually have dementia rather than Alzheimer's disease.

There are two classes of drugs available at present to treat Alzheimer's disease: glutamate regulators and cholinesterase inhibitors. The former blocks the death of brain cells, and the latter improves symptoms, or possibly only reduces unwanted behaviors. The glutamate regulators are prescribed to patients in moderate-to-severe stages of Alzheimer's disease, and cholinesterase inhibitors are given to patients in early-to-moderate stages. Both drugs have some side effects, though they are considered minor. Ironically, a potential side effect of the class of glutamate regulators is confusion.

8. Based on the last sentence in paragraph 1, we can infer that
   A. there is no way to distinguish dementia from Alzheimer's disease.
   B. dementia is a complication of Alzheimer's disease.
   C. dementia and Alzheimer's disease are unrelated conditions.
   D. dementia and Alzheimer's disease have similar symptoms.

9. *Definitive* in the first paragraph means
   A. differential.
   B. death-related.
   C. decisive.
   D. debatable.

10. We may infer from the last sentence of the article that
    A. confusion is a symptom of Alzheimer's disease that the medication is intended to alleviate.
    B. glutamate regulators are not effective in alleviating the symptoms of Alzheimer's disease.
    C. glutamate regulators are less effective than cholinesterase inhibitors in alleviating symptoms.
    D. most people who take glutamate regulators experience confusion as a side effect.

STOP

IF YOU FINISH BEFORE TIME IS CALLED, YOU MAY CHECK YOUR WORK ON THIS SECTION ONLY. DO NOT TURN TO ANY OTHER SECTION IN THE TEST.

Judgment and Comprehension in Practical Nursing

10 Questions • 5 Minutes

Directions: For questions 1–10, carefully read the question and then choose the correct response.

1. Your nursing supervisor has a bad temper and sometimes curses at you when you make even minor mistakes. This behavior really stresses you out. The best way for you to respond is to:

   A. submit a written complaint to your human resources manager.

   B. ask a coworker for advice on how to handle the situation.

   C. start practicing yoga to alleviate the stress.

   D. tell your supervisor you will quit if she doesn't stop yelling at you.

2. You observe a registered nurse on your unit taking some medications from a cabinet and stuffing them in a purse just before leaving for the day. Your best response is to:

   A. inform your supervisor.

   B. confront the nurse about the theft.

   C. call the police.

   D. watch the nurse closely over the next few shifts to see if it happens again.

3. A 30-year-old patient expresses distress to you over the decision of whether to pursue chemotherapy or palliative care for advanced cancer. Your best response is to say:

   A. "You're still so young; I'd choose the chemotherapy, if I were you."

   B. "My grandmother had hospice care before she died, and it was wonderful."

   C. "I know that must be hard for you. Do you have any questions about your treatment options?"

   D. "Sorry. I can't help you with that. I'm just here to take your vitals."

4. You are greeting a new patient to the unit, Grace Sanderson, who is 86 years old. The most appropriate way to address this patient would be to say:

   A. "Hi there, sweetie! I'm your nurse, and I'll be taking good care of you."

   B. "Hello, Grace. I'll be taking care of you today."

   C. "Hi there. Don't mind me. I'm just here to take your vitals."

   D. "Hello, Mrs. Sanderson. I'm your nurse for this shift."

5. A patient's 6-year-old son is playing a game on a tablet computer. The music from the game is getting on your nerves, but the patient doesn't seem bothered by it. Your best response is to:

   A. tell the child to turn off the game and find something else to do.

   B. ignore the music and go on about your work.

   C. complain to the patient about the music.

   D. inform your supervisor.

6. A 10-year-old girl who is about to undergo an appendectomy tells you she's afraid something bad will happen. Your best response is to say:

   A. "You have nothing to worry about. Nothing will go wrong."

   B. "Stop being a worry-wort! Everything will be fine."

   C. "I know it can be scary. But we have a great team here who will be taking good care of you."

   D. "So, what's your favorite subject in school?"

7. You enter the room of a patient with Alzheimer's disease to confirm that the patient has no drug allergies. The best approach would be to:

   A. ask the patient directly whether she has any drug allergies.

   B. ask the patient's husband, who is standing next to her, whether she has any drug allergies.

   C. find the attending physician to confirm that the patient's record is accurate.

   D. double-check the patient's record and then administer any needed medications.

8. A frustrated patient who has just been admitted tells you, "I don't even know why I'm having this surgery." Your best response would be to say:

   A. "Don't worry. Your surgeon is excellent and has performed many of these procedures."

   B. "Are you saying that you don't want to have the surgery?"

   C. "Then don't go through with it. I'll contact the surgeon and let him know."

   D. "Your surgery is necessary. Relax. It will all be over quickly."

9. A 92-year-old man tells you he can't wait for his wife to come visit him in the hospital. You are aware that the man's wife died 10 years ago. What is your best response?

   A. "Your wife died years ago."

   B. "Tell me about your wife."

   C. "I look forward to meeting her."

   D. "When are you expecting her to arrive?"

10. A patient has just been admitted who speaks only Spanish. She seems upset and is speaking to you rapidly in Spanish, but you do not speak Spanish. What is your best response?

    A. Explain that you do not speak Spanish and go on about your business.

    B. Ask the woman's 8-year-old son, who is bilingual, to translate for you.

    C. Arrange to have an interpreter come and assist the patient.

    D. Try to communicate with the patient using hand gestures.

STOP

IF YOU FINISH BEFORE TIME IS CALLED, YOU MAY CHECK YOUR WORK ON THIS SECTION ONLY. DO NOT TURN TO ANY OTHER SECTION IN THE TEST.

ANSWER KEYS AND EXPLANATIONS

Verbal Ability

1. D	3. D	5. D	7. C	9. C
2. A	4. E	6. D	8. B	10. C

1. **The correct answer is D.** *Contraindicated* and *inadvisable* are synonyms. You can eliminate *warranted* (choice B), which means "justified" or "called for," because the word "but" in the sentence indicates that the healthcare provider's response contradicts the woman's desire to have the surgery. Choices A and C are incorrect because although *ineffective* and *unavailable* make sense, they aren't synonyms for *contraindicated*. (SYNONYMS)

2. **The correct answer is A.** *Taxonomy* and *classification* are synonyms. Choice B is incorrect because *origin* refers to source or beginning, not classification. Choice C is incorrect because *adaptability*, which means "the ability to change to meet the demands of one's environment," is not a synonym of *taxonomy*. Choice D is incorrect because *similarity* refers to the ways in which things are alike, whereas *taxonomy* refers to a classification of things based on similarities and differences. (SYNONYMS)

3. **The correct answer is D.** *Perceive* means "to know, to understand." The words *presume*, *guess*, *conjecture*, and *suppose* are incorrect because they are synonyms and indicate a lack of full knowledge, which is the opposite of *perceive*. (ANTONYMS)

4. **The correct answer is E.** *Detached* means "objective, impartial." The words *subjective*, *biased*, *intuitive*, and *instinctive* are incorrect because they all relate to subjectivity, which is the opposite of *detached*. (ANTONYMS)

5. **The correct answer is D.** This is a place analogy. The city of *Chicago* is located on the continent of *North America*, and the city of *Beijing* is located on the continent of *Asia*. Choice A is incorrect because China is the country, not the continent, in which Beijing is located. Choice B is incorrect because the Eastern hemisphere is the hemisphere, not the continent, in which Beijing is located. Choice C is incorrect because Hebei Province is the province, not the continent, in which Beijing is located. (PLACE ANALOGY)

6. **The correct answer is D.** This is a degree analogy. *Risky* is a degree of, or step to being, *life-threatening*, and *proficient* is a degree of, or step to being, *masterful*. Choice A is incorrect because *competent* is a synonym, not a degree, of *proficient*. Choices B and C are incorrect because *bungling* and *amateurish* are antonyms, not degrees, of *proficient*. (DEGREE ANALOGY)

7. **The correct answer is C.** This is a characteristic analogy. *Intelligence* is a characteristic of *professors* as *agility* is characteristic of *acrobats*. Choice A is incorrect because *nimbleness* is a synonym, not a characteristic of *agility*. Choice B is incorrect because *training* is a cause of *agility*; *agility* is not a characteristic of *training*. Choice D is incorrect because *agility* is not a characteristic, in general, of *accountants* in the same way that *intelligence* is of *professors*. (CHARACTERISTIC ANALOGY)

8. **The correct answer is B.** The pronouns needed in this sentence are objects of the preposition *between* and thus must be in the objective case; *you* and *me* (choice B) are both in the objective case. Choices A and D are incorrect because *I* is in the subjective case. Choice C is incorrect because *we* is in the subjective case. (GRAMMAR)

9. **The correct answer is C.** What is needed in this sentence is an adjective to modify *exam* that is in the comparative form; *easier* meets these qualifications. Choice A is incorrect because *easy* is not the comparative form of this adjective. Choice B is incorrect because *more easier* is a double comparison and thus nonstandard. Choice D is incorrect because *easiest* is the superlative, not comparative, form of this adjective and thus does not make sense in this sentence. (GRAMMAR)

10. **The correct answer is C.** Introductory adverb clauses, such as *because you are my friend*, should be followed by a comma. Choice A is incorrect because semicolons should be used to separate independent clauses, not dependent clauses from independent clauses. Choice B is incorrect because introductory adverb clauses, such as *because you are my friend*, should be followed by a comma. Choice D is incorrect because adverb clauses, such as *because you are my friend*, are dependent clauses and may not stand alone as sentences. (GRAMMAR)

Mathematics

1. B	3. C	5. B	7. C	9. A
2. D	4. D	6. D	8. B	10. D

1. **The correct answer is B.**

$$\frac{1}{2} + \frac{3}{5} + \frac{7}{10} = \frac{5}{10} + \frac{6}{10} + \frac{7}{10}$$

$$= \frac{18}{10}$$

$$= 1\frac{8}{10}$$

$$= 1\frac{4}{5}$$

(ADDITION OF FRACTIONS)

2. **The correct answer is D.**

$$
\begin{array}{r}
7.19 \\
\times\ 3.68 \\
\hline
5752 \\
4314 \\
2137 \\
\hline
26.4592
\end{array}
$$

(MULTIPLICATION OF DECIMALS)

3. **The correct answer is C.**

$$
\begin{array}{r}
743.2200 \\
-72.3047 \\
\hline
670.9153
\end{array}
$$

(SUBTRACTION OF DECIMALS)

4. **The correct answer is D.**

$$
0.05\overline{)31.187} = 5\overline{)3118.70}
$$

$$
\begin{array}{r}
623.74 \\
\end{array}
$$

$$
\begin{array}{r}
30 \\
\hline
11 \\
10 \\
\hline
18 \\
15 \\
\hline
37 \\
35 \\
\hline
20 \\
20 \\
\hline
0
\end{array}
$$

(DIVISION OF DECIMALS)

5. **The correct answer is B.**

$$\frac{48}{100} = \frac{48 \div 4}{100 \div 4} = \frac{12}{25}$$

(CONVERSION OF PERCENTAGE TO FRACTION IN LOWEST TERMS)

6. **The correct answer is D.**

$$6:11 = \frac{6}{11}$$

(CONVERSION OF RATIOS TO FRACTIONS)

7. **The correct answer is C.**

$$\frac{5}{7} - \frac{6}{21} = \frac{15}{21} - \frac{6}{21}$$

$$= \frac{9}{21}$$

$$= \frac{3}{7}$$

(SUBTRACTION OF FRACTIONS)

8. **The correct answer is B.**

$$\frac{33}{2} = \frac{x}{12.8}$$

$$\frac{33(12.8)}{2} = x$$

$$\frac{422.4}{2} = x$$

$$211.2 = x$$

(ARITHMETIC: PROPORTIONS, PROBLEM SOLVING)

9. The correct answer is A.

$$2\frac{1}{4} + 2\frac{3}{8} + \frac{1}{3} = \frac{9}{4} + \frac{19}{8} + \frac{1}{3}$$
$$= \frac{54}{24} + \frac{57}{24} + \frac{8}{24}$$
$$= \frac{119}{24}$$
$$= 4\frac{23}{24}$$

(ADDITION OF COMPLEX FRACTIONS)

10. The correct answer is D.

$$\frac{x}{63} = \frac{8}{9}$$
$$x = \frac{63(8)}{9}$$
$$x = \frac{504}{9}$$
$$x = 56$$

(PROPORTIONS: PROBLEM SOLVING)

Spelling

1. A	**3.** A	**5.** A	**7.** B	**9.** C
2. C	**4.** B	**6.** B	**8.** C	**10.** A

1. **The correct answer is A.** The correct spelling is *microorganism*.

2. **The correct answer is C.** The correct spelling is *hemorrhage*.

3. **The correct answer is A.** The correct spelling is *obstetrics*.

4. **The correct answer is B.** The correct spelling is *intravenous*.

5. **The correct answer is A.** The correct spelling is *carbohydrate*.

6. **The correct answer is B.** The correct spelling is *laboratory*.

7. **The correct answer is B.** The correct spelling is *phlebotomy*.

8. **The correct answer is C.** The correct spelling is *esophagus*.

9. **The correct answer is C.** The correct spelling is *ventricle*.

10. **The correct answer is A.** The correct spelling is *integumentary*.

Nonverbal Ability

1. D	**3.** D	**5.** E	**7.** E	**9.** A
2. A	**4.** B	**6.** C	**8.** B	**10.** D

1. **The correct answer is D.** The relationship between the first two shapes is that the second is a mirror image of the first. You could also say that the second image is the same as the first only rotated 90 degrees to the right. So, in the second pair, we begin with a perpendicular line segments figure and are looking for its mirror image or the same figure only rotated 90 degrees to the right. Therefore, triangle is to mirror image of triangle as perpendicular line segments figure is to mirror image of perpendicular line segments figure.

2. **The correct answer is A.** The relationship between the first two shapes is that the second consists of only the circumscribed portion (the part inside the circle) of the first. So, in the second pair, we begin with a circle with a multiplication sign circumscribed within it and are looking for just the multiplication sign. Therefore, circle with a plus sign circumscribed within it is to plus sign as circle with a multiplication sign circumscribed within it is to multiplication sign.

3. **The correct answer is D.** The relationship between the first two shapes is that the second is a thicker version of the first. So, in the second pair, we begin with a thin multiplication sign and are looking for a thick multiplication sign. Therefore, thin plus sign is to thick plus sign as thin multiplication sign is to thick multiplication sign (choice D). Although the multiplication sign in choice A is slightly thicker than the thin multiplication sign shown in the second pair, the one in choice D more accurately represents the degree of increase in thickness that occurs in the first two shapes.

4. **The correct answer is B.** The relationship between the first two shapes is that the second has one more point than the first. So, in the second pair, we begin with a triangle, which has three points, and are looking for a shape that has one more point, or four, which is a square. Therefore, three-pointed star is to four-pointed star as triangle is to square.

5. **The correct answer is E.** The relationship between the first two shapes is that the second is an inversion, or 180-degree rotation, of the first. So, in the second pair, we begin with a square and are looking for an inversion of the square, which is simply the same square. Therefore, up-pointing triangle is to down-pointing triangle as square is to square.

6. **The correct answer is C.** The relationship between the first two shapes is that the second is a mirror image of the first and opposite in color. So, in the second pair, we begin with a right-pointing black triangle and are looking for its opposite-color mirror image, which is a left-pointing white triangle. Therefore, right-pointing white triangle is to left-pointing black triangle as right-pointing black triangle is to left-pointing white triangle.

7. **The correct answer is E.** The relationship between the first two shapes is that the second shape includes a same-size, opposite-color (negative-image) version

of the first enveloped by and concentric with a larger, same-color version of the first. So, in the second pair, we begin with a small black square and are looking for a large black square containing a concentric small white square. Therefore, small black circle is to large black circle containing a concentric small white circle as small black square is to large black square containing a concentric small white square.

8. **The correct answer is B.** The relationship between the first two shapes is that they are opposite and complementary halves of a whole. Another way of viewing the relationship is that the second shape is the same as the first, only rotated 180 degrees. So, in the second pair, we begin with the left half of a black circle and are looking for the right half of a black circle. Therefore, top half of black circle is to bottom half of black circle as left half of black circle is to right half of black circle.

9. **The correct answer is A.** The relationship between the first two shapes is that the first is the left half of the second. That is, if you were to take the second shape and divide it in half along its vertical axis, the left half would be equivalent to the first shape. So, in the second pair, we begin with a left-pointing isosceles right triangle and are looking for the shape that would be formed by combining this triangle with its mirror image, which is a square rotated 45 degrees from horizontal. Therefore, left-pointing semicircle is to circle as left-pointing isosceles right triangle is to square rotated 45 degrees from horizontal.

10. **The correct answer is D.** The relationship between the first two shapes is that the second is the upper right quarter of the first. That is, if you were to take the cross (the first shape in the first pair) and divide it in half along both its vertical and horizontal axes, producing quarters, the upper right quarter would be equivalent to L, the second shape in the first pair. So, in the second pair, we begin with a square rotated 45 degrees from horizontal and are looking for the shape that forms its upper right quarter, which is the triangle that is pointing down and left. Therefore, cross formed by four L's is to the L that forms its upper right quarter as square rotated 45 degrees from horizontal is to the triangle that forms its upper right quarter.

Science

| 1. D | 3. D | 5. B | 7. A | 9. B |
| 2. B | 4. C | 6. A | 8. D | 10. B |

1. **The correct answer is D.** Veins are the blood vessels that carry blood from all over the body back to the heart. Choice A is incorrect because the function of arteries is to carry blood away from the heart to the rest of the body. Choice B is incorrect because the bronchioles are small branching structures in the lungs through which air travels, not blood vessels. Choice C is incorrect because capillaries are the tiny blood vessels that participate in gas exchange in the lungs and cells throughout the body. (RESPIRATORY SYSTEM)

2. **The correct answer is B.** The ventricles are the two lower chambers of the heart. Choice A is incorrect because the atria are the upper chambers of the heart. Choice C is incorrect because arteries are blood vessels that carry blood away from the heart. Choice D is incorrect because valves are structures that separate the upper and lower chambers of the heart to ensure that blood does not flow from the lower chamber back into the upper chamber. (CARDIOVASCULAR SYSTEM)

3. **The correct answer is D.** The spleen is the largest single mass of lymphatic tissue in the body and contains lymphocytes and macrophages, which are involved in immune response. Choice A is incorrect because the thymus is the site of maturation of T cells, which, when mature, leave the thymus and populate other organs, including the spleen. Choice B is incorrect because lymph nodes are tiny, bean-shaped structures located throughout the body and are responsible for filtering foreign substances out of the lymph. Choice C is incorrect because the liver, although the largest organ in the body, is not composed of lymphoid tissue but of specialized epithelial cells known as hepatocytes. (LYMPHATIC SYSTEM)

4. **The correct answer is C.** The liver produces and releases a mixture called bile, which is stored in the gallbladder. The bile acts to break down fats into small droplets. Choice A is incorrect because bile breaks down fat into small easily digestible droplets. It does not break down proteins. Choice B is incorrect because fats, not carbohydrates, are broken down by bile stored in the gallbladder. Choice D is incorrect because fats, not sugars, are broken down by bile. (DIGESTIVE SYSTEM)

5. **The correct answer is B.** The nephron is the functional unit of the kidney, numbering about one million in each kidney. The nephrons filter the blood plasma and form urine with the filtered wastes to be excreted from the body. Choice A is incorrect because the neuron is the primary functional unit of the nervous system and is involved in transmitting signals to and from the brain. Choice C is incorrect because the hepatocyte is a functional unit of the liver and is involved in secreting bile, which aids in digesting fats. Choice D is incorrect because the osteocyte is a functional unit of bone tissue and is involved in bone tissue's metabolism. (URINARY SYSTEM)

6. **The correct answer is A.** Tendons are cords of dense regular connective tissue that attach muscles to bone. Choice B is incorrect because ligaments are tough

flexible strands of connective tissue that connect bones to one another. Ligaments hold joints between bones together and allow for movement and flexibility of the body. Choice C is incorrect because joints are the places where bones connect to each other. Choice D is incorrect because cartilage provides smooth surfaces for movement at joints, flexibility, and support. (MUSCULOSKELETAL SYSTEM)

7. **The correct answer is A.** During weeks 1 to 4 of gestation, the heart forms and begins to beat. Choice B is incorrect because it is during weeks 5 to 8 of gestation that limbs become more distinct and digits become visible. Choice C is incorrect because it is during weeks 9 to 12 of gestation that gender becomes distinguishable on the basis of external genitalia. Choice D is incorrect because it is during weeks 17 to 20, roughly, when the mother typically begins to feel fetal movements for the first time. (REPRODUCTION)

8. **The correct answer is D.** Carbohydrates, specifically glucose, are the body's primary source for producing ATP, the form of energy required by the body to function. Choice A is incorrect because vitamins provide no energy to the body, although they do serve many other important functions in the body. Choice B is incorrect because although protein is an energy source for the body, it is not the body's primary energy source. Choice C is incorrect because although lipids are an energy source for the body, they are not the body's primary energy source. (NUTRITION–CHEMICAL ENERGY)

9. **The correct answer is B.** Phosphorous is an essential mineral, required for formation of bones and teeth, buffering of blood, muscle contraction, nerve activity, and building of DNA and RNA. Choice A is incorrect because tocopherol is an essential vitamin, also known as vitamin E, not an essential mineral. Choice C is incorrect because biotin is an essential vitamin, not an essential mineral. Choice D is incorrect because omega-3 is an essential fatty acid, not an essential mineral. (NUTRITION)

10. **The correct answer is B.** LDL is known as the "bad" cholesterol because of its contribution to the accumulation of fatty plaques in the arteries and increased risk for heart disease. Choice A is incorrect because HDL, the "good" cholesterol, helps prevent accumulation of cholesterol in the blood. Choice C is incorrect because VLDLs transport triglycerides made in the liver to adipose cells for storage. They are eventually converted to LDLs. Choice D is incorrect because amino acids are the building blocks of proteins and are not associated with fatty plaque accumulation. (FACTORS AFFECTING HEALTH)

Reading Comprehension

1. C	3. A	5. D	7. B	9. C
2. C	4. B	6. B	8. D	10. A

1. **The correct answer is C.** The answer is stated in paragraph 1, sentence 2.

2. **The correct answer is C.** The answer is stated in paragraph 3, sentence 6.

3. **The correct answer is A.** The answer may be inferred from paragraph 3, sentence 5, by process of elimination.

4. **The correct answer is B.** *Indispensable* means "essential."

5. **The correct answer is D.** The answer may be inferred from paragraph 2, sentence 3.

6. **The correct answer is B.** A title reflects the main idea, or theme, of a piece of writing, so it must be broad enough to include the main points of the passage. Only choice B accomplishes this. Choice A is incorrect because it is too specific. Although job boards are mentioned in the article, other resources are mentioned, as well. Choice C is incorrect because the article is not primarily about deciding on a career path but on finding jobs in one's field of interest, although it does mention that information on different careers may also be found on job search websites. Choice D is incorrect because the article is not primarily about how technology has changed the job search process, although this is briefly mentioned at the beginning of the article.

7. **The correct answer is B.** *Per diem*, a Latin term, literally means "per day" but in the context of this article most likely refers to employment in which the employer calls the employee in to work as needed, which typically results in an irregular schedule and inconsistent number of hours worked per week.

8. **The correct answer is D.** Although the article does not explicitly state that dementia and Alzheimer's disease have similar symptoms, it does imply that it can be difficult to distinguish between patients who have dementia and those who have Alzheimer's disease. From this we may infer that the conditions produce similar symptoms in patients. Choice A is incorrect because although the article implies that the two conditions can be difficult to distinguish, it does not state or imply that there is no way to distinguish them. Choice B is incorrect because the article does not state or imply that dementia is a complication of Alzheimer's disease. Choice C is incorrect because the article does not state or imply that the two conditions are unrelated.

9. **The correct answer is C.** *Definitive* means "decisive, clear-cut, definite."

10. **The correct answer is A.** The word *ironically* in the last sentence of the article implies that glutamate regulators having confusion as a potential side effect is the opposite of what we would expect. The opposite of causing confusion is alleviating confusion, and because the medication is designed to alleviate the symptoms of Alzheimer's disease, we may infer that confusion is a symptom of Alzheimer's disease. The other answer choices are not valid inferences based on the last sentence.

Judgment and Comprehension in Practical Nursing

1. A	3. C	5. B	7. A	9. B
2. A	4. D	6. C	8. B	10. C

1. **The correct answer is A.** Abusive behavior is unacceptable in the workplace and should be addressed. The best response is to submit a written complaint to the human resources manager, who is trained to address such problems. Choice B is incorrect because although it might be a good idea to get advice from a coworker, the better response is to submit a complaint to the human resources manager. Choice C is incorrect because practicing yoga, though it may help alleviate some stress, does not address the root problem, which is the supervisor's abusive behavior. Choice D is incorrect because threatening to quit is more likely to further agitate the supervisor rather than stop the abusive behavior.

2. **The correct answer is A.** The best response is to notify the supervisor, who can take the appropriate steps to address the suspected drug diversion. Choice B is incorrect because the supervisor or another manager should be the one to confront the nurse. Choice C is incorrect, as the practical nurse should follow the facility's internal protocol for reporting drug diversion, which typically calls for notifying the supervisor. Choice D is incorrect because waiting for it to happen again does not address the problem and gives the registered nurse more opportunities to divert drugs.

3. **The correct answer is C.** The best response is to show empathy to the patient and to make sure the patient has all of the needed information about treatment options to help make the decision. Even if the practical nurse does not have the answer, they can make sure the patient's questions are communicated to the appropriate member of the healthcare team. Choices A and B are incorrect because a practical nurse should not try to persuade the patient by expressing a personal opinion or life experience. Choice D is incorrect because it lacks empathy and does nothing to help address the patient's concern.

4. **The correct answer is D.** With older patients, it is better to err on the side of formality when addressing them, referring to them as "Mr." or "Ms." or "Mrs.," as appropriate, plus their last name. If they indicate a preference to be called by their first name, then the nurse may do so. Choice A is incorrect because it is patronizing and possibly insulting to refer to patients by such nicknames as "sweetie" or "honey." Choice B is incorrect because it is more respectful to refer to the patient by her last name, at least initially. Choice C is incorrect because the nurse should address the patient by name.

5. **The correct answer is B.** Unless the child's behavior is truly disruptive, the best response would be to ignore the game and continue working. Choices A and C are incorrect because there's no good reason to have the child stop playing the game. Choice D is incorrect because there is no need to inform your supervisor.

6. **The correct answer is C.** The best response would be to show empathy and provide appropriate reassurance, as in choice C. Choices A and B are incorrect because the nurse is providing false reassurance and trivializing the child's concern. Choice D is

incorrect because changing the subject just ignores the child's concern.

7. **The correct answer is A.** The best response would be to ask the patient directly whether a patient has any drug allergies. Just because they have Alzheimer's disease doesn't mean that you shouldn't address the patient directly with questions. Choices B and C are incorrect because you should first address the patient directly. Choice D is incorrect because you should verbally confirm with the patient that there are no drug allergies, not just rely on what is in the patient's record.

8. **The correct answer is B.** The best response is to clarify what the patient means, as the patient's comment could indicate confusion over the purpose or necessity of the surgery or simply reluctance to undergo the surgery. Choice A is incorrect because the nurse is trivializing and not addressing the patient's concern. Choice C is incorrect because the nurse should first clarify what the patient means and should not be urging the patient to not have the surgery.

Choice D is incorrect because the nurse is dismissing the patient's concern.

9. **The correct answer is B.** The best response is to shift the conversation to reality without emotionally upsetting the patient or encouraging false expectations. Choice A, although true, is incorrect because it is likely to be emotionally upsetting to the patient. Choices C and D are incorrect because they encourage the patient's false expectations.

10. **The correct answer is C.** The best response would be to arrange to have an interpreter come and assist the patient, as such a professional will be the best equipped to facilitate communication with her. Choice A is incorrect because it does not address the patient's concern and need to communicate. Choice B is incorrect because though he is bilingual, the woman's son may not developmentally be able to communicate fully what the woman's concern is. Choice D is incorrect because communicating with hand gestures is not likely to be effective.

PART III
PRACTICE FOR REGISTERED NURSING SCHOOL ENTRANCE EXAMINATIONS

Verbal and Nonverbal Ability

OVERVIEW

- What Is Verbal Ability?
- Measuring Verbal Ability
- Extending Your Vocabulary
- Etymology—Key to Word Recognition
- Know Your Roots (or Stems)
- Prefixes and Suffixes
- Increased Word Power from Beginning to End
- Synonyms
- Test 1: Synonyms Answer Sheet
- Test 1: Synonyms
- Antonyms
- Test 2: Antonyms Answer Sheet
- Test 2: Antonyms
- Skill with Verbal Analogies
- Test 3: Analogy Relationships Answer Sheet
- Test 3: Analogy Relationships
- Test 4: Verbal Analogies Answer Sheet
- Test 4: Verbal Analogies
- English Grammar and Usage
- Test 5: English Grammar and Usage Answer Sheet
- Test 5: English Grammar and Usage
- Spelling
- Test 6: Spelling Answer Sheet
- Test 6: Spelling
- Nonverbal Ability
- Test 7: Nonverbal Ability Answer Sheet
- Test 7: Nonverbal Ability

- **Answer Keys and Explanations**
- **Let's Put You to the Test**
- **Final Verbal and Nonverbal Ability Examination Answer Sheet**
- **Final Verbal and Nonverbal Ability Examination**
- **Final Answer Keys and Explanations**

The purpose of this section is to provide you with practice exercises representative of the five most common kinds of verbal ability test items—synonyms, antonyms, verbal analogies, English grammar and usage, and spelling—as well as nonverbal ability test items. This section covers these question types in six separate subsections.

An explanation of each kind of test item, helpful study hints, and test-taking strategies precede each subsection. Subsections also include multiple-choice tests. Answer Keys and Explanations follow the sample tests to help you evaluate your performance and determine areas of weakness. You may wish to use the answer keys and explanations to compile a word study list.

Remember that this section is not meant for easy reading. It is a guide to a program of study that will prove invaluable if you do your part. Do not try to absorb too much at one time. If you can put in a half-hour every day, your study will yield better results.

After you have done your preliminary work and have a better idea of how words are formed in English, attempt the various vocabulary tests we have provided. They cover a wide variety of the vocabulary questions commonly encountered on examinations. These lengthy tests are not meant to be taken all at once. Space them out. Adhere closely to the directions, which differ depending on the test. Keep an honest record of your scores. Study your corrected mistakes and look them up in your dictionary. Concentrate closely on each sample test, and watch your scores improve.

WHAT IS VERBAL ABILITY?

Verbal ability may be defined as skill with word usage and comprehension. It is often evaluated in the form of written vocabulary tests. These vocabulary tests measure the test-taker's ability to recall and produce *lexical units*. A lexical unit is a word or group of words possessing a specific meaning. A single word can have a variety of meanings in different contexts (that is, phrases or sentences). For this reason, a single word may represent several lexical units. Consider the following example:

> Her answer to the question was *right*.
>
> She handed the paper to the person on her *right*.
>
> She has a *right* to know the results of the test.
>
> She felt compelled to help *right* the wrong that was done.

MEASURING VERBAL ABILITY

Measurement of verbal skill encompasses many elements. Although vocabulary test items may or may not appear on your test, it is advisable to study and practice with the kind of material presented in this verbal ability section. Words and their meanings are vital for good scores on tests of reading comprehension, effective writing, and current usage. Expanding your vocabulary will result in a marked improvement in your scores in these and similar subjects.

The vocabulary test usually includes words from your *active* vocabulary—words that you see, hear, and use frequently—and words from your *passive* vocabulary—words that you have heard and seen, and might comprehend, but that you rarely, if ever, use. It also includes words that may be common in written language but are not often used in spoken expression, and vice versa.

EXTENDING YOUR VOCABULARY

A good command of words is essential to most aspects of your life. Words can broaden your horizons and reveal new interests in your daily environment and activities. Such discoveries may never be accessible to you if your vocabulary remains restricted or too specialized.

Effective expression is essential to making and maintaining meaningful social relationships. An extensive vocabulary will help you to convey ideas, desires, and information. If you are enrolled in school, regardless of the level, you will learn faster and enjoy the process more if you are "fortified" with a large, effective vocabulary. Your comprehension of a broad range of words will help you to determine what you do *not* understand and will help you remedy the situation by posing intelligent questions.

Your word power directly affects your work. If you are seeking to improve your occupational status through a job change or a promotion from your present position, a better command of words will undoubtedly help you to succeed. This fact has been proven time and again through scientific studies conducted by educators, psychologists, sociologists, and personnel specialists. Many employers require a battery of tests, the results of which are used in determining which applicants are best suited to an available position. Frequently these tests incorporate a number of items designed to measure verbal ability.

Attaining a leadership role depends on, among other things, the extent of your vocabulary. Leadership tasks demand that you get your ideas across, that you speak and are heard. You will need to use all your expressive powers to voice your opinion with conviction. Articulation can furnish you with an astonishing amount of persuasive power. A larger vocabulary will help you feel secure and competent in every undertaking.

Let's explore the means by which this vocabulary may be acquired. The following strategies are designed to increase your vocabulary and help you achieve word mastery. Word mastery implies reaching a level of verbal ability at which you can both recognize and comprehend words—and use them frequently and appropriately.

- **Read as much as you can, taking care not to confine yourself to one kind of reading material.** Seek variety in what you read—periodicals, newspapers, nonfiction, novels and other fiction, poetry, prose, essays, etc. Reading from a broad range of material will accelerate your vocabulary growth. You will learn the meaning of words by context. This means that at times you will not know the definition of an isolated word, but the words or phrase within which this word appears will be familiar and therefore provide a clue to its meaning.

- **Take vocabulary tests.** There are many practice books containing word tests. These tests are challenging and make an enjoyable leisure-time activity. More important, they are fast vocabulary builders.

- **Listen to lectures, discussions, and talks given by people who speak well.** TV and radio are excellent means of learning new terminology coming into common usage in the English language. A word of caution: You cannot always rely on a speaker's pronunciation. Always check your dictionary for proper pronunciation.

- **Use a dictionary when you are not certain of a word's meaning.** If you do not have access to a dictionary when you encounter the word, make a note of it (and its context) and research it at your earliest convenience. Find out how it is pronounced, what words are related to it, its finer shades of meaning, and its correct usage. A good dictionary is a must!

- **Crossword puzzles, anagrams, and similar word games provide a relaxing method of acquiring new vocabulary.** Most of these puzzles are published in varying degrees of difficulty. Start with the easy level and progress to the expert level. You will find it a challenging learning experience.

- **Review the etymological charts and diagrams in this book, which explain word derivations.** A knowledge of roots, or stems, of words will enable you to infer the meaning of new words having roots similar to words you already know.

- **Study words by central ideas.** It is difficult to study and retain isolated words. Even context clues sometimes are not enough to help you remember a word, its meaning, or its appropriate use. Studying vocabulary by central idea encourages you to consider groups of related words. As you learn each term, you associate it with some other word. For example: The words *ingest, devour, consume, voracious, edible, delectable,* and *palatable* are all tied to the principal idea of eating. The central idea strategy of studying words will not only provide you with a basis for remembering the word but will also motivate you to use the word in your everyday oral and written expression. Frequent use of the word will in turn ensure your ability to recall its meaning in a testing situation. This word study method also fosters comprehension of jargon or word usage particular to specific fields. A number of workbooks and study materials present words according to a central idea and feature exercises formatted to this method. Such books may be found in the "study aids" section of most bookstores.

Be sure to record all new words in a notebook dedicated to that purpose. Make notes alongside each entry that include a simple definition or synonym, finer shades of meaning, related forms, and sample sentences of the word in context. Finally, make these words your own. Use them in your writing and speaking. Remember—verbal ability is a skill you can improve at any age.

ETYMOLOGY—KEY TO WORD RECOGNITION

Etymology is the study of the history and origin of words. It explains how a word came into being, the place of its beginning, and how it has been used through the ages. The etymology of a word also outlines alterations in its meaning, usage, and spelling through the years.

Although the term *etymology* sounds somewhat complex and weighty, the science itself is not difficult to understand. Etymologies may be simple and concise or lengthy and intricate. To find them, use your dictionary. Etymologies are usually found at the beginning of a definition of a principal entry (the word you are looking up, usually printed in bold type), enclosed in brackets and placed directly before the definition.

Example

> **a͞rris** ar ə s\n, pl arris or **arrises** [probably modif. of MF *areste,* lit., fishbone, fr LL *arista,* ear of grain]: the sharp edge or salient angle formed by the meeting of two surfaces, esp. in moldings.

To familiarize yourself with the abbreviations used to denote the origin of words, consult the front pages of your dictionary, where you will find a guide to the use of that particular publication. Look for a heading that refers to etymologies or abbreviations and symbols used in etymologies. These keys will help you interpret a word's entry. In the example shown, the abbreviations MF and LL indicate that the entry *a͞rris* is derived from Middle French or Late Latin.

Many English words have their origin in Greek and Roman myths and legends. If you are well-read, you may already have an edge in using the etymological method of determining word meaning. For instance, if you have read the story of the mythical king Tantalus, you would understand the derivation of the verb *tantalize.* King Tantalus, after his death, was punished for his wickedness by being placed in water up to his chin. When he stooped to drink, the water would recede out of reach. Above his head, branches laden with fruit bobbed out of his reach. So from the name Tantalus came the word *tantalize,* meaning "to tease."

A great many of the words we use daily came into our language from the Latin and Greek. Approximately half the words in the dictionary are derived from Latin. Many Latin words and phrases have been borrowed and adopted by other languages. European languages such as French and Spanish came directly from Latin and are known as Romance languages. Consequently, if you are or have been a student of Latin, you will find it easier to build your vocabulary.

Many foreign terms were absorbed into English as parts of several different words related in meaning to each other. These parts of words fall into three groups.

> *Roots (or stems)*—These carry the basic meaning and are combined with each other and with prefixes and suffixes to create other words with related meanings.

> *Prefixes*—Letter combinations with their own particular meaning that appear at the beginning of a word.

> *Suffixes*—Letter combinations with their own particular meaning that appear at the end of a word.

The lists of roots, prefixes, and suffixes in this section are accompanied by words in which the letter combinations appear. Use the dictionary to look up any words that are not clear in your mind.

KNOW YOUR ROOTS (OR STEMS)

The root, or stem, is that part of the word that conveys the basic meaning of the word. For example, in the word *introduction, duct* is the root. It means "lead." *Intro-* means *within, into,* and *-tion* is a noun ending. Hence, the meaning of introduction—a "leading into."

Below is a chart of common stems. See how well you "know your roots."

Common Stems

Stem	Meaning	Example
ag, ac	do	agenda, action
agri	farm	agriculture
aqua	water	aquatic
auto	self	automatic
biblio	book	bibliography
bio	life	biography
cad, cas	fall	cadence, casual
cap, cep, cept	take	captive, accept
capit	head	capital, decapitate
ced, cede, ceed, cess	go	intercede
celer	speed	accelerate
chrom	color	monochromatic
chron	time	chronological
cide, cis	cut	incision
clude, clud, clus	close, close in	include, cluster
cog, cogn	knowledge of	recognize
cur, curs	run	recur, cursive
ded	give	dedicate
dent, dont	tooth	dental
duce, duct	lead	induce, deduct
fact, fect, fict	make, do	perfect, fiction, factory
fer, late	carry	refer, dilate, transfer, translate
flect, flex	bend, turn	reflect
fring, fract	break	infringe, refract
graph, gram	picture, writing	graphic, telegram
greg	group, gather	gregarious, congregation
gress, grad	step, walk	progress, degrade
hydr	water	hydrate
ject	throw	inject
jud	right	judicial

Stem	Meaning	Example
junct	join	conjunction
juris	law, justice	jurist
lect, leg	read, choose	collect, legible
logue	speech, speaking	dialogue
logy	study of	psychology
loq, loc	speak	elocution
lude, lus	play, perform	elude, ludicrous
manu	by hand	manuscript
mand	order	demand
mar	sea	maritime
med	middle	intermediate
ment, mem	mind, memory	mention
meter	measure	thermometer
micro	small	microscope
min	lessen	miniature
mis, miss, mit	send	remit, dismiss
mot, mov	move	remote, remove
mute	change	commute, mutation
naut	sailor, sail	nautical
nounce, nunci	declare, state	announce, enunciate
ped, pod	foot	pedal
pel, pulse	drive, push	dispel, impulse
pend, pense	hang	depend, dispenser
plac	please	placate
plic	fold	implicate
port	carry	portable
pose, pone	put, place	depose, component
reg, rect	rule	regulate, direct
rupt	break	disruption
sec, sect	cut	bisect
sed	remain	sedentary
sert	weave, bind	insert
serve	keep, save	preserve
scend, scent	climb	ascent
scribe, script	write	describe, transcript
sist	stand, set	insist
spect	look	inspect
spire, spirat	breath, breathe	perspire
strict	tighten	restrict

Stem	Meaning	Example
tain	hold	detain
term	end	terminate
tract	draw, drag	detract
tort	twist	distort
vene, vent	come	intervene, invent
vict	overcome, conquer	evict
volve, volu	roll, turn	evolve, evolution

PREFIXES AND SUFFIXES

Prefixes and suffixes are the "beginning and end." A prefix is a letter-combination attached to the beginning of a word; it usually carries a meaning independent of the word to which it is attached. For example, the prefix *semi* means "half." It can be added to many words—*semicircle, semilunar, semiprofessional, semiformal*. Attaching a prefix sometimes requires the placement of a hyphen between the prefix and the root word. A hyphen is used when the prefix is attached to a proper noun: *all-American, pro-British, anti-Fascist, un-Christian*.

A suffix is a combination of letters attached to the end of a word and usually possesses a meaning separate from the word to which it is affixed, for example, *-less* (without)—*careless, hopeless, meaningless*. Usually, affixing a suffix to a word changes its part of speech, for example, *assert* (verb)—*assertion* (noun), *beautiful* (adjective)—*beautifully* (adverb).

Study the following prefix and suffix charts to increase your understanding of related words and inflected (changed) forms.

Prefixes

Prefix	Meaning	Example
a	not	amoral
ab, a	away from	absent
ad, ac, ag, at	to	advent, accrue, attract, aggressive
an	without	anarchy
ante	before	antedate
anti	against	antipathy
aud, audit	hear	auditor
bene	well	beneficent
bi	two	bicameral
cap, capt, cept	take, seize, hold	capture
ced, cess	go, yield	rescind, recess
circum	around	circumspect
com, con, col	together	commit, confound, collate
contra	against	contraband

Prefix	Meaning	Example
cred, credit	believe	credible
de	from, down	descend
dic, dict	say	dictionary
dis, di	apart	distract, divert
dom	home, rule	domicile, dominate
duc, duct	lead	induce
ex, e	out	exit, emit
extra	beyond	extracurricular
fac, fact	make	facsimile
in, im, ir, il	not	inept, irregular, illegal
in, im	in, into	interest, imbibe
inter	between	interscholastic
intra, intro	within	intramural
mal	bad	malcontent
mis	wrong	misnomer
non	not	nonentity
ob	against	obstacle
omni	all	omnivorous
per	through	permeate
peri	around	periscope
poly	many	polytheism
post	after	postmortem
pre	before	premonition
pro	forward	propose
re	again	review
se	apart	seduce
semi	half	semicircle
sub	under	subvert
sui	self	suicide
super	above	superimpose
sur	on, upon	surcharge
trans	across	transpose
un	not	unwelcome
vice	instead of	vice-president

Suffixes

Suffix	Meaning	Example
able, ible	capable of being	capable, reversible
age	state of	storage
al	pertaining to	instructional
ance	relating to	reliance
ary	relating to	dictionary
ate	act	confiscate
ation	action	radiation
cy	quality	democracy
ed	past action	subsided
ence	relating to	confidence
er, or	one who	adviser, actor
ic	pertaining to	democratic
ing	present action	surmising
ious	full of	rebellious
ish	like, as	childish
ive	having the quality of	creative
ize	to make like	harmonize
less	without	hopeless
ly	the quality of	carefully
ment	result	amusement
ness	the quality of being	selfishness
ty	condition	sanity

INCREASED WORD POWER FROM BEGINNING TO END

Using the etymological approach can simplify the process by which you attack the monumental feat of learning medical terminology. By knowing that the suffix *itis* implies inflammation and *ectomy* means "the cutting out or removal of," you can easily deduce that the term *appendicitis* means "inflammation of the appendix" and *appendectomy* means "the cutting out or removal of the appendix."

Now that you have studied the various letter combinations or word components, see if you can make an educated guess at the meanings of the terms listed below. Start with the root or stem. Next, add the suffix and/or prefix to the interpretation in the order that provides a clear definition. The result will be increased word power from "beginning to end." It's as challenging as a jigsaw puzzle! Be sure to compare your definitions with those in the dictionary.

decapitate	colloquy	emissary	aggregation	incursion
retractable	involuted	implacable	convocation	celerity

SYNONYMS

The Name's the Same

Synonyms are words that share meanings. The English language abounds in synonyms. In your effort to acquire word mastery, you must learn to express your ideas without redundancy and constant use of overworked words. Effective writing and speaking may be achieved through the precise use of synonyms.

Words such as *brave* and *courageous*, which may allude to an identical quality, can be used interchangeably. Some synonyms, however, differ in definition or usage. For example, *fewer* refers to number, while *less* refers to quantity: John has *fewer* books and *less* money than his brother. These words are indeed similar in meaning, but one cannot be substituted for the other.

The adjectives *beautiful* and *handsome* both describe someone or something attractive or pleasing to the eye. Nevertheless, you would not usually speak of a "beautiful man" or a "handsome young lady." In our society, common usage would cause one to reverse these expressions to a "beautiful young lady" and a "handsome man."

A study of the finer shades of the meaning of synonyms will help you be more precise when you convey your feelings or mental picture of an object or scene. For instance, if you were to say, "The *bottom* of the lamp is made of Indian brass and features intricate carvings," one might simply envision the underside of the lamp. However, if you were to substitute *base* for the word *bottom*, one would instead get a visual image of something highly decorative that supports the upper structure of the lamp. So even though the "name" appears to be the same, an investigation into finer shades of definition will assist you in distinguishing variations in usage.

Familiar Surroundings?

The most common way of testing vocabulary on a standardized test is in context, that is, to present the items in a sentence or phrase so that you can see how a word is used. You can then determine whether the word is used as a noun, a verb, an adjective, etc. The test, therefore, is designed to encourage the extraction of word meaning from context; however, the context will not be so explicit that you can easily infer the meaning of a word.

More specifically, the synonym test item is usually a multiple-choice item that appears in one of three formats:

Type A

Given an underlined or italicized word in a complete sentence, the test-taker is required to identify which of the four other words is a synonym for the underlined or italicized word.

Example

The disinterested witness was able to give a *candid* account of the incident.

A. complete

B. impartial

C. biased

D. candescent

Type B

Given an underlined or italicized word in a phrase, the test-taker is required to identify which of the four other words is a synonym for the underlined or italicized word.

Example

The *emaciated* patient

A. discharged

B. emancipated

C. emotional

D. shriveled

Type C

Given a sentence with a missing word, the test-taker is required to identify which of the four other words best completes the sentence.

Example

An *apology* is appropriate when a person feels

A. sorry.

B. apathetic.

C. rejected.

D. elated.

OR

Example

He is a *staunch* supporter of the presidential candidate. Staunch means

A. stubborn.

B. faithful.

C. inflexible.

D. hopeful.

Context Clues

Examining the various types of context clues is another means of understanding how to extract the meaning of a word from the words surrounding it. The fourteen sample sentences below illustrate the different kinds of context clues.

1. Since the *litigation* would be costly, the lawyers advised that such a suit should be settled out of court. (**DEFINITION**)

2. The crumbling *edifice*, a building located on the north side of town, is targeted for implosion early in June. (**DEFINITION**)

3. He exhibits his *sloth* by resting on the couch while his wife and elderly father shovel snow. (**DESCRIPTION**)

4.   She had indeed turned into a *shrew* with her screaming, nagging, and quarrelsome manner. (**DESCRIPTION**)

5.   Tyler was anything but *amenable* to the proposal of another coed dorm on campus; on the contrary, he vehemently protested the board's recommendation for such action. (**CONTRAST**)

6.   Crestville was a *quaint*, little town until the relocation of several large corporations turned it into a bustling metropolis. (**CONTRAST**)

7.   Charles, like his brave and *dauntless* father, was fearless in the face of trouble. (**COMPARISON**)

8.   She was stricken with the disease at an early age; her daughter likewise was *infirm* while very young. (**COMPARISON**)

9.   The sentence of five years in prison hardly seemed adequate *retribution* for this dreadful crime. (**EXAMPLES**)

10. Peas and beans are two kinds of *legumes*. (**EXAMPLES**)

11. The disease is considered *infectious*, or contagious. (**SYNONYMS**)

12. The *cardiologist*, or heart specialist, ordered several tests for his patient. (**SYNONYMS**)

13. Karin was *elated* at the news of her job transfer; however, her mother appeared sad. (**ANTONYMS**)

14. The *arid* climate was a welcome change from the dampness I experienced in London. (**ANTONYMS**)

Especially Special: Scientific Terms

When preparing for an entrance exam for programs leading to science-related careers, it is beneficial to familiarize yourself with the specialized vocabulary of this discipline. Remember, even though the general public considers scientific jargon confusing, technical terms are imperative for scientific communication. If you plan to study science, your ability to comprehend the terminology of the field could indicate how well you will do in the related course work. Your entrance exam may measure your scientific vocabulary skills.

Mastery of specialized vocabulary—or any vocabulary for that matter—can best be achieved by learning words as you encounter them in your reading. However, when preparing for an entrance exam, you may want to employ the following nine strategies:

1.   Review "Know Your Roots (or Stems)" and "Prefixes and Suffixes" on pages 118-122 of this publication.

2.   Read a variety of scientific articles, science textbook chapters, etc.

3.   Try to understand the unfamiliar words that you encounter in these readings as they are used in context.

4.   If you cannot grasp the meaning from context, then put your knowledge of roots and affixes to work. Take the word apart and see if you can determine a meaning that fits the context (or if you are in the testing situation, a meaning that comes close to one of the multiple-choice items).

5. If Step 4 does not yield a reasonable definition, then check the footnotes, glossary, or index of the text you are reading. If you find the word in the index, skim the pages listed for that word, checking for either its definition or its contextual usage.

6. If you cannot find a definition of the word in the material that you are reading, look it up in a dictionary. It would be best to use a scientific dictionary or encyclopedia. There are dictionaries that are for specific areas of study, such as geography, modern history, politics, and biology.

7. Once you have come up with a definition for the word, you may want to write it on an index card (word on one side, definition on the other). After accumulating a number of these vocabulary cards, carry them in your pocket or book bag. Flip through them when you have a spare moment (commuting by train or bus, sitting in the waiting room of the dentist or doctor, etc.).

8. Become accustomed to recognizing words that stand for concepts rather than facts. To a scientist, a concept is a generalization or an idea based on information or knowledge that explains a phenomenon. Read the following paragraph and underline those words which you feel represent scientific concepts. *Karotyping is a process that enables scientists to study the chromosomes of human beings. Sometimes the study can be made even before birth. Chromosomes can best be observed during metaphase in mitosis. At this point they are coiled. Skin cells are good to use in making a Karyotype because they divide frequently. Some genetic disorders can be identified just by looking at the Karyotype of a person.* If you underlined *Karyotype process, metaphase, mitosis,* and *genetic disorders,* you would be correct. These words represent ideas. They cannot be touched and they have no exact physical form or boundaries, yet they are real because they represent scientific facts.

9. Finally, learn to connect symbols to words. A scientific symbol is an abbreviation that stands for a word or concept.

Example

$C_6H_{12}O_6$ represents glucose, a chemical compound.

You will have the opportunity to practice your use of these vocabulary expansion strategies as you encounter scientific terms on the verbal ability tests in this book. The answers to several of the questions in the reading comprehension test involve scientific terms. These questions are indicated by asterisks.

In completing a synonym test item, remember to look for a word that means the same, or almost the same, as the target word in the item (the underlined or italicized word). Do not be distracted by a word that is a look-alike, that is, one that looks similar or begins with the same three or four letters but is unrelated in meaning. When possible, apply the etymological approach of interpreting roots, prefixes, and suffixes.

TEST 1: SYNONYMS ANSWER SHEET

answer sheet

1. Ⓐ Ⓑ Ⓒ Ⓓ	16. Ⓐ Ⓑ Ⓒ Ⓓ	31. Ⓐ Ⓑ Ⓒ Ⓓ	46. Ⓐ Ⓑ Ⓒ Ⓓ	61. Ⓐ Ⓑ Ⓒ Ⓓ
2. Ⓐ Ⓑ Ⓒ Ⓓ	17. Ⓐ Ⓑ Ⓒ Ⓓ	32. Ⓐ Ⓑ Ⓒ Ⓓ	47. Ⓐ Ⓑ Ⓒ Ⓓ	62. Ⓐ Ⓑ Ⓒ Ⓓ
3. Ⓐ Ⓑ Ⓒ Ⓓ	18. Ⓐ Ⓑ Ⓒ Ⓓ	33. Ⓐ Ⓑ Ⓒ Ⓓ	48. Ⓐ Ⓑ Ⓒ Ⓓ	63. Ⓐ Ⓑ Ⓒ Ⓓ
4. Ⓐ Ⓑ Ⓒ Ⓓ	19. Ⓐ Ⓑ Ⓒ Ⓓ	34. Ⓐ Ⓑ Ⓒ Ⓓ	49. Ⓐ Ⓑ Ⓒ Ⓓ	64. Ⓐ Ⓑ Ⓒ Ⓓ
5. Ⓐ Ⓑ Ⓒ Ⓓ	20. Ⓐ Ⓑ Ⓒ Ⓓ	35. Ⓐ Ⓑ Ⓒ Ⓓ	50. Ⓐ Ⓑ Ⓒ Ⓓ	65. Ⓐ Ⓑ Ⓒ Ⓓ
6. Ⓐ Ⓑ Ⓒ Ⓓ	21. Ⓐ Ⓑ Ⓒ Ⓓ	36. Ⓐ Ⓑ Ⓒ Ⓓ	51. Ⓐ Ⓑ Ⓒ Ⓓ	66. Ⓐ Ⓑ Ⓒ Ⓓ
7. Ⓐ Ⓑ Ⓒ Ⓓ	22. Ⓐ Ⓑ Ⓒ Ⓓ	37. Ⓐ Ⓑ Ⓒ Ⓓ	52. Ⓐ Ⓑ Ⓒ Ⓓ	67. Ⓐ Ⓑ Ⓒ Ⓓ
8. Ⓐ Ⓑ Ⓒ Ⓓ	23. Ⓐ Ⓑ Ⓒ Ⓓ	38. Ⓐ Ⓑ Ⓒ Ⓓ	53. Ⓐ Ⓑ Ⓒ Ⓓ	68. Ⓐ Ⓑ Ⓒ Ⓓ
9. Ⓐ Ⓑ Ⓒ Ⓓ	24. Ⓐ Ⓑ Ⓒ Ⓓ	39. Ⓐ Ⓑ Ⓒ Ⓓ	54. Ⓐ Ⓑ Ⓒ Ⓓ	69. Ⓐ Ⓑ Ⓒ Ⓓ
10. Ⓐ Ⓑ Ⓒ Ⓓ	25. Ⓐ Ⓑ Ⓒ Ⓓ	40. Ⓐ Ⓑ Ⓒ Ⓓ	55. Ⓐ Ⓑ Ⓒ Ⓓ	70. Ⓐ Ⓑ Ⓒ Ⓓ
11. Ⓐ Ⓑ Ⓒ Ⓓ	26. Ⓐ Ⓑ Ⓒ Ⓓ	41. Ⓐ Ⓑ Ⓒ Ⓓ	56. Ⓐ Ⓑ Ⓒ Ⓓ	71. Ⓐ Ⓑ Ⓒ Ⓓ
12. Ⓐ Ⓑ Ⓒ Ⓓ	27. Ⓐ Ⓑ Ⓒ Ⓓ	42. Ⓐ Ⓑ Ⓒ Ⓓ	57. Ⓐ Ⓑ Ⓒ Ⓓ	72. Ⓐ Ⓑ Ⓒ Ⓓ
13. Ⓐ Ⓑ Ⓒ Ⓓ	28. Ⓐ Ⓑ Ⓒ Ⓓ	43. Ⓐ Ⓑ Ⓒ Ⓓ	58. Ⓐ Ⓑ Ⓒ Ⓓ	73. Ⓐ Ⓑ Ⓒ Ⓓ
14. Ⓐ Ⓑ Ⓒ Ⓓ	29. Ⓐ Ⓑ Ⓒ Ⓓ	44. Ⓐ Ⓑ Ⓒ Ⓓ	59. Ⓐ Ⓑ Ⓒ Ⓓ	74. Ⓐ Ⓑ Ⓒ Ⓓ
15. Ⓐ Ⓑ Ⓒ Ⓓ	30. Ⓐ Ⓑ Ⓒ Ⓓ	45. Ⓐ Ⓑ Ⓒ Ⓓ	60. Ⓐ Ⓑ Ⓒ Ⓓ	75. Ⓐ Ⓑ Ⓒ Ⓓ

TEST 1: SYNONYMS

75 Questions • 35 Minutes

Directions: In each of the sentences below, one word is italicized. Following each sentence are four words or phrases. For each sentence, choose the word or phrase that most nearly corresponds in meaning with the italicized word.

1. The *diction* acceptable in speech is usually more informal than that required in writing.
   - A. conviction
   - B. language
   - C. discourse
   - D. denunciation

2. It is apparent that Gina Smith is the most *sedulous* and active member of the group.
   - A. hideous
   - B. generous
   - C. infirm
   - D. industrious

3. During the hockey game several *altercations* took place.
   - A. fracases
   - B. substitutions
   - C. alterations
   - D. plays

4. The carrot is a perfect illustration of a *biennial*.
   - A. occurring quarterly
   - B. occurring once in two years
   - C. perennial
   - D. bisection

5. He has run the *gamut* of clerical jobs in this office.
   - A. periphery
   - B. margin
   - C. range
   - D. imperception

6. His deeds amounted to nothing more than those of a *sanctimonious* hypocrite.
   - A. parsimonious
   - B. perpetual
   - C. intrinsic
   - D. self-righteous

7. He displayed the manners of an *urbane* gentleman.
   - A. suave
   - B. poignant
   - C. spasmodic
   - D. pensive

8. The *slogan* is appropriate for both the product and its service.
   - A. catchword
   - B. sample
   - C. design
   - D. passage

9. The man was *vociferous* in his complaints about his dinner.
   A. strident
   B. muted
   C. insistent
   D. importunate

10. He was determined to *foil* the scheme of his opponent.
    A. heighten
    B. secure
    C. disencumber
    D. thwart

11. The examiner *purported* to be an official representative.
    A. addressed
    B. claimed
    C. propitiated
    D. conciliated

12. The ships carried happy vacationers *bent* on having a good time.
    A. flexible
    B. determined
    C. inclined
    D. endowed

13. The child could not *recollect* the incident.
    A. remember
    B. doubt
    C. interrogate
    D. illumine

14. The governor *rescinded* the state of emergency as soon as the roads were cleared of snow.
    A. negated
    B. maneuvered
    C. revoked
    D. accepted

15. The implementation of the plan was given *scant* consideration.
    A. audacious
    B. fervid
    C. little
    D. clothed

16. The key speaker, in his lengthy presentation, *scoffed at* the notion of marketing as a public service.
    A. exonerated
    B. amplified
    C. confuted
    D. mocked

17. She completed the *sprint* with a sudden surge of energy.
    A. relaxation
    B. adventure
    C. run
    D. convergence

18. The content of the message was *urgent*.
    A. privileged
    B. amendable
    C. pressing
    D. absolved

19. A *simulated* rescue mission was conducted by the forest rangers.
    A. pretended
    B. superficial
    C. stimulated
    D. simultaneous

20. Through the course of the day, she became more *agitated* by the noise of the demolition and less focused on her work.
    A. worried
    B. upset
    C. convulsed
    D. composed

21. Her quickening gait seemed regulated by the *pulse* of the big city.
    A. utility
    B. pace
    C. reverence
    D. solace

22. The language of the publication is *unsophisticated* but informative.
    A. ponderous
    B. elaborate
    C. simple
    D. artificial

23. All the evidence presented pointed to *willful* execution of a crime.
    A. deliberate
    B. eminent
    C. amicable
    D. remorseful

24. There is no *provision* for deadlines in the contract.
    A. improvement
    B. convenience
    C. aggregation
    D. stipulation

25. The furnishings *impart* an air of elegance to the room.
    A. communicate
    B. indemnify
    C. reinforce
    D. disguise

26. She exhibited great *valor* in handling the emergency.
    A. ingeniousness
    B. courage
    C. discretion
    D. optimism

27. Various courses were *fused* in the revision of the curriculum.
    A. required
    B. implicated
    C. combined
    D. involved

28. He was able to *duplicate* his work even though his hard drive with all his data had died.
    A. replicate
    B. synthesize
    C. fixate
    D. replenish

29. The task of choosing one from so many qualified applicants *bewildered* the employer.
    A. perplexed
    B. aggravated
    C. subdued
    D. infuriated

30. The revision of the city plan incorporated adjustments in the projected *modes* of transportation.
    A. increments
    B. expenditures
    C. means
    D. modifications

31. The politician sought to *aggrandize* himself at the expense of the people.
    A. exhaust
    B. subjugate
    C. sacrifice
    D. enrich

32. The newcomer made an effort to *mingle* with the crowd.
    A. argue
    B. mix
    C. disrupt
    D. flout

33. If an organization's programs were described as *philanthropic*, the programs would be
    A. primitive.
    B. deleterious.
    C. extraneous.
    D. benevolent.

34. If the traits of a nation's leader were *covetous*, they were
    A. greedy.
    B. exemplary.
    C. disparate.
    D. adventitious.

35. Rabbits *breed* offspring rapidly.
    A. raise
    B. gather
    C. propagate
    D. destroy

36. He *reiterated* the need to document the procedures in the experiment.
    A. adjusted
    B. defended
    C. fermented
    D. repeated

37. A shadow of a man *loomed* ominously in the dimly lit corridor.
    A. asserted
    B. yielded
    C. appeared
    D. rebuffed

38. Alcohol consumption often exerts *an adverse* influence on an individual.
    A. an ecstatic
    B. an injurious
    C. a luminous
    D. a gloomy

39. The girl is reported to have left of her own *volition*.
    A. flight
    B. will
    C. repudiation
    D. recognizance

40. The one-sided score was *an anomaly* in a Division 1 game.
    A. an anachronism
    B. a change
    C. an embarrassment
    D. an aberration

41. The *similitude* between the original painting and the reproduction is remarkable.
    A. incongruity
    B. connection
    C. resemblance
    D. relationship

42. A *prudent* individual will save some portion of his or her wage.
    A. judicious
    B. terse
    C. audacious
    D. laconic

43. His decision to return home was *instinctive*.
    A. spontaneous
    B. turgid
    C. premeditated
    D. irrelevant

44. It seemed as if the sky opened and a *torrent* of rain poured down on unprepared pedestrians.
    A. slide
    B. avalanche
    C. deluge
    D. air

45. The self-portrait *embodies* the true spirit of the artist.

   A. combats

   B. eliminates

   C. abjures

   D. symbolizes

46. Her sudden decision is typical of her *impetuous* behavior.

   A. contemptible

   B. sophisticated

   C. impulsive

   D. fallacious

47. It is fitting that we *eulogize* one who has contributed so greatly to our society.

   A. promulgate

   B. praise

   C. denigrate

   D. append

48. The convention hall swelled with the *vociferation* of various campaign groups.

   A. clamor

   B. taciturnity

   C. oblivion

   D. discernment

49. The blackmailer has placed her in a *precarious* position.

   A. mellifluous

   B. intrusive

   C. unusual

   D. unstable

50. Her neighbor's display of so much fine china was too *ostentatious*.

   A. pretentious

   B. inconspicuous

   C. ascribable

   D. candid

51. To *manifest* interest

   A. conceal

   B. diminish

   C. augment

   D. display

52. *Banter* and laughter

   A. discourse

   B. singing

   C. toasting

   D. raillery

53. *Aesthetic* value

   A. practical

   B. artistic

   C. monetary

   D. estimable

54. Confirmed his *apostasy*

   A. defiance

   B. defection

   C. belief

   D. inference

55. The *cryptic* message

   A. cynical

   B. mysterious

   C. critical

   D. censorious

56. New witnesses *emerged*

   A. deviated

   B. divested

   C. declined

   D. appeared

57. The *contumacious* youngster

   A. exuberant

   B. rebellious

   C. awkward

   D. mischievous

58. *Cognizant* of the ill will
    A. ignorant
    B. aware
    C. insensitive
    D. remorseful

59. *Glacial* region
    A. glass-like
    B. illiberal
    C. frigid
    D. reticent

60. *Instigated* the rebellion
    A. quelled
    B. incited
    C. assisted
    D. depressed

61. A fight *ensued*
    A. followed
    B. terminated
    C. was avoided
    D. culminated

62. *Retrospect* of events
    A. review
    B. concept
    C. knowledge
    D. awareness

63. *Malice* toward my friend
    A. adoration
    B. sympathy
    C. ill will
    D. apathy

64. *Saturated* with moisture
    A. void (of)
    B. mixed
    C. soaked
    D. replaced

65. *Debilitating* to people
    A. invigorating
    B. stimulating
    C. tolerable
    D. weakening

66. Ten years' *servitude*
    A. freedom
    B. lethargy
    C. vicissitude
    D. bondage

67. *Relish* the thought
    A. enjoy
    B. dread
    C. spread
    D. implant

68. A *lackadaisical* attitude
    A. enthusiastic
    B. complacent
    C. profound
    D. indifferent

69. To *hoist* the sails
    A. cast
    B. raise
    C. prepare
    D. repair

70. *Asperse* the family's good name
    A. slander
    B. fathom
    C. extol
    D. palliate

71. *Sordid* details
    A. bizarre
    B. wretched
    C. primordial
    D. exaggerated

72. Sudden *alienation*
    A. agitation
    B. inception
    C. subsistence
    D. isolation

73. *Dereliction* of duty
    A. neglect
    B. expansion
    C. attainment
    D. fulfillment

74. *Accede* to the request
    A. attend
    B. refer
    C. adjust
    D. agree

75. The *proximity* of the lake
    A. worthlessness
    B. nearness
    C. level
    D. ebullition

STOP

IF YOU FINISH BEFORE TIME IS CALLED, YOU MAY CHECK YOUR WORK ON THIS SECTION ONLY. DO NOT TURN TO ANY OTHER SECTION IN THE TEST.

ANTONYMS

The Turnabouts

Thus far, emphasis has been placed on synonyms, or words with similar or identical meanings. You are now ready to increase your word power from a contrasting point of view. Antonyms are words that are opposite in meaning. Some simple examples are: *hot/cold, strong/weak, sit/stand, night/day,* and *lazy/industrious.*

Antonyms are extremely useful to express contrast. The use of certain antonyms can result in the verbal creation of a universal portrait or concept. For instance, everyone associates the name "Scrooge" with *penny-pinching* or *miserly* traits. The Dickens character was anything but philanthropic, a term that characterizes people or agencies who devote themselves to helping and giving to humanity. Therefore, if you read that "a former Scrooge has transformed himself into a philanthropist," you would surmise that the person being described has had a complete change of heart. The term *philanthropist* has been contrasted with a symbol of *miserly* and *penny-pinching* traits.

When taking a test measuring your comprehension of verbal contrasts, be certain to select a response that is the same part of speech as the term in question. Although *discourtesy* and *insolent* share the same shade of meaning, one could not be substituted for the other—the former is a noun and the latter an adjective. Therefore, they could not play identical roles in a sentence.

If you are stumped by any one test item, move on quickly to the next. When you have completed the test, and if time permits, return to any test item(s) you have skipped. Mentally put the various word choices, including the test item, in a sentence. Then remove the test item again.

Example

Polite

A. desperate

B. discourtesy

C. insolent

D. discriminate

For the above example, make up a sentence using the word *polite* and then substitute the choices, such as "The boy is *discourtesy*" and "The boy is *insolent*." Obviously, *insolent* is the correct response, as it is the word opposite in meaning to *polite* and best fits the sentence pattern "The boy is . . ."

Using Prefixes

Another helpful technique in taking antonym tests is the close examination of prefixes. Review the etymological information before attempting the sample antonym test, and pay special attention to prefixes. Prefixes can often be the key to contrast in meaning. For example, the prefixes *un, im,* and *in* frequently denote the opposite meaning of the word to which they are affixed: *happy/unhappy; adequate/inadequate; polite/impolite.* These examples make it apparent that the actual meaning of the prefixes is "not." The prefixes *in* and *ex* are opposite in meaning. *In* means, "in," "into," "inside"; and *ex* means "out," "outside of."

If the target word is *internal,* which of the following words would you select as its antonym?

A. interior

B. ephemeral

C. illegal

D. external

Of course, *external* is the correct response. Study the list of contrasting prefixes below. Then try your hand at making the "turnabout."

Contrasting Prefixes

ad, ac, ag, at (to)	*ab, a* (away from)
ante (before)	*post* (after)
anti, contra (against)	*pro* (for)
bene (well, good)	*mal* (bad)
corn, con, col (together)	*dis, di* (apart)
con, com (with)	*an* (without)
eu (good)	*dys* (bad)
in, im (in)	*e, ex* (out)
hypo (under)	*hyper* (over)
pro (forward)	*retro* (backward)
sub (under)	*super, sur* (above)

TEST 2: ANTONYMS ANSWER SHEET

1. Ⓐ Ⓑ Ⓒ Ⓓ	16. Ⓐ Ⓑ Ⓒ Ⓓ	31. Ⓐ Ⓑ Ⓒ Ⓓ	46. Ⓐ Ⓑ Ⓒ Ⓓ	61. Ⓐ Ⓑ Ⓒ Ⓓ Ⓔ
2. Ⓐ Ⓑ Ⓒ Ⓓ	17. Ⓐ Ⓑ Ⓒ Ⓓ	32. Ⓐ Ⓑ Ⓒ Ⓓ	47. Ⓐ Ⓑ Ⓒ Ⓓ	62. Ⓐ Ⓑ Ⓒ Ⓓ Ⓔ
3. Ⓐ Ⓑ Ⓒ Ⓓ	18. Ⓐ Ⓑ Ⓒ Ⓓ	33. Ⓐ Ⓑ Ⓒ Ⓓ	48. Ⓐ Ⓑ Ⓒ Ⓓ	63. Ⓐ Ⓑ Ⓒ Ⓓ Ⓔ
4. Ⓐ Ⓑ Ⓒ Ⓓ	19. Ⓐ Ⓑ Ⓒ Ⓓ	34. Ⓐ Ⓑ Ⓒ Ⓓ	49. Ⓐ Ⓑ Ⓒ Ⓓ	64. Ⓐ Ⓑ Ⓒ Ⓓ Ⓔ
5. Ⓐ Ⓑ Ⓒ Ⓓ	20. Ⓐ Ⓑ Ⓒ Ⓓ	35. Ⓐ Ⓑ Ⓒ Ⓓ	50. Ⓐ Ⓑ Ⓒ Ⓓ	65. Ⓐ Ⓑ Ⓒ Ⓓ Ⓔ
6. Ⓐ Ⓑ Ⓒ Ⓓ	21. Ⓐ Ⓑ Ⓒ Ⓓ	36. Ⓐ Ⓑ Ⓒ Ⓓ	51. Ⓐ Ⓑ Ⓒ Ⓓ	66. Ⓐ Ⓑ Ⓒ Ⓓ Ⓔ
7. Ⓐ Ⓑ Ⓒ Ⓓ	22. Ⓐ Ⓑ Ⓒ Ⓓ	37. Ⓐ Ⓑ Ⓒ Ⓓ	52. Ⓐ Ⓑ Ⓒ Ⓓ	67. Ⓐ Ⓑ Ⓒ Ⓓ Ⓔ
8. Ⓐ Ⓑ Ⓒ Ⓓ	23. Ⓐ Ⓑ Ⓒ Ⓓ	38. Ⓐ Ⓑ Ⓒ Ⓓ	53. Ⓐ Ⓑ Ⓒ Ⓓ	68. Ⓐ Ⓑ Ⓒ Ⓓ Ⓔ
9. Ⓐ Ⓑ Ⓒ Ⓓ	24. Ⓐ Ⓑ Ⓒ Ⓓ	39. Ⓐ Ⓑ Ⓒ Ⓓ	54. Ⓐ Ⓑ Ⓒ Ⓓ	69. Ⓐ Ⓑ Ⓒ Ⓓ Ⓔ
10. Ⓐ Ⓑ Ⓒ Ⓓ	25. Ⓐ Ⓑ Ⓒ Ⓓ	40. Ⓐ Ⓑ Ⓒ Ⓓ	55. Ⓐ Ⓑ Ⓒ Ⓓ	70. Ⓐ Ⓑ Ⓒ Ⓓ Ⓔ
11. Ⓐ Ⓑ Ⓒ Ⓓ	26. Ⓐ Ⓑ Ⓒ Ⓓ	41. Ⓐ Ⓑ Ⓒ Ⓓ	56. Ⓐ Ⓑ Ⓒ Ⓓ	71. Ⓐ Ⓑ Ⓒ Ⓓ Ⓔ
12. Ⓐ Ⓑ Ⓒ Ⓓ	27. Ⓐ Ⓑ Ⓒ Ⓓ	42. Ⓐ Ⓑ Ⓒ Ⓓ	57. Ⓐ Ⓑ Ⓒ Ⓓ	72. Ⓐ Ⓑ Ⓒ Ⓓ Ⓔ
13. Ⓐ Ⓑ Ⓒ Ⓓ	28. Ⓐ Ⓑ Ⓒ Ⓓ	43. Ⓐ Ⓑ Ⓒ Ⓓ	58. Ⓐ Ⓑ Ⓒ Ⓓ	73. Ⓐ Ⓑ Ⓒ Ⓓ Ⓔ
14. Ⓐ Ⓑ Ⓒ Ⓓ	29. Ⓐ Ⓑ Ⓒ Ⓓ	44. Ⓐ Ⓑ Ⓒ Ⓓ	59. Ⓐ Ⓑ Ⓒ Ⓓ	74. Ⓐ Ⓑ Ⓒ Ⓓ Ⓔ
15. Ⓐ Ⓑ Ⓒ Ⓓ	30. Ⓐ Ⓑ Ⓒ Ⓓ	45. Ⓐ Ⓑ Ⓒ Ⓓ	60. Ⓐ Ⓑ Ⓒ Ⓓ	75. Ⓐ Ⓑ Ⓒ Ⓓ Ⓔ

answer sheet

TEST 2: ANTONYMS

75 Questions • 35 Minutes

Directions: For each of the following questions, select the word opposite in meaning to the word printed in capital letters.

1. DEFACE
   A. defame
   B. embellish
   C. vilify
   D. disfigure

2. SUPERFLUOUS
   A. coarse
   B. transient
   C. insufficient
   D. abundant

3. ASSUAGE
   A. presume
   B. agitate
   C. alleviate
   D. absorb

4. AUGURY
   A. gentility
   B. relentlessness
   C. supremacy
   D. science

5. TERMINATE
   A. withhold
   B. construe
   C. repel
   D. initiate

6. VITIATE
   A. liquidate
   B. revive
   C. validate
   D. slander

7. JUBILANT
   A. lugubrious
   B. irrepressible
   C. discernible
   D. jocular

8. HOSTILE
   A. affable
   B. awkward
   C. judicious
   D. politic

9. TACITURN
   A. tactful
   B. talkative
   C. crucial
   D. impetuous

10. LAGGARDLY
    A. laboriously
    B. languidly
    C. briskly
    D. cowardly

11. PHLEGMATIC
    A. vital
    B. apparent
    C. conversant
    D. apprehensive

12. LOATHSOME
    A. alluring
    B. mournful
    C. indifferent
    D. preposterous

13. EXALT
    A. degrade
    B. gratify
    C. expose
    D. desiderate

14. PACIFY
    A. conciliate
    B. palliate
    C. quell
    D. exasperate

15. SUBSEQUENT
    A. worthless
    B. inactive
    C. preceding
    D. demeaning

16. ULTIMATE
    A. initial
    B. equitable
    C. irrefutable
    D. turbid

17. LEEWAY
    A. relevance
    B. restriction
    C. protection
    D. satisfaction

18. PRETENTIOUS
    A. flagrant
    B. diabolical
    C. officious
    D. modest

19. QUANDARY
    A. certainty
    B. mediocrity
    C. ruthlessness
    D. criterion

20. SAGACIOUS
    A. obtuse
    B. scurrilous
    C. indulgent
    D. impertinent

21. SAVANT
    A. uncivilized
    B. master
    C. neophyte
    D. constituent

22. SQUALID
    A. staunch
    B. stately
    C. avaricious
    D. equivocal

23. EXQUISITE
    A. exorbitant
    B. obscure
    C. extraneous
    D. ordinary

24. FACILITATE
    A. falsify
    B. delude
    C. hinder
    D. assimilate

25. FLAWLESS
    A. pertinent
    B. conventional
    C. defective
    D. complacent

26. RECOMPENSE
    A. renovate
    B. embezzle
    C. retribution
    D. sanction

27. FERVENT
    A. nonchalant
    B. lenient
    C. meager
    D. liable

28. AVERT
    A. pursue
    B. forestall
    C. reject
    D. relinquish

29. ARID
    A. fragrant
    B. moist
    C. parched
    D. odoriferous

30. IMPERATIVE
    A. conceivable
    B. illustrative
    C. speculative
    D. optional

31. SUCCINCT
    A. corporeal
    B. graphic
    C. princely
    D. loquacious

32. JEOPARDY
    A. security
    B. discernment
    C. curiosity
    D. tedium

33. SOMBER
    A. insipid
    B. congruous
    C. festive
    D. voluminous

34. EXOTIC
    A. inveterate
    B. erotic
    C. common
    D. harmonious

35. AFFILIATE
    A. annihilate
    B. disassociate
    C. proffer
    D. disparage

36. SINISTER
    A. auspicious
    B. immaculate
    C. fanatical
    D. transitory

37. INEXTRICABLE
    A. intricate
    B. judicious
    C. disentangled
    D. desperate

38. PROFLIGATE
    A. insolvent
    B. virtuous
    C. redundant
    D. incessant

39. TURBULENT
    A. diaphanous
    B. tranquil
    C. formidable
    D. diffident

40. UNWARRANTED
    A. justifiable
    B. baneful
    C. depleted
    D. contemplated

41. PLAINTIVE
   A. embellished
   B. poignant
   C. rational
   D. gleeful

42. ORNATE
   A. unadorned
   B. deft
   C. subtle
   D. conspicuous

43. ABROGATE
   A. ratify
   B. reconcile
   C. abridge
   D. alleviate

44. ABASE
   A. cede
   B. dignify
   C. repudiate
   D. engulf

45. RENOUNCE
   A. claim
   B. deride
   C. conceive
   D. alienate

46. SABOTAGE
   A. compensate
   B. reinforce
   C. restrain
   D. release

47. OBLIVIOUS
   A. latent
   B. integrant
   C. repugnant
   D. cognizant

48. SUBMISSIVE
   A. offensive
   B. tactless
   C. incompliant
   D. manifest

49. NURTURE
   A. distinguish
   B. impart
   C. neglect
   D. disclose

50. PRUDENCE
   A. compunction
   B. dilemma
   C. anticipation
   D. recklessness

51. LAMENT
   A. rejoice
   B. acclaim
   C. surmise
   D. deceive

52. GRUELING
   A. relaxing
   B. satisfying
   C. taming
   D. suppressing

53. TRIVIAL
   A. nugatory
   B. ungainly
   C. critical
   D. solicitous

54. ZENITH
   A. vitality
   B. rage
   C. reverence
   D. nadir

55. UNOBTRUSIVE

   A. resonant

   B. prominent

   C. controlled

   D. subjective

56. REFRACTIVE

   A. cryptic

   B. interruptive

   C. applicable

   D. direct

57. REBUFF

   A. exclusion

   B. disturbance

   C. recall

   D. encouragement

58. ADVERSARY

   A. opponent

   B. administrator

   C. accomplice

   D. enemy

59. OPTIMIST

   A. rival

   B. pessimist

   C. analyst

   D. protagonist

60. PERVASIVE

   A. limited

   B. universal

   C. ubiquitous

   D. common

Directions: In the following sets of words, choose the word that is most different in meaning from the others.

---

61. A. erudite

   B. learned

   C. scholarly

   D. savvy

   E. ignorant

62. A. paramount

   B. essential

   C. inconsequential

   D. momentous

   E. supreme

63. A. surreptitious

   B. secretive

   C. candid

   D. clandestine

   E. covert

64. A. mendacious

   B. duplicitous

   C. deceptive

   D. prevaricating

   E. creditable

65. A. unctuous

   B. awkward

   C. charming

   D. slick

   E. urbane

66. A. impetuous

   B. cautious

   C. rash

   D. impulsive

   E. capricious

67. A. penurious
    B. frugal
    C. extravagant
    D. parsimonious
    E. thrifty

68. A. odious
    B. abhorrent
    C. loathsome
    D. winsome
    E. repugnant

69. A. ostensible
    B. ulterior
    C. alleged
    D. purported
    E. overt

70. A. deleterious
    B. insalubrious
    C. beneficial
    D. toxic
    E. pernicious

71. A. ignominy
    B. honor
    C. shame
    D. humiliation
    E. disgrace

72. A. compatible
    B. complementary
    C. simpatico
    D. incongruous
    E. harmonious

73. A. premeditated
    B. plotted
    C. calculated
    D. improvised
    E. developed

74. A. pernicious
    B. restorative
    C. calamitous
    D. detrimental
    E. baneful

75. A. umbrage
    B. offense
    C. resentment
    D. chagrin
    E. amity

STOP

IF YOU FINISH BEFORE TIME IS CALLED, YOU MAY
CHECK YOUR WORK ON THIS SECTION ONLY. DO NOT
TURN TO ANY OTHER SECTION IN THE TEST.

SKILL WITH VERBAL ANALOGIES

The verbal analogy is one variation of the vocabulary question often encountered on nursing school tests. It tests your understanding of word meanings and your ability to grasp relationships between words and ideas. This practice in mental agility will help you do better with all the other questions on the test.

In addition to their simple meanings, words carry subtle shades of implication that depend in some degree upon the relationship they bear to other words. There are various classifications of relationship, such as similarity (synonyms) and opposition (antonyms). Careful students will try to examine each shade of meaning they encounter.

The ability to detect the exact nature of the relationship between words is a function of your intelligence. In a sense, the verbal analogy test is a vocabulary test. But it is also a test of your ability to analyze meanings, think things out, and see the relationships between ideas and words. In mathematics, this kind of situation is expressed as a proportion problem: 3:5::6:X. Sometimes, verbal analogies are written in this mathematical form:

CLOCK : TIME :: THERMOMETER :

- **A.** hour
- **B.** degrees
- **C.** climate
- **D.** temperature

Or the question may be put:

CLOCK is to TIME as THERMOMETER is to

- **A.** hour
- **B.** degrees
- **C.** climate
- **D.** temperature

The challenge is to determine which one of the lettered words has the same relationship to *thermometer* as *time* has to *clock*. The best way to determine the correct answer is to provide a word or phrase that shows the relationship between these words. In the above example, "measures" is a word expressing the relationship. However, this may not be enough. The analogy must be exact. *Climate* or *weather* would not be exact enough. *Temperature*, of course, is the correct answer.

You will find that many of the choices have some relationship to the third word. Select the one with a relationship that *best* approximates the relationship between the first two words.

Three Examples of Verbal Analogy Questions

Some standardized tests provide four answer choices (A,B,C,D) and some, five (A,B,C,D,E).

Example 1

From the four pairs of words that follow, select the pair related in the same way as are the words of the first pair.

SPELLING: PUNCTUATION ::

A. pajamas : fatigue

B. powder : shaving

C. bandage : cut

D. biology : physics

Spelling and *punctuation* are elements of the mechanics of English; *biology* and *physics* are two of the subjects that make up the field of science. The other choices do not possess this part : part relationship. Therefore, **D** is the correct answer.

Example 2

Another popular format gives two words followed by a third word. The latter is related to one word in a group of choices in the same way that the first two words are related.

WINTER : SUMMER :: COLD :

A. wet

B. future

C. hot

D. freezing

Winter and *summer* bear an opposite relationship. *Cold* and *hot* have the same kind of opposite relationship. Therefore, choice **C** is the correct answer.

Example 3

Still another analogy format has a variable construction. Any one of the four relationship elements may not be specified. From choices offered—regardless of position—you are to select the one choice that completes the relationship with the other three items. In this example, the third relationship element is not specified.

SUBMARINE: FISH :: ___ : BIRD

A. kite

B. limousine

C. feather

D. chirp

Both a *submarine* and a *fish* are usually found in the water; both a *kite* and a *bird* are customarily seen in the air. Consequently, choice **A** is the correct answer.

TEST 3: ANALOGY RELATIONSHIPS ANSWER SHEET

1. Ⓐ Ⓑ Ⓒ Ⓓ   4. Ⓐ Ⓑ Ⓒ Ⓓ   7. Ⓐ Ⓑ Ⓒ Ⓓ   10. Ⓐ Ⓑ Ⓒ Ⓓ   13. Ⓐ Ⓑ Ⓒ Ⓓ

2. Ⓐ Ⓑ Ⓒ Ⓓ   5. Ⓐ Ⓑ Ⓒ Ⓓ   8. Ⓐ Ⓑ Ⓒ Ⓓ   11. Ⓐ Ⓑ Ⓒ Ⓓ   14. Ⓐ Ⓑ Ⓒ Ⓓ

3. Ⓐ Ⓑ Ⓒ Ⓓ   6. Ⓐ Ⓑ Ⓒ Ⓓ   9. Ⓐ Ⓑ Ⓒ Ⓓ   12. Ⓐ Ⓑ Ⓒ Ⓓ   15. Ⓐ Ⓑ Ⓒ Ⓓ

answer sheet

TEST 3: ANALOGY RELATIONSHIPS

15 Questions • 8 Minutes

Directions: In the following questions, determine the relationship between the first pair of capitalized words and then decide which pair of words among the answer choices shares a similar relationship.

1. GLOVE : BALL ::
   A. hook : fish
   B. winter : weather
   C. game : pennant
   D. stadium : seats

2. RACE : FATIGUE ::
   A. track : athlete
   B. ant : bug
   C. fast : hunger
   D. walking : running

3. SNAKE : REPTILE ::
   A. patch : thread
   B. removal : snow
   C. struggle : wrestle
   D. hand : clock

4. GILL : FIN ::
   A. plasma display : electrodes
   B. instrument : violin
   C. sea : fish
   D. salad : supper

5. KICK : FOOTBALL ::
   A. kill : bomb
   B. break : pieces
   C. question : team
   D. smoke : pipe

6. STEAK : BROIL ::
   A. bread : bake
   B. food : eat
   C. pour : wine
   D. spill : sugar

7. ENORMOUS : HUGE ::
   A. rogue : rock
   B. muddy : unclear
   C. purse : kitchen
   D. black : white

8. PURITY : EVIL ::
   A. suavity : bluntness
   B. north : climate
   C. angel : horns
   D. boldness : victory

9. MIAMI : FLORIDA ::
   A. Chicago : United States
   B. New York : Albany
   C. United States : Chicago
   D. Albany : New York

10. WARM : HOT ::
    A. glue : paste
    B. climate : weather
    C. fried egg : boiled egg
    D. bright : genius

11. SKILL : PRACTICE ::
    A. blood : wound
    B. money : dollar
    C. schools : elevators
    D. education : stupidity

12. SPRING : SUMMER ::
    A. Thursday : Wednesday
    B. Wednesday : Monday
    C. Monday : Sunday
    D. Wednesday : Thursday

13. RESTORE : CLIMB ::
    A. segregation : seem
    B. into : nymph
    C. precipice : although
    D. overpower : seethe

14. DEVIL : WRONG ::
    A. color : sidewalk
    B. slipper : state
    C. ink : writing
    D. picture : bed

15. 4 : 12 ::
    A. 10 : 16
    B. 9 : 27
    C. 3 : 4
    D. 12 : 6

Points to Remember

In many analogy questions, the incorrect choices may be related in some way to the first two words. Don't let this association mislead you. For example, in number four (part : part relationship), choice A, *plasma display : electrodes* is the correct answer. Choice C, *sea : fish*, is incorrect, although these two latter words are associated in a general sense with the first two words (*gill : fin*).

Often, the relationship of the first two words may apply to *more than one* of the choices given. In such a case, you must narrow down the initial relationship in order to get the correct choice. For example, in number six (object: action relationship), a *steak* is something that you *broil*. Now let us consider the choices: *bread* is something that you *bake*; *food* is something that you *eat*; *wine* is something that you *pour;* and *sugar* is something that you (can) *spill.* Thus far, each choice seems correct. Let us now narrow down the relationship: a *steak* is something that you *broil* with *heat*. The only choice that fulfills this *complete* relationship is choice A, *bread*—something that you bake with *heat*. It follows that choice A is the correct answer.

Remember that the two keys to analogy success are:

Step One: Determine the relationship between the first two words.

Step Two: Find the same relationship among the choices that follow the first two words.

TEST 4: VERBAL ANALOGIES ANSWER SHEET

Part A

1. Ⓐ Ⓑ Ⓒ Ⓓ   6. Ⓐ Ⓑ Ⓒ Ⓓ   11. Ⓐ Ⓑ Ⓒ Ⓓ   16. Ⓐ Ⓑ Ⓒ Ⓓ   21. Ⓐ Ⓑ Ⓒ Ⓓ
2. Ⓐ Ⓑ Ⓒ Ⓓ   7. Ⓐ Ⓑ Ⓒ Ⓓ   12. Ⓐ Ⓑ Ⓒ Ⓓ   17. Ⓐ Ⓑ Ⓒ Ⓓ   22. Ⓐ Ⓑ Ⓒ Ⓓ
3. Ⓐ Ⓑ Ⓒ Ⓓ   8. Ⓐ Ⓑ Ⓒ Ⓓ   13. Ⓐ Ⓑ Ⓒ Ⓓ   18. Ⓐ Ⓑ Ⓒ Ⓓ   23. Ⓐ Ⓑ Ⓒ Ⓓ
4. Ⓐ Ⓑ Ⓒ Ⓓ   9. Ⓐ Ⓑ Ⓒ Ⓓ   14. Ⓐ Ⓑ Ⓒ Ⓓ   19. Ⓐ Ⓑ Ⓒ Ⓓ   24. Ⓐ Ⓑ Ⓒ Ⓓ
5. Ⓐ Ⓑ Ⓒ Ⓓ   10. Ⓐ Ⓑ Ⓒ Ⓓ   15. Ⓐ Ⓑ Ⓒ Ⓓ   20. Ⓐ Ⓑ Ⓒ Ⓓ   25. Ⓐ Ⓑ Ⓒ Ⓓ

Part B

1. Ⓐ Ⓑ Ⓒ Ⓓ Ⓔ   6. Ⓐ Ⓑ Ⓒ Ⓓ Ⓔ   11. Ⓐ Ⓑ Ⓒ Ⓓ Ⓔ   16. Ⓐ Ⓑ Ⓒ Ⓓ Ⓔ   21. Ⓐ Ⓑ Ⓒ Ⓓ Ⓔ
2. Ⓐ Ⓑ Ⓒ Ⓓ Ⓔ   7. Ⓐ Ⓑ Ⓒ Ⓓ Ⓔ   12. Ⓐ Ⓑ Ⓒ Ⓓ Ⓔ   17. Ⓐ Ⓑ Ⓒ Ⓓ Ⓔ   22. Ⓐ Ⓑ Ⓒ Ⓓ Ⓔ
3. Ⓐ Ⓑ Ⓒ Ⓓ Ⓔ   8. Ⓐ Ⓑ Ⓒ Ⓓ Ⓔ   13. Ⓐ Ⓑ Ⓒ Ⓓ Ⓔ   18. Ⓐ Ⓑ Ⓒ Ⓓ Ⓔ   23. Ⓐ Ⓑ Ⓒ Ⓓ Ⓔ
4. Ⓐ Ⓑ Ⓒ Ⓓ Ⓔ   9. Ⓐ Ⓑ Ⓒ Ⓓ Ⓔ   14. Ⓐ Ⓑ Ⓒ Ⓓ Ⓔ   19. Ⓐ Ⓑ Ⓒ Ⓓ Ⓔ   24. Ⓐ Ⓑ Ⓒ Ⓓ Ⓔ
5. Ⓐ Ⓑ Ⓒ Ⓓ Ⓔ   10. Ⓐ Ⓑ Ⓒ Ⓓ Ⓔ   15. Ⓐ Ⓑ Ⓒ Ⓓ Ⓔ   20. Ⓐ Ⓑ Ⓒ Ⓓ Ⓔ   25. Ⓐ Ⓑ Ⓒ Ⓓ Ⓔ

Part C

1. Ⓐ Ⓑ Ⓒ Ⓓ Ⓔ   6. Ⓐ Ⓑ Ⓒ Ⓓ Ⓔ   11. Ⓐ Ⓑ Ⓒ Ⓓ Ⓔ   16. Ⓐ Ⓑ Ⓒ Ⓓ Ⓔ   21. Ⓐ Ⓑ Ⓒ Ⓓ Ⓔ
2. Ⓐ Ⓑ Ⓒ Ⓓ Ⓔ   7. Ⓐ Ⓑ Ⓒ Ⓓ Ⓔ   12. Ⓐ Ⓑ Ⓒ Ⓓ Ⓔ   17. Ⓐ Ⓑ Ⓒ Ⓓ Ⓔ   22. Ⓐ Ⓑ Ⓒ Ⓓ Ⓔ
3. Ⓐ Ⓑ Ⓒ Ⓓ Ⓔ   8. Ⓐ Ⓑ Ⓒ Ⓓ Ⓔ   13. Ⓐ Ⓑ Ⓒ Ⓓ Ⓔ   18. Ⓐ Ⓑ Ⓒ Ⓓ Ⓔ   23. Ⓐ Ⓑ Ⓒ Ⓓ Ⓔ
4. Ⓐ Ⓑ Ⓒ Ⓓ Ⓔ   9. Ⓐ Ⓑ Ⓒ Ⓓ Ⓔ   14. Ⓐ Ⓑ Ⓒ Ⓓ Ⓔ   19. Ⓐ Ⓑ Ⓒ Ⓓ Ⓔ   24. Ⓐ Ⓑ Ⓒ Ⓓ Ⓔ
5. Ⓐ Ⓑ Ⓒ Ⓓ Ⓔ   10. Ⓐ Ⓑ Ⓒ Ⓓ Ⓔ   15. Ⓐ Ⓑ Ⓒ Ⓓ Ⓔ   20. Ⓐ Ⓑ Ⓒ Ⓓ Ⓔ   25. Ⓐ Ⓑ Ⓒ Ⓓ Ⓔ

answer sheet

TEST 4: VERBAL ANALOGIES

75 Questions • 30 Minutes

Directions: In the following questions, determine the relationship between the first pair of capitalized words and then decide which of the answer choices shares a similar relationship with the third capitalized word. Parts A and B of this test are written in mathematical form (expressed as proportion problems). The questions for Part A have four answer choices, and the questions for Parts B and C have five. Part C is written so that relationships are expressed with "is to" and "as."

Part A

25 Questions • 10 Minutes

1. GUN : SHOOTS :: KNIFE :
   A. run
   B. cuts
   C. sharpen
   D. poke

2. EAR : HEAR :: EYE :
   A. table
   B. hand
   C. see
   D. foot

3. FUR : MAMMAL :: FEATHERS :
   A. bird
   B. neck
   C. feet
   D. bill

4. HANDLE : HAMMER :: KNOB :
   A. key
   B. room
   C. shut
   D. door

5. SHOE : FOOT :: COAT :
   A. hat
   B. buttons
   C. body
   D. head

6. WATER : DRINK :: BREAD :
   A. cake
   B. coffee
   C. eat
   D. pie

7. FOOD : HUMAN :: GASOLINE :
   A. lube
   B. oil
   C. automobile
   D. spark

8. EAT : FAT :: STARVE :
   A. thin
   B. food
   C. bread
   D. thirsty

9. HUMAN : HOUSE :: BIRD :
   A. tree
   B. insect
   C. limb
   D. nest

10. GO : COME :: SELL :
    A. leave
    B. buy
    C. money
    D. pawn

11. PENINSULA : LAND :: BAY :
   A. boat
   B. inlet
   C. water
   D. harbor

12. HOUR : MINUTE :: MINUTE :
   A. hour
   B. week
   C. second
   D. short

13. ABIDE : DEPART :: STAY :
   A. over
   B. home
   C. play
   D. leave

14. JANUARY : FEBRUARY :: JUNE :
   A. July
   B. May
   C. month
   D. year

15. BOLD : TIMID :: ADVANCE :
   A. proceed
   B. retreat
   C. campaign
   D. soldiers

16. ABOVE : BELOW :: TOP :
   A. spin
   B. bottom
   C. surface
   D. side

17. LION : ANIMAL :: ROSE :
   A. smell
   B. leaf
   C. plant
   D. thorn

18. TIGER : CARNIVOROUS :: HORSE :
   A. cow
   B. nervous
   C. omnivorous
   D. herbivorous

19. SAILOR : NAVY :: SOLDIER :
   A. gun
   B. cap
   C. hill
   D. army

20. PICTURE : SEE :: SOUND :
   A. noise
   B. music
   C. hear
   D. bark

21. SUCCESS : JOY :: FAILURE :
   A. sadness
   B. enthusiasm
   C. fault
   D. work

22. HOPE : DESPAIR :: HAPPINESS :
   A. frolic
   B. fun
   C. joy
   D. misery

23. PRETTY : UGLY :: ATTRACT :
   A. fine
   B. repel
   C. nice
   D. draw

24. PUPIL : TEACHER :: CHILD :
   A. parent
   B. doll
   C. youngster
   D. obey

25. CITY : MAYOR :: ARMY :
    A. navy
    B. soldier
    C. general
    D. private

Part B

25 Questions • 10 Minutes

1. REMUNERATIVE : PROFITABLE ::
   FRAUDULENT :
   A. liar
   B. slander
   C. fallacious
   D. plausible
   E. reward

2. AX : WOODSMAN :: WRENCH :
   A. cut
   B. hew
   C. technician
   D. plumber
   E. cobbler

3. SURGEON : SCALPEL :: BUTCHER :
   A. mallet
   B. cleaver
   C. chisel
   D. screwdriver
   E. medicine

4. CAT : FELINE :: HORSE :
   A. equine
   B. tiger
   C. quadruped
   D. carnivore
   E. vulpine

5. ADVERSITY : HAPPINESS ::
   VEHEMENCE :
   A. misfortune
   B. gaiety
   C. troublesome
   D. petulance
   E. serenity

6. NECKLACE : ADORNMENT ::
   MEDAL :
   A. jewel
   B. metal
   C. bravery
   D. bronze
   E. decoration

7. MINER : SHOVEL :: PIRATE :
   A. treasure
   B. sword
   C. ship
   D. flag
   E. gold

8. ARCHAEOLOGIST : ANTIQUITY ::
   ICHTHYOLOGIST :
   A. theology
   B. ruins
   C. horticulture
   D. marine life
   E. mystic

9. SHOE : LEATHER :: HIGHWAY :
   - A. passage
   - B. road
   - C. asphalt
   - D. trail
   - E. journey

10. SERFDOM : FEUDALISM ::
    ENTREPRENEUR :
    - A. liberal
    - B. captain
    - C. radical
    - D. agriculture
    - E. capitalism

11. FIN : FISH :: PROPELLER :
    - A. wing
    - B. plane
    - C. air
    - D. water
    - E. canoe

12. SATISFIED : SATIETY :: POOR :
    - A. destitute
    - B. subsistence
    - C. sustainable
    - D. lesser
    - E. abandoned

13. SKIN : HUMAN :: HIDE :
    - A. scales
    - B. fur
    - C. animal
    - D. hair
    - E. fish

14. RAIN : DROP :: SNOW :
    - A. ice
    - B. cold
    - C. zero
    - D. flake
    - E. sleet

15. WING : BIRD :: HOOF :
    - A. dog
    - B. foot
    - C. horse
    - D. girl
    - E. horseshoe

16. CONSTELLATION : STAR ::
    ARCHIPELAGO :
    - A. continent
    - B. peninsula
    - C. country
    - D. island
    - E. river

17. INTERNET : EMAILING ::
    SMARTPHONE :
    - A. fast
    - B. messaging
    - C. calling
    - D. landline
    - E. snail mail

18. ABSENCE : PRESENCE :: STABLE :
    - A. steady
    - B. secure
    - C. safe
    - D. changeable
    - E. influential

19. RUBBER : FLEXIBILITY :: PIPE :
    - A. iron
    - B. copper
    - C. pliability
    - D. elasticity
    - E. rigidity

20. SAFETY VALVE : BOILER :: SPARK
    PLUG :
    - A. engine
    - B. house
    - C. wire
    - D. city
    - E. factory

21. SCHOLARLY : UNSCHOLARLY ::
    LEARNED :
    A. ignorant
    B. wise
    C. skilled
    D. educated
    E. literary

22. IMMIGRANT : ARRIVAL ::
    EMIGRANT :
    A. departure
    B. alienation
    C. native
    D. welcoming
    E. travel

23. GOVERNOR : STATE :: ADMIRAL :
    A. lieutenant
    B. army
    C. navy
    D. captain
    E. general

24. TROUBLESOME : DISASTROUS ::
    COSTLY :
    A. cheap
    B. extravagant
    C. gorgeous
    D. valuable
    E. turbulent

25. WOOL : COAT :: COTTON :
    A. tablecloth
    B. cover
    C. washable
    D. dress
    E. cleaner

Part C

25 Questions • 10 Minutes

1. BOAT is to DOCK as AIRPLANE is to
   A. wing
   B. strut
   C. engine
   D. wind
   E. hangar

2. OAT is to BUSHEL as DIAMOND is to
   A. gram
   B. hardness
   C. usefulness
   D. carat
   E. ornament

3. MEDICINE is to EXAMINATION as
   LAW is to
   A. jurist
   B. court
   C. interrogation
   D. contract
   E. suit

4. PARENT is to GUIDE as SOLDIER
   is to
   A. serve
   B. obedience
   C. participate
   D. fly
   E. achieve

5. CAPTAIN is to VESSEL as DIRECTOR is to
   A. football team
   B. board
   C. cheerleader squad
   D. orchestra
   E. musician

6. FATHER is to DAUGHTER as UNCLE is to
   A. son
   B. daughter
   C. son-in-law
   D. niece
   E. aunt

7. PISTOL is to TRIGGER as MOTOR is to
   A. wire
   B. dynamo
   C. amperes
   D. barrel
   E. switch

8. CUBE is to PYRAMID as SQUARE is to
   A. box
   B. solid
   C. pentagon
   D. triangle
   E. cylinder

9. PROFIT is to SELLING as FAME is to
   A. buying
   B. cheating
   C. publicity
   D. praying
   E. loving

10. PRINTING is to BOOK as WELDING is to
    A. door
    B. tank
    C. chair
    D. wire
    E. pencil

11. GYMNASIUM is to HEALTH as SCHOOL is to
    A. sick
    B. study
    C. books
    D. knowledge
    E. library

12. RIGHT is to WRONG as SUCCESS is to
    A. aid
    B. profit
    C. failure
    D. error
    E. gain

13. EIGHT is to OCTAGON as SEVEN is to
    A. polygon
    B. polyhedron
    C. hexagon
    D. quadrilateral
    E. heptagon

14. IDIOM is to EXPRESSION as PARAPHRASE is to
    A. version
    B. translation
    C. statement
    D. dialect
    E. language

15. BOTTLE is to BRITTLE as TIRE is to
   A. elastic
   B. scarce
   C. rubber
   D. spheroid
   E. automobile

16. SOPRANO is to HIGH as BASS is to
   A. violin
   B. good
   C. low
   D. fish
   E. soft

17. OLFACTORY is to NOSE as TACTILE
   is to
   A. tacit
   B. bloody
   C. finger
   D. handkerchief
   E. stomach

18. STREET is to HORIZONTAL as
   BUILDING is to
   A. tall
   B. brick
   C. broad
   D. vertical
   E. large

19. ALLEGIANCE is to LOYALTY as
   TREASON is to
   A. obedience
   B. rebellion
   C. murder
   D. felony
   E. homage

20. CANVAS is to PAINT as MOLD is to
   A. clay
   B. cloth
   C. statue
   D. art
   E. aesthetic

21. ABRUPT is to SUDDEN as
   INCESSANT is to
   A. ceaseless
   B. occasional
   C. irregular
   D. brutal
   E. concise

22. CONQUEST is to ASCENDANCY as
   DEFEAT is to
   A. omission
   B. frustration
   C. censure
   D. subjugation
   E. mastery

23. SOLUTION is to MYSTERY as
   COMPLETION is to
   A. puzzle
   B. books
   C. college
   D. school
   E. detective

24. ALUMNUS is to ALUMNA as PRINCE
   is to
   A. castle
   B. king
   C. knight
   D. country
   E. princess

25. OCCULT is to OVERT as SECRET
is to
A. abstract
B. outward
C. science
D. tarry
E. concealed

STOP

IF YOU FINISH BEFORE TIME IS CALLED, YOU MAY
CHECK YOUR WORK ON THIS SECTION ONLY. DO NOT
TURN TO ANY OTHER SECTION IN THE TEST.

ENGLISH GRAMMAR AND USAGE

The Pre-Admission Exam (PAX) and the Test of Essential Academic Skills (TEAS) both include questions related to English grammar and usage. On the PAX, such questions appear in the Word Knowledge subsection of the Verbal section of the exam. On the TEAS, these questions appear in the English and Language Usage section. Although a thorough review of grammar and usage is beyond the scope of this book, some related topics that commonly appear on these exams are provided below to help you prepare for this type of question.

Subject and Verb Agreement

One tricky aspect of English usage that often appears on entrance exams is matching the correct form of a verb with its subject. A verb must agree with its subject in number. In simple sentences, whether the subject is a noun or pronoun, finding such agreement is typically easy. In the present tense, most verbs end in *s* in the third person singular and not in *s* in all other forms:

> I *am* hungry. I *eat* some fruit.
>
> You *are* hungry. You *eat* a salad.
>
> The boy *is* hungry. The boy *eats* a sandwich. He *eats* a sandwich.
>
> The girl *is* hungry. The girl *eats* a cookie. She *eats* a cookie.
>
> The dog *is* hungry. The dog *eats* the rest of the boy's sandwich. It *eats* a sandwich.
>
> We *are* hungry. We *eat* a big meal.
>
> You all *are* hungry. You all *eat* spaghetti.
>
> The dancers *are* hungry. The dancers *eat* ice cream. They *eat* ice cream.

Making the verb agree is trickier, however, when a phrase comes between the subject and verb. Keep in mind that the verb always agrees with the subject, not with any phrases that follow it:

> He, along with his dog, *walks* to the park.
>
> The woman, as well as her three children, *goes* into the bank.

The indefinite pronouns *each*, *either*, and *neither* and those ending in *-one* (i.e., *one, no one, every one, anyone, someone, everyone*) or *–body* (i.e., *anybody, somebody, everybody*) are singular:

> Each of the cats *has* its own collar.
>
> Everybody *loves* Raymond.
>
> Either of the restaurants *is* fine with me. Neither *is* bad.

The words *some*, *any*, *none*, *all*, and *most* may be singular or plural, depending on whether they are referring to a singular or plural word:

> Some of my pie *is* missing.
>
> Some of my chocolates *are* missing.
>
> All of the house *is* hot.
>
> All of the rooms *are* hot.

Subjects joined by *and* are plural:

> The boy and his cousin *like* to go fishing.

But singular subjects joined by *or* or *nor* take a singular verb:

> Either Elaine or Jill *is* going with us. Neither Elaine nor Jill *knows* how to swim.

When a singular and a plural subject are joined by *or* or *nor*, the subject nearer the verb determines whether it is singular or plural:

> Neither the cats nor the dog *likes* to be ignored.

> Either the dog or the cats *tear* up the furniture when I'm away too long.

Pronoun Cases

Using the correct case of a pronoun can also be challenging. Recall that that personal pronouns have different forms for each of the three cases: nominative, objective, and possessive.

Number	Person	Case		
		Nominative	**Objective**	**Possessive**
Singular	First	I	me	my, mine
	Second	you	you	your, yours
	Third	he, she, it	him, her, it	his, her, hers, its
Plural	First	we	us	our, ours
	Second	you	you	your, yours
	Third	they	them	their, theirs

Subjects in the **nominative case**:

> *I* work at the pharmacy.

> *He* works at the hospital.

> *We* work in our garden.

> *They* work at the train station.

Predicate nominatives, which are nouns or pronouns that follow linking verbs (such as *to be*), and which rename the subject, are also in the nominative case:

> It is *I* who am speaking.

> The woman on the street was *she*.

> The smartest ones in the class are *we*.

> The people who are moving next door are *they*.

The **objective case** is used for both direct and indirect objects of action verbs:

> The boss paid *me*.

> The family watched *her* perform in the recital.

The Australians gave *us* a warm welcome.

The company promoted *them* last year.

The objective case is also used for objects of prepositions:

Between you and *me*, there's no chance it will snow.

Would you like to go to the party with *her*?

The lodge was above *us*, on the side of the mountain.

Among *them*, they had only $10.

Verb Use

Verbs are likely the most complex part of speech in English and thus are often the source of errors in writing and speech. Below are some of the common areas related to verbs that will help you prepare for your exam.

Verb Form

Verbs all have four primary forms that are used in different situations. They are called principle parts and include the **infinitive**, **present participle**, **past**, and **past participle**. The infinitive is the stem or base form, which is modified to produce the other forms. For regular verbs, the present participle is formed by adding *–ing* to the infinitive and the past and past participle are formed by adding *–ed* to the infinitive, as shown below.

Infinitive	Present Participle	Past	Past Participle
(to) walk	(is) walking	walked	(have) walked

Note that the present participle and past participle must be accompanied by the correct form of the helping verb *be*.

Unfortunately, many verbs in English are irregular, meaning that they form their past and past participle in ways other than adding *–ed* to the infinitive. These verbs and their principle parts must be memorized. Below is a table showing some of the more common irregular verbs and their past and past participle forms.

Infinitive	Past	Past Participle
begin	began	(have) begun
bite	bit	(have) bitten
break	broke	(have) broken
bring	brought	(have) brought
catch	caught	(have) caught
choose	chose	(have) chosen
come	came	(have) come
do	did	(have) done

Infinitive	Past	Past Participle
drink	drank	(have) drunk
drive	drove	(have) driven
eat	ate	(have) eaten
get	got	(have) got *or* gotten
give	gave	(have) given
go	went	(have) gone
know	knew	(have) known
lay	laid	(have) laid
lie	lay	(have) lain
run	ran	(have) run
say	said	(have) said
see	saw	(have) seen
shake	shook	(have) shaken
sing	sang	(have) sung
sit	sat	(have) sat
speak	spoke	(have) spoken
swim	swam	(have) swum
take	took	(have) taken
wear	wore	(have) worn
write	wrote	(have) written

Tense

The tense of a verb indicates when an action occurred. There are six verb tenses in English: present, past, future, present perfect, past perfect, and future perfect.

The **present tense** is used to communicate an action that is taking place now, in the present. It is formed using the infinitive. A variant known as the present progressive is formed using the appropriate form of *be* plus the present participle.

> I *play* chess with my friend.

> I *am playing* chess with my friend.

The **past tense** is used to communicate an action that occurred in the past and that did not continue into the present. It is formed using the principle part known as *past*, or, in regular verbs, by adding –*ed* to the infinitive.

> She *parked* the car on the street.

> The student *dove* into the pool and *swam* to the other side.

The **future tense** is used to communicate an action that is expected to occur at some point in the future. It is formed using *will* plus the infinitive.

> Next year, they *will travel* to France.

The **present perfect tense** is used to communicate an action that occurred in the past and is continuing or may be continuing in the present. It is formed using *have* or *has* plus the past participle.

We *have lived* in this house for 5 years.

The patient *has visited* often for the same complaint.

The **past perfect tense** is used to communicate an action that occurred in the past before some other past action or event. It is formed using *had* plus the past participle.

He *had left* the building by the time I arrived.

The **future perfect tense** is used to communicate an action that is expected to occur in the future before some other future action or event. It is formed using *will have* plus the past participle.

By midnight, they *will have finished* all of their homework.

Adjective and Adverb Use

Adjectives modify nouns and pronouns, and **adverbs** modify verbs, adjectives, and other adverbs.

Distinguishing Adjectives and Adverbs

Avoid using an adjective where an adverb is called for and vice versa. Most adverbs end in *–ly*, making it easy to distinguish them from adjectives, but many do not, and some adjectives end in *–ly*. These variations can make it difficult to distinguish the two groups and to know when it is appropriate to use certain words. To complicate matters even more, some words may function as either an adjective or an adverb, as shown below.

That was a *fast* train. (adjective) The horse ran *fast*. (adverb)

He was wearing a *hard* hat. (adjective) I studied *hard* for that test. (adverb)

The following four tips may help you to decide when to use an adjective and when to use an adverb.

1. Adjectives *typically* precede the nouns they are modifying.

   Our basketball team consisted of a *tall* kid, a *short* kid, a *fast* kid, a *slow* kid, and a *bored* kid.

2. Adjectives, rather than adverbs, *typically* follow linking verbs (i.e., appear, be, feel, look, seem, smell, sound, stay, taste).

   Dinner smells *delicious*.

   I feel *sick*.

   You seem *happy*.

3. Adverbs *often* end in –ly and *often* follow action verbs.

   My grandmother walks *briskly* around her neighborhood.

   That car drives *smoothly*.

4. When modifying a noun or pronoun, choose an adjective. When modifying a verb, adjective, or adverb, choose an adverb.

Comparative and Superlative Forms

Adjectives and adverbs have special forms when they are used for making comparisons. These forms are known as **comparative** and **superlative**. The comparative is used to indicate which of two people or things possesses a trait to a greater degree than does the other. The superlative is used to indicate which of three or more people or things possesses a trait to a greater degree than does any of the others, or to the greatest degree within the group considered.

Most one-syllable adjectives and adverbs form the comparative by adding *–er* and the superlative by adding *–est*.

> His bicycle is *faster* than mine. Of the five trains I've been on, this one is the *fastest*.

> As usual, I arrived *later* than everyone else. It's embarrassing to always arrive *latest*.

Some two-syllable adjectives form the comparative by adding *–er* and the superlative by adding *–est*, others form the comparative by using *more* and the superlative by using *most*, and yet others can follow either approach.

> The kitchen is *smokier* than it was a few minutes ago. It's the *smokiest* I've ever seen it.

> Their meal was *more meager* than ours. In fact, it was the *most meager* meal in the camp.

> That coffee grinder is *quieter* (or *more quiet*) than mine. It's the *quietest* (or *most quiet*) coffee grinder there is.

Adjectives of more than two syllables and adverbs ending in *–ly* typically form the comparative by using *more* and the superlative by using *most*.

> She was a *more formidable* competitor than was her father. She was the *most formidable* competitor on her team.

> The sun is shining *more brightly* today than it did yesterday. The sun shines *most brightly* at the equator.

To indicate a lesser degree, adjectives and adverbs form the comparative by using *less* and the superlative by using *least*.

> Matthew is *less fit* to run in the marathon than his cousin. In fact, he's the *least fit* runner out there.

> You are *less likely* to do well on the exam than she. If you don't study, you will be the student in your class *least likely* to pass the exam.

Some adjectives and adverbs have irregular comparative and superlative forms; these must be memorized.

Adjective or Adverb	Comparative	Superlative
bad	worse	worst
good, well	better	best
many, much	more	most

The following tips may help you when using comparatives and superlatives.

1. Use the comparative form when comparing two items; use the superlative form when comparing more than two items.

2. Avoid double comparisons (using both *–er* or *–est* and *more* or *most* in one comparison).

    He is *more quieter* than she.

Sentence Use

Sentence Fragments and Run-on Sentences

A sentence should contain both a subject and verb and express a complete thought. A phrase or dependent clause set off as if it were a sentence is known as a *sentence fragment* and should be avoided.

> The rain down from the sky.

> Poured down from the sky.

Run-on sentences are another common grammatical error. A run-on sentence is one in which two or more independent clauses are improperly joined, typically without any punctuation (with or without a coordinating conjunction) or with a comma alone.

> The building caught on fire it burned down.

> She rented the car, he drove it to the beach.

> The concrete workers poured the foundation and the carpenters framed the walls and the plumbers laid the pipe and the electricians installed the wiring.

Independent clauses should be joined by either a comma and a coordinating conjunction or with a semicolon. Run-on sentences may be corrected by following one of these approaches or by setting apart each of the independent clauses as a separate sentence.

> She rented the car; he drove it to the beach.

> She rented the car, and he drove it to the beach.

> She rented the car. He drove it to the beach.

Capitalization and Punctuation

You may also be tested on use of proper capitalization and punctuation on an entrance exam.

Capitalization

Follow the 5 rules below for proper capitalization.

1. Capitalize the first word in any sentence.

2. Capitalize the first word in a direct quotation.

3. Capitalize proper nouns and proper adjectives.

4. Capitalize the title of a person when it comes before the person's name.

5. Capitalize the first word and all important words in titles of books, magazine or journal articles, and other written works.

Punctuation

Rules governing punctuation are many, and using punctuation correctly can be challenging. You are likely to see questions related to punctuation on your entrance exam. Although covering all of the rules of punctuation is beyond the scope of this book, below is a list of some of the most common rules.

1. End every sentence with the proper punctuation: a period for statements and requests, a question mark for questions, and an exclamation mark for exclamations and commands.

2. Use a comma after every item in a series except the last, unless the item is immediately preceded by a coordinating conjunction (and, but, or, nor, for, so, yet).

3. Use a comma to separate two or more adjectives that precede a noun.

4. Use a comma just before a coordinating conjunction when it joins two independent clauses.

5. Use a comma to set off a nonessential phrase or clause within a sentence.

6. Use a comma after an introductory word, phrase, or clause.

7. Use a comma to separate items in dates and addresses.

8. Avoid using unnecessary commas.

9. Use a semicolon to join two independent clauses when a coordinating conjunction is not used.

10. Use a semicolon between items in a series if the items contain commas.

11. Use a colon to mean "note what follows."

12. Use quotation marks to set off direct quotations; place commas and periods inside closing quotation marks, semicolons and colons outside, and question marks and exclamation points inside if they apply to the quotation and outside if they apply to the sentence as a whole.

13. Use an apostrophe and an *s* after a singular noun, even if the noun ends in an *s* (e.g., the octopus's suckers) and after a plural noun that does not end in an *s* (e.g., children's) to show possession.

14. Use an apostrophe alone after a plural noun that ends in an *s* to show possession (e.g., the Smiths' house).

15. Do not use an apostrophe to show possession with a pronoun in the possessive case (e.g., its leash).

16. Use an apostrophe in a contraction to indicate where a letter or letters have been omitted (e.g., don't, it's, they're).

17. Use a dash to set off an interrupting phrase or clause within a sentence.

TEST 5: ENGLISH GRAMMAR AND USAGE
ANSWER SHEET

1. Ⓐ Ⓑ Ⓒ Ⓓ   4. Ⓐ Ⓑ Ⓒ Ⓓ   7. Ⓐ Ⓑ Ⓒ Ⓓ   10. Ⓐ Ⓑ Ⓒ Ⓓ   13. Ⓐ Ⓑ Ⓒ Ⓓ

2. Ⓐ Ⓑ Ⓒ Ⓓ   5. Ⓐ Ⓑ Ⓒ Ⓓ   8. Ⓐ Ⓑ Ⓒ Ⓓ   11. Ⓐ Ⓑ Ⓒ Ⓓ   14. Ⓐ Ⓑ Ⓒ Ⓓ

3. Ⓐ Ⓑ Ⓒ Ⓓ   6. Ⓐ Ⓑ Ⓒ Ⓓ   9. Ⓐ Ⓑ Ⓒ Ⓓ   12. Ⓐ Ⓑ Ⓒ Ⓓ   15. Ⓐ Ⓑ Ⓒ Ⓓ

answer sheet

TEST 5: ENGLISH GRAMMAR AND USAGE

15 Questions • 10 Minutes

In the following questions, select the answer that completes the sentence in a grammatically correct manner or that represents the most grammatically correct of all options.

---

1. Which of the following sentences is grammatically correct?
   A. Each of the horses has its own stall.
   B. Each of the horses has it's own stall.
   C. Each of the horses have their own stall.
   D. Each of the horses have they're own stall.

2. Neither Tillie _____ Maxine _____ how to properly bake a quiche.
   A. or; knows
   B. or; know
   C. nor; knows
   D. nor; know

3. It was _____ who left the front door open; I was in a hurry and forgot to close it behind _____.
   A. I; I
   B. me; I
   C. me; me
   D. I; me

4. By the time we finally sent our proposal to them, they already _____ to go with another company.
   A. chose
   B. had chose
   C. had choosed
   D. had chosen

5. Before the end of this year, Hector _____ at more than 100 concerts.
   A. will sing
   B. will have sung
   C. sang
   D. has sung

6. Identify the part of speech of the italicized word in the following sentence: Heather likes to drive *fast*.
   A. Adverb
   B. Adjective
   C. Verb
   D. Preposition

7. Of the three bands that performed at the concert, the Endoplasmic Reticulum was the _____.
   A. most lamely
   B. lamer
   C. lamest
   D. lamelier

8. Gabriella can rebuild an engine _____ than anyone I've ever known.
   A. most rapidly
   B. more rapidly
   C. rapidlier
   D. more rapid

9. Which of the following sentences is grammatically correct?

   A. The tide slowly rolling in and out; a light breeze gently rocking the beach umbrella.

   B. The tide slowly rolls in and out, a light breeze gently rocks the beach umbrella.

   C. The tide slowly rolls in and out, and a light breeze gently rocks the beach umbrella.

   D. The tide slowly rolls in and out a light breeze gently rocks the beach umbrella.

10. Which of the following sentences is grammatically correct?

   A. their names are Sebastian and Marie; they are from Toulouse, in southern France.

   B. Their names are sebastian and marie; they are from Toulouse, in southern France.

   C. Their names are Sebastian and Marie; they are from Toulouse, in Southern France.

   D. Their names are Sebastian and Marie; they are from Toulouse, in southern France.

11. Which of the following sentences is grammatically correct?

   A. Anthony said, "Are you sure about that?"

   B. Anthony said "Are you sure about that?"

   C. Anthony said, "are you sure about that?"

   D. Anthony said, "Are you sure about that"?

12. Which of the following sentences is grammatically correct?

   A. I disagree Alex with your assessment of him; I think he's a funny, smart guy.

   B. I disagree, Alex with your assessment of him; I think he's a funny, smart guy.

   C. I disagree, Alex, with your assessment of him; I think he's a funny, smart guy.

   D. I disagree, Alex, with your assessment of him; I think he's a funny smart guy.

13. In the following sentence, identify the *most appropriate* punctuation mark to include in the blank: The investigation revealed one thing _____ he was not the person everyone had thought he was.

   A. ;

   B. ,

   C. :

   D. .

14. In the following sentence, identify the *most appropriate* punctuation marks to include in the blanks: Yesterday my sister ate the following: chocolate chip cookies for breakfast _____ leftover pizza, potato chips, and a milkshake for lunch _____ and a bowl of cereal for dinner.

   A. ; ;

   B. , ,

   C. , ;

   D. , —

15. No, my parents aren't in town this weekend; _____ in Boston, visiting my brother.

   A. theyr'e

   B. they're

   C. their

   D. there

SPELLING

The Psychological Service Bureau (PSB) exams include a section on spelling, and the other entrance exams often integrate spelling questions into their Verbal and English Language sections. Below are some basic rules on spelling, along with a couple of lists of commonly misspelled words—general and medical—to help you prepare for questions of this type.

1. In general, *i* comes before *e* except after *c* or when pronounced like the letter *a*, as in weigh.

    -   *i* before *e*: achieve, believe, chief, fierce, grief, niece, piece, relieve, thief, wield

    -   *e* before *i* after *c*: ceiling, conceited, conceive, deceive, perceive, receive

    -   *e* before *i* when pronounced like *a*: eight, freight, neighbor, sleigh, vein, weigh

    -   Some exceptions: either, financier, height, leisure, neither, seize, weird

2. Adding a prefix to a word does not change its spelling.

    -   dis + satisfied = dissatisfied

    -   il + legal = illegal

    -   im + movable = immovable

    -   mis + spell = misspell

    -   mis + understand = misunderstand

    -   un + necessary = unnecessary

3. Drop the final *e* of a word before adding a suffix beginning with a vowel but not before adding a suffix beginning with a consonant.

    -   *e* dropped: dare + -ing = daring; locate + -ion = location; use + -able = usable

    -   *e* retained: announce + -ment = announcement; care + -ful = careful; late + -ly = lately; sure + -ly = surely

    -   Some exceptions: argument, awful, changeable, judgment, noticeable, truly

4. Change the final *y* of a word to an *i* before adding a suffix, except when the suffix begins with *i*.

    -   eighty + -eth = eightieth

    -   heavy + -est = heaviest

    -   play + -ing = playing

    -   rely + -ance = reliance

5. Double the final consonant of a word before adding a suffix that begins with a vowel if (a) the word has only one syllable or the accent is on the last syllable and (b) the word ends in a single consonant preceded by a single vowel.

    -   Final consonant doubled: drop + -ing = dropping; forget + -able = forgettable; submit + -ed = submitted

    -   Final consonant not doubled: cancel + -ed = canceled; droop + -ing = drooping; travel + -ing = traveling

6. Add *-s* to most singular nouns to form the plural; add *-es* to singular nouns ending in *-s*, *-sh*, *-ch*, and *-x* to form the plural.

   • Examples: book/books, box/boxes, church/churches, dish/dishes, glass/glasses

7. In singular nouns that end in *y* preceded by a consonant, form the plural by changing the *y* to *i* and adding *-es*.

   • Examples: body/bodies, fly/flies, nursery/nurseries, spy/spies

8. In singular nouns that end in *y* preceded by a vowel, form the plural by just adding *-s*.

   • Examples: day/days, donkey/donkeys, guy/guys, key/keys, monkey/monkeys

9. In singular nouns that end in *o* preceded by a consonant, form the plural by adding *-es*.

   • Examples: hero/heroes, mosquito/mosquitoes, potato/potatoes, tomato/tomatoes

   • Exceptions: piano/pianos, solo/solos, soprano/sopranos

10. Many nouns form their plurals in irregular ways; these forms must be memorized.

   • Examples: child/children, man/men, mouse/mice, ox/oxen, tooth/teeth, woman/women

Commonly Misspelled General Words*				
absence	accommodate	achieve	acquire	across
address	advice	among	apparent	argument
awful	balance	basically	becoming	before
beginning	believe	benefit	breathe	brilliant
business	calendar	careful	ceiling	certain
chief	citizen	coming	competition	convenience
criticize	decide	definite	deposit	describe
desperate	develop	difference	disappear	disappoint
discipline	does	during	easily	eight
embarrass	environment	equipped	exaggerate	excellent
except	exercise	existence	expect	experience
explanation	familiar	fascinating	finally	foreign
forty	forward	friend	fundamental	generally
guarantee	guidance	happiness	heroes	humorous
identity	imaginary	imitation	immediately	incidentally
independent	intelligent	interesting	interfere	interpretation
interruption	invitation	irrelevant	irritable	judgment
knowledge	laboratory	length	license	loneliness
losing	lying	mathematics	medicine	miniature
minute	naturally	necessary	neighbor	neither
noticeable	occasion	occurred	official	often
omission	operate	optimism	original	ought
paid	parallel	particularly	peculiar	perceive

Commonly Misspelled General Words*				
perform	permanent	persevere	personally	persuade
picture	piece	planning	pleasant	possess
possible	practical	prefer	prejudice	presence
privilege	probably	professional	promise	proof
psychology	quantity	quarter	quiet	quit
quite	realize	receive	recognize	recommend
reference	religious	repetition	rhythm	ridiculous
sacrifice	safety	scissors	separate	shining
similar	sincerely	speech	stopping	strength
studying	succeed	successful	surely	surprise
temperature	temporary	through	toward	tries
truly	until	unusual	using	usually
weird	welcome	weather	whether	writing

* Adapted from Nordquist, R. (2018). The 201 most commonly misspelled words in English. Available at https://www.thoughtco.com/commonly-misspelled-words-in-english-1692761.

Commonly Misspelled Medical Words**				
accommodation	afferent	ascites	aphagia	anuresis
aphasia	asymmetry	auscultation	basilar	barbiturates
brachial	branchial	callous	callus	catheterization
chalazion	circumferential	chlamydia	cord	cor
debridement	dependent	diaphragm	dyspareunia	efferent
elicit	enuresis	epididymis	erythematosus	exacerbated
gamma	gaseous	hemoptysis	hemorrhage	humerus
hygiene	ileum	ilium	inoculate	insufflate
malacia	mucous	mucus	myxedema	occur
occurrence	occurring	oophorectomy	ophthalmology	palliative
paroxysmal	perfusion	profusion	perineal	peroneal
persistent	petechia	petechiae	plain	plane
pleurisy	polyposis	prostate	pruritus	pterygium
regime	regimen	rhythm	sagittal	scalene
scarring	seborrheic	serotonin	senile	suppuration
symmetry	tonsil	trachea	vesicle	xerosis

** Adapted from Meditech™. (2018). Commonly misspelled words. Available at https://www.meditec.com/resourcestools/medical-words/commonly-misspelled-words/

TEST 6: SPELLING

1. Ⓐ Ⓑ Ⓒ	4. Ⓐ Ⓑ Ⓒ	7. Ⓐ Ⓑ Ⓒ	10. Ⓐ Ⓑ Ⓒ	13. Ⓐ Ⓑ Ⓒ
2. Ⓐ Ⓑ Ⓒ	5. Ⓐ Ⓑ Ⓒ	8. Ⓐ Ⓑ Ⓒ	11. Ⓐ Ⓑ Ⓒ	14. Ⓐ Ⓑ Ⓒ
3. Ⓐ Ⓑ Ⓒ	6. Ⓐ Ⓑ Ⓒ	9. Ⓐ Ⓑ Ⓒ	12. Ⓐ Ⓑ Ⓒ	15. Ⓐ Ⓑ Ⓒ

answer sheet

TEST 6: SPELLING

15 Questions • 5 Minutes

Directions: In the following sets of words, choose the word that is spelled correctly.

1. A. afasia
   B. aphasia
   C. aphazia

2. A. ascultation
   B. oscultation
   C. auscultation

3. A. beleive
   B. beileve
   C. believe

4. A. catheterization
   B. cathreization
   C. cathrization

5. A. definate
   B. definite
   C. defenite

6. A. ellicit
   B. elicit
   C. elissit

7. A. hygene
   B. higiene
   C. hygiene

8. A. immediately
   B. imediately
   C. immediutley

9. A. liscense
   B. licence
   C. license

10. A. ocurrence
    B. occurrence
    C. occurence

11. A. pirfusion
    B. perfusion
    C. parfusion

12. A. rhythm
    B. ryhthm
    C. rhithym

13. A. symmetry
    B. symetry
    C. simmetry

14. A. trackea
    B. trachia
    C. trachea

15. A. wierd
    B. weird
    C. weard

NONVERBAL ABILITY

Nonverbal ability questions are included only on the PSB exams. This type of question tests your ability to understand logical relationships between different geometric shapes or forms. Typically, these questions are presented as analogies, similar to the ones you've already encountered in the Verbal Ability section except using geometric shapes rather than words.

The nonverbal ability questions that appear on the PSB exams and throughout this book typically consist of three shapes or groups of shapes in the question stem presented in the following format:

> *First shape* is to *second shape* as *third shape* is to?

The question stem is followed by five answer options, A to E, each containing a shape or group of shapes. Below is an example of a nonverbal ability question.

○ is to ● as □ is to?

A. ○
B. □
C. ■
D. △
E. ▲

The strategy for solving these nonverbal analogies is similar to that for solving verbal analogies, as described earlier, except that you are analyzing relationships between shapes rather than words. It involves two steps:

> *Step One:* Determine the relationship between the first two shapes or groups of shapes.

> *Step Two:* Find the shape among the answer options that bears this same relationship with the third shape.

Using the example question above, let's practice solving a nonverbal analogy using these steps. First, determine the relationship between the first two shapes. One way to analyze the relationship is to consider how the two shapes are similar and how they are different. In this case, we note that both shapes are circles of the same size. How are they different? The first is white, whereas the second is black. So the relationship between the first two shapes is that they are both of the same shape but opposite in color.

Now that we've determined the relationship between the first two shapes, let's see which shape among the answer options bears this same relationship with the third shape. The third shape is a white square. We are looking for a form that is of the same shape but opposite in color, which means we are looking for a black square. Thus, the correct answer to this question is C.

Another way to analyze the relationship between two shapes is to determine what change has occurred to the first shape that would produce the second shape. For instance, in the example above, we might conclude that the white circle switched to its opposite color. The element that changes is color. Many other elements related to the shape can be manipulated.

A summary of these elements, along with examples, is provided in the table below. Study these elements and learn to recognize them so that you can more easily determine the relationships between shapes in the nonverbal ability questions.

Element	Example
Shape Position	
Rotation of the shape	△ is to ▷
Inversion of the shape (turning upside-down)	△ is to ▽
Reflection of the shape (mirror image)	▷ is to ◁
Movement of the shape relative to another	● △ is to △ ●
Composition of the Shape	
Division/bisection of the shape	☐ is to ⊟
Fragmentation of the shape	● is to ◖
Other Elements	
Shape color	△ is to ▲
Shape size	▲ is to ▲
Object embedded within the shape	◇ is to ◈
Object circumscribing the shape	● is to ⊙
Line patterns within the shape	☐ is to ⦀
Duplication of the shape	⟨ is to ⟪
Shape sequence	▲ is to ■
Numerical representation of the shape	△ is to 3

TEST 7: NONVERBAL ABILITY ANSWER SHEET

1. Ⓐ Ⓑ Ⓒ Ⓓ Ⓔ   4. Ⓐ Ⓑ Ⓒ Ⓓ Ⓔ   7. Ⓐ Ⓑ Ⓒ Ⓓ Ⓔ   10. Ⓐ Ⓑ Ⓒ Ⓓ Ⓔ   13. Ⓐ Ⓑ Ⓒ Ⓓ Ⓔ

2. Ⓐ Ⓑ Ⓒ Ⓓ Ⓔ   5. Ⓐ Ⓑ Ⓒ Ⓓ Ⓔ   8. Ⓐ Ⓑ Ⓒ Ⓓ Ⓔ   11. Ⓐ Ⓑ Ⓒ Ⓓ Ⓔ   14. Ⓐ Ⓑ Ⓒ Ⓓ Ⓔ

3. Ⓐ Ⓑ Ⓒ Ⓓ Ⓔ   6. Ⓐ Ⓑ Ⓒ Ⓓ Ⓔ   9. Ⓐ Ⓑ Ⓒ Ⓓ Ⓔ   12. Ⓐ Ⓑ Ⓒ Ⓓ Ⓔ   15. Ⓐ Ⓑ Ⓒ Ⓓ Ⓔ

answer sheet

TEST 7: NONVERBAL ABILITY

15 Questions • 15 Minutes

Directions: In the following questions, determine the relationship between the first pair of shapes and then decide which of the answer choices shares a similar relationship with the third shape.

1. ■ is to □ as ▲ is to?
   A. ○
   B. □
   C. △
   D. ●
   E. ■

2. ▯ is to ▭ as △ is to?
   A. ▽
   B. ▷
   C. ▮
   D. ▯
   E. ▶

3. ◉ is to ○ as ◈ is to?
   A. ◇
   B. ◎
   C. ●
   D. ▣
   E. ⬜

4. ⊐ is to ⊏ as ⊃ is to?
   A. ⊓
   B. ⊑
   C. ⊔
   D. ⋂
   E. ∪

5. ⌐ is to □ as ` is to?
   A. ○
   B. ⌒
   C. ⌣
   D. ◡
   E. ⌣

6. ⊗ is to ⊕ as ⊘ is to?
   A. ◵
   B. ⊞
   C. ⊟
   D. ◎
   E. ⊖

7. ⬗ is to ◉ as ∪ is to?
   A. ⬤
   B. ⬓
   C. ⌢
   D. ○
   E. ⬒

8. ▱ is to ▭ as ◣ is to?
   A. ▪
   B. ▯
   C. ▬
   D. ◇
   E. ▮

9. ⬟ is to ⬠ as ■ is to?
   A. ⬤
   B. ▲
   C. ●
   D. ◆
   E. ◆

10. ◖ is to ● as ◕ is to?
    A. ○
    B. ◉
    C. □
    D. ◎
    E. ▣

11. △ is to ▵ as ▲ is to?

A. □

B. ▶

C. ▲

D. ■

E. ●

12. ⑪ is to ◯ as ⚏ is to?

A. ▤

B. ◉

C. ◎

D. ▨

E. □

13. ⋈⋈ is to ⋈|⋈ as ●—○ ○—● is to?

A. ●—○ ○—○

B. ○—●—● ○

C. —○ ○—●

D. ⋈|⋈

E. ○—●—● ○

14. ❮ is to •⋀ as ⋃ is to?

A. ⊂+

B. +∩

C. +∪

D. +⊂

E. ⊃+

15. ✖ is to ⸫ as ✚ is to?

A. ∶∶

B. +

C. ×

D. □

E. ⬦

ANSWER KEYS AND EXPLANATIONS

Test 1: Synonyms

1. B	16. D	31. D	46. C	61. A
2. D	17. C	32. B	47. B	62. A
3. A	18. C	33. D	48. A	63. C
4. B	19. A	34. A	49. D	64. C
5. C	20. B	35. C	50. A	65. D
6. D	21. B	36. D	51. D	66. D
7. A	22. C	37. C	52. D	67. A
8. A	23. A	38. B	53. B	68. D
9. A	24. D	39. B	54. B	69. B
10. D	25. A	40. D	55. B	70. A
11. B	26. B	41. C	56. D	71. B
12. B	27. C	42. A	57. B	72. D
13. A	28. A	43. A	58. B	73. A
14. C	29. A	44. C	59. C	74. D
15. C	30. C	45. D	60. B	75. B

1. **The correct answer is B.** *Diction* and *language* are synonyms. Choice A is incorrect because *conviction* makes no sense and is not a synonym. Choice C is incorrect because *discourse* means "conversation, expressing one's self in writing or speaking" and isn't specific enough to be a synonym in this case. Choice D is incorrect because, while *denunciation* might tempt you into thinking it has something to do with words, it means "a public condemnation or accusation of someone" and has nothing to do with language.

2. **The correct answer is D.** *Sedulous* and *industrious* both mean "hard working" and so are synonyms. *Hideous, generous,* and *infirm* (choices A, B, and C) have no relation to *sedulous*.

3. **The correct answer is A.** An *altercation* is a fight, quarrel, or argument, and a *fracas* is a noisy fight or quarrel. Choice B is incorrect, but might tempt you because

substitutions makes sense in the sentence; however, it is not a synonym for *altercation*. Choice C might also look like the answer if you think of *alterations* as changes, but remember you're looking for the synonym for *altercations*, not what makes sense in the sentence. Choice D is incorrect because *plays* is not a synonym.

4. **The correct answer is B.** If you didn't know what *biennial* means, remember that *bi-* means "two," which narrows the choices to choice B. Choice A is incorrect because a biennial blooms once every two years, not once a quarter. Choice C is incorrect because a plant can't be a biennial and a *perennial*, which is a plant that blooms every year. Choice D is incorrect because *bisection* has no relation to *biennial*.

5. **The correct answer is C.** *Gamut* means "range or extent," so *range* is a synonym. Choice A is incorrect because *periphery* means "outside boundary." Choice B is

incorrect because *margin,* meaning "a boundary line," is a synonym for *periphery,* not *gamut.* Choice D is incorrect because *imperception* means "lack of perception."

6. **The correct answer is D.** *Sanctimonious* means "making a show of being holy or pious," so *self-righteous,* meaning "excessively or hypocritically pious," is a synonym. Choice A is incorrect because *parsimonious* means "stingy, miserly." Choice B is incorrect because *perpetual* means "for all eternity" or "lasting for an indefinite period." Choice C is incorrect because *intrinsic* means "essential to something, belonging to something by its nature."

7. **The correct answer is A.** *Urbane* means "characterized by sophistication" or "polite, refined," and *suave* means "having sophistication and charm" or "urbane, courteous." Choice B is incorrect because *poignant* means "very moving, distressing." Choice C is incorrect because *spasmodic* means "intermittently," "relating to a spasm," or "excitable," none of which indicates that *spasmodic* is a synonym for *urbane.* Choice D is incorrect because *pensive* means "very thoughtful, serious."

8. **The correct answer is A.** A slogan is a phrase used in advertising to describe a product or service; groups and organizations may also have slogans. A *catchword* is a favorite saying of a group. *Sample, design,* and *passage* all make sense if they were substituted into the sentence, but these words are not synonyms for *slogan.*

9. **The correct answer is A.** *Vociferous* means "very loud, noisy, vehement," and *strident* means "loud, vehement." Choice B is incorrect because *muted,* meaning "silent," is the opposite. Choice C is incorrect because *insistent,* meaning "demanding," has no relation to *vociferous.* Choice D is incorrect because *importunate* means "insistent, demanding."

10. **The correct answer is D.** To *foil* is "to stop, prevent," which are meanings of *thwart.* Choice A is incorrect because *heighten* has no relation to *foil,* nor does choice B, *secure.* Choice C is incorrect because *disencumber* means "to relieve of burdens" or "to free from difficulties."

11. **The correct answer is B.** *Purported* means "to have claimed to be something, usually falsely," so *claimed* is a synonym. Choice A is incorrect because the word *addressed* is not a synonym for *purported.* It doesn't make sense to substitute *addressed* in the sentence ("addressed to be an official"). Choice C is incorrect because *propitiated* means "to make peace with someone, to appease." Choice D is incorrect because *conciliated* means "to overcome distrust, to appease," so *propitiated* and *conciliated* are synonyms for each other, but not *purported.*

12. **The correct answer is B.** *Bent* in this context means "determined, disposed to," so *determined* is a synonym. Choice A is incorrect because *flexible* means "able to be bent," which is not the same as being *determined.* Choice C is incorrect because *inclined* does not relate to this meaning of *bent.* Choice D is incorrect because *endowed* means "having been given certain qualities or abilities."

13. **The correct answer is A.** *Remember* is a synonym for *recollect.* None of the other words makes sense in the context. *Illumine,* choice D, means "to shed light on" and might tempt you, but it doesn't have the same or a similar meaning as *recollect.* Sometimes the simplest answer is the right answer.

14. **The correct answer is C.** To *rescind* is "to *revoke.*" Choice A is incorrect because typically an official order such as a declaration of a state of emergency is *revoked,* not *negated.* Choice B is incorrect because *maneuver* means "to carry out a military

action," "to change tactics," or "to alter the placement of troops," and none of these meanings equate to *maneuver* being a synonym of *rescind*. Choice D is incorrect because the governor is ending the state of emergency, not *accepting* it.

15. **The correct answer is C.** *Scant* means "little." Choice A is incorrect because *audacious* means "bold, fearless, spirited." Choice B is incorrect because *fervid* means "impassioned, intense emotion." Choice D is incorrect because *clothed* makes no sense, even in a metaphorical sense.

16. **The correct answer is D.** To *scoff at* is "to mock or make fun of." Choice A makes no sense because *exonerate* is "to free someone from blame or responsibility." Choice B is incorrect because *amplify* is "to increase," "to exaggerate," or "to make complete." Choice C, *confute*, is "to prove something or someone wrong."

17. **The correct answer is C.** *Run* and *sprint* can be synonyms and are in this case. Choice A makes no sense because you don't need a surge of energy to *relax*. Choice B is incorrect because, while *adventure* makes some sense, it is not a synonym for *sprint*. Choice D, *convergence*, meaning "where two things come together," makes no sense.

18. **The correct answer is C.** *Pressing* means "demanding immediate attention," in other words, *urgent*. Choice A, *privileged*, meaning "confidential," isn't correct. Choice B, *amendable*, meaning "capable of being changed," is also incorrect. Choice D, *absolved*, meaning "pronounced not guilty," is also incorrect.

19. **The correct answer is A.** *Simulated* is something made to resemble something else; in other words, it is *pretended*. Choice B is incorrect because something *superficial* is something that may be frivolous, perfunctory, or on the surface, none of

which is the same as *simulated*. Choice C is incorrect because *stimulated* means "aroused or excited emotionally." Choice D is incorrect because *simultaneous* means "at the same time."

20. **The correct answer is B.** Both *worried* and *upset* can be synonyms of *agitated*, but in this sentence, *upset* fits the context better. Choice C is incorrect because *convulsed* means "shaking violently"; it can be a synonym of *agitated*, but not in this context. Choice D is incorrect because *composed*, meaning "calm," is the opposite of *agitated*.

21. **The correct answer is B.** A *pulse* is beat or pace. Choice A is incorrect because *utility* means either "usefulness" or "a power company." Choice C is incorrect because *reverence* is a feeling of profound awe or respect and makes no sense; it is also not a synonym of *pulse*. Choice D is incorrect because *solace* is the same as comfort, not a *pulse*.

22. **The correct answer is C.** One synonym for *unsophisticated* is *simple*. Choice A is incorrect because *ponderous* means "heavy, dull, tedious," none of which is the same as *unsophisticated*. Choice B is incorrect because *elaborate* tends to mean the opposite of *unsophisticated*. Choice D is incorrect because *artificial* means "contrived, inauthentic, forced, affected," in other words, the opposite of *unsophisticated*.

23. **The correct answer is A.** *Willful* and *deliberate* are synonyms. Choice B is incorrect because *eminent* means "prominent, great, well-known"; don't confuse it with *imminent*, meaning "about to happen." Choice C, *amicable*, means "friendly" and makes no sense. Choice D is incorrect because *remorseful* means "sorry," and while someone caught for a crime may feel remorseful, it is not a synonym for *willful* and makes no sense.

24. **The correct answer is D.** *Stipulation* is a synonym for *provision*, meaning "arrangement or plan." Choice A is incorrect because *improvement* is not the same as a *stipulation* and doesn't fit the sense. Choice B is incorrect because *convenience* means "benefit, advantage" or "suitability." Choice C is incorrect because *aggregation* means "a collection of several things taken as a whole."

25. **The correct answer is A.** *Impart* and *communicate* are synonyms. Choice B is incorrect because *indemnify* means "to protect against damage or loss." Choice C, *reinforce*, may seem like a good choice, and, in terms of context, could work, except that *impart* and *reinforce* aren't synonyms. Choice D is incorrect because *disguise* isn't a synonym for transmitting information, in this case, a feeling or sense of style.

26. **The correct answer is B.** *Valor* and *courage* are the same thing. Choice A is incorrect because *ingeniousness* is cleverness, inventiveness, and creative thinking. Choice C is incorrect because *discretion* is tactfulness. Choice D is incorrect because *optimism* means "expecting that the best will happen."

27. **The correct answer is C.** To *fuse* is "to mix together," but also "to unite, to join," and, among the answer choices, *combine* is the closest in meaning. Choice A is incorrect because *required* is not a synonym for joining, though courses can be required. Choice B is incorrect because *implicated*, meaning "to involve or incriminate someone," makes no sense. Choice D is incorrect because, while *involved* may make sense in the context, it is not a synonym for *fuse*.

28. **The correct answer is A.** To *duplicate* is "to replicate" or "to make an exact copy." Choice B is incorrect because *synthesize* means "to combine pieces to form something new."

Choice C is incorrect because "to *fixate*" is "to make something stable" or "to focus attention on something or someone." Choice D, *replenish*, means "to make something full or complete again."

29. **The correct answer is A.** To *bewilder* is "to *perplex*," meaning "to confuse." Choice B is incorrect because *aggravated* means "made angry" or "made something worse." Choice C is incorrect because *subdued* means "conquered, brought under control." Choice D is incorrect because *infuriated* means "angry, enraged."

30. **The correct answer is C.** *Means* can be a synonym of *modes* when they both mean "method, way, or variety," which fits the context of the sentence. Choice A is incorrect because *increments* means "the process of increasing in number, size, or quantity." Choice B is incorrect because *expenditures* refer to the disbursement of money. Choice D is incorrect because *modifications* refer to changes.

31. **The correct answer is D.** One meaning of *aggrandize* is "to *enrich* one's self." Choice A is incorrect because *exhaust*, "to tire," is not a synonym and doesn't make sense since the politician would be exhausting himself, not the people. Choice B is incorrect because *subjugate* means "to conquer, to make subservient" and is not only not a synonym, but the politician isn't about to subjugate himself. Choice C is incorrect because *sacrifice* is not a synonym and a politician aggrandizing himself is the opposite of one sacrificing himself for his constituents.

32. **The correct answer is B.** To *mingle* is "to mix." Choice A is incorrect because *argue* is not the same as *mingle*. Choice C is incorrect because to *disrupt* is "to interrupt" or "to break up." Choice D is incorrect because to *flout* is "to show contempt for" or "to brush off, to ignore."

33. **The correct answer is D.** *Philanthropic* programs are *benevolent,* meaning "generous in helping others, showing kindness." Choice A is incorrect because *primitive* means "basic, simple." Choice B is incorrect because *deleterious* means "harmful," the opposite of *philanthropic.* Choice C is incorrect because *extraneous* means "not essential, unnecessary."

34. **The correct answer is A.** A *covetous* person is a *greedy* person. Choice B is incorrect because *exemplary* means "worthy of being imitated, a model." Choice C is incorrect because *disparate* means "something that is very different, unlike." Choice D is incorrect because *adventitious* means "added to something by chance or accidentally."

35. **The correct answer is C.** To *breed* is "to *propagate,*" or reproduce. Choice A is incorrect because *raise* is not the same as reproduce. Choice B, *gather,* is not only not a synonym, but makes no sense. Choice D, *destroy,* is the opposite of breeding.

36. **The correct answer is D.** To *reiterate* is "to *repeat.*" Choice A is incorrect because *adjusted* is not a synonym for *reiterate,* nor is choice B, *defended,* even though it would make sense in the sentence. Choice C is incorrect because *fermented* means "having been broken down into simpler substances."

37. **The correct answer is C.** To *loom* is "to appear in one's view, seemingly threateningly," so *appeared* is a synonym. Choice A is incorrect because *assert* means "to state something positively, to insist." Choice B is incorrect because *yield* means "to give up, to give in." Choice D is incorrect because *rebuff* means "to reject" or "to drive back."

38. **The correct answer is B.** *Adverse* means "harmful, *injurious.*" Choice A is incorrect because *ecstatic* means "joyful, feeling great delight." Choice C is incorrect because *luminous* means "full of light, radiant." Choice D is incorrect because *gloomy* is not a synonym for *adverse.*

39. **The correct answer is B.** *Volition* means "conscious decision, doing something willingly," so *will* is a synonym. Choice A is incorrect because *flight* has no relation to *volition* and doesn't make sense in the sentence either. Choice C is incorrect because *repudiation* means "rejection or disowning something as invalid." Choice D is incorrect because *recognizance* means "an obligation entered into as a result of court order, typically to go free on condition of appearing in court for a hearing."

40. **The correct answer is D.** An *anomaly* is a departure from the normal, or something that is abnormal or irregular, and an *aberration* is a departure from the normal or typical. Choice A is incorrect because an *anachronism* is someone or something that seems to belong to another time period. It's similar to *anomaly,* but *aberration* is closer in meaning to *anomaly* in this sentence. Choice B is incorrect because a *change* is not the same as an *anomaly.* Choice C is incorrect because the score may have been an embarrassment, but *embarrassment* is not a synonym for *anomaly.*

41. **The correct answer is C.** *Similitude* means "similarity in appearance," so *resemblance* is a synonym. Choice A is incorrect because *incongruity* means "lacking congruity," that is, "being unsuitable or inappropriate." Choice B is incorrect because a *connection* is not the same as being similar. Choice D is incorrect because a similarity in appearance shows some *relationship* between things, but it's not a synonym.

42. **The correct answer is A.** *Prudent* means "wise, careful and sensible, using good judgment," so *judicious,* meaning "prudent,

showing good judgment," is a synonym. Choice B is incorrect because *terse* means "brief, to the point." Choice C is incorrect because *audacious* means "bold, fearless, spirited" and can be considered an antonym for *prudent*. Choice D is incorrect because *laconic* means "using few words, terse, to the point" and is a synonym for *terse*, but not *prudent*.

43. **The correct answer is A.** *Instinctive* means "impulsive, *spontaneous*, and unthinking." Choice B is incorrect because *turgid* means "pompous, lofty in style." Choice C is incorrect because *premeditated* means "thought out in advance," making it an antonym for *instinctive*. Choice D is incorrect because *irrelevant* means "not important, not having a connection with something."

44. **The correct answer is C.** A *torrent* is "a fast-flowing stream or water" or "a deluge, a heavy downpour," so *deluge* is a synonym. Choice A is incorrect because a *slide* has no relation to a torrent. Choice B is incorrect because an *avalanche* is a fall or slide of snow, not water. Choice D is incorrect because *air* has no relation to *torrent*.

45. **The correct answer is D.** To *embody* is "to represent or express something" or "to symbolize something," so *symbolize* is a synonym. Choice A is incorrect because *combat* has no relation to *embody*, nor has choice B, *eliminate*. Choice C is incorrect because *abjure* means "to renounce, to repudiate."

46. **The correct answer is C.** To be *impetuous* is "to be *impulsive*." Choice A is incorrect because *contemptible* means "worthy of contempt, shameful, despicable." Choice B is incorrect because *sophisticated* means "refined or cultured in tastes and habits" as well as "complex." Choice D is incorrect

because *fallacious* means "deceptive" or "erroneous."

47. **The correct answer is B.** *Eulogize* means "to praise, acclaim, usually in a speech," so *praise* is a synonym. Choice A is incorrect because *promulgate* means "to make known, to announce, to proclaim." Choice C is incorrect because *denigrate* is the opposite of *eulogize*. Choice D is incorrect because *append* means "to add, to attach." Think of an *appendix* to a book.

48. **The correct answer is A.** *Vociferation* means "a loud outcry, often in protest," so *clamor* meaning "a loud outcry" or "a vehement expression of protest" is a synonym. Choice B is incorrect because *taciturnity* means "silent, a habit of not being communicative," so this can be considered an antonym. Choice C is incorrect because *oblivion* means "the condition of being forgotten or disregarded." Choice D is incorrect because *discernment* means "evidence of keen judgment or insight."

49. **The correct answer is D.** To be *precarious* is "to be *unstable*." Choice A is incorrect because *mellifluous* means "pleasing to the ear." Choice B is incorrect because *intrusive* means "tending to intrude, to interfere." Choice C is incorrect because *unusual* has no relation to *precarious*.

50. **The correct answer is A.** *Ostentatious* means "showy, pretentious, meaning to attract attention and impress others," so *pretentious* is a synonym. Choice B is incorrect because *inconspicuous* means "not very noticeable," so it's actually an antonym. Choice C is incorrect because *ascribable* means "able to be attributed to something" or "able to assign a quality or characteristic to someone." Choice D is incorrect because *candid* means "frank, outspoken, open, unreserved."

51. **The correct answer is D.** To *manifest* interest is to show, that is, to *display*, interest. Choice A is incorrect because *conceal* is an antonym for *manifest*. Choice B is incorrect because to *diminish* is to lessen. Choice C is incorrect because to *augment* is to add.

52. **The correct answer is D.** *Banter* is good-natured teasing, which is also what *raillery* is. Choice A is incorrect because *discourse* is conversation. Choices B and D are incorrect because *singing* and *toasting* are not synonyms for *banter*.

53. **The correct answer is B.** *Aesthetic* means "artistic" as well as "characterized by an appreciation of beauty." Choices A and C are incorrect because neither *practical* nor *monetary* relates to *aesthetic*. Choice D is incorrect because *estimable* means "admirable."

54. **The correct answer is B.** *Apostasy* means "abandoning one's faith, political party, or similar loyalty," so *defection*, meaning "abandonment of principles, duty, and the like," is a synonym. Choice A is incorrect because *defiance* means "boldly resisting." Choice C is incorrect because *belief* is what an apostate abandons, not the act of abandonment. Choice D is incorrect because an *inference* is "a conclusion reached by interpreting information."

55. **The correct answer is B.** *Cryptic* means "having a hidden meaning," in other words, *mysterious*. Choice A is incorrect because *cynical* means "believing the worst of people, distrustful." Choice C is incorrect because *critical* is not related to *cryptic*. Choice D is incorrect because *censorious* means "highly critical, fault finding" and is a synonym for *critical*, but not *cryptic*.

56. **The correct answer is D.** To *emerge* is "to *appear*." Choice A is incorrect because

deviated means "to have departed or moved away from the norm or purpose." Choice B is incorrect because *divested* means "to have disposed of" or "to have taken something away from someone." Choice C is incorrect because *declined* means "to have refused politely."

57. **The correct answer is B.** *Contumacious* means "disobedient, rebellious," so *rebellious* is a synonym. Choice A is incorrect because *exuberant* means "unrestrained, high-spirited." Choices C and D are incorrect because *awkward* and *mischievous* have no relation to *contumacious*.

58. **The correct answer is B.** *Cognizant* means "aware" and "having knowledge," so *aware* is a synonym. Choice A is incorrect because *ignorant* is the opposite of *cognizant*. Choice C is incorrect because *insensitive* has no relation to *cognizant*. Choice D is incorrect because *remorseful* means "feeling sorrow or pain for having done something."

59. **The correct answer is C.** A *glacial* region is one that has a glacier, making it *frigid*. Choice A is incorrect because *glass-like* may be tempting, but *frigid* is closer in meaning to *glacial*. Choice B is incorrect because *illiberal*, meaning not liberal, has no relation to glacial. Choice D is incorrect because *reticent* means "reluctant, unwilling" or "reserved, quiet."

60. **The correct answer is B.** *Instigate* means the same as *incite*, "to stir up, to urge, to provoke." Choice A is incorrect because to *quell* is "to stop, to put down a rebellion." Choice C is incorrect because, while *assisted* is close in meaning, *incite* is the same meaning, so it's a better choice. Choice D is incorrect because *depressed*, meaning either "gloomy, dejected" or "to press down," doesn't fit as a synonym.

61. **The correct answer is A.** *Ensued* means "*followed*." Choice B is incorrect because *terminated* means "ended." Choice C is incorrect because *was avoided* is the reverse of *ensued*. Choice D is incorrect because *culminated* means "ended in" and is a synonym for *terminated*, rather than *ensued*.

62. **The correct answer is A.** *Retrospect* means "*review*, contemplation of past events." Choice B is incorrect because a *concept* is a general idea, usually an abstract idea. *Knowledge* and *awareness* (choices C and D) are incorrect because they have no relation to *retrospect*.

63. **The correct answer is C.** *Malice* means "*ill will*, desire to harm." Choice A is incorrect because *adoration* is the opposite. Choice B is incorrect because *sympathy*, meaning "sharing another's feeling or emotions," has no relation to *malice*. Choice D is incorrect because *apathy* means "lack of interest, feelings, or emotion,"

64. **The correct answer is C.** *Saturated* means "*soaked*." Choice A is incorrect because *void of* means "empty of." *Mixed* and *replaced* (choices B and D) are incorrect because neither have any relation to *saturated*.

65. **The correct answer is D.** *Debilitating* means "draining the strength from, *weakening*." Choice A is incorrect because *invigorating*, meaning "giving energy or strength, making lively," is an antonym. Choice B is incorrect because *stimulating* means "exciting or invigorating someone," so it's a synonym for *invigorating* and another antonym for *debilitating*. Choice C is incorrect because *tolerable* means "able to be tolerated or endured" and has no relation to *debilitating*.

66. **The correct answer is D.** *Servitude* is similar to *bondage* in the sense of forced labor—slavery or serfdom. Choice A is incorrect because *freedom* is the opposite. Choice B is incorrect because *lethargy* means "slowness, sluggishness" or "being inactive." Choice C is incorrect because *vicissitude* means "sudden change in circumstances."

67. **The correct answer is A.** *Relish* in this sense means *enjoy*. Choice B is incorrect because *dread* means "fear, terror." *Spread* and *implant* (choices C and D) have no relation to *relish*.

68. **The correct answer is D.** *Lackadaisical* means "lazy" and "lacking in liveliness," so *indifferent* is a synonym. Choice A is incorrect because *enthusiastic* is an antonym. Choice B is incorrect because *complacent* means "self-satisfied, pleased with one's self." Choice C is incorrect because *profound* means "intense" and "showing great intellectual depth."

69. **The correct answer is B.** To *hoist* is "to *raise*." *Cast*, *prepare*, and *repair* are incorrect because they are not synonyms.

70. **The correct answer is A.** *Asperse* is "to spread false rumors," and *slander* means "to spread false information." Choice B is incorrect because *fathom* means "to understand"; it is also a unit of measurement. Choice C is incorrect because *extol* means "to praise greatly," so it's an antonym. Choice D is incorrect because *palliate* means "to relieve pain, make pain less intense."

71. **The correct answer is B.** *Sordid* means "dirty, filthy," and *wretched* means "miserable, in pitiful circumstances." Of the entries in the list, *wretched* is the nearest in meaning. Choice A is incorrect because *bizarre* means "odd, unusual." Choice C is incorrect because *primordial* means "fundamental, existing from the beginning." Choice D is incorrect because *exaggerated* has no relation to *sordid*.

72. **The correct answer is D.** *Alienation* means "*isolation,* a turning away." Choice A is incorrect because *agitation* means "being in a state of excitement or worry." Choice B is incorrect because *inception* means "the beginning of something." Choice C is incorrect because *subsistence* means "means of surviving, the least needed to live on."

73. **The correct answer is A.** *Dereliction* of duty is *neglect* of duty. Choice B is incorrect because *expansion* may make sense, but is not a synonym. *Attainment* and *fulfillment* (choices C and D) are antonyms of *dereliction.*

74. **The correct answer is D.** *Accede* means "to agree." *Attend, refer,* and *adjust* (choices A, B, and C) have no relation to *accede.*

75. **The correct answer is B.** *Proximity* means "*nearness.*" Choice A is incorrect because *worthlessness* has no relation to *proximity.* Choice C is incorrect because, although *level* makes sense, it is not a synonym. Choice D is incorrect because *ebullition* means either "a sudden outburst" or "the process of boiling."

Test 2: Antonyms

1. B	16. A	31. D	46. B	61. E
2. C	17. B	32. A	47. D	62. C
3. B	18. D	33. C	48. C	63. C
4. D	19. A	34. C	49. C	64. E
5. D	20. A	35. B	50. D	65. B
6. C	21. C	36. A	51. A	66. B
7. A	22. B	37. C	52. A	67. C
8. A	23. D	38. B	53. C	68. D
9. B	24. C	39. B	54. D	69. B
10. C	25. C	40. A	55. B	70. C
11. A	26. B	41. D	56. D	71. B
12. A	27. A	42. A	57. D	72. D
13. A	28. A	43. A	58. C	73. D
14. D	29. B	44. B	59. B	74. B
15. C	30. D	45. A	60. A	75. E

1. **The correct answer is B.** *Deface* means "to *disfigure*" so that makes choice D incorrect because we are looking for the antonym. *Embellish* (choice B) means "to decorate, to beautify," so it's the correct answer. Choice A is incorrect because *defame* means "to attack the reputation of someone, to accuse a person falsely with the intent to damage his or her good name." Choice C is incorrect because *vilify* means "to make vicious statements about someone, to degrade," which is similar to *defame*.

2. **The correct answer is C.** *Superfluous* means "more than enough, *abundant*" so choice D is incorrect because it's a synonym. *Insufficient* (choice C) is the opposite of *superfluous* so it's the correct answer. *Coarse* (choice A) has no relation to *superfluous*. *Transient* (choice B) is incorrect because it means "for a short time" or "a person who moves around a lot, who stays for just a short time."

3. **The correct answer is B.** To *assuage* is "to soothe, to relieve," so *agitate*, meaning "to excite," is its opposite. Choice A is incorrect because *presume* is "to take something for granted" or "to take something as true without evidence." Choice C is incorrect because *alleviate* is similar in meaning to *assuage*, rather than being an antonym. Choice D is incorrect because *absorb* means "to soak up," "to occupy one's interest or attention," or "to take in, assimilate," none of which is an antonym for *assuage*.

4. **The correct answer is D.** *Augury* is foretelling the future by means of signs. It is an art, not a *science*. Choice A is incorrect because *gentility* means "refinement, fine manners." Choice B is incorrect because *relentlessness*, meaning "never giving up, being persistent," has no relation to *augury*, and neither does choice C, *supremacy*, meaning "supreme power or authority."

5. **The correct answer is D.** *Terminate* means "to end," so its antonym is *initiate*, meaning "to begin." Choice A is incorrect because *withhold* has no relation to *terminate*. Choice B is incorrect because *construe* means "to interpret, to make sense of." Choice C is

incorrect because *repel* means "to force back," "to fight against," and "to reject."

6. **The correct answer is C.** *Vitiate* means "to corrupt," "to undermine," and "to destroy the legal force of something," so its antonym is *validate*, meaning "to declare legally valid." Choice A is incorrect because *liquidate* means "to pay off as debts" and "to end business operations." Choice B is incorrect because *revive* means "to bring back to life" and "to restore to use." Choice D is incorrect because *slander* means "to spread false information."

7. **The correct answer is A.** A *jubilant* person is an *irrepressible* person, so choice B is incorrect. *Irrepressible* means "impossible to control" in a happy, ebullient way, so it's a synonym of *jubilant*. Choice A is correct because a *lugubrious* person is a dismal, gloomy person, the opposite of *jubilant*. Choice C is incorrect because *discernible* means "able to be perceived, obvious." Choice D is incorrect because *jocular* means "joking."

8. **The correct answer is A.** The opposite of *hostile* in this list is *affable*, meaning "pleasant, easy." Choice B is incorrect because *awkward* has no relation to hostile, and neither does *judicious* (choice C), meaning "having good judgment." Choice D is incorrect because *politic* means "showing shrewdness or cunning" and "judicious," making it a synonym of *judicious*, but not an antonym of *hostile*.

9. **The correct answer is B.** *Taciturn* means "not talkative by nature," so *talkative* is an antonym. Choice A is incorrect because *tactful* means "showing concern in dealing with others, diplomatic, thoughtful." Choice C is incorrect because *crucial* means "very important." Choice D is incorrect because *impetuous* means "impulsive, lacking in thought, hasty."

10. **The correct answer is C.** *Laggardly* means "hanging back, lingering," whereas *briskly* is the opposite. Choice A is incorrect because *laboriously* means "hard working, industrious." Choice B is incorrect because *languidly* means "listlessly" or "lacking energy." Choice D is incorrect because *cowardly* has no relation to *laggardly*.

11. **The correct answer is A.** *Phlegmatic* means "calm, showing little emotion," whereas *vital* means "full of life, lively" in this case. Choice B is incorrect because *apparent* has no relation to *phlegmatic*. Choice C is incorrect because *conversant* means "knowledgeable, skilled in, familiar with." Choice D is incorrect because *apprehensive* means "anxious, fearful."

12. **The correct answer is A.** *Loathsome* means "hateful, disgusting, revolting," so *alluring*, meaning "attractive" or "fascinating," is its opposite. Choices B and C are incorrect because *mournful*, meaning "sad," and *indifferent*, have no relation to *loathsome*. Choice D is incorrect because *preposterous* means "absurd, ridiculous."

13. **The correct answer is A.** *Exalt* means "to glorify, to praise," or "to raise in rank or status," so *degrade*, which means "to reduce in rank or status or "to dishonor or disgrace," is an antonym. Choice B is incorrect because *gratify* means "to please or satisfy." Choice C is incorrect because *expose* has no relation to *exalt*. Choice D is incorrect because *desiderate* means "to wish for" or "to miss."

14. **The correct answer is D.** *Pacify* means "to calm" or "in military terms to restore peace or order," so *exasperate*, meaning "to make angry," is an antonym. Choice A is incorrect because *conciliate* means "to reconcile" or "to overcome distrust" and is close in meaning to *pacify*. Choice B is incorrect because *palliate* means "to

make something less serious" or "to lessen physical pain." Choice C is incorrect because *quell* means "to pacify" or "to suppress or put down something like a riot," so it's a synonym, not an antonym.

15. **The correct answer is C.** *Subsequent* means "following in order, succeeding," so *preceding*, meaning "previous," is an antonym. Choices A and B are incorrect because *worthless* and *inactive* have no relation to *subsequent*. Choice D is incorrect because *demeaning* means "lacking in honor or integrity" or "humiliating or shaming one's self."

16. **The correct answer is A.** *Ultimate* means "last or final in a series" as well as "most significant," so *initial* is an antonym. Choice B is incorrect because *equitable* means "fair, just." Choice C is incorrect because *irrefutable* means "impossible to deny." Choice D is incorrect because *turbid* means "muddy."

17. **The correct answer is B.** *Leeway* means "amount of freedom of movement, both physical and abstract, margin of error," so *restriction* is an antonym. Choice A is incorrect because *relevance* means "connection or relation to something." Choices C and D are incorrect because *protection* and *satisfaction* have no relation to *leeway*.

18. **The correct answer is D.** *Pretentious* means "trying to be something that one isn't, claiming a distinction or importance that is not deserved," whereas *modest* is the opposite. Choice A is incorrect because *flagrant* means "outrageous, shocking." Choice B is incorrect because *diabolical* means "evil." Choice C is incorrect because *officious* means "unnecessarily or excessively eager" or "intruding in an offensive way."

19. **The correct answer is A.** A *quandary* is something difficult to get out of, in other words, a predicament, but it can also be

a state of uncertainty, so *certainty* is an antonym. Choice B is incorrect because *mediocrity* means "ordinary, moderate to inferior." Choice C is incorrect because *ruthlessness* has no relation to *quandary*. Choice D is incorrect because a *criterion* is a standard or rule by which something is judged.

20. **The correct answer is A.** A *sagacious* person is a wise person, and an *obtuse* person is one who is dull, slow, or stupid, sometimes deliberately. Choice B is incorrect because *scurrilous* means "using vulgar or abusive language." Choice C is incorrect because *indulgent* means "lenient, giving in to someone's wishes," or "easygoing." Choice D is incorrect because *impertinent* means "rude."

21. **The correct answer is C.** A *savant* is a person of great learning, so a *neophyte*, one who is new to something, is an antonym. Choice A might tempt you, but *uncivilized* is an adjective and *savant* is a noun, so you can rule out *uncivilized* immediately. Choice B is incorrect because *master* is a near synonym of *savant*. Choice D is incorrect because *constituent*, meaning "a person represented by an elected official," has no relation to *savant*.

22. **The correct answer is B.** A *squalid* place is filthy, often because of extreme poverty, so a *stately* place is its opposite. *Stately* means "impressive, large, and orderly in appearance." Choice A is incorrect because *staunch* means "dependable, loyal." Choice C is incorrect because *avaricious* means "greedy." Choice D is incorrect because *equivocal* means "doubtful" or "deliberately vague."

23. **The correct answer is D.** *Exquisite*, meaning "unusually fine and delicate in design" as well as "very beautiful," and *ordinary* are opposites. Choice A is

incorrect because *exorbitant* means "very expensive." Choice B is incorrect because *obscure* means "unclear, vague" or "hidden, secret." Choice C is incorrect because *extraneous* means "unnecessary, irrelevant."

24. **The correct answer is C.** To *facilitate* is "to make easier" or "to be of use," so *hinder*, or "to get in the way of," is an antonym. Choice A is incorrect because *falsify* means "to misrepresent, to make a false statement." Choice B is incorrect because *delude* means "to mislead, to deceive." Choice D is incorrect because *assimilate* is "to incorporate."

25. **The correct answer is C.** *Flawless* means "having no flaws or imperfections," whereas *defective* is the condition of having flaws or defects, that is, being faulty in some way. Choice A is incorrect because *pertinent* means "relevant." Choice B is incorrect because *conventional* means "generally agreed on" or "following accepted practice." Choice D is incorrect because *complacent* means "self-satisfied, pleased with one's self."

26. **The correct answer is B.** To *recompense* someone is "to pay someone, to compensate a person" or "the payment itself." To *embezzle* is "to steal from someone," so choice B is an antonym. Choice A is incorrect because *renovate* is "to restore of good condition, to repair." Choice C is incorrect because *retribution* means "something given or demanded in payment"; it's a synonym for *recompense* used as a noun. Choice D is incorrect because a *sanction* is "authorization to do something" or "a penalty or punishment."

27. **The correct answer is A.** *Fervent* means "showing great emotion," whereas *nonchalant* means "indifferent, unconcerned." Choice B is incorrect because *lenient* means "generous, not harsh." Choice C is incorrect

because *meager* means "very little, stingy." Choice D is incorrect because *liable* means "legally responsible" or "likely, probable."

28. **The correct answer is A.** To *avert* is "to prevent from happening," whereas to *pursue* is "to seek to do or get something." Choice B is incorrect because *forestall* is "to delay, hinder, or prevent," so it's a synonym, not an antonym. Choice C is incorrect because *reject* has no relation to *avert*, and neither does *relinquish* (choice D), meaning "to give up" or "surrender."

29. **The correct answer is B.** Something that is *arid* is very dry, so *moist* is an antonym. Choice A is incorrect because *fragrant* has no relation to *arid*, and neither does *odoriferous* (choice D), meaning "having an odor." Choice C is incorrect because *parched* is a synonym for *arid*.

30. **The correct answer is D.** *Imperative* means "very urgent"; a person must do what is being ordered. On the other hand, *optional* indicates something that may or not be done; it's up to the person to decide. Choice A is incorrect because *conceivable* means "capable of conceiving." Choice B is incorrect because *illustrative* means "something used as an example." Choice C is incorrect because *speculative* means "not financially safe" or "not based on evidence."

31. **The correct answer is D.** *Succinct* means "brief, concise," whereas *loquacious*, meaning "very wordy," is the opposite. Choice A is incorrect because *corporeal* means "of the body" or "something that is tangible, can be touched." Choice B is incorrect because *graphic* means "something described in great and vivid detail" or "relating to a representation, either written or pictorial." Choice C is incorrect because *princely* has no relation to *succinct*.

32. **The correct answer is A.** *Jeopardy* means "in danger of injury, death, risk, loss, damage," so *security* is the opposite. Choice B is incorrect because *discernment* means "evidence of keen judgment or interest." Choice C is incorrect because *curiosity* has no relation to *jeopardy*. Choice D is incorrect because *tedium* means "boredom, monotony."

33. **The correct answer is C.** *Somber* means "dark, gloomy" or "melancholy, grave," so *festive* is an antonym. Choice A is incorrect because *insipid* means "lacking in flavor" or "lacking in anything that excites or stimulates." Choice B is incorrect because *congruous* means "appropriate, in harmony with, suitable." Choice D is incorrect because *voluminous* means "large in size, fullness, or number."

34. **The correct answer is C.** *Exotic* means "foreign" or "very unusual, strange or bizarre beauty," so *common* is an antonym. Choice A is incorrect because *inveterate* means "deep-seated" or "habitual." Choice B is incorrect because *erotic* means "of or concerning sexual desire." Choice D is incorrect because *harmonious*, being in agreement, has no relation to *exotic*.

35. **The correct answer is B.** To *affiliate* is "to associate or join with," so *disassociate* is an antonym. Choice A is incorrect because *annihilate* is to "kill all, to destroy." Choice C is incorrect because *proffer* is "to offer or propose something for acceptance or rejection." Choice D is incorrect because *disparage* is "to speak disrespectfully or in a belittling way about something or someone."

36. **The correct answer is A.** *Sinister* means "evil, treacherous" or "ominous, foretelling harm," so *auspicious*, meaning "foretelling favorable conditions," is an antonym. Choice B is incorrect because *immaculate* means "spotless." Choice C is incorrect because *fanatical* means "beyond normal enthusiasm, intense devotion to something or someone." Choice D is incorrect because *transitory* means "temporary, lasting only a short time."

37. **The correct answer is C.** *Inextricable* means "not able to untangle or escape from," so *disentangle* is an antonym. Choice A is incorrect because *intricate* means "complex, elaborate." Choice B is incorrect because *judicious* means "having good judgment, being prudent." Choice D is incorrect because *desperate* has no relation to *inextricable*.

38. **The correct answer is B.** *Profligate* means "shamelessly immoral" or "extremely wasteful," and *virtuous* is the opposite. Choice A is incorrect because *insolvent* means "bankrupt, unable to pay one's debts," which is what a profligate person may be, so it's not an antonym. Choice C is incorrect because *redundant* means "more than is needed or required" or "repetitive." Choice D is incorrect because *incessant* means "having no interruption, continual."

39. **The correct answer is B.** *Turbulent* and *tranquil* are opposites, unrest and disorder versus calm. Choice A is incorrect because *diaphanous* means "transparent, flimsy." Choice C is incorrect because *formidable* means "inspiring awe or admiration" or "arousing fear or dread." Choice D is incorrect because *diffident* means "timid, shy" or "reserved, modest."

40. **The correct answer is A.** *Unwarranted* means "lacking authorization or justification," so *justifiable* is an antonym. Choice B is incorrect because *baneful* means "very harmful." Choice C is incorrect because *depleted* means "drained, used up, no longer sufficient." Choice D is incorrect because *contemplated* means "thought about, considered."

41. **The correct answer is D.** *Plaintive* means "mournful" or "sorrowful," so *gleeful* is an antonym. Choice A is incorrect because *embellished* means "made more interesting or beautiful by adding decoration." Choice B is incorrect because *poignant* means "very moving or touching, at times causing painful feelings." Choice C is incorrect because *rational* has no relation to *plaintive*.

42. **The correct answer is A.** Something that is *ornate* is highly decorated or adorned, so something that is *unadorned* is the opposite. Choice B is incorrect because *deft* means "skillful, expert." Choice C is incorrect because *subtle* means "not immediately obvious" or "the ability to perceive small differences." Choice D is incorrect because *conspicuous* means "obvious, easy to see," so it is an antonym for *subtle*, but not for *ornate*.

43. **The correct answer is A.** To *abrogate* is "to do away with, revoke, cancel," so *ratify*, to approve, is an antonym. Choice B is incorrect because *reconcile* means "to settle or resolve." Choice C is incorrect because *abridge* is "to cut short" or "reduce the length of a written work by rewriting." Choice D is incorrect because *alleviate* is "to relieve, lessen, especially pain."

44. **The correct answer is B.** *Abase* means "to belittle, humiliate," so *dignify* is an antonym. Choice A is incorrect because *cede* means "to surrender, relinquish." Choice C is incorrect because *repudiate* means "to reject, refuse to acknowledge someone or something as legitimate or valid." Choice D is incorrect because *engulf* means "to overwhelm."

45. **The correct answer is A.** To *renounce* is "to give up" or "to reject," whereas to *claim* is the opposite. Choice B is incorrect because *deride* is "to ridicule, to treat or speak about with contempt." Choice C is incorrect

because *conceive* has no relation to *renounce*. Choice D is incorrect because *alienate* is "to arouse indifference or hostility in a former friend."

46. **The correct answer is B.** To *sabotage* is "to destroy, to damage," whereas to *reinforce* is "to strengthen or give more support to." Choice A is incorrect because *compensate* is "to pay for." Choice C is incorrect because *restrain* is "to hold back, to control" or "to limit." Choice D is incorrect because *release* has no relation to *sabotage*.

47. **The correct answer is D.** *Oblivious* means "forgetful, unaware," so *cognizant*, meaning "aware" or "having knowledge of," is the opposite. Choice A is incorrect because *latent* means "not obvious, concealed." Choice B is incorrect because *integrant* means "part of a whole, that is, integral." Choice C is incorrect because *repugnant* means "offensive, distasteful."

48. **The correct answer is C.** *Submissive* means "willing to submit to another's wishes, obedient, passive," whereas *incompliant* means "not willing to comply or yield." Choices A and B, *offensive* and *tactless*, are incorrect because they have no relation to *submissive*. Choice D is incorrect because *manifest* means "very apparent, obvious."

49. **The correct answer is C.** To *nurture* is "to help grow" or "to help raise," whereas to *neglect* is an antonym. Choice A is incorrect because *distinguish* is "to notice as different" or "to see, to perceive." Choice B is incorrect because *impart* is "to communicate" or "to give." Choice D is incorrect because *disclose* has no relation to *nurture*.

50. **The correct answer is D.** *Prudence* is discretion or caution, whereas *recklessness* is the lack of prudence and, thus, an antonym. Choice A is incorrect because *compunction* means "feeling of remorse or guilt."

Choice B is incorrect because a *dilemma* may require prudence, but it is neither a synonym nor an antonym for *prudence*. Choice C is incorrect because *anticipation* has no relation to *prudence*.

51. **The correct answer is A.** To *lament* is "to express grief, to mourn," so to *rejoice* is its opposite. Choice B is incorrect because *acclaim* is "to honor or praise." Choice C is incorrect because *surmise* is "to guess" or "to infer." Choice D is incorrect because *deceive* has no relation to *lament*.

52. **The correct answer is A.** *Grueling* means "activity to the point of exhaustion," whereas *relaxing* is its opposite. Choices B and C are incorrect because *grueling* has no relation to *satisfying* or *taming*. Choice D is incorrect because *suppressing* means "putting an end to, often by force" or "restraining."

53. **The correct answer is C.** *Trivial*, meaning "of little significance," and *critical*, meaning "essential," are antonyms. Choice A is incorrect because *nugatory* is a synonym for *trivial*. Choice B is incorrect because *ungainly* means "awkward." Choice D is incorrect because *solicitous* means "anxious, concerned, showing anxiety or concern for someone."

54. **The correct answer is D.** The *zenith* is the highest point, the peak of something such as a career, whereas the *nadir* is the lowest point. Choice A is incorrect because *vitality*, meaning "liveliness, full of life," has no relation to *zenith*. Choice B is incorrect because *rage* has no relation to *zenith*, nor does choice C, *reverence*.

55. **The correct answer is B.** *Unobtrusive* means "not noticeable, not easily seen," so the opposite is *prominent*, meaning "immediately noticeable, conspicuous." Choice A is incorrect because *resonant* means "bringing to mind, reminiscent" as well as

"producing a deep, full sound." Choice C is incorrect because *controlled* has no relation to *unobtrusive*, nor does choice D, *subjective*.

56. **The correct answer is D.** *Refractive* means "capable of changing or bending the direction of light or sound," so *direct* is an antonym. Choice A is incorrect because *cryptic* means "hidden, secret." Choice B is incorrect because *interruptive* is not an antonym for *refractive*, nor is *applicable* (choice C).

57. **The correct answer is D.** A *rebuff* is a refusal or rejection, so *encouragement* is an antonym. Choice A is incorrect because *exclusion* means "a deliberate omission." Choices B and C are incorrect because *disturbance* and *recall* have no relation to *rebuff*.

58. **The correct answer is C.** An *adversary* is an *opponent* and so is an *enemy*, so choices A and D are incorrect. Choice C is correct because an *accomplice* aids someone in committing a crime. Choice B is incorrect because *administrator* has no relation to an adversary.

59. **The correct answer is B.** An *optimist* is a person who sees things in a favorable way, in other words, who believes that good things will happen, whereas a *pessimist* is just the opposite. Choices A, C, and D are all incorrect because an *optimist* has no relation to a *rival*, an *analyst*, or a *protagonist*. The last is the main character in a play or work of fiction or nonfiction.

60. **The correct answer is A.** *Pervasive* means "widespread," so *limited* is an antonym. Choices B and C are incorrect because both *universal* and *ubiquitous* are synonyms for *pervasive*. Choice D is incorrect because *common* may also be a synonym for *pervasive*.

61. **The correct answer is E.** *Ignorant*, which means "lacking knowledge," is the word

most different in meaning from the others. *Erudite, learned, scholarly,* and *savvy* all pertain to being knowledgeable.

62. **The correct answer is C.** *Paramount, essential, momentous,* and *supreme* all mean "important," whereas *inconsequential* (choice C) means "unimportant," and therefore is the word most different from the others.

63. **The correct answer is C.** *Surreptitious, secretive, clandestine,* and *covert* all refer to something that is done in secret, so *candid,* meaning "frank, outspoken, open, unreserved," is the word most different from the others.

64. **The correct answer is E.** *Mendacious, duplicitous, deceptive,* and *prevaricating* all mean "untruthful, lying," whereas *creditable* (choice E) means "admirable, praiseworthy, honorable" and so is the word most different from the others.

65. **The correct answer is B.** *Unctuous, charming, slick,* and *urbane* all mean "suave" or "socially smooth," whereas *awkward* (choice B) means the opposite—clumsy, embarrassed, not elegant—making it the word most different from the others.

66. **The correct answer is B.** *Impetuous, rash, impulsive,* and *capricious* all refer to someone who acts on impulse, without thinking first, whereas *cautious* refers to a person who is slow to act and tends to think before acting. Therefore, choice B is the word most different from the others.

67. **The correct answer is C.** *Penurious, frugal, parsimonious,* and *thrifty* all refer to someone who is stingy, destitute, and/or thrifty, whereas *extravagant* (choice C) refers to someone who spends liberally and thus is the word most different from the others.

68. **The correct answer is D.** *Odious, abhorrent, loathsome,* and *repugnant* all mean "arousing

strong dislike," so *winsome,* which means "attractive, charming," is the word most different from the others.

69. **The correct answer is B.** *Ostensible, alleged, purported,* and *overt* all mean "apparent, seeming," whereas *ulterior* means "secret, hidden" and so choice B is the word most different from the others.

70. **The correct answer is C.** *Deleterious, insalubrious, toxic,* and *pernicious* all mean "injurious, harmful," whereas *beneficial* (choice C) means "causing good" and thus is the most different from the others.

71. **The correct answer is B.** *Ignominy, shame, humiliation,* and *disgrace* all mean something degrading or painful, so *honor* is the word most different from the others.

72. **The correct answer is D.** *Compatible, complementary, simpatico,* and *harmonious* all refer to people or things that get along well with one another. *Incongruous,* meaning to be "incompatible, not in agreement with principles, inconsistent with" is the word most different from the others.

73. **The correct answer is D.** *Premeditated, plotted, calculated,* and *developed* all mean "planned, marked by prior thought," so *improvised,* meaning "invented with little forethought or preparation," is the word most different from the others.

74. **The correct answer is B.** *Pernicious, calamitous, detrimental,* and *baneful* all mean "disastrous, tending to cause harm or injury," whereas *restorative* means "tending to restore" and therefore is the word most different from the others.

75. **The correct answer is E.** *Umbrage, offense, resentment,* and *chagrin* all refer to displeasure, whereas *amity* means "friendship" and so is the word most different from the others.

Test 3: Analogy Relationships

1. A	4. A	7. B	10. D	13. D
2. C	5. D	8. A	11. A	14. C
3. D	6. A	9. D	12. D	15. B

1. **The correct answer is A.** In this purpose relationship, a *glove* is used to catch a *ball* and a *hook* is used to catch a *fish*. Choice B is incorrect because *winter* is a season, not a type of *weather*. Choice C is incorrect because a single *game* is not a way to win a *pennant*, that is, a championship. Choice D is incorrect because the purpose of a *stadium* is not to provide *seats*, but to provide a place for events.

2. **The correct answer is C.** In this cause-and-effect relationship, a person is *fatigued*, that is, tired, after running a *race*. A person is *hungry* as a result of *fasting*, that is, not eating. Choice A is incorrect because a *track* doesn't result in an *athlete*. Choice B is incorrect because an *ant* is a type of *bug*, or insect; there is no cause-and-effect relationship. Choice D is incorrect because *walking* and *running* are both types of activities; there is no cause-and-effect relationship between them.

3. **The correct answer is D.** In this part-to-whole relationship, a *snake* is one of the category *reptile*, and a *hand* is part of a *clock*. Choice A is incorrect because a *patch* is not a type of *thread*. Choice B is incorrect because *removal* is not a part of *snow*, though it is a way to get rid of snow. A snowball would be a part of snow. Choice C is incorrect because *struggle* is not a part of *wrestle; wrestle* would be a part of sports.

4. **The correct answer is A.** In this part-to-part relationship, a *gill* and a *fin* are both parts of a fish as a *plasma display* and *electrodes* are both parts of flat screen TVs. Choice B is incorrect because a *violin* is

an *instrument*, not part of an instrument. Choice C is incorrect because a *sea* is home to many *fish;* it's not a part of something shared with fish. Choice D is incorrect because *salad* is part of a *supper*, which is a whole, not a part.

5. **The correct answer is D.** In this action-to-object relationship, *kicking* is the action and the object that is kicked is a *football*. The action is *smoking* and the object that is smoked is a *pipe*. Choice A is incorrect because the action is to *kill*, but the object is not a *bomb;* a bomb is a means to kill; people would be the object. Choice B is incorrect because the action is *breaking*, and *pieces* aren't the object, but the result. The object would be something like a plate or bowl. Choice C is incorrect because *question* and *team* aren't related. The object for question would be answer.

6. **The correct answer is A.** This is the reverse of the previous question. *Steak* is what receives the action, *broiling*, in this object-to-action relationship, so the second analogy is *bread*, the object, to *baking*, the action. Choice B is incorrect because *food* is the object and *eat* is the action, but the analogy is set up backwards. The same is true for choices C and D, *pour* and *wine*, and *spill* and *sugar*.

7. **The correct answer is B.** In this synonym relationship, you're looking for the two words that are alike. *Enormous* means the same as *huge*, and *muddy* means the same as *unclear*. Choice A is incorrect because *rogue* is a deceitful and unreliable person, which has no relation to *rock*. Choice C is

incorrect because *purse* and *kitchen* are not synonyms, and neither are *black* and *white,* choice D.

8. **The correct answer is A.** This question asks for an antonym pair. *Evil* is the opposite of *purity* as *bluntness* is the opposite of *suavity,* meaning "smoothly agreeable, graciously polite." Choice B is incorrect because *north* and *climate* have no relation. Choice C is incorrect because *angel* and *horns* have no relation; it would have to be *devil* rather than *horns* to be an antonym pair. Choice D is incorrect because *boldness* and *victory* have no relation.

9. **The correct answer is D.** The place relationship is city to state—the city of *Miami* to its state of *Florida.* The only pair that follows this model is the city of *Albany* to its state of *New York.* This makes choice B incorrect because here, the relationship is reversed. Choices A and C are incorrect because the *United States* is not a state.

10. **The correct answer is D.** *Warm* is a degree of, or step to being, *hot* in this degree relationship. *Bright* is a degree of, or step in being, a *genius.* Choice A is incorrect because *glue* and *paste* are comparable materials; there is no degree relationship between them. Choice B is incorrect because *climate* is not a degree of *weather.* Choice C is incorrect because a *fried egg* and a *boiled egg* have no degree relationship; both are cooked eggs.

11. **The correct answer is A.** In this characteristic relationship, *skill* is a characteristic gained from *practice. Blood* is a characteristic of a *wound,* that is, a wound bleeds. Choice B is incorrect because a *dollar* is *money;* it's not a characteristic of money,

such as, for example, value and portability. Choice C is incorrect because *schools* are not characteristics of *elevators,* though schools may have elevators. Choice D is incorrect because *education* is not a characteristic of *stupidity.*

12. **The correct answer is D.** In this sequence relationship, *summer* follows *spring* and *Wednesday* follows *Thursday.* Choice A is incorrect because the sequence is reversed. Choice B is incorrect because the sequence is reversed and one day is missing between the days. Choice C is incorrect because the sequence is reversed.

13. **The correct answer is D.** Both words— *restore* and *climb*—are verbs, so you need to find the answer with a pair of verbs. Only choice D includes two verbs—*overpower* and *seethe.* Choice A is incorrect because *segregation* is a noun and *seem* is a verb. Choice B is incorrect because *into* is a preposition and *nymph* is a noun. Choice C is incorrect because *precipice* is a noun and *although* is a conjunction.

14. **The correct answer is C.** In this association relationship, *devil* is to *wrong* as *ink* is to *writing.* Choice A is incorrect because a *color* and a *sidewalk* have no relation. Choice B is incorrect because a *slipper* and a *state* have no relation. Choice D is incorrect because a *picture* and a *bed* have no relation.

15. **The correct answer is B.** The connection in this numerical relationship is multiplication by 3: $4 \times 3 = 12$ and $9 \times 3 = 27$. Choice A is incorrect because $10 \times 3 = 30$, not 16. Choice C is incorrect because $3 \times 3 = 9$, not 4. Choice D is incorrect because $12 \times 3 = 36$, not 6.

Test 4: Verbal Analogies

Part A

1. B	6. C	11. C	16. B	21. A
2. C	7. C	12. C	17. C	22. D
3. A	8. A	13. D	18. D	23. B
4. D	9. D	14. A	19. D	24. A
5. C	10. B	15. B	20. C	25. C

1. **The correct answer is B.** In this object-to-use analogy, a *knife cuts* as a *gun shoots.* Choice C, *sharpen,* may tempt you, but sharpening is done to a knife, not done by a knife. A knife may be used to *poke* someone, but that is not the usual use for a knife, so eliminate choice D.

2. **The correct answer is C.** This is also an object-to-use analogy, an *eye sees* as an *ear hears.* None of the other answers makes sense with *eye.*

3. **The correct answer is A.** In this object-to-use analogy, *feathers* cover *birds* and *fur* covers some *mammals.* None of the other answers makes sense with feathers.

4. **The correct answer is D.** In this part-to-whole analogy, a *hammer* has a *handle* as a *door* has a *knob.* None of the other answers makes sense with a knob.

5. **The correct answer is C.** In this object-to-use analogy, a *foot* wears a *shoe* as a *body* wears a *coat.* Don't be fooled by the typical use of *coat* and *hat* together as a phrase, so eliminate choice A. A coat may have *buttons* (choice B), but that relationship of whole to part is not the relationship set up in the question.

6. **The correct answer is C.** This is another object-to-use analogy. *Water* is *drunk* as *bread* is *eaten.* You might have thought that the initial pair was setting up a relationship between near synonyms, water as a drink, but *bread* is not a *cake* or a *pie* (choices A and D), so that relationship couldn't be correct.

7. **The correct answer is C.** In this object-to-use relationship, *food* fuels a *human* as *gasoline* fuels an *automobile.* Choices A and B are incorrect because *lube* and *oil* are what's done to an engine but are not uses of gasoline. Neither is a *spark* (choice D).

8. **The correct answer is A.** This question sets up an action-to-quality relationship. *Eating* leads to being *fat,* and *starving* leads to being *thin.* Food and bread (choices B and C) are things, not qualities. Choice D is a quality, but not *necessarily* related to starving.

9. **The correct answer is D.** This is a person-to-place analogy. A *human* lives in a *house* and a *bird* lives in a *nest.* Birds may also be found in *trees* and on *limbs* (choices A and B) but neither is as specific to birds as *house* is for humans. Choice B is a *meal,* not a place to live.

10. **The correct answer is B.** This is an antonym analogy. The opposite of *go* is *come,* and the opposite of *sell* is *buy.* Choice A relates to the first pair in the question, not the second. Choice C is incorrect because *money* is what you hope to get when you sell something, but is not antonym for *sell.* Choice D is incorrect because it's a near synonym for *sell,* not an antonym.

11. **The correct answer is C.** In this example-to-category analogy, a *peninsula* is a type of *landform* and a *bay* is a type of *body of water*. Choice A is incorrect because a bay is not a *boat* type. Choices B and D are incorrect because both an *inlet* and a *harbor* are other types of bodies of water.

12. **The correct answer is C.** In this whole-to-part analogy, a *minute* is part of an *hour* and a *second* is part of a *minute*. None of the other answer choices fits this whole-to-part relationship.

13. **The correct answer is D.** You can tell by the first pair that this is an antonym relationship. "To *abide*" is "to remain or *stay*," so *depart* is an antonym. An antonym for *stay* is *leave*. None of the other answer choices fits an antonym relationship.

14. **The correct answer is A.** "*January* is to *February*" sets up a sequence relationship, so the missing month is *July*, that is, as "*June* is to *July*." Choices C and D can't be correct because they are not the names of months. Choice B is incorrect because May precedes June, not follows it as February follows January.

15. **The correct answer is B.** This is an antonym analogy. *Bold* and *timid* are antonyms, so you're looking for an antonym for *advance*. Instead of advancing, or moving forward, an army falls back, or *retreats*. Choice A is incorrect because, although *proceed* also means "to move forward," it doesn't fit the military connotation of *advance*. Choice C is incorrect because a *campaign* is a series of military operations, not a single advance or retreat, and so doesn't fit the sense. Choice D is incorrect because *soldiers* in its verb form means "to push doggedly forward," which would be a synonym for *advance*.

16. **The correct answer is B.** This is another antonym relationship. The opposite of *above* is *below*, and the opposite of *top* is *bottom*. Either choice C or choice D might tempt you, but neither is the opposite of *top*.

17. **The correct answer is C.** This is an example-to-category analogy. A *lion* is a type of *animal*, and a *rose* is a type of *plant*. All the other choices characterize a rose, but each is a quality, not the category to which roses belong.

18. **The correct answer is D.** Consider this an object-to-quality relationship. A *tiger* is *carnivorous*, that is, a meat eater, and a *horse* is *herbivorous*, a plant eater. You can fairly easily eliminate choices A and B, but you may be stumped by choices C and D. This is where prefixes help. *Omni-* means "all," so an animal that is an omnivore eats plants and animals. *Herb* is not a prefix, but think of herbs as green leafy plants to help you remember that herbivores are plant eaters.

19. **The correct answer is D.** In this part-to-whole relationship, a *sailor* is part of the *navy* and a *soldier* is part of the *army*. None of the other answers fits this part-to-whole relationship.

20. **The correct answer is C.** This is a form of an object-to-use analogy. You *see* a *picture*, and you *hear* a *sound*. A clue here is that *see* is a verb, and the only answer choice that is a verb is choice C, *hear*.

21. **The correct answer is A.** Consider this a cause-and-effect relationship. *Success* causes *joy*, and *failure* causes *sadness*; both are effects. Choice C may tempt you, but a *fault* can be the cause of failure, not an effect. It's also incorrect because *joy* is an abstract quality and a fault is not.

22. **The correct answer is D.** In this antonym analogy, *hope* is the opposite of *despair*, so the opposite of *happiness* is *misery*. On a

quick read if you're running out of time, you might be confused into choosing one of the other choices, which are synonyms for *happiness*. So remember to read quickly, but carefully.

23. **The correct answer is B.** This is an antonym analogy with a twist. The first pair is adjectives, but *attract* is a verb, so you'll need to find the answer choice that is both an antonym and a verb. The only one that fits is *repel* (choice B) since it is the opposite of *attract*. *Fine* (choice A) could be a noun or a verb, but it doesn't fit as an antonym for attract. *Draw* (choice D) is a verb and may mean "to cause to move toward," but that would be a synonym for *attract*, not an antonym.

24. **The correct answer is A.** This is another association analogy. A *pupil* and a *teacher* have a superior-subordinate relationship as a *child* and a *parent* have. Choice B is incorrect because a *doll* and a *child* may have a relationship, but it's not of the same superior-subordinate relationship and one part of the relationship isn't living. Choice C is incorrect because *child* and *youngster* are synonymous. Choice D is incorrect because, while *obey* indicates the type of relationship between a superior and a subordinate, it doesn't name a person.

25. **The correct answer is C.** This is a person-to-occupation analogy. A *mayor* runs a *city*, and a *general* runs the *army*. None of the other answer choices fits the concept of operating or managing.

Part B

1. C	**6.** E	**11.** B	**16.** D	**21.** A
2. D	**7.** B	**12.** A	**17.** B	**22.** A
3. B	**8.** D	**13.** C	**18.** D	**23.** C
4. A	**9.** C	**14.** D	**19.** E	**24.** B
5. E	**10.** E	**15.** C	**20.** A	**25.** D

1. **The correct answer is C.** This is a synonym analogy. *Remunerative* means "profitable, paying," so *profitable* is a synonym. *Fraudulent* means "deceitful," so *fallacious,* "tending to mislead or deceptive," is a synonym. Choices A and B are incorrect because both *liar* and *slander* are nouns, and the analogy requires an adjective. Choice D is incorrect because *plausible* means "likely, apparently reasonable." Choice E is incorrect because *reward* is both a noun and a synonym for *remunerative,* not *fraudulent.*

2. **The correct answer is D.** This is a tool-to-worker analogy. A *woodsman* uses an *ax,* and a *plumber* uses a *wrench. Cut* and *hew* (choices A and B) are actions that a woodsman might do, but you need a person to complete the partial analogy. Choice C is incorrect because a *technician* works on electronic equipment. Choice E is incorrect because a *cobbler* is a person who mends shoes.

3. **The correct answer is B.** This analogy reverses the tool-to-worker analogy in question 2 and is a worker-to-tool analogy. A *surgeon* uses a *scalpel* to cut and a *butcher* cuts with a *cleaver,* a large broad-bladed knife or hatchet. Choices A, C, D, and E are incorrect because a *mallet,* a *chisel,* a *screwdriver,* and *medicine* are not tools a butcher uses.

4. **The correct answer is A.** The initial analogy sets up an example-to-category relationship. A *cat* belongs to the category of *feline* (or the family Felidae), and a *horse* belongs to the category of *equine* (or family Equidae). Even if you didn't know the Latin names, you might have recognized that a cat is a feline, so the missing word would be similar. Choice B is incorrect because a *tiger* isn't a horse. Choice C is incorrect because, although a horse has four legs and so does a cat, the first pair in the analogy isn't about leg number. Choice D is incorrect because horses aren't meat-eaters, the meaning of *carnivore.* Choice E is incorrect because *vulpine* means "resembling a fox."

5. **The correct answer is E.** This analogy is looking for antonyms. *Adversity* means "misfortune, hardship," so *happiness* is an antonym. An antonym for *vehemence,* meaning "forcefulness, violence" as well as "energy, passion," is *serenity,* "great calmness." Choices A and C are incorrect because *misfortune* is a synonym for *adversity,* and *troublesome,* meaning "worrisome" and "turbulent, violent," is also a synonym. Choice B is incorrect because *gaiety* has no relation to *vehemence.* Choice D is incorrect because *petulance* means "characterized by being irritable, impatient, ill humored" and is closer in meaning to *vehemence* than an antonym.

6. **The correct answer is E.** This is a characteristic relationship. A *necklace* is an *adornment* as a *medal* is a *decoration.* The correct answer is based on what is essential about a medal. Choices A, B, and D are

incorrect because a medal is still a medal whether it has a *jewel*, or is made of some *metal*, including *bronze*. Choice C is incorrect because a medal may be given for *bravery*, but bravery is not an essential characteristic of medals.

7. **The correct answer is B.** This is a worker-to-tool analogy. A *miner* uses a *shovel*, and a *pirate* uses a *sword* in his line of work. Both a miner and a pirate want *treasure*, including *gold* possibly, but gold is not a tool, so choices A and E are incorrect. Choice C is incorrect because a pirate sails a *ship*, but it's not a tool in the same way that a sword is. Choice D is incorrect because, although a pirate ship may fly a *flag*, a flag is not a tool for a pirate.

8. **The correct answer is D.** This is a person-to-occupation relationship. An *archaeologist* studies *antiquity*, and an *ichthyologist* studies *marine life*. If you didn't know the answer, you could at least eliminate some answer choices as incorrect. Someone who studies *theology* (choice A) is a theologian. Choice B is incorrect because *ruins* are what archaeologists study; always check to make sure that an answer doesn't relate to the initial pair to confuse you. Choice C is incorrect because *horticulture* is studied by a horticulturalist. Choice E is incorrect because a *mystic* practices mysticism.

9. **The correct answer is C.** In this characteristic analogy, you're looking for what *highways* are made of because *shoes* are made of *leather* (or at least some shoes are). *Passage*, *road*, and *trail* (choices A, B, and D) can be near synonyms of *highway*, but this isn't what is required to answer the analogy. Choice E is incorrect because a *journey* is a trip and not a characteristic of a highway.

10. **The correct answer is E.** *Serfdom* is a characteristic of the *feudal system*, and *entrepreneurship* is a characteristic of *capitalism*.

None of the other answer choices relates to *entrepreneurship*.

11. **The correct answer is B.** This is a part-to-whole analogy. A *fin* is part of a *fish* as a *propeller* is part of a *plane*. Choice A is incorrect because a *wing* is also part of a plane, not the whole plane. Choices C and D are incorrect because neither is the whole of which a propeller is part, though a propeller may be used in both. Choice E is incorrect because *canoes* don't have propellers.

12. **The correct answer is A.** This is a quality-to-extreme, or degree, analogy. *Satiety* means "being full beyond just being satisfied," and *destitute* is more than being poor; it is being impoverished, without any resources. Choice B is incorrect because *subsistence* means "a small amount of resources needed to survive," whereas being destitute is having no resources. Choice C is incorrect because *sustainable* means "able to supply with resources," or "able to be maintained." Choice D is incorrect because *lesser* has no relation with *poor*, and neither does choice E, *abandoned*.

13. **The correct answer is C.** This is a characteristic analogy. *Skin* is the external covering of *humans*, and *hide* is a similar external covering of *animals*. Choice A is incorrect because *scales* are the covering of fish. Choice B is incorrect because *fur* covers some animals' hides. Choice D is incorrect because *hair* covers some parts of humans' skin. Choice E is incorrect because a *fish* is not covered by a hide.

14. **The correct answer is D.** This is a whole-to-part analogy. A *drop* is single particle of *rain*, and a *flake* is a single particle of *snow*. Choice A is incorrect because snow is not the same as *ice*. Choices B and C are incorrect because, while it may be *cold*, even *zero* degrees, when it snows, neither is a particle of snow. The same is true of *sleet* (choice E).

15. **The correct answer is C.** This is a part-to-whole analogy. A *wing* is part of a *bird*, and of the choices listed, only a *horse* has a *hoof*.

16. **The correct answer is D.** This is another whole-to-part analogy. A *constellation* is a collection of *stars*, and an *archipelago* is a collection of *islands*. Choices A, B, and C are all landforms, but not the correct landform. *River* (choice E) has no relation to an archipelago.

17. **The correct answer is B.** In this object-to-use relationship, the *internet* is used for *emailing* and *smartphones* are used for *messaging*. Choice A is incorrect because *fast* doesn't parallel *emailing* in meaning. It's a characteristic, not a use. Choice C is incorrect because, while you can make calls on a smartphone, it's not as similar of an innovative use of a smartphone as using the internet is to send emails. Making calls is an old use for a new invention. Choice D is incorrect because *landlines* are things, not uses. Choice E is incorrect because smartphones don't send *snail mail*.

18. **The correct answer is D.** This is an antonym analogy. Being *absent* is the opposite of being *present*, and *stable* is the opposite of *changeable*. *Steady*, *secure*, and *safe* (choices A, B, and C) are similar in meaning to *stable*, so all are incorrect. Choice E is incorrect because *influential* has no relation to *stable*.

19. **The correct answer is E.** In this object-to-quality analogy, *flexibility* is a quality of *rubber*, and *rigidity* is a quality of a *pipe*. Choice A is incorrect because *iron* can be a type of pipe, but it is not a characteristic related to movement—or lack of movement. This is also true for *copper* (choice B). Choices C and D are incorrect because both *pliability* and *elasticity* are qualities related to flexibility, which is not a quality of pipes.

20. **The correct answer is A.** This is a part-to-whole analogy. A *safety valve* is part of a *boiler*, and a *spark plug* is part of an *engine*. *House*, *wire*, *city*, and *factory* have no relation to *spark plug*.

21. **The correct answer is A.** This is an antonym analogy. The opposite of *scholarly* is *unscholarly*, and the opposite of *learned* is *ignorant*. *Wise*, *skilled*, and *educated* (choices B, C, and D) are incorrect because they are similar in meaning to *scholarly* rather than being antonyms. Choice E is incorrect because *literary* has no relation to *learned*.

22. **The correct answer is A.** This is a person-to-behavior analogy. An *immigrant arrives*, and an *emigrant departs*. Choice B is incorrect because *alienation* means "state or condition of isolation." Choice C is incorrect because *native* has no relation to *emigrant*. If you weren't sure if choice D was incorrect, you can eliminate it because *welcoming* is an adjective and you need a noun to match the second word in the first pair, *arrival*. Choice E is incorrect because *travel* is not specific enough to an emigrant.

23. **The correct answer is C.** This is a person-to-place analogy. A *governor* runs a *state*, and an *admiral* runs the *navy*. Choices A, D, and E are incorrect because each is an officer in the military, and the analogy established by the first pair requires one of the armed services as the answer. Choice B is incorrect because an admiral runs the navy, not the army.

24. **The correct answer is B.** This is a quality-to-extreme or degree analogy. *Disastrous* is an extreme form of *troublesome*, and *extravagant* is an extreme form of *costly*. Choice A is incorrect because *cheap* is an antonym for *extravagant*, not an extreme version of the word. Choice C is incorrect because *gorgeous* relates to looks, not price. Choice D is incorrect because *valuable* is

not an extreme version of *costly*. Choice E is incorrect because *turbulent* has no relation to *costly*.

25. **The correct answer is D.** This is a category analogy. A *coat* can be made out of *wool*, and a *dress* can be made out of *cotton*.

Choice A is incorrect because a *tablecloth* isn't a piece of clothing. Choice B is incorrect because a *cover* isn't a specific type of clothing. Choice C is incorrect because *washable* is not a type of clothing, and neither is a *cleaner*, choice E.

Part C

1. E	6. D	11. D	16. C	21. A
2. D	7. E	12. C	17. C	22. D
3. C	8. D	13. E	18. D	23. A
4. A	9. C	14. A	19. B	24. E
5. B	10. B	15. A	20. A	25. B

1. **The correct answer is E.** This is a place analogy. A *boat* is kept at a *dock,* and an *airplane* is kept in a *hangar.* All the other answer choices are parts of a plane, not a place to keep one.

2. **The correct answer is D.** In this association analogy, *oats* are measured in *bushels,* and *diamonds* are measured in *carats.* Choice A is incorrect because *gram* has no relation to diamonds. Choices B, C, and E are incorrect because they are characteristics or uses of diamonds, but not how diamonds are measured.

3. **The correct answer is C.** In this characteristic analogy, an *examination* is a normal practice or part of *medicine,* and an *interrogation* is a normal practice or part of *law.* All the other answer choices are things associated with the law, but are not a practice. For example, for choice D to be correct, the answer would need to be "write a contract," and for choice E to be correct, the answer would need to be "sue."

4. **The correct answer is A.** This is a person-to-action analogy. A *parent guides* children, and a *soldier serves* in the army. Choice B is incorrect because *obedience* is a noun, and the answer, based on the first pair, requires a verb. Choice C is incorrect because *participate* in relation to a soldier in the army is not typical usage. Choice D is incorrect because the typical job of a soldier is not *flying.* Choice E is incorrect because *achieve* is not typical usage with the word *soldier.*

5. **The correct answer is B.** This is a person/worker-to-place analogy. A *captain* serves on a *vessel,* or ship, and a *director* serves on a *board.* Choice A is incorrect because a *football team* is led by a coach. Choice C is incorrect because a *cheerleader squad* is led by a captain. Choice D is incorrect because an *orchestra* has a conductor, not a director. Choice E is incorrect because a *musician* is not a director.

6. **The correct answer is D.** This is a category-to-example relationship. Having a *daughter* (or son) makes a man a *father,* and having a *niece* (or nephew) makes a man an *uncle.* Choices A and B are incorrect because having a *son* or a *daughter* would make a man a father, not an uncle. Choice C is incorrect because a *son-in-law* has no bearing on whether a man is an uncle, and neither does having an *aunt* (choice E).

7. **The correct answer is E.** Pull the *trigger* and the *pistol* fires; turn the *switch* and the *motor* starts in this object-to-action analogy. Choices A, B, and C are incorrect because *wire, dynamo,* and *amperes* may all relate to some aspect of motors, but they are not what turns it on. Choice D is incorrect because *barrel* relates to a gun, not a motor.

8. **The correct answer is D.** This is a characteristic analogy. A *cube* is a three-dimensional figure based on a *square.* A *pyramid* is a three-dimensional figure based on a *triangle.* Choices A and B are incorrect because both a *box* and a *solid*

are three-dimensional figures, but you are looking for a two-dimensional figure. Choice C is incorrect because even though a *pentagon* is a two-dimensional figure, it is not the base for a pyramid. Choice E is incorrect because a *cylinder* is a three-dimensional figure based on a circle.

9. **The correct answer is C.** In this cause-and-effect analogy, *profit* is the end product of *selling* and *fame* is the end product, or result, of *publicity*. Choice A is incorrect because *buying* refers to the first pair in the analogy, not to *fame*. Choice B is incorrect because *cheating* has no relation to the analogy. Choices D and E are incorrect because *praying* and *loving* have no relation to the analogy.

10. **The correct answer is B.** In this action-to-object relationship, a *book* is *printed* and a *tank* is *welded*. *Door*, *chair*, and *pencil* (choices A, C, and E) have no relation to welding and are, therefore, incorrect. Choice D may tempt you, but if you think about it, *wires* aren't welded.

11. **The correct answer is D.** This is a cause-and-effect analogy. The end product or result of going to the *gym* is being *healthy* and the end product of going to *school* is gaining *knowledge*. Choice A is incorrect because *sick* has no relation to *school*. Choices B, C, and E are incorrect because, although they may relate to school, they are not the desired end product.

12. **The correct answer is C.** This is a straightforward antonym analogy. The opposite of *right* is *wrong*, and the opposite of *success* is *failure*. *Aid*, *profit*, and *gain* (choices A, B, and E) are incorrect because they are somewhat similar in meaning to *success*. Choice D is incorrect because *error* is a synonym of *wrong*, not an antonym for *success*.

13. **The correct answer is E.** This is a characteristic analogy. An *octagon* is an *eight-sided figure*, and a *heptagon* is a *seven-sided figure*. Knowledge of prefixes and geometry could help you answer this question. A *polygon* (choice A) is a closed two-dimensional figure composed of line segments that are not curved; therefore, a heptagon is a polygon, but *polygon* is not as specific as heptagon, so it doesn't fit in the analogy as well as heptagon. Choice B is incorrect because a *polyhedron* is a three-dimensional solid with many faces. A heptagon is not a polyhedron because it isn't three-dimensional. Choice C is incorrect because a *hexagon* has only six sides. Choice D is incorrect because a *quadrilateral* has four sides.

14. **The correct answer is A.** This is a grammatical analogy. An *idiom* is an *expression*, and a *paraphrase* is a *version* of a piece of writing or speech. Choice B is incorrect because a *translation* is typically a near restatement of a piece of writing or speech from one language to another, whereas a paraphrase expresses the same idea in different words in the same language. Choice C is incorrect because a paraphrase is not a *statement*, but a restatement. Choice D is incorrect because a *dialect* is a set of usages and pronunciations used by a particular group or region. Choice E is incorrect because *language* is too broad a term to fit with *paraphrase*.

15. **The correct answer is A.** This is an object-to-quality relationship. A *bottle* is *brittle*, or likely to break or snap, and a *tire* is flexible, or *elastic*. Choice B is incorrect because *scarce* has no relation to *tire*. Choice C is incorrect, although it might confuse you into choosing it. Tires are made of *rubber*, but that is not a quality of a tire, and neither is *spheroid*, choice D. Choice E is incorrect because, while a tire is part of an *automobile*, that is not a quality of a tire.

16. **The correct answer is C.** This is a person/worker-to-abstraction or quality relationship. A *soprano* has a *high* voice, and a *bass* has a *low* voice. *Violin, good, fish,* and *soft* do not relate to the voice of a bass singer. Don't be confused by choice D, which wants you to think that *bass* is pronounced with a short "a" and is the name of a fish.

17. **The correct answer is C.** This is a characteristic analogy. The sense of smell is characteristic of the *nose,* and *olfactory* relates to the sense of smell. The sense of touch is characteristic of the *finger,* and *tactile* relates to the sense of touch. Choice A is incorrect because *tacit* means "implied, understood, unspoken." *Bloody, handkerchief,* and *stomach* do not relate to a part of the body with the sense of touch.

18. **The correct answer is D.** In this object-to-quality analogy, the missing word refers to direction. A *street* is *horizontal,* and a *building* is *vertical.* While the words *tall, brick, broad,* and *large* may describe a building, these words do not relate to direction.

19. **The correct answer is B.** This is a synonym analogy. *Allegiance* and *loyalty* are synonyms, just as *treason* and *rebellion* are synonyms. Choice A is incorrect because *obedience* is the opposite of *rebellion.* Choice C is incorrect because, while treason may involve *murder,* murder doesn't necessarily involve treason, so it isn't a synonym for *treason.* For the same reason, choice D, *felony,* is not a synonym. Choice E is incorrect because *homage* means "honor, respect paid to someone."

20. **The correct answer is A.** In this association analogy, *paint* is used on a *canvas* and *clay* may be used in a *mold.* Choice B is incorrect because *cloth* has no relation to a mold. Choice C is incorrect because a *statue* may be the finished product of clay and a mold, but it doesn't fit the analogy. Paint is not a finished product of a canvas; a painting is. Choice D is incorrect because a clay figure may result in *art,* yet art is not an ingredient in a mold. Choice E is incorrect because *aesthetic* is the appreciation of art.

21. **The correct answer is A.** The initial pair sets up a synonym relationship. *Incessant* means "uninterrupted, unending, unceasing," so *ceaseless* is a synonym. Choices B and C are incorrect because *occasional* and *irregular* are antonyms for *incessant.* Choice D is incorrect because *brutal* has no relation to *incessant,* and neither has *concise,* choice E, meaning "brief, to the point."

22. **The correct answer is D.** This is a sequence relationship. A *conquest* leads to *ascendancy,* or control, on one side, and *defeat* on the other side leads to *subjugation,* or being controlled. Choice A is incorrect because *omission* has no relation to *defeat.* Choice B is incorrect because being defeated may be *frustrating,* but it's not a typical usage for the word. Choice C is incorrect because *censure* means "to strongly disapprove, criticize harshly." Choice E is incorrect because *mastery* means "having great skill, expertise."

23. **The correct answer is A.** The first pair of words sets up an action-to-object analogy. A *solution* ends a *mystery,* and *completion* ends a *puzzle.* Choices B, C, and D are incorrect because completing a *book, college,* or *school* has no element of problem solving to them that both a mystery and a puzzle have. Choice E is incorrect because a *detective* isn't completed, which is how the analogy is set up.

24. **The correct answer is E.** In this association analogy, an *alumnus,* a male graduate, and an *alumna,* a female graduate, are linked as

equals, and a *prince* and *princess* are linked because they belong to the same rank of royalty. Choice A is incorrect because a *castle* is a thing, and the answer requires a person. For the same reason *country* (choice D) is incorrect. Choice B is incorrect because a *king* is one rank above a prince; the answer also requires a woman. Choice C is incorrect because a *knight* is a man and is at a lower rank than a *prince*.

25. **The correct answer is B.** The first pair set up an antonym relationship. *Occult* means "hidden, not apparent to the senses, mysterious," whereas *overt* means "not hidden, able to be seen." Among the answer choices, only *outward* is the opposite of *secret*. Choice A is incorrect because *abstract* means "theoretical, difficult to understand." Choice C is incorrect because *science* has no relation to being secretive. Choice D is incorrect because *tarry* is "to delay." Choice E is incorrect because *concealed* is a synonym for *secret*, not an antonym.

Test 5: English Grammar and Usage

1. A	**4.** D	**7.** C	**10.** D	**13.** C
2. C	**5.** B	**8.** B	**11.** A	**14.** A
3. D	**6.** A	**9.** C	**12.** C	**15.** B

1. **The correct answer is A.** The indefinite pronoun *each* is third-person singular and thus requires in this sentence a third-person singular verb form (*has*) and third-person singular possessive pronoun (*its*). This makes choices C and D incorrect because they feature a third-person plural verb form (*have*). Choice C is additionally incorrect because a third-person plural possessive pronoun (*their*) is used. Choice D is additionally incorrect because the contraction *they're* is incorrectly used rather than a possessive pronoun. Choice B is incorrect for the same reason; the contraction *it's* is used instead of the possessive pronoun *its*.

2. **The correct answer is C.** *Neither* functions in this sentence as a correlative conjunction joining the words *Tillie* and *Maxine*, which serve as the compound subject. As a correlative conjunction, *neither* is always paired with *nor*. This allows us to rule out choices A and B as correct answers. Singular subjects joined by *or* or *nor* take a singular verb, which allows us to rule out choice D as a correct answer.

3. **The correct answer is D.** *Was* is a linking verb and therefore calls for a predicate nominative in this sentence rather than a direct object. As predicate nominatives, as their name implies, are in the nominative case, the correct choice for the first blank is *I*, which allows us to rule out choices B and C. *Behind* is a preposition, and therefore the word needed in the second blank is an object of the preposition, which, as its name implies, must be in the objective case. Therefore, choice A is incorrect.

4. **The correct answer is D.** In this sentence, the act of choosing occurred in the past before another past event, which was the sending of the proposal. This means that the past perfect tense of the verb *choose* is needed, which is *had chosen*. Choice A is incorrect because *chose* is in the past tense, not the past perfect tense. Choices B and C are incorrect because the past participle (the form of a verb that is used together with *had* to express the past perfect tense) of *choose* (an irregular verb) is *chosen*, not *chose* or *choosed*.

5. **The correct answer is B.** In this sentence, Hector's singing at more than 100 concerts occurs in the future before another future event, which is the end of the year. This means that the future perfect tense is needed, which is formed by using *will have* plus the past participle of the verb in question. The past participle of *sing* (an irregular verb) is *sung*.

6. **The correct answer is A.** In this sentence, *fast* modifies the verb *drive* and thus is an adverb. Fast can also function as an adjective (e.g., a *fast* car), a verb (e.g., *to fast* [go without food] before having blood drawn), and even a noun (e.g., an overnight *fast*), but none of these is its role in this sentence. *Fast* cannot function as a preposition.

7. **The correct answer is C.** When comparing three or more items, use the superlative form of an adjective or adverb. In this

sentence, a form of the adjective *lame* modifies a noun, the Endoplasmic Reticulum, in the context of comparing three different bands, and thus its superlative form should be used. The superlative form of *lame* is *lamest*.

8. **The correct answer is B.** A form of the word *rapid* modifies the word *rebuild* in this sentence. Because *rebuild* is a verb, the adverb form of *rapid* is needed, which is *rapidly*. Choice D is incorrect because it is the adjective form. Also, the subject, *Gabriella*, is being compared with the indefinite pronoun *anyone*, which is singular. Because just two items, essentially, are being compared, the comparative form of *rapidly* should be used. This allows us to rule out choice A, which is the superlative form. Adverbs usually form their comparatives by using *more* plus the adverb, so the correct answer is *more rapidly*.

9. **The correct answer is C.** Choice C shows two independent clauses joined properly by a comma followed by a coordinating conjunction. Choice A is incorrect because neither clause is independent (each lacks a verb, because a participle, such as *rolling* or *rocking*, does not constitute a verb when used alone) and thus the sentence as a whole is incomplete. Choice B is incorrect because the two independent clauses are improperly joined by a comma alone, an error known as a "comma splice." Choice D is incorrect because the two independent clauses have no coordinating conjunction or punctuation and thus are improperly joined.

10. **The correct answer is D.** The first word in a sentence and all proper nouns (names of particular people or places) should be capitalized, as in choice D. Choice A is incorrect because the first word in the sentence (*their*) is not capitalized. Choice

B is incorrect because the proper names *Sebastian* and *Marie* are not capitalized. Choice C is incorrect because the common noun *southern* is capitalized.

11. **The correct answer is A.** A direct quotation is set off from the rest of the sentence with a comma or commas, the first word of a direct quotation is capitalized, and a question mark that applies only to the direct quotation, not the sentence as a whole, should be placed inside the closing quotation mark, as shown in choice A. Choice B is incorrect because a comma is needed after *said* to set off the direct quotation from the rest of the sentence. Choice C is incorrect because the first word in the direct quotation, *are*, should be capitalized. Choice D is incorrect because the question mark, which applies only to the direct quotation, is placed outside of the closing quotation mark.

12. **The correct answer is C.** In a sentence that directly addresses someone, the person's name should be set off by commas from the rest of the sentence as shown in choice C. In addition, two or more adjectives preceding a noun should be separated by a comma, also shown in choice C. Choice A is incorrect because the direct address to Alex is not set off from the rest of the sentence by commas. Choice B is incorrect because another comma, following Alex, is needed to set off the direct address. Choice D is incorrect because a comma is needed to separate the two adjectives preceding *guy*, which are *funny* and *smart*.

13. **The correct answer is C.** The first independent clause in this sentence builds the expectation for what will be conveyed in the second part; thus a colon, which is used to mean "note what follows," is the most appropriate choice. Choice A is incorrect because, although a semicolon would be

grammatically correct, it is not the most appropriate choice. Choice B is incorrect because a comma may not join two independent clauses (comma splice). Choice D is incorrect because a period may not join two independent clauses. If the *he* immediately following the blank were capitalized, indicating two separate sentences, then the period would be correct.

14. **The correct answer is A.** When any item in a series contains within it one or more commas, semicolons should be used to separate all items in the series, to avoid confusion. Choices B and C are incorrect because only semicolons may be used to separate the items in this series, as one of the items contains commas within it. Choice D is incorrect because neither the comma nor the dash is appropriate for separating items in this series.

15. **The correct answer is B.** In this sentence, the subject and verb are missing in the second independent clause. Therefore, the contraction *they're*, which supplies both, is the correct answer. Choice A is incorrect because in contractions the apostrophe should appear where the missing letter or letters should be. The missing letter in the contraction *they're*, which stands for *they are*, is the *a* in *are*; thus, the apostrophe should appear between *y* and *r*, not between *r* and *e*. Choice C is incorrect because *their* is the third-person plural possessive pronoun and does not make sense here. Choice D is incorrect because *there* is an adverb and does not make sense here.

Test 6: Spelling

1. B	4. A	7. C	10. B	13. A
2. C	5. B	8. A	11. B	14. C
3. C	6. B	9. C	12. A	15. B

1. **The correct answer is B.** The correct spelling is *aphasia*.

2. **The correct answer is C.** The correct spelling is *auscultation*.

3. **The correct answer is C.** The correct spelling is *believe*.

4. **The correct answer is A.** The correct spelling is *catheterization*.

5. **The correct answer is B.** The correct spelling is *definite*.

6. **The correct answer is B.** The correct spelling is *elicit*.

7. **The correct answer is C.** The correct spelling is *hygiene*.

8. **The correct answer is A.** The correct spelling is *immediately*.

9. **The correct answer is C.** The correct spelling is *license*.

10. **The correct answer is B.** The correct spelling is *occurrence*.

11. **The correct answer is B.** The correct spelling is *perfusion*.

12. **The correct answer is A.** The correct spelling is *rhythm*.

13. **The correct answer is A.** The correct spelling is *symmetry*.

14. **The correct answer is C.** The correct spelling is *trachea*.

15. **The correct answer is B.** The correct spelling is *weird*.

Test 7: Nonverbal Ability

1. C	4. B	7. D	10. A	13. E
2. B	5. A	8. C	11. C	14. D
3. A	6. E	9. B	12. E	15. A

1. **The correct answer is C.** The relationship between the first two shapes is that they are both squares but the first is black whereas the second is white. So, in the second pair, we begin with a black triangle and are looking for a white triangle. Therefore, black square is to white square as black triangle is to white triangle.

2. **The correct answer is B.** The relationship between the first two shapes is that they are both rectangles but the second is rotated 90 degrees to either the left or the right in relation to the first. So, in the second pair, we begin with a triangle pointing up and are looking for a triangle rotated 90 degrees to either the left or the right. Answers B and E are the only options that show the triangle rotated 90 degrees in either direction. Because there is no change in color in the first two shapes, the white triangle in choice B is correct.

3. **The correct answer is A.** The relationship between the first two shapes is that they are both white circles but the first has a smaller black circle embedded within it and the second doesn't. So, in the second pair, we begin with a white diamond with a smaller black diamond embedded within it and are looking for a plain white diamond. Therefore, white circle with a smaller black circle embedded within it is to white circle as white diamond with a smaller black diamond embedded within it is to white diamond.

4. **The correct answer is B.** The relationship between the first two shapes is that the second is the mirror image of the first. So,

in the second pair, we begin with a black U pointing left and are looking for its mirror image, which is a black U pointing right. Therefore, open black rectangle pointing left is to open black rectangle pointing right as black U pointing left is to black U pointing right.

5. **The correct answer is A.** The relationship between the first two shapes is that the first is the upper right portion of the second. So, in the second pair, we begin with an upper right quadrant circular arc and are looking for the whole shape of which it is a part, which is a circle. Therefore, upper right square corner is to square as upper right quadrant circular arc is to circle.

6. **The correct answer is E.** The relationship between the first two shapes is that they are both circles bisected by two line segments perpendicular to one another but the second is rotated 45 degrees to the right or left in relation to the first. So, in the second pair, we begin with a circle bisected by one diagonal line segment and are looking for a circle similarly bisected but rotated 45 degrees to the right or left in relation to the first. The most appropriate choice is a circle bisected by one horizontal line segment (choice E). You might be tempted to choose choice A, but note that it is rotated 90 degrees to the right or left of the first circle in this pair.

7. **The correct answer is D.** The relationship between the first two shapes is the first is the lower half of the second. So, in the second pair, we begin with a lower half circular arc and are looking for the whole

circle of which it is a part, which is a white circle. Therefore, lower half of black square with circumscribed white ring is to black square with circumscribed white ring as lower half circular arc is to white circle.

8. **The correct answer is C.** The relationship between the first two shapes is that they are both horizontal white parallelograms (quadrilaterals with two pairs of parallel sides), but the first is a rhomboid (a parallelogram with unequal adjacent sides and without right angles) and the second is a rectangle (a parallelogram with four right angles) with unequal adjacent sides. So, in the second pair, we begin with a horizontal black rhomboid and are looking for a horizontal black rectangle with unequal adjacent sides. Only choice C is a horizontal black rectangle with unequal adjacent sides. Choice A is incorrect because it is a square (a parallelogram with all equal sides and right angles). Choice B is incorrect because it is a vertical white rectangle with unequal adjacent sides. Choice D is incorrect because it is a white diamond (a parallelogram with all equal sides but without right angles). While choice E is a rather tempting choice, it is incorrect because it is a *vertical* black rectangle with unequal adjacent sides.

9. **The correct answer is B.** The relationship between the first two shapes is that the first has one more side than the second. So, in the second pair, we begin with a square, which has four sides, and are looking for a shape with one less side, or three sides, which is a triangle. Therefore, hexagon is to pentagon as square is to triangle.

10. **The correct answer is A.** The relationship between the first two shapes is that the first is the negative image, or total inversion, of the second. So, in the second pair, we begin with a negative image of a white circle and

are looking for a white circle. Therefore, negative image of black circle is to black circle as negative image of white circle is to white circle.

11. **The correct answer is C.** The relationship between the first two shapes is that they are both white triangles pointing up but the first is larger than the second. So, in the second pair, we begin with a large black triangle pointing up and are looking for a small black triangle pointing up. Large white triangle is to small white triangle as large black triangle is to small black triangle.

12. **The correct answer is E.** The relationship between the first two shapes is that the second is the same as the first except that it doesn't have vertical stripes. So, in the second pair, we begin with a square with vertical stripes and are looking for a plain square. Therefore, circle with vertical stripes is to circle as square with vertical stripes is to square.

13. **The correct answer is E.** The first set of shapes consists of an open hourglass pointing right and an open hourglass pointing left. The second set of shapes consists of an open hourglass pointing left and an open hourglass pointing right. The third set of shapes consists of a line segment connecting a black circle to a white circle and a line segment connecting a white circle to a black circle. Choice E is the most appropriate answer because it consists of a line segment connecting a white circle to a black circle and a line segment connecting a black circle to a white circle. The relationship between the first two pairs of shapes is that both contain an object and its mirror image, but in the second pair, the objects from the first pair have each been rotated 180 degrees. So, in the second pair, we begin with the line segment connecting

a black circle to a white circle and a line segment connecting a white circle to a black circle and are looking for a line segment connecting a white circle to a black circle and a line segment connecting a black circle to a white circle.

14. **The correct answer is D.** The relationship between the first two images is that both contain a V and a circle, but in the second image, the circle has moved out of and to the left of the V and has grown larger and the V has rotated 90 degrees to the right. So, in the second pair, we begin with a U pointed up with a small plus sign embedded within it and are looking for a large plus sign to the left of a U that has rotated 90 degrees to the right. Therefore, V pointed right with small circle embedded within it is to large circle and V pointed down as U pointed up with small plus sign embedded within it is to large plus sign and U pointed right (choice D). You might be tempted to choose choice B because it resembles the second image in the first pair, but this would mean that the U had rotated 180 degrees from its original position rather than 90 degrees. Remember that it is the *relationships* you are attempting to match, not necessarily the appearance of the images.

15. **The correct answer is A.** Multiplication sign surrounded by four dots that form a diamond is to four dots that form a diamond as plus sign surrounded by four dots that form a square is to four dots that form a square. The relationship between the first two images is that the second is the same as first except it has no multiplication sign. So, in the second pair, we begin with a plus sign surrounded by four dots that form a square and are looking for the same image except without the plus sign, which is four dots that form a square (choice A).

LET'S PUT YOU TO THE TEST

Now that you have thoroughly reviewed the various kinds of verbal ability items and are familiar with the test-taking strategies associated with them, let's put you to the test.

Pay strict attention to the time allotted for each section of the test and do your best to adhere to these time limits. Read the directions for each part of the test before attempting to answer any of the questions.

This test has six parts: A—Synonyms; B—Antonyms; C—Verbal Analogies; D—English Grammar and Usage; E—Spelling; F—Nonverbal Ability. The total time allotted for this test is 70 minutes. Have extra pencils available in case of point breakage, so as not to lose testing time.

Answer Keys and Explanations are provided at the end of the test so that you can evaluate your performance. Remember, this is a simulation of the "real thing," so be honest with yourself and look at the answer keys and explanations only after you have completed the test.

FINAL VERBAL AND NONVERBAL ABILITY EXAMINATION ANSWER SHEET

Part A: Synonyms

1. Ⓐ Ⓑ Ⓒ Ⓓ   8. Ⓐ Ⓑ Ⓒ Ⓓ   15. Ⓐ Ⓑ Ⓒ Ⓓ   22. Ⓐ Ⓑ Ⓒ Ⓓ   29. Ⓐ Ⓑ Ⓒ Ⓓ
2. Ⓐ Ⓑ Ⓒ Ⓓ   9. Ⓐ Ⓑ Ⓒ Ⓓ   16. Ⓐ Ⓑ Ⓒ Ⓓ   23. Ⓐ Ⓑ Ⓒ Ⓓ   30. Ⓐ Ⓑ Ⓒ Ⓓ
3. Ⓐ Ⓑ Ⓒ Ⓓ   10. Ⓐ Ⓑ Ⓒ Ⓓ   17. Ⓐ Ⓑ Ⓒ Ⓓ   24. Ⓐ Ⓑ Ⓒ Ⓓ   31. Ⓐ Ⓑ Ⓒ Ⓓ
4. Ⓐ Ⓑ Ⓒ Ⓓ   11. Ⓐ Ⓑ Ⓒ Ⓓ   18. Ⓐ Ⓑ Ⓒ Ⓓ   25. Ⓐ Ⓑ Ⓒ Ⓓ   32. Ⓐ Ⓑ Ⓒ Ⓓ
5. Ⓐ Ⓑ Ⓒ Ⓓ   12. Ⓐ Ⓑ Ⓒ Ⓓ   19. Ⓐ Ⓑ Ⓒ Ⓓ   26. Ⓐ Ⓑ Ⓒ Ⓓ   33. Ⓐ Ⓑ Ⓒ Ⓓ
6. Ⓐ Ⓑ Ⓒ Ⓓ   13. Ⓐ Ⓑ Ⓒ Ⓓ   20. Ⓐ Ⓑ Ⓒ Ⓓ   27. Ⓐ Ⓑ Ⓒ Ⓓ   34. Ⓐ Ⓑ Ⓒ Ⓓ
7. Ⓐ Ⓑ Ⓒ Ⓓ   14. Ⓐ Ⓑ Ⓒ Ⓓ   21. Ⓐ Ⓑ Ⓒ Ⓓ   28. Ⓐ Ⓑ Ⓒ Ⓓ   35. Ⓐ Ⓑ Ⓒ Ⓓ

Part B: Antonyms

1. Ⓐ Ⓑ Ⓒ Ⓓ   9. Ⓐ Ⓑ Ⓒ Ⓓ   17. Ⓐ Ⓑ Ⓒ Ⓓ   25. Ⓐ Ⓑ Ⓒ Ⓓ   33. Ⓐ Ⓑ Ⓒ Ⓓ Ⓔ
2. Ⓐ Ⓑ Ⓒ Ⓓ   10. Ⓐ Ⓑ Ⓒ Ⓓ   18. Ⓐ Ⓑ Ⓒ Ⓓ   26. Ⓐ Ⓑ Ⓒ Ⓓ   34. Ⓐ Ⓑ Ⓒ Ⓓ Ⓔ
3. Ⓐ Ⓑ Ⓒ Ⓓ   11. Ⓐ Ⓑ Ⓒ Ⓓ   19. Ⓐ Ⓑ Ⓒ Ⓓ   27. Ⓐ Ⓑ Ⓒ Ⓓ   35. Ⓐ Ⓑ Ⓒ Ⓓ Ⓔ
4. Ⓐ Ⓑ Ⓒ Ⓓ   12. Ⓐ Ⓑ Ⓒ Ⓓ   20. Ⓐ Ⓑ Ⓒ Ⓓ   28. Ⓐ Ⓑ Ⓒ Ⓓ   36. Ⓐ Ⓑ Ⓒ Ⓓ Ⓔ
5. Ⓐ Ⓑ Ⓒ Ⓓ   13. Ⓐ Ⓑ Ⓒ Ⓓ   21. Ⓐ Ⓑ Ⓒ Ⓓ   29. Ⓐ Ⓑ Ⓒ Ⓓ   37. Ⓐ Ⓑ Ⓒ Ⓓ Ⓔ
6. Ⓐ Ⓑ Ⓒ Ⓓ   14. Ⓐ Ⓑ Ⓒ Ⓓ   22. Ⓐ Ⓑ Ⓒ Ⓓ   30. Ⓐ Ⓑ Ⓒ Ⓓ   38. Ⓐ Ⓑ Ⓒ Ⓓ Ⓔ
7. Ⓐ Ⓑ Ⓒ Ⓓ   15. Ⓐ Ⓑ Ⓒ Ⓓ   23. Ⓐ Ⓑ Ⓒ Ⓓ   31. Ⓐ Ⓑ Ⓒ Ⓓ Ⓔ   39. Ⓐ Ⓑ Ⓒ Ⓓ Ⓔ
8. Ⓐ Ⓑ Ⓒ Ⓓ   16. Ⓐ Ⓑ Ⓒ Ⓓ   24. Ⓐ Ⓑ Ⓒ Ⓓ   32. Ⓐ Ⓑ Ⓒ Ⓓ Ⓔ   40. Ⓐ Ⓑ Ⓒ Ⓓ Ⓔ

Part C: Verbal Analogies

1. Ⓐ Ⓑ Ⓒ Ⓓ   6. Ⓐ Ⓑ Ⓒ Ⓓ   11. Ⓐ Ⓑ Ⓒ Ⓓ   16. Ⓐ Ⓑ Ⓒ Ⓓ   21. Ⓐ Ⓑ Ⓒ Ⓓ
2. Ⓐ Ⓑ Ⓒ Ⓓ   7. Ⓐ Ⓑ Ⓒ Ⓓ   12. Ⓐ Ⓑ Ⓒ Ⓓ   17. Ⓐ Ⓑ Ⓒ Ⓓ   22. Ⓐ Ⓑ Ⓒ Ⓓ
3. Ⓐ Ⓑ Ⓒ Ⓓ   8. Ⓐ Ⓑ Ⓒ Ⓓ   13. Ⓐ Ⓑ Ⓒ Ⓓ   18. Ⓐ Ⓑ Ⓒ Ⓓ   23. Ⓐ Ⓑ Ⓒ Ⓓ
4. Ⓐ Ⓑ Ⓒ Ⓓ   9. Ⓐ Ⓑ Ⓒ Ⓓ   14. Ⓐ Ⓑ Ⓒ Ⓓ   19. Ⓐ Ⓑ Ⓒ Ⓓ   24. Ⓐ Ⓑ Ⓒ Ⓓ
5. Ⓐ Ⓑ Ⓒ Ⓓ   10. Ⓐ Ⓑ Ⓒ Ⓓ   15. Ⓐ Ⓑ Ⓒ Ⓓ   20. Ⓐ Ⓑ Ⓒ Ⓓ   25. Ⓐ Ⓑ Ⓒ Ⓓ

Part D: English Grammar and Usage

1. Ⓐ Ⓑ Ⓒ Ⓓ   3. Ⓐ Ⓑ Ⓒ Ⓓ   5. Ⓐ Ⓑ Ⓒ Ⓓ   7. Ⓐ Ⓑ Ⓒ Ⓓ   9. Ⓐ Ⓑ Ⓒ Ⓓ
2. Ⓐ Ⓑ Ⓒ Ⓓ   4. Ⓐ Ⓑ Ⓒ Ⓓ   6. Ⓐ Ⓑ Ⓒ Ⓓ   8. Ⓐ Ⓑ Ⓒ Ⓓ   10. Ⓐ Ⓑ Ⓒ Ⓓ

Part E: Spelling

1. Ⓐ Ⓑ Ⓒ   3. Ⓐ Ⓑ Ⓒ   5. Ⓐ Ⓑ Ⓒ   7. Ⓐ Ⓑ Ⓒ   9. Ⓐ Ⓑ Ⓒ

2. Ⓐ Ⓑ Ⓒ   4. Ⓐ Ⓑ Ⓒ   6. Ⓐ Ⓑ Ⓒ   8. Ⓐ Ⓑ Ⓒ   10. Ⓐ Ⓑ Ⓒ

Part F: Nonverbal Ability

1. Ⓐ Ⓑ Ⓒ Ⓓ Ⓔ   3. Ⓐ Ⓑ Ⓒ Ⓓ Ⓔ   5. Ⓐ Ⓑ Ⓒ Ⓓ Ⓔ   7. Ⓐ Ⓑ Ⓒ Ⓓ Ⓔ   9. Ⓐ Ⓑ Ⓒ Ⓓ Ⓔ

2. Ⓐ Ⓑ Ⓒ Ⓓ Ⓔ   4. Ⓐ Ⓑ Ⓒ Ⓓ Ⓔ   6. Ⓐ Ⓑ Ⓒ Ⓓ Ⓔ   8. Ⓐ Ⓑ Ⓒ Ⓓ Ⓔ   10. Ⓐ Ⓑ Ⓒ Ⓓ Ⓔ

FINAL VERBAL AND NONVERBAL ABILITY EXAMINATION

130 Questions • 70 Minutes

Part A: Synonyms

35 Questions • 20 Minutes

Directions: In each of the sentences below, one word is in italics. Following each sentence are four words or phrases. For each sentence, select the word or phrase that best corresponds in meaning to the italicized word.

1. The chart *classifies* these organisms.
   - A. fuses
   - B. categorizes
   - C. controls
   - D. camouflages

2. On many teams, a player may face a *penalty* for irresponsible or unruly behavior.
   - A. arrangement
   - B. gratification
   - C. punishment
   - D. precaution

3. He used the *allotted* study time to complete his assignments.
   - A. authorized
   - B. designated
   - C. agreed
   - D. alerted

4. In examining the patient, the doctor noted his *pallor*.
   - A. paleness
   - B. ruddiness
   - C. fever
   - D. rigidity

5. It was apparent that he had attempted to *concoct* an alibi.
   - A. inculcate
   - B. conceal
   - C. reveal
   - D. fabricate

6. The City Council *sanctioned* as a responsible option the hiring of an outside firm to oversee the health department.
   - A. positioned
   - B. appeased
   - C. rejected
   - D. approved

7. The claim was *substantiated* by the evidence offered by the attorney.
   - A. repealed
   - B. ineffective
   - C. applied
   - D. supported

8. The soldiers retreated to a position of *comparative* safety.
   - A. objective
   - B. relative
   - C. subjective
   - D. scientific

9. Geologists *assure* us that our Earth is a few billion years old.
   A. guarantee
   B. instruct
   C. deny
   D. assail

10. It has been said that he is a *connoisseur* of fine wines.
    A. expert on
    B. taster of
    C. procurer of
    D. vendor of

11. He *spurned* the offer to run for office after the party's first three choices declined.
    A. accepted
    B. extolled
    C. acclaimed
    D. rejected

12. The well-dressed gentleman bowed *ceremoniously*.
    A. without ritual
    B. disrespectfully
    C. serenely
    D. formally

13. His diet was marked by *inordinate* amounts of carbohydrates and fats.
    A. redundant
    B. excessive
    C. reasonable
    D. exuberant

14. The annual parade *traversed* this magnificent city from the east to the west side.
    A. was patronized
    B. extended
    C. crossed
    D. augmented

15. *Enraptured* by the beauty of the mountains, they had not spoken for 20 minutes.
    A. summoned
    B. impeded
    C. exonerated
    D. entranced

16. The results of the experiment upheld the *contention* of those who supported the hypothesis.
    A. realization
    B. contiguity
    C. argument
    D. exhilaration

17. The *consensus* of the group was that the lawsuit had no merit.
    A. stipulation
    B. regulation
    C. conviction
    D. collective opinion

18. Arthritis is a *chronic* disease that results from a faulty immune system.
    A. long-lasting
    B. serious
    C. contagious
    D. infectious

19. Mayan magnificence *abounds* in the small resort village of Kailuum.
    A. is remote
    B. is abundant
    C. is significant
    D. is inadequate

20. As enthusiasm for the project *waxed* under the direction of a newly appointed administrator, the level of excitement
    A. stirred.
    B. waned.
    C. vanished.
    D. increased.

21. The conversation was *void* of intellectual stimuli.
    A. composed
    B. in excess
    C. empty
    D. full

22. The injuries sustained resulted in paralysis in two of the four *appendages*.
    A. chambers
    B. muscles
    C. limbs
    D. tubes

23. Security was *risked* to attain maximum career satisfaction.
    A. ventured
    B. squandered
    C. exhausted
    D. wasted

24. The fruit was *pared* and sliced for the salad.
    A. divided
    B. rinsed
    C. peeled
    D. sectioned

25. The hospital reorganization was an *initiative* of the new board chair.
    A. enterprise
    B. energy
    C. zeal
    D. leadership

26. The introduction *delineates* the book's content and format.
    A. discredits
    B. describes
    C. disproves
    D. endorses

27. The X-ray clearly showed the torn *cartilage* in the knee.
    A. tissue
    B. ligament
    C. tendon
    D. membrane

28. The receptionist *confirmed* the appointment.
    A. canceled
    B. rescheduled
    C. verified
    D. recorded

29. Her license was *invalidated* because she made a misstatement on her application.
    A. authorized
    B. canceled
    C. contradicted
    D. modified

30. If the engine was *malfunctioning* at the time, it was
    A. operative.
    B. operating incorrectly.
    C. firing.
    D. igniting.

31. The clients were shocked at the *fraudulent* practices of the contractors.
    A. thorough
    B. extensive
    C. legal
    D. deceitful

32. The employer questioned the *competence* of his staff. The employer was not sure about their
    A. honesty.
    B. punctuality.
    C. credibility.
    D. ability.

33. The reading list included an *anthology* by a famous author.
    A. collection of literary selections
    B. annotated bibliography
    C. archaeological study
    D. autobiography

34. Some bacteria are *mobile* because of their flagellum.
    A. movement
    B. deadly
    C. migratory
    D. motile

35. He smiled *wryly*.
    A. deceptively
    B. nastily
    C. ironically
    D. delightedly

Part B: Antonyms

40 Questions • 15 Minutes

Directions: For each of the following test items, select the word that is opposite in meaning to the term printed in capital letters.

1. IMPERIOUS
   A. submissive
   B. valuable
   C. pointed
   D. positive

2. CAPRICIOUS
   A. whimsical
   B. judicious
   C. steadfast
   D. tranquil

3. CANTANKEROUS
   A. pleasant
   B. dubious
   C. effective
   D. awkward

4. FORBEARANCE
   A. indulgence
   B. pliancy
   C. politeness
   D. impatience

5. HAPHAZARD
   A. inefficient
   B. premeditated
   C. unsatisfactory
   D. blundering

6. The *efficacy* of the procedure was in doubt until the study was completed.
   A. ineffectiveness
   B. efficiency
   C. value
   D. success

7. CHIMERICAL
   A. philosophical
   B. elite
   C. factual
   D. unimpressive

8. REPRESS
   A. reserve
   B. liberate
   C. thrust
   D. precipitate

9. ABOMINABLE
   A. agreeable
   B. loathsome
   C. sufficient
   D. degrading

10. UNETHICAL
    A. vulgar
    B. feasible
    C. pompous
    D. scrupulous

11. ANTECEDENT
    A. previous
    B. subsequent
    C. foregoing
    D. propitious

12. PONDEROUS
    A. delicate
    B. potent
    C. supportive
    D. massive

13. SUPPLICATION
    A. worship
    B. compassion
    C. entreaty
    D. disdain

14. POSITIVE
    A. negative
    B. sensitive
    C. diplomatic
    D. popular

15. RENEGADE
    A. constant
    B. extricate
    C. loyal
    D. heretical

16. DISREGARD
    A. disown
    B. attend to
    C. revoke
    D. recover

17. WRATH
    A. delight
    B. travail
    C. frivolity
    D. detriment

18. TEDIOUS
    A. ungainly
    B. imperative
    C. stimulating
    D. suitable

19. EMBODY
    A. impel
    B. fuse
    C. dissociate
    D. collect

20. DEFERRABLE
    A. urgent
    B. furtive
    C. inclined
    D. deniable

21. HOMOGENOUS
    A. invariable
    B. homosexual
    C. importunate
    D. heterogeneous

22. ADHERENT
    A. disciple
    B. repudiator
    C. soothsayer
    D. hypocrite

23. CRUDE
    A. barbarous
    B. refined
    C. obscure
    D. covetous

24. IRRATIONAL
    A. cynical
    B. sharp
    C. prevalent
    D. sensible

25. GRAPHIC
    A. vague
    B. illustrative
    C. forcible
    D. glacial

26. DEVASTATE
    A. tolerate
    B. obstruct
    C. renovate
    D. promote

27. STRINGENT
    A. exacting
    B. tough
    C. influential
    D. flexible

28. ACQUIESCE
    A. contest
    B. invest
    C. dismiss
    D. supply

29. BREVITY
    A. abbreviation
    B. lengthy
    C. ramification
    D. delusion

30. FLAUNT
    A. disavow
    B. conserve
    C. blight
    D. astonish

Directions: In the following sets of words, choose the word that is most different in meaning from the others.

31. A. cultivate
    B. restore
    C. stifle
    D. reinstate
    E. nurture

32. A. dilate
    B. distend
    C. augment
    D. constrict
    E. amplify

33. A. befitting
     B. suitable
     C. apropos
     D. inappropriate
     E. proper

34. A. coherent
     B. illogical
     C. rational
     D. reasonable
     E. sensible

35. A. paltry
     B. pathetic
     C. trifling
     D. underwhelming
     E. impressive

36. A. bucolic
     B. urban
     C. rural
     D. rustic
     E. agrarian

37. A. extravagant
     B. lavish
     C. prodigal
     D. frugal
     E. indulgent

38. A. leniency
     B. indulgence
     C. severity
     D. mercy
     E. permissiveness

39. A. manifest
     B. latent
     C. divulged
     D. glaring
     E. apparent

40. A. plebeian
     B. vulgar
     C. ignoble
     D. common
     E. patrician

Part C: Verbal Analogies

25 Questions • 15 Minutes

> **Directions:** In the following questions, determine the relationship between the first pair of capitalized words and then decide which of the choices share a similar relationship with the third capitalized word.

1. CAT is to DOG as CUP is to
   A. knife
   B. coffee
   C. saucer
   D. cream

2. SALTY is to SALINE as SUGARY is to
   A. sweet
   B. stale
   C. bread
   D. insipid

3. FLANNEL is to WOOL as BRICK is to
   A. wood
   B. clay
   C. stone
   D. mortar

4. CONTEMPORARY is to PRESENT as FUTURE is to
   A. past
   B. posterior
   C. eventual
   D. ancient

5. MOON is to EARTH as EARTH is to
   A. space
   B. moon
   C. sky
   D. sun

6. ACUTE is to CHRONIC as INTENSE is to
   A. sardonic
   B. tonic
   C. persistent
   D. pretty

7. PEAK is to MOUNTAIN as FLOOR is to
   A. ceiling
   B. canyon
   C. river
   D. cliff

8. EAST is to WEST as NORTHWEST is to
   A. southeast
   B. southwest
   C. north
   D. northeast

9. GASOLINE is to PETROLEUM as SUGAR is to
   A. oil
   B. cane
   C. plant
   D. sweet

10. DEFERENCE is to RESPECT as CONTEMPT is to
    A. esteem
    B. capitulation
    C. discourtesy
    D. tendency

11. SLOPE is to INCLINE as PLANE is to
    A. dimensional
    B. flat
    C. square
    D. rectangular

12. EDGE is to CENTER as EFFUSIVE is to
    A. unemotional
    B. exuberant
    C. eclectic
    D. eccentricity

13. PROCRASTINATOR is to DELAY as MENTOR is to
    A. trusted
    B. teacher
    C. advice
    D. measure

14. SOPHISTICATION is to FINESSE as INEPTITUDE is to
    A. inefficiency
    B. artistry
    C. trickiness
    D. insatiability

15. CAPTAIN is to STEAMSHIP as PRINCIPAL is to
    A. interest
    B. school
    C. agent
    D. concern

16. DIME is to SILVER as PENNY is to
    A. mint
    B. copper
    C. currency
    D. value

17. REVERT is to REVERSION as SYMPATHIZE is to
    A. sympathetic
    B. symposium
    C. sympathy
    D. sympathizing

18. REGRESSIVE is to REGRESS as STERILE is to
    A. sterilization
    B. sterilize
    C. sterility
    D. sterilizer

19. DOWN is to UP as AGE is to
    A. year
    B. youth
    C. snow
    D. date

20. I is to MINE as MAN is to
    A. men
    B. man's
    C. his
    D. hers

21. DISLOYAL is to FAITHLESS as IMPERFECTION is to
    A. faithful
    B. depression
    C. foible
    D. decrepitude

22. NECKLACE is to PEARLS as CHAIN is to
    A. locket
    B. prisoner
    C. links
    D. clasp

23. DRIFT is to SNOW as DUNE is to
    A. hill
    B. rain
    C. sand
    D. hail

24. BANK is to DEPOSITS as HOSPITAL is to
    A. blood
    B. care
    C. surgery
    D. tests

25. SCHOONER is to VESSEL as PERSIMMON is to
    A. machine
    B. fruit
    C. engine
    D. vehicle

Part D: English Grammar and Usage

10 Questions • 5 Minutes

Directions: In the following questions, select the answer that completes the sentence in a grammatically correct manner or that represents the most grammatically correct of all options.

1. The rower, accompanied by three of her teammates, _____ into the coach's office to speak with _____.
    A. walk; her
    B. walks; her
    C. walk; she
    D. walks; she

2. Either Anna or the twins _____ on _____ way to pick _____ up.
    A. is; their; us
    B. is; her; we
    C. are; their; us
    D. are; their; we

3. By the time practice ended, we _____ over 100 laps in the pool.
    A. have swum
    B. have swam
    C. had swum
    D. had swam

4. Tomorrow, we _____ to the store to buy some tomatoes.
    A. went
    B. had gone
    C. will have gone
    D. will go

5. Identify the part of speech of the italicized word in the following sentence: This coffee tastes *delicious*.
    A. Conjunction
    B. Preposition
    C. Adverb
    D. Adjective

6. Of the two movies, which do you think is _____?
    A. better
    B. best
    C. more better
    D. more good

7. Which of the following sentences is grammatically correct?

    A. My car ran out of gas I had to walk 2 miles in the pouring rain to the nearest gas station, it was not fun.

    B. My car ran out of gas, I had to walk 2 miles in the pouring rain to the nearest gas station it was not fun.

    C. My car ran out of gas, and I had to walk 2 miles in the pouring rain to the nearest gas station; it was not fun.

    D. My car ran out of gas and I had to walk 2 miles in the pouring rain to the nearest gas station and it was not fun.

8. Which of the following sentences is grammatically correct?

    A. My favorite president is Abraham Lincoln; did you know he was born on February 12th, 1809, in Kentucky?

    B. My favorite President is Abraham Lincoln; did you know he was born on February 12th, 1809, in Kentucky?

    C. My favorite president is Abraham Lincoln; did you know he was born on february 12th, 1809, in Kentucky?

    D. My favorite president is Abraham Lincoln; did you know he was born on February 12th, 1809, in kentucky?

9. Candace is smart and diligent _____ therefore _____ she will do well on her entrance exam.

    A. , ;

    B. ; ,

    C. , :

    D. , ,

10. As we drove away, Amber's mother yelled at us, "Don't forget to fill up the gas tank _____

    A. "!

    B. !"

    C. !".

    D. !

Part E: Spelling

10 Questions • 5 Minutes

Directions: In the following sets of words, choose the word that is spelled correctly.

1. A. acommodate
    B. acomodate
    C. accommodate

2. A. assites
    B. ascites
    C. acites

3. A. basically
    B. basicly
    C. basickly

4. A. callace
    B. callus
    C. callice

5. A. diaphram
   B. diafram
   C. diaphragm

6. A. guarantee
   B. guerantee
   C. garantee

7. A. knowledge
   B. knowlege
   C. knowlage

8. A. paliative
   B. palliative
   C. pallative

9. A. sagital
   B. sagittal
   C. sajittol

10. A. vennus
    B. venis
    C. venous

Part F: Nonverbal Ability

10 Questions • 10 Minutes

Directions: In the following questions, determine the relationship between the first pair of shapes and then decide which of the answer choices shares a similar relationship with the third shape.

1. ⟋ is to ⟍ as ◣ is to?
   A. ◢
   B. ▲
   C. ▼
   D. ◤
   E. ▶

2. ✕ is to ⊗ as ✛ is to?
   A. ⊞
   B. ◯
   C. #
   D. ⊠
   E. ⊕

3. ✖ is to ✕ as ✛ is to?
   A. ✚
   B. +
   C. ⊠
   D. ✦
   E. ✕

4. ■ is to ▲ as ✚ is to?
   A. ●
   B. ▼
   C. ⋋
   D. ▶
   E. ⬟

5. ⬠ is to ⬟ as ▲ is to?
   A. ▼
   B. ◀
   C. ▶
   D. ◥
   E. ■

6. ◁ is to ▶ as ◀ is to?
   A. ▶
   B. ◁
   C. △
   D. ▷
   E. ▽

7. ▢ is to ▪ as ⬤ is to?
   A. ◉
   B. ◯
   C. ●
   D. •
   E. ▣

8. ◖ is to ◗ as ⌒ is to?
   A. ●
   B. ◉
   C. ▼
   D. ◆
   E. ◗

9. ◆ is to ◀ as ● is to?
   A. ◼
   B. ◖
   C. ◖
   D. ◖
   E. ◖

10. ◆ is to ◣ as ╫ is to?
    A. ∟
    B. Γ
    C. ⌐
    D. ⌐
    E. ╥

STOP

IF YOU FINISH BEFORE TIME IS CALLED, YOU MAY
CHECK YOUR WORK ON THIS SECTION ONLY. DO NOT
TURN TO ANY OTHER SECTION IN THE TEST.

FINAL ANSWER KEYS AND EXPLANATIONS

Part A: Synonyms

1. B	8. B	15. D	22. C	29. B
2. C	9. A	16. C	23. A	30. B
3. B	10. A	17. D	24. C	31. D
4. A	11. D	18. A	25. A	32. D
5. D	12. D	19. B	26. B	33. A
6. D	13. B	20. D	27. A	34. D
7. D	14. C	21. C	28. C	35. C

1. **The correct answer is B.** *Classify* and *categorize* both mean "sort, file, arrange by class or category." Choice A is incorrect because *fuse* means "to merge, to combine." Choice C is incorrect because *control* is not a synonym for *classify*. *Camouflage* (choice D) means "to conceal by using a disguise or color."

2. **The correct answer is C.** A *penalty* is a *punishment*. *Arrangement* (choice A) has no relation to *penalty*. Choice B is incorrect because *gratification* means "the state of being satisfied, satisfaction." Choice D is incorrect because *precaution* is not a synonym for *penalty*.

3. **The correct answer is B.** *Designated* means "allocated, assigned" and so is a synonym for *allotted*. Nothing indicates that someone gave the person permission to use his study time to do the assignment, so eliminate choice A. *Agreed* (choice C) can be eliminated because there is no indication that the person had *agreed* with someone to use the study time for the assignment. *Alerted* (choice D) makes no sense.

4. **The correct answer is A.** All of the answer choices make sense, but only *paleness* is an antonym for *pallor*. Choice B, *ruddiness*, means "flushed, reddish" and is an antonym for *pallor*.

5. **The correct answer is D.** *Concoct* means "to make up," and so does *fabricate*. Choice A, *inculcate*, means "to instill or drill something into someone's mind by forceful repetition" and doesn't make sense. The same goes for *conceal* (choice B) meaning "to hide." *Reveal* (choice C) might be tempting, but the word is not a synonym for *concoct*.

6. **The correct answer is D.** *Sanction* may mean "to approve" or it may mean "to penalize," though, as the latter, *sanction* is typically used in terms of legal activity, especially international law. In this case, it means "to approve," so choice D is correct. Choice A is incorrect because *position* has no relation to *sanction*, and neither does *appease* (choice B), meaning "to calm, to quiet." *Reject* (choice C) is incorrect because it is the opposite of *approve*, so it's an antonym.

7. **The correct answer is D.** To *substantiate* is "to *support*, to verify." Choice A is incorrect because *repeal* is used in reference to laws and legal orders, not evidence. Choice B is incorrect because the question requires a verb and *ineffective* is an adjective. Choice C is incorrect because *applied* is not a synonym and doesn't make sense in this sentence.

8. **The correct answer is B.** *Comparative* means "relating to, based on, or involving comparison," and one meaning of *relative* is "in comparison." Choices A, C, and D are incorrect because *objective*, *subjective*, and *scientific* have no relation to *comparative*.

9. **The correct answer is A.** To *assure* is "to promise or guarantee." Choice B is incorrect because, while *instruct* makes sense, it's not a synonym for *assure*, and neither is *deny* (choice C). Choice D is incorrect because *assail* means "to attack with words, to criticize."

10. **The correct answer is A.** A *connoisseur* is an *expert*. Choice B is incorrect because, while a connoisseur *tastes* wine, it's not a synonym, and neither is a *procurer* (choice C), meaning "a person who obtains things." Choice D is incorrect because *vendor*, or seller of goods and services, is not a synonym either.

11. **The correct answer is D.** To *spurn* is "to reject, to refuse, to decline." Choice A is incorrect because *accept* is the opposite of *spurn*. Choice B is incorrect because *extol* means "to praise," as does *acclaim* (choice C). If you're not sure about an answer, but two of the choices are similar in meaning, you can eliminate them both.

12. **The correct answer is D.** *Ceremoniously* means "formally, with ceremony and ritual." Choice A is incorrect because *without ritual* is the opposite of *ceremoniously*. Choice B is incorrect because *disrespectfully* is closer in meaning to that of an antonym for *ceremoniously* than a synonym. Choice C is incorrect because *serenely* may describe someone who is acting ceremoniously, but it is not a synonym.

13. **The correct answer is B.** *Inordinate* and *excessive* are synonyms. Choice A is incorrect because *redundant* means "more than is needed or required" or "repetitive." Choice C is incorrect because *reasonable* is the opposite of *inordinate*. Choice D is incorrect because *exuberant* is a synonym for *excessive*, depending on the context, but not for *inordinate*.

14. **The correct answer is C.** To *traverse* is "to cross." Choice A is incorrect because *patronized* makes no sense and is not a synonym for *traverse*, and neither is *extended* (choice B). Choice D is incorrect because *augment* means "to add to, to enlarge."

15. **The correct answer is D.** Pronunciation may make all the difference in finding the correct answer. *Entranced* doesn't mean "entered" in this context; it means "in a trance," that is, "delighted, enchanted." Choices A and B are incorrect because *summoned* and *impeded* are not synonyms for *enraptured*. Choice C is incorrect because *exonerated* means "freed from blame, accusation, or suspicion."

16. **The correct answer is C.** *Contention* and *argument*, meaning "a line of reasoning," are synonyms. Choice A is incorrect because *realization* is not a synonym for *contention*. Choice B is incorrect because *contiguity* means "being adjacent, being so near as to be touching." Choice D is incorrect because *exhilaration* means "feeling joyful."

17. **The correct answer is D.** *Consensus* is the same as a *collective opinion*. Choice A is incorrect because *stipulation* means "a condition, an agreement reached by contending parties." Choice B is incorrect because *regulation* has no relation to *consensus*. Choice C is incorrect because *conviction*, meaning "strong belief," is not a synonym for *consensus*.

18. **The correct answer is A.** A *chronic* disease is a *long-lasting* one. Choices B, C, and D are incorrect because, although each one—*serious, contagious, infectious*—refers to diseases, none is a synonym for *chronic*.

19. The correct answer is B. To *abound* is "to *be abundant*." Choice A is incorrect because *remote* means "far away, isolated." Choices C and D, *is significant* and *is inadequate*, are not synonyms for *abounds*.

20. The correct answer is D. To *wax* is "to *increase* in size, intensity, etc." Choice A is incorrect because, although *stirred* can mean "to excite strong feelings" and, therefore, may confuse you, it's not a synonym for *wax*. Choice B is incorrect because *wane* means "to decrease gradually in size, intensity, etc.," so it is an antonym of *waxed*. Choice C is incorrect because *vanished* means "to disappear."

21. The correct answer is C. Something that is *void* is *empty*. The other choices are antonyms for *void*.

22. The correct answer is C. An *appendage* is a body part that extends from the body, that is, not an internal part. Answer choices A, B, and D are internal parts of the body.

23. The correct answer is A. To *risk* is "to *venture*." To *squander* is to "waste" which makes choices B and D (*squandered* and *wasted*) incorrect. *Exhausted* (choice C) is incorrect because *exhausted* has no relation to *risked*.

24. The correct answer is C. To *pare* is "to remove the outer skin," that is, to *peel* a fruit. The other choices all relate to preparing fruit for consumption, but they are not synonyms for *pare*. Note that choices A and D are themselves synonyms, and since both can't be right, both must be incorrect.

25. The correct answer is A. An *initiative*, meaning "the opening or first step in a series of actions," and an *enterprise*, meaning "a readiness to begin a new venture," are near synonyms. Choices B and D, *energy* and *leadership*, can be synonyms for *initiative*, but not in this context. Choice C

is incorrect because *zeal*, meaning "enthusiasm," is not a synonym.

26. The correct answer is B. *Delineate* means "to describe in great detail," so *describe* is its synonym. Choice A is incorrect because *discredit* means "to damage the reputation of someone" or "to cause distrust or disbelief." Choice C is incorrect because *disprove* means "to show something to be in error or false." *Endorses* (choice D) is incorrect because it means "to approve."

27. The correct answer is A. *Cartilage* is *tissue*. Though *ligament*, *tendon*, and *membrane* are related to the body, they are not the same as *cartilage*.

28. The correct answer is C. To *confirm* is "to *verify*, to show to be true." *Canceled*, *rescheduled*, and *recorded* are not synonyms for *confirm*.

29. The correct answer is B. To *invalidate* something is "to *cancel*" it. Choice A is incorrect because *authorize* means "to approve" and is the opposite of *invalidate*. Choice C is incorrect because *contradict* means "to deny something" or "to express the opposite." Choice D is incorrect because *modify* is "to change in some way," but is not the same as *invalidating*.

30. The correct answer is B. A *malfunction* is a problem, so the correct synonym is "*operating incorrectly*." Choice A is incorrect because if the engine was not working properly, it probably wasn't *operative*. Choices C and D, *firing* and *igniting*, can be applied to engines, but neither is a synonym for *malfunctioning*.

31. The correct answer is D. *Fraudulent* means "*deceitful*." Choice A is incorrect because *thorough* has no relation to *fraudulent*, and neither does choice B, *extensive*. Choice C, *legal*, is the opposite of *fraudulent*.

32. **The correct answer is D.** *Competence* and *ability* are synonyms. Choice A is incorrect because *honesty* has no relation to *competence*. Choice B is incorrect because *punctuality* refers to being on time. Choice C is incorrect because *credibility* refers to trustworthiness and reliability.

33. **The correct answer is A.** An *anthology* is a *collection of literary selections*. An anthology may contain an *annotated bibliography*, choice B, but that is not an anthology. Choices C and D are not synonyms for *anthology*.

34. **The correct answer is D.** *Mobile* and *motile*, meaning "having the power to move," are synonyms. Choice A is incorrect because *movement* is a noun, and the question requires an adjective. Choice B is incorrect because, while bacteria can be *deadly*, that is not a synonym for *mobile*. Choice C is incorrect because *migratory* means "nomadic," and this is not correct usage for *mobile*.

35. **The correct answer is C.** *Wryly* means "dryly humorous, often using *irony*." Choice A is incorrect because *deceptively*, meaning "dishonestly," is not a synonym. Choice B is incorrect because wry humor is not the same as being *nasty*. Choice D is incorrect because *delightedly*, meaning "very pleased," is not a synonym.

Part B: Antonyms

1. A	9. A	17. A	25. A	33. D
2. C	10. D	18. C	26. C	34. B
3. A	11. B	19. C	27. D	35. E
4. D	12. A	20. A	28. A	36. B
5. B	13. D	21. D	29. B	37. D
6. A	14. A	22. B	30. A	38. C
7. C	15. C	23. B	31. C	39. B
8. B	16. B	24. D	32. D	40. E

1. **The correct answer is A.** *Imperious* means "overbearing, domineering," so the opposite is *submissive*, meaning "passive, compliant, obedient." None of the other choices has any relation to *imperious*.

2. **The correct answer is C.** *Capricious* means "given to whims, unpredictable, unstable," so *steadfast*, meaning "steady, firm and dependable," is the opposite. Choice A is incorrect because *whimsical* is a synonym. *Judicious* (choice B) is incorrect because it means "having good judgment, prudent." Choice D is incorrect because *tranquil* means "peaceful, serene."

3. **The correct answer is A.** A *cantankerous* person is a disagreeable and difficult person, whereas the opposite is a *pleasant* person. Choice B is incorrect because *dubious* means "doubtful." Choices C and D are incorrect because *effective* and *awkward* are not antonyms.

4. **The correct answer is D.** *Forbearance* means "tolerance, patience," so *impatience* is an antonym. *Indulgence* (choice A) is incorrect because it's a synonym. Choice B is incorrect because *pliancy* means "easily influenced" or "adaptable." Choice C is incorrect because *politeness* has no relation to *forbearance*.

5. **The correct answer is B.** Something that is *haphazard* is done without care, in a casual or careless way. The opposite is something that is *premeditated*, or done with purpose and at least some planning. Choice A is incorrect because *inefficient* means "unable to do something effectively or competently" and is closer in meaning to haphazard than to its opposite. Choice C, *unsatisfactory*, is incorrect because it may be the result of something done haphazardly, but it's not an antonym. Choice D is incorrect because *blundering* means "making a stupid and often serious mistake."

6. **The correct answer is A.** *Efficacy* means "effectiveness, efficiency," so *ineffectiveness* is an antonym. Choice B, *efficiency*, is incorrect because it's a synonym. Choices C and D are incorrect because *value* and *success* are near synonyms for *efficacy*.

7. **The correct answer is C.** Something that is *chimerical* is highly imaginative or fanciful, and something that is *factual* is the opposite. Choice A is incorrect because *philosophical* has no relation to *chimerical*, and neither does *elite* (choice B) meaning "a group of people with some superior quality or position in society." Choice D is incorrect because *unimpressive* has no relation to *chimerical*.

8. **The correct answer is B.** To *repress* is "to restrain, to keep under control," so *liberate*, meaning "to free," is the opposite. Choice

A is incorrect because *reserve* is "to keep back for future use" or "to set something apart for a particular use." Choice C, *thrust,* means "to push with force" or "to impose on something." Choice D is incorrect because "to precipitate" is "to cause to happen."

9. **The correct answer is A.** *Abominable* means "completely unpleasant or disagreeable," so *agreeable* is the opposite. Choice B is incorrect because *loathsome* is a synonym for *abominable.* Choice C is incorrect because *sufficient* has no relation to *abominable,* and neither does choice D, *degrading,* meaning "humiliating someone, shaming."

10. **The correct answer is D.** *Unethical,* that is, having no ethics or code of right and wrong, is the opposite of *scrupulous,* "having principles, being moral." Choice A is incorrect because *vulgar* means "crude, lacking good manners." Choice B is incorrect because *feasible* means "possible, able to be achieved." Choice C is incorrect because *pompous* means "self-important, exaggerated sense of self."

11. **The correct answer is B.** *Antecedent* as an adjective indicates something that comes before, and *subsequent* indicates something that comes after. Choice A is incorrect because *previous* indicates something occurring before. Choice C is incorrect because *foregoing* means "previous." Choice D is incorrect because *propitious* means "favorable."

12. **The correct answer is A.** Something that is *ponderous* is heavy, awkward, and dull, so *delicate* is an antonym. Choice B is incorrect because *potent* means "powerful." Choice C is incorrect because *supportive* has no relation to *ponderous.* Choice D is incorrect because *massive* is a synonym for *ponderous.*

13. **The correct answer is D.** *Supplication* means "a humble request, a plea," so *disdain,* meaning "scorn, a feeling or show of contempt" is an antonym. Choice A is incorrect because *worship* can be a near synonym for *supplication* when the latter means "prayer." *Compassion* (choice B) is incorrect because it has no relation to *supplication.* Choice C is incorrect because *entreaty,* meaning "a plea," is a synonym for *supplication.*

14. **The correct answer is A.** The opposite of *positive* is *negative.* None of the other choices has a relation to *positive.*

15. **The correct answer is C.** *Renegade* as an adjective means "disloyal," so an antonym is *loyal.* Choice A is incorrect because *constant* has no relation to *renegade.* Choice B is incorrect because *extricate,* meaning "to disentangle, to get out of a difficulty," is a verb, and the answer requires an adjective. Choice D is incorrect because *heretical* is a near synonym for *renegade.*

16. **The correct answer is B.** To *disregard* is "to pay no attention to, to ignore," so "to *attend to*" is an antonym. *Disown, revoke,* and *recover* are incorrect because they are not antonyms for *disregard.*

17. **The correct answer is A.** *Wrath* is anger, so *delight,* meaning "extreme pleasure or joy," is an antonym. Choice B is incorrect because *travail* means "very hard work." Choice C is incorrect because *frivolity* means "not being serious, silliness." Choice D is incorrect because *detriment* means "damage, harm" or "something that causes damage or harm."

18. **The correct answer is C.** *Tedious* means "tiresome, boring, dull," so *stimulating* is an antonym. *Ungainly* (choice A) is incorrect because it means "awkward." Choice B is incorrect because *imperative* means

"urgent." Choice D is incorrect because *suitable* is not an antonym for *tedious*.

19. **The correct answer is C.** To *embody* is "to be an example of, to give form to an idea," so *dissociate*, meaning "to separate, to differentiate," is the only possible antonym in the list. Choice A is incorrect because *impel* means "to force." Choice B is incorrect because *fuse* means "to merge, to combine." Choice D is incorrect because *collect* has no relation to *embody*.

20. **The correct answer is A.** *Deferrable* means "able to be put off or postponed," so *urgent* is an antonym. Choice B is incorrect because *furtive* means "secretive." Choice C is incorrect because *inclined* means "having a preference or tendency." Choice D is incorrect because *deniable* means "possible to contradict, able to be denied."

21. **The correct answer is D.** *Homogenous* means "consisting of elements that are all the same," whereas *heterogeneous* means "consisting of elements that are different." Choice A is incorrect because *invariable* means "unchanging." Choice B is incorrect because *homosexual* refers to a sexual orientation. Choice C is incorrect because *importunate* means "insistent, demanding."

22. **The correct answer is B.** An *adherent* is a supporter or follower of a cause, whereas a *repudiator* is one who rejects authority. Choice A is incorrect because a *disciple* is a follower, so it is a synonym for *adherent*. Choice C is incorrect because a *soothsayer* is one who predicts the future. Choice D is incorrect because a *hypocrite* is a person who pretends to be something he or she is not or to hold beliefs and opinions that the person does not.

23. **The correct answer is B.** The opposite of *crude* is *refined*. Choice A is incorrect because *barbarous* is similar to *crude*.

Choice C is incorrect because *obscure* means "unclear, vague" or "secret, hidden." Choice D is incorrect because *covetous* means "greedy."

24. **The correct answer is D.** The opposite of *irrational* is *sensible*. Choice A is incorrect because *cynical* means "believing the worst of people." Choice B is incorrect because *sharp* has no relation to *irrational*. Choice C is incorrect because *prevalent* means "widespread" or "predominant."

25. **The correct answer is A.** *Graphic* has several meanings, but the one that works in this question is "describes in detail" because the only word that works as an antonym is *vague*. Choice B is incorrect because *illustrative* means "acting as an example or illustration of something," so it's similar in meaning to *graphic*. Choice C is incorrect because *forcible* has no relation to *graphic*. Choice D is incorrect because *glacial* refers to glaciers.

26. **The correct answer is C.** To *devastate* is "to destroy," so "to *renovate*," meaning "to restore, to repair, to remodel," is an antonym. Choices A, B, and D—*tolerate*, *obstruct*, and *promote*—have no relation to *devastate*.

27. **The correct answer is D.** *Stringent* means "exacting," so rule out choices A and B, *exacting* and *tough*. Choice C is incorrect because *influential* has no relation to *stringent*. Choice D, *flexible*, is the only possible answer.

28. **The correct answer is A.** To *acquiesce* is "to agree," so *contest*, meaning "to argue, to dispute," is an antonym. Choice B is incorrect because *invest* has no relation to *acquiesce*. Choice C is incorrect because *dismiss* means "to discharge, to let go." Choice D is incorrect because *supply* is not an antonym for *acquiesce*.

29. **The correct answer is B.** *Brevity* refers to being concise or of short duration, so *lengthy* is an antonym. Choice A is incorrect because an abbreviation is a shortened form of a word or phrase. Choice C is incorrect because *ramification* means "consequence of an action or event." Choice D is incorrect because *delusion* means "a misconception, mistaken idea or opinion."

30. **The correct answer is A.** To *flaunt* is "to show off," whereas *disavow* is "to deny knowledge of something, to refuse to acknowledge." Choice B is incorrect because *conserve* is "to save." Choice C is incorrect because *blight* is "to have a bad effect on something." Choice D is incorrect because *astonish* is not an antonym for *flaunt*.

31. **The correct answer is C.** *Cultivate* and *nurture* (choices A and E) relate to encouraging growth in something, and *restore* and *reinstate* (choices B and D) pertain to returning something to a state of health or power. Thus, all of these words have a connotation of promoting the healthy state of something. Conversely, *stifle* (choice C) means "to suppress" or "to restrain," and thus is the word most different from the others.

32. **The correct answer is D.** *Dilate*, *distend*, *augment*, and *amplify* all relate to making or becoming larger, whereas *constrict* (choice D) relates to making or becoming smaller, and so is the word most different from the others.

33. **The correct answer is D.** *Befitting*, *suitable*, *apropos*, and *proper* all mean "appropriate," whereas *inappropriate* (choice D) clearly means the opposite.

34. **The correct answer is B.** *Coherent*, *rational*, *reasonable*, and *sensible* are all synonyms for *logical*, so *illogical* (choice B) is the word most different from the others.

35. **The correct answer is E.** *Paltry*, *pathetic*, *trifling*, and *underwhelming* all mean "meager, insignificant," so *impressive* (choice E) is the word most different from the others.

36. **The correct answer is B.** *Bucolic*, *rural*, *rustic*, and *agrarian* all mean "having to do with the country," so *urban* (choice B), meaning "having to do with cities," is the opposite.

37. **The correct answer is D.** *Extravagant*, *lavish*, *prodigal*, and *indulgent* all mean "excessive, unrestrained, wasteful," so *frugal*, meaning "thrifty," is the word most different from the others.

38. **The correct answer is C.** *Leniency*, *indulgence*, *mercy*, and *permissiveness* mean "mercifulness, compassion," so *severity* (choice C) is an antonym and the word most different from the others.

39. **The correct answer is B.** *Manifest*, *divulged*, *glaring*, and *apparent* mean "clear, obvious," so *latent*, meaning "not evident, potential," is an antonym and the word most different from the others.

40. **The correct answer is E.** *Plebeian*, *vulgar*, *ignoble*, and *common* all mean "of the common people," whereas *patrician* (choice E) refers to the aristocracy or elite, or having good manners and upbringing.

Part C: Verbal Analogies

1. C	6. C	11. B	16. B	21. C
2. A	7. B	12. A	17. C	22. C
3. B	8. A	13. C	18. B	23. C
4. C	9. B	14. A	19. B	24. B
5. D	10. C	15. B	20. C	25. B

1. **The correct answer is C.** This is an association analogy. *Cat* and *dog* are often associated and so are *cup* and *saucer*. Choice A is incorrect because a *knife* is associated with a fork, but not a cup. Choices B and D are incorrect because *coffee* and *cream* may be found in a cup, but they are not associated with *cup* the way a saucer is.

2. **The correct answer is A.** *Saline* is *salty* and *sugary* is *sweet* in this characteristic analogy. Choice B is incorrect because *stale* isn't a quality of sugar. Choice C is incorrect because the answer requires a quality, or adjective, and *bread* is a thing. Choice D is incorrect because *insipid*, meaning "not tasty," isn't a quality of associated with sugar.

3. **The correct answer is B.** *Flannel* is made out of *wool*, and *bricks* are made out of *clay*. Choice D is incorrect because *mortar* is used to hold bricks in place, but bricks are not made of mortar. *Wood* and *stone* (choices A and C) have no relation to bricks.

4. **The correct answer is C.** This is a synonym analogy. *Contemporary*, meaning "current," is similar to *present*, and *future* is similar to *eventual*, meaning "at some indefinite time in the future." *Past* (choice A)and *posterior* (choice B) are incorrect because this is not an antonym analogy.

5. **The correct answer is D.** The first pair sets up an analogy. The *moon* revolves around *Earth*, and *Earth* revolves around the *sun*.

None of the other answer choices fulfills this association of Earth with an action.

6. **The correct answer is C.** This is an antonym analogy. *Acute* pain is pain that begins abruptly and is of short duration, whereas *chronic* pain is long lasting. The word *intense* mirrors *acute*, so the answer must be similar to *chronic*. The only answer choice that is similar is *persistent*. Choice A is incorrect because *sardonic* means "bitterly mocking, sarcastic." Choice B is incorrect because *tonic* means "a kind of medicine" or "producing and restoring normal muscle or tissue tone." Choice D is incorrect because *pretty* has no relation to *intense*.

7. **The correct answer is B.** This is a part-to-whole analogy. A *peak* is the top of a *mountain*, and a *floor* is the bottom of a *canyon*. Choice A is incorrect because a *ceiling* has nothing to do with topography, that is, physical geography. Choice C is incorrect because the bottom of a *river* is a riverbed. Choice D is incorrect because a *cliff* is a steep, rugged, high face of rock.

8. **The correct answer is A.** The first pair sets up an antonym analogy. *East* is the opposite of *west* as *northwest* is the opposite of *southeast*. *Northeast* (choice D) is tempting, but not the better answer when compared to southeast, which is both south and east of northwest. Choice C is incorrect because *north* is not as specific as the other answers.

9. **The correct answer is B.** This is a cause-and-effect analogy. *Gasoline* is made from *petroleum*, and *sugar* is made from *cane*, that is, sugar cane. Choice A is incorrect because *oil* relates to petroleum, not sugar. Choices C and D are incorrect because, although sugar comes from a *plant* and is *sweet*, there is no cause and effect involved in either answer.

10. **The correct answer is C.** In this synonym analogy, *deference*, meaning "courtesy regard, submission or courteous compliance with another's wishes," and *respect* are synonyms. A synonym for *contempt* is *discourtesy*. Choice A is incorrect because *esteem*, meaning "holding someone in high regard," is a synonym for *deference* and an antonym for *contempt*. Choice B is incorrect because *capitulation* means "giving up, surrendering." Choice D is incorrect because *tendency* means "attitude, a leaning toward someone or something, an inclination."

11. **The correct answer is B.** This is a characteristic or object-to-quality analogy. A *slope* has an *incline*, and a *plane* is *flat*. It is true that a plane is *dimensional* (choice A) in that it is one-dimensional, but choice B is a better answer because it is more specific to what a plane is—flat. Choices C and D are incorrect because a plane may be any of several one-dimensional shapes, including *square* and *rectangular*.

12. **The correct answer is A.** This is an antonym analogy. An *edge* is the opposite of a *center*, and *effusive*, meaning "unrestrained, exuberant," is the opposite of *unemotional*. Choice B is incorrect because *exuberant* is a synonym for *effusive*. Choice C is incorrect because *eclectic* means "choosing from a variety of ideas or styles." Choice D is incorrect because *eccentricity* means "unconventional behavior, nonconformity."

13. **The correct answer is C.** The first pair sets up a person-to-action relationship. A *procrastinator delays* and a *mentor advises*. Choices A and B are incorrect because even though a mentor advises a mentee and may be a kind of *teacher*, the answer requires a verb, not a noun. Choice D is incorrect because *measuring* is not a particular action of a mentor.

14. **The correct answer is A.** This is a synonym analogy. *Sophistication* means "worldliness, possessing finesse," and *finesse* means "skillful, tactful" as well as "elegant, polished in style and manners." Among the list, the only synonym for *ineptitude*, meaning "lacking in skill or ability, clumsiness, incompetence" is *inefficiency*. Choice B is incorrect because *artistry* might be considered an antonym for *ineptitude*. Choice C is incorrect because *trickiness* has no relation to *ineptitude*. Choice D is incorrect because *insatiability* means "impossible to satisfy."

15. **The correct answer is B.** This is a straightforward person-to-occupation relationship. A *captain* runs a *steamship*, and a *principal* runs a *school*.

16. **The correct answer is B.** This is a characteristic analogy. A dime is made out of silver and a penny is made out of *copper*. Though *mint*, *currency*, and *value* relate to a penny in some way, they are not a characteristic of a penny.

17. **The correct answer is C.** This is a grammatical analogy. *Reversion* is a noun related to the verb *revert*, meaning "to return to a former condition, practice, belief, etc." *Sympathy* is a noun related to the verb *sympathize*. Choice A is incorrect because *sympathetic* is an adjective, and the question requires a noun. Choice B is incorrect because *symposium*, meaning "conference," has no relation to *sympathize*. Choice D

is incorrect because *sympathizing* is an adjective, and the question requires a noun.

18. **The correct answer is B.** This is another grammatical analogy. *Regressive* is an adjective related to the verb *regress*, meaning "to go backward." *Sterile* is an adjective related to the verb *sterilize*. Choice A is incorrect because *sterilization* is a noun, just like *sterility* and *sterilizer* (choices C and D).

19. **The correct answer is B.** In this antonym analogy, *down* is the opposite of *up* and *age* is the opposite of *youth*. None of the other choices is related to age.

20. **The correct answer is C.** In this grammar analogy, *mine* is the possessive pronoun for *I* and *his* is the possessive pronoun for *man*. Choice A is incorrect because *men* is a plural noun, and the question requires a possessive pronoun. Choice B is incorrect because *man's* could be a possessive adjective or a possessive noun, and the answer requires a possessive pronoun to parallel the first pair. Choice D is incorrect because *hers* is a possessive pronoun for a female antecedent, and the question offers a male antecedent in *man*.

21. **The correct answer is C.** This is a synonym analogy. *Disloyal* and *faithless* are synonyms, and *imperfection* and *foible*, meaning "minor weakness of character, an eccentricity" are synonyms. Choice A is incorrect because *faithful* has no relation to *imperfection*, and neither does *depression* (choice B). Choice

D is incorrect because *decrepitude* means "being worn out, deteriorated because of old age or use."

22. **The correct answer is C.** This is an object-to-use analogy. A *necklace* is made of pearls, and a chain is made of *links*. Choice B is incorrect because a *prisoner* has no relation to a jewelry analogy. Choices A and D are incorrect because a *locket* and a *clasp* are found on a chain, but they are not what a chain is made of.

23. **The correct answer is C.** This is a part-to-whole analogy. A *drift* is made of *snow,* and a *dune* is made of *sand.* Choice A is incorrect because a dune is a small *hill;* a dune isn't made out of a hill. *Rain* and *hail* (choices B and D) have no relation to a dune.

24. **The correct answer is B.** This is a purpose analogy. The primary purpose of a *bank* is to hold *deposits,* and the primary purpose of a *hospital* is to provide *care.* Choices A, C, and D are incorrect because *blood, surgery,* and *tests* are ways that hospitals provide care, which is the primary purpose.

25. **The correct answer is B.** In this category-to-example analogy, a *schooner* is type of *vessel,* or ship, and a *persimmon* is a type of *fruit.* Choices A, C, and D are incorrect because a *machine,* an *engine,* and a *vehicle* have no relation to a *persimmon.* If you weren't sure what a *persimmon* is, you could figure out that because choices A, C, and D are similar, the odd answer must be the correct one.

Part D: English Grammar and Usage

1. B	3. C	5. D	7. C	9. B
2. C	4. D	6. A	8. A	10. B

1. **The correct answer is B.** The subject of the sentence, *the rower*, is singular and thus takes a singular verb, *walks*. Note that the phrase that comes between the subject and the verb in this sentence does not affect the number of the verb. This eliminates choices A and C. *With* is a preposition, and the word following it is an object of this preposition and so should be in the objective case (*her*), not the subjective case (*she*), making choice D incorrect.

2. **The correct answer is C.** When a singular and a plural subject are joined by *or* or *nor*, the subject nearer the verb determines whether it is singular or plural. In this sentence, *twins*, which is closer to the verb, is plural and thus requires a plural verb and, by extension, a plural possessive pronoun (which refers back to the subject). This makes choices A and B incorrect. The word following *pick* is the direct object of the verb phrase *pick up* and so should be in the objective case (*us*), not the subjective case (*we*). This makes choice D incorrect.

3. **The correct answer is C.** This sentence refers to an event (swimming over 100 laps) that was completed before some other past event (the ending of practice). So the past perfect tense of the verb *swim* is needed. The past perfect tense is formed by using *had* plus a verb's past participle. The past participle of *swim* is *swum*, so the correct answer is *had swum* (choice C). Note that *swam* is the simple past tense of *swim*.

4. **The correct answer is D.** The word *tomorrow* in this sentence indicates that we are referring to something in the future. This eliminates choices A and B, which

represent the past tense and past perfect tense, respectively. Because the sentence is not referring to some future event that is completed before some other future event, the future perfect tense is not appropriate, thus making choice C incorrect.

5. **The correct answer is D.** In this sentence, *delicious* modifies the noun *coffee* and so is an adjective. Recall that adjectives modify nouns and pronouns and that adverbs modify verbs, adjectives, and other adverbs. You might be tempted to identify *delicious* as an adverb, thinking that it modifies the verb *tastes*. However, *taste* is a linking verb and so merely serves to link *coffee* to *delicious*. It could easily be replaced with another linking verb without affecting the meaning of the sentence (e.g., "This coffee is delicious."). When an adjective follows a linking verb like this, it is known as a *predicate adjective*.

6. **The correct answer is A.** In this sentence, we are comparing just two things. This means that we should use the comparative form of an adjective. This allows us to rule out choice B, which is the superlative form of the adjective *good*. *More better* is a double comparison and should be avoided, which makes choice C incorrect. *Good* has irregular comparative and superlative forms—*better* and *best*, respectively—so *more good* (choice D) is incorrect.

7. **The correct answer is C.** Two independent clauses should be joined by a comma with a coordinating conjunction or by a semicolon. Choice A is incorrect because the first and second independent clauses have no coordinating punctuation between

them and the second and third have only a comma (an error known as a comma splice). Choice B is incorrect because the first and second independent clauses have only a comma (comma splice) and the second and third have no coordinating punctuation between them. Choice D is incorrect because the three independent clauses are joined only by *and*, without any commas (an error known as a run-on sentence).

8. **The correct answer is A.** The focus of this question is proper capitalization. Proper nouns—such as *Abraham Lincoln*, *February*, and *Kentucky*—should be capitalized. Choice B is incorrect because *president* is a common noun in this sentence and thus should be in lower case. Only when a personal title immediately precedes a proper name should it be capitalized (e.g., "President Abraham Lincoln is my favorite president."). Choice C is incorrect because *February* should be capitalized. Choice D is incorrect because *Kentucky* should be capitalized.

9. **The correct answer is B.** The semicolon is the correct mark of punctuation (when used alone) to join two independent clauses, and introductory words such as *therefore* should be set off by a comma. Thus, a semicolon should appear following *diligent* to join the two independent clauses in this sentence, and a comma should appear after *therefore*, which introduces the second independent clause. Choice A is incorrect because the semicolon should come before *therefore* and the comma should come after it; the current punctuation does not make sense. Choice C is incorrect because stronger coordination is needed following *diligent* and because a colon does not make sense following *therefore*. Choice D is incorrect because stronger coordination is needed following *diligent*.

10. **The correct answer is B.** When a question mark or an exclamation point is used in a sentence with a direct quotation, it should be included inside the closing quotation mark if it applies only to the quotation and outside the closing quotation mark if it applies to the sentence as a whole. In this sentence, the exclamation point clearly applies only to the quotation and so should be included inside the closing quotation mark. Choice A is incorrect because the exclamation point should appear inside, not outside, the closing quotation mark. Choice C is incorrect because only one ending punctuation mark is needed for the sentence, regardless of whether it is inside or outside the closing quotation mark; thus, the period following the closing quotation mark is not necessary. Choice D is incorrect because no closing quotation mark is provided.

Part E: Spelling

1. C	3. A	5. C	7. A	9. B
2. B	4. B	6. A	8. B	10. C

1. **The correct answer is C.** The correct spelling is *accommodate*.

2. **The correct answer is B.** The correct spelling is *ascites*.

3. **The correct answer is A.** The correct spelling is *basically*.

4. **The correct answer is B.** The correct spelling is *callus*.

5. **The correct answer is C.** The correct spelling is *diaphragm*.

6. **The correct answer is A.** The correct spelling is *guarantee*.

7. **The correct answer is A.** The correct spelling is *knowledge*.

8. **The correct answer is B.** The correct spelling is *palliative*.

9. **The correct answer is B.** The correct spelling is *sagittal*.

10. **The correct answer is C.** The correct spelling is *venous*.

Part F: Nonverbal Ability

1. A	**3.** B	**5.** A	**7.** D	**9.** B
2. E	**4.** C	**6.** D	**8.** E	**10.** A

1. **The correct answer is A.** The relationship between the first two shapes is that the second is a mirror image of the first. You could also say that the second image is the same as the first only rotated 90 degrees to the right. So, in the second pair, we begin with a triangle and are looking for its mirror image, or the same figure only rotated 90 degrees to the right. Therefore, perpendicular line segments figure is to mirror image of perpendicular line segments figure as triangle is to mirror image of triangle.

2. **The correct answer is E.** The relationship between the first two shapes is that the second is a circle that is circumscribing the first. So, in the second pair, we begin with a plus sign and are looking for a circle with a plus sign circumscribed within it. Therefore, multiplication sign is to circle with a multiplication sign circumscribed within it as plus sign is to circle with a plus sign circumscribed within it.

3. **The correct answer is B.** The relationship between the first two shapes is that the second is a thinner version of the first. So, in the second pair, we begin with a thick plus sign and are looking for a thin plus sign. Therefore, thick multiplication sign is to thin multiplication sign as thick plus sign is to thin plus sign. Although the plus sign in choice A is slightly thinner than the thick plus sign, the one in choice B more accurately represents the degree of decrease in thickness that occurs in the first two shapes.

4. **The correct answer is C.** The relationship between the first two shapes is that the second is a similar shape only with one less point or vertex than the first. So, in the second pair, we begin with a four-pointed star and are looking for a similar shape that has one less point, or a three-pointed star. Therefore, square is to triangle as four-pointed star is to three-pointed star.

5. **The correct answer is A.** The relationship between the first two shapes is that the second is an inversion, or 180-degree rotation, of the first. So, in the second pair, we begin with an up-pointing triangle and are looking for its inversion, which is a down-pointing triangle. Therefore, up-pointing pentagon is to down-pointing pentagon as up-pointing triangle is to down-pointing triangle.

6. **The correct answer is D.** The relationship between the first two shapes is that the second is a mirror image of the first and opposite in color. So, in the second pair, we begin with a left-pointing black triangle and are looking for its opposite-color mirror image, which is a right-pointing white triangle. Therefore, left-pointing white triangle is to right-pointing black triangle as left-pointing black triangle is to right-pointing white triangle.

7. **The correct answer is D.** The relationship between the first two shapes is that the first shape includes a same-size, opposite-color (negative-image) version of the second enveloped by and concentric with a larger, same-color version of the second. So, in the second pair, we begin with a large black circle containing a concentric small white circle and are looking for a small black circle. Therefore, large black square

containing a concentric small white square is to small black square as large black circle containing a concentric small white circle is to small black circle.

8. **The correct answer is E.** The relationship between the first two shapes is that they are opposite and complementary halves of a whole. Another way of viewing the relationship is that the second shape is the same as the first, only rotated 180 degrees. So, in the second pair, we begin with the top half of a black circle and are looking for the bottom half of a black circle. Therefore, left half of black circle is to right half of black circle as top half of black circle is to bottom half of black circle.

9. **The correct answer is B.** The relationship between the first two shapes is that the second is the left half of the first. That is, if you were to take the first shape and divide it in half along its vertical axis, the left half would be equivalent to the second shape. So, in the second pair, we begin with a circle and are looking for the left half of this circle. Therefore, diamond is to left half of diamond as circle is to left half of circle.

10. **The correct answer is A.** The relationship between the first two shapes is that the second is the upper right quarter of the first. That is, if you were to take the first shape (the diamond) and divide it in half along both its vertical and horizontal axes, producing quarters, the upper right quarter would be equivalent to the second shape (the triangle). So, in the second pair, we begin with a cross formed by four L's and are looking for the shape that forms its upper right quarter. Therefore, diamond is to the triangle that forms its upper right quarter as cross formed by four L's is to the L that forms its upper right quarter.

Mathematics

OVERVIEW

This section's review of mathematics and the numerical ability tests include the following: basic quantitative problems involving addition, subtraction, multiplication, and division; calculations including decimals, fractions, percentages, and measurements; basic operations in algebra and geometry; and quantitative comparison questions. Throughout the exercises, emphasis is placed on verbal problems to prepare you for the interpretations and methods required for problem solving. The explanatory answers and problem solutions provide a variety of opportunities to review or to learn the numerical processes included on the pre-nursing examinations.

Study the guidelines listed below; they provide the major concepts needed for successful performance on your mathematics examination.

TIPS FOR STUDYING MATHEMATICS

To perform well on mathematics tests, it is important to be well prepared. To prepare, you must know what material will be covered on the test. The mathematics guidelines and practice exercises in this book provide a review of materials that are covered on the mathematics section of the nursing school entrance examination. You can maximize your performance on the test by following these eight steps:

1. Choose a place to study where you won't be distracted.

2. Set aside adequate time to study. Try to set aside at least one hour for each study session. Study and practice each day if possible. Make a study schedule and stick to it.

3. Give your full focus and attention to your studies.

4. Read the explanatory material before doing any practice tests. Make sure that you understand what you're reading. Review information that you don't understand, and use other references when necessary.

5. Take the practice tests under test conditions. Read the instructions carefully. Complete tests in the amount of time suggested.

6. Compare your answers with those provided in the book. Carefully review answers to questions that you missed.

7. Seek help if you don't understand a problem after several tries.

8. Review regularly, and practice, practice, practice.

Test-Taking Tips

- Read test instructions carefully. Note the amount of time allotted for completion of the test and pace yourself accordingly.

- Read each problem carefully. Make sure you understand the concepts and terms being used. Try to restate the problem in your own words.

- Simplify the problem by breaking it down into smaller parts.

- Determine what information is given and what is to be solved.

- Determine whether there is enough information given to solve the problem.

- Eliminate extraneous information.

- Choose a strategy for solving the problem.

- Express your answer in the number of units requested. You may be asked to express your answer in terms of minutes, feet, or hours, or you may be asked to write your answer as a decimal or fraction.

- Check your solution to determine if it is reasonable. Does your answer appear to be unreasonably large or small?

- Don't spend too much time on a question that you find difficult. Move on to the next question and return to questions you have skipped after you complete the other test questions.

- Try an alternative strategy if the one you used didn't work.

- Review your answers if you finish before time is up. Check your computations very carefully.

MATHEMATICS REVIEW

Whole Numbers

Digits in whole numbers have **place-value** based on units of ten (decimal system). Therefore, it is important that all digits, including zeros, are lined up correctly in columns when adding and subtracting whole numbers.

Example:

- Place values for the whole number 5,264 are illustrated below.

  $5{,}264 = (5 \times 1{,}000) + (2 \times 100) + (6 \times 10) + (4 \times 1)$

- Numbers are lined up according to place values in the following **addition** and **subtraction** examples.

$$\begin{array}{r} 5{,}264 \\ +\,478 \\ \hline 5{,}742 \end{array} \qquad \begin{array}{r} 5{,}264 \\ -\,478 \\ \hline 4{,}786 \end{array}$$

Use **multiplication** to determine the value of several quantities with the same value if the value of one quantity is given.

Example: If one loaf of bread costs $0.80, how much will three loaves of bread cost? Multiply $0.80 times 3. The answer is $2.40 ($0.80 is the multiplicand, 3 is the multiplier, and the product is $2.40).

When multiplying, be certain to include all zeros and to keep the columns in line.

Example:

$$\begin{array}{r} 3{,}600 \\ \times\quad 507 \\ \hline 25{,}200 \\ 0000 \\ 18{,}000 \\ \hline 1{,}825{,}200 \end{array}$$

Use **division** to determine the value of one quantity when the value of several quantities is given.

Example: Three loaves of bread cost $2.40. How much will one loaf cost? Divide $2.40 by 3. The answer is $0.80 (3 is the divisor, $2.40 is the dividend, and the quotient is $0.80).

Divisibility Tips

- If the last digit of a number is 0, 2, 4, 6, or 8, the number is divisible by 2.
- If the last digit of a number ends in 0 or 5, the number is divisible by 5.
- If the sum of the digits of a number is divisible by 3, the number is divisible by 3.

Example: The sum of the digits of 234 is 2 + 3 + 4 = 9. Since 9 is divisible by 3, we know that 234 is also divisible by 3 (234 ÷ 3 = 78).

- If the sum of the digits of a number is divisible by 9, the number is divisible by 9. In the previous example, it was shown that the sum of the digits of 234 is 9. By the same rule, we know that 234 is divisible by 9.

- If the number represented by the last two digits of a number is divisible by 4, the number is divisible by 4.

  Example: 32 is the number represented by the last two digits of 232. Since 32 is divisible by 4, the number 232 is divisible by 4.

- Note that it is not possible to divide by zero.

- A **prime number** is any whole number other than 0 or 1 that is divisible only by itself and by 1.

  Example: 17 is a prime number since it is divisible only by 1 and 17. The whole numbers 2, 3, 5, 7, and 11 are the first five prime numbers.

- Divisibility rules can be used to find the prime factors of whole numbers.

  Example: 24 is divisible by 2 (last digit is 4) and is divisible by 3 (sum of digits is 6).

  $$24 = 2 \times 2 \times 2 \times 3$$
  $$= 2^3 \times 3$$

  Two methods for determining the prime factors of a number are illustrated below. In each method, keep dividing until your quotient is a prime number.

- The **average** of a set of numbers is the sum of the numbers divided by the number of numbers added.

  Example: The average of the numbers 10, 14, 17, and 23 is

  $$\frac{10 + 14 + 17 + 23}{4} = \frac{64}{4} = 16.$$

- The **square** of a number is the product obtained when a number is multiplied by itself.

  Example: $4^2 = 4 \times 4 = 16$

- The **square root** ($\sqrt{\ }$) of a given number is the number that yields the given number when multiplied by itself.

  Example: $\sqrt{16} = 4$, since $4 \times 4 = 16$

- The square of any whole number is called a **perfect square.** Conversely, the square root of a perfect square is a whole number.

  Example: $4^2 = 16$ (a perfect square); thus $\sqrt{16} = 4$.

- If a number is not a perfect square, you can **approximate the square root** of the number when a calculator is not available.

  Example: Approximate the square root of $90 \left(\sqrt{90} \right)$.

  1. Estimate the square root of the given number. Since 90 is between 81 ($= 9^2$) and 100 ($= 10^2$), the square root of 90 will be between 9 and 10. A possible estimate is 9.30.

  2. Divide the given number by the estimated square root.

  $$90 \div 9.30 = 9.68$$

  3. Find the average of the resulting quotient and the estimated square root.

  $$\frac{9.68 + 9.30}{2} = 9.49 \left(9.49 \text{ is the first approximation for } \sqrt{90} \right)$$

  4. Divide the given number by the average (first approximation) found above.

  $$90 \div 9.49 = 9.48$$

  5. Find the **average of the divisor** (first approximation) and the quotient found in step 3.

  $$\frac{9.49 + 9.48}{2} = 9.485$$

  6. The approximate square root of 90 is 9.485.

  7. This process may be repeated to get a more accurate estimate of the square root of a number.

- To add or subtract **radicals** (numbers expressed as square roots), the **radicands** (numbers under the radical) must be the same.

  Example: $4\sqrt{12} + 3\sqrt{12} = 7\sqrt{12}$

  Example: If the radicands are not the same, simplify the radicals and then see if they can be combined.

  $$
  \begin{aligned}
  3\sqrt{12} - 8\sqrt{3} &= 3(\sqrt{4} \times \sqrt{3}) - 8\sqrt{3} \quad (\text{12 can be factored as } 4 \times 3) \\
  &= 3 \times 2\sqrt{3} - 8\sqrt{3} \quad (\text{take } \sqrt{4}, \text{ which equals 2}) \\
  &= 6\sqrt{3} - 8\sqrt{3} \\
  &= -2\sqrt{3}
  \end{aligned}
  $$

Fractions

A fraction is a part of something. A fraction is expressed using two terms: a **numerator**, which is the number above the fraction line, and a **denominator**, which is the number below the fraction line. In the fraction $\frac{3}{4}$, the numerator is 3 and the denominator is 4.

A **proper fraction** is one in which the numerator is less than its denominator. An **improper fraction** has a numerator that is equal to or greater than its denominator.

$\frac{4}{5}$ is a proper fraction, and $\frac{7}{3}$ is an improper fraction.

An improper fraction can be expressed as a **mixed number,** which has both a whole and a fractional part. Divide the denominator into the numerator to get the whole part. The remainder will be the numerator, and the divisor will be the denominator of the fractional part.

Example: $\frac{7}{3} = 2\frac{1}{3}$

7 divided by 3 gives a quotient of 2 and a remainder of 1.

Reducing Fractions

Factor the numerator and denominator into prime factors and divide the numerator and denominator by the common factors. (The value of a fraction is unchanged when the numerator and denominator are multiplied or divided by the same number.)

Example: $\frac{35}{55} = \frac{7 \times 5}{11 \times 5} = \frac{7}{11}$

Note that the numerator and denominator were divided by 5.

Multiplying Fractions

To multiply two fractions, multiply the two numerators to get the numerator of the product of the two fractions, and multiply the two denominators to get the denominator of the product of the fractions. Then simplify the resulting fraction by reducing it to lowest terms and/or by changing it to a mixed number.

Example: $\frac{6}{9} \times \frac{3}{8} = \frac{18}{72} = \frac{2 \times 3 \times 3}{2 \times 2 \times 2 \times 3 \times 3} = \frac{1}{4}$

Dividing Fractions

To divide two fractions, invert the divisor, then multiply the two fractions and simplify.

Examples: $\frac{9}{20} \div \frac{3}{4} = \frac{9}{20} \times \frac{4}{3} = \frac{36}{60} = \frac{2 \times 2 \times 3 \times 3}{2 \times 2 \times 3 \times 5} = \frac{3}{5}$

$2\frac{2}{3} \div 4 = \frac{8}{3} \div \frac{4}{1} = \frac{8}{3} \times \frac{1}{4} = \frac{8}{12} = \frac{2 \times 2 \times 2}{2 \times 2 \times 3} = \frac{2}{3}$

Note that the mixed number $2\frac{2}{3}$ was changed to the improper fraction $\frac{8}{3}$, and

that the inversion of the whole number 4, which equals $\frac{4}{1}$, is $\frac{1}{4}$.

Adding and Subtracting Fractions

To add or subtract fractions with the **same**, or common, denominator, keep the common denominator and add or subtract the numerators of the fractions.

Examples: $\dfrac{7}{9} + \dfrac{4}{9} = \dfrac{11}{9} = 1\dfrac{2}{9}$

$\dfrac{15}{32} - \dfrac{5}{32} = \dfrac{10}{32} = \dfrac{5}{16}$

To add or subtract fractions with different denominators, express the fractions as equivalent fractions with a common denominator. The **lowest common denominator** is the smallest number that can be divided evenly by the denominators of the given fractions. To find the lowest common denominator of two fractions, first express each denominator as a product of its prime factors. The lowest common denominator will be the number formed by multiplying each prime factor the largest number of times it occurs in the factorization of the denominators.

Example: $\dfrac{5}{9} + \dfrac{7}{12} = \dfrac{20}{36} + \dfrac{21}{36} = \dfrac{41}{36} = 1\dfrac{5}{36}$

Since $9 = 3 \times 3$ and $12 = 3 \times 4$, the lowest common denominator of 9 and 12 is

$3 \times 3 \times 4 = 36.$

Example: $\dfrac{7}{24} - \dfrac{9}{150}$

$24 = 2 \times 2 \times 2 \times 3$
$150 = 2 \times 3 \times 5 \times 5$

The largest number of times that 2 appears as a factor is 3 (in 24) and the largest number of times that 5 appears as a factor is 2 (in 150). 3 appears as a factor only once in each of the factorizations.

Thus, the lowest common denominator of the two fractions is 600.

$2 \times 2 \times 2 \times 3 \times 5 \times 5 = 600$

$\dfrac{7}{24} - \dfrac{9}{150} = \dfrac{7}{24} \times \dfrac{25}{25} - \dfrac{9}{150} \times \dfrac{4}{4} = \dfrac{175}{600} - \dfrac{36}{600} = \dfrac{139}{600}$

Thus, $\dfrac{7}{24} - \dfrac{9}{150} = \dfrac{175}{600} - \dfrac{36}{600} = \dfrac{139}{600}$

TIP

To add or subtract fractions quickly, remember that a sum can be found by adding the two cross-products and putting this answer over the denominator product.

Example: $4\frac{2}{3} - 1\frac{3}{4}$

$$4\frac{2}{3} - 1\frac{3}{4} = 4\frac{8}{12} - 1\frac{9}{12}$$

Since $\frac{9}{12}$ is greater than $\frac{8}{12}$, $4\frac{8}{12}$ is changed to $3 + 1 + \frac{8}{12}$.

Note that $1 = \frac{12}{12}$.

$$= 3 + \frac{12}{12} + \frac{8}{12}$$

$$= 3 + \frac{20}{12} \text{ or } 3\frac{20}{12}$$

then $4\frac{2}{3} - 1\frac{3}{4}$

$$= 4\frac{8}{12} - 1\frac{9}{12}$$

$$= 3\frac{20}{12} - 1\frac{9}{12}$$

$$= 2\frac{11}{12}$$

Comparison of Fractions

To determine which of two fractions is larger, change the two fractions to equivalent fractions with a common denominator and then compare the numerator of the fractions. The fraction with the larger numerator is the larger fraction.

Example: Which is larger, $\frac{5}{6}$ or $\frac{7}{8}$?

24 is a common denominator for the two fractions, hence $\frac{5}{6} = \frac{20}{24}$ and $\frac{7}{8} = \frac{21}{24}$.

Since $\frac{21}{24}$ is larger than $\frac{20}{24}$, $\frac{7}{8}$ is larger than $\frac{5}{6}$.

Decimals

A common fraction can be expressed as a decimal. For example: $\frac{1}{2} = \frac{5}{10} = 0.5$. Each common fraction has an equivalent decimal form.

To change a common fraction to a decimal, divide the numerator of the fraction by the denominator.

Example: $\frac{3}{8} = .375$

$$
\begin{array}{r}
.375 \\
8)\overline{3.000} \\
\underline{24} \\
60 \\
\underline{56} \\
40 \\
\underline{40} \\
0
\end{array}
$$

When a decimal is changed to a fraction, the digits after the decimal point become the numerator. The denominator is 1 followed by as many zeros as there are decimal places. (The denominator can also be determined by raising 10 to a power. The power is the number of decimal places in the number.)

An alternate method for changing a decimal to a common fraction is to count the number of decimal places after the decimal. One decimal place represents tenths; two decimal places, hundredths; three decimal places, thousandths; and so on. The digits of the decimal indicates how many tenths, hundredths, thousandths, etc., there are.

Example: $0.540 = \dfrac{540}{1,000}$

(Note that $1,000 = 10^3$. There are 3 decimal places in the number so the power is 3.)

Example: $0.48 = \dfrac{48}{100}$ (There are 48 hundredths.)

Rounding Decimals

To round a decimal number to one decimal place, first observe the digit two places to the right of the decimal point. If that digit is 0, 1, 2, 3, or 4, then simply remove that digit and all digits to the right. If the second digit after the decimal point is 5, 6, 7, 8, or 9, then round up by increasing the digit immediately to the right of the decimal point by one and removing all the digits to its right. When rounding up, if the digit you must increase by one is 9, change the 9 to 0 and increase the digit to its left by one.

Example: Round 1.333… to one decimal place:

1.333… = 1.3

Example: Round 6.3480 to two decimal places:

$$\overset{5}{6.34\cancel{80}} = 6.35$$

Example: Round 126.95 to one decimal place:

$$\overset{7\ 0}{12\cancel{6.95}} = 127.0$$

Adding and Subtracting Decimals

Arrange the decimals vertically with the decimal points aligned under each other. (Express whole numbers as decimals by appending a decimal point at the end of the number and adding as many zeros as desired, e.g., 23 = 23.0.)

Example: Subtract 2.715 from 4

$$\begin{array}{r} 4.000 \\ -\ 2.715 \\ \hline 1.285 \end{array}$$

Example: Add 11.3 + 0.968 + 0.24 + 3

$$
\begin{array}{r}
11.300 \\
.968 \\
.240 \\
+\ \ 3.000 \\
\hline
15.508
\end{array}
$$

Multiplying Decimals

To multiply decimals, multiply as you would with whole numbers. The number of decimal places in the product is the sum of the number of decimal places in the two numbers being multiplied.

Example: Multiply 2.47 times 0.315

$$
\begin{array}{r}
2.47 \\
\times\ .315 \\
\hline
1235 \\
247\ \ \\
741\ \ \ \ \\
\hline
.77805
\end{array}
$$

There are two decimal places in 2.47 and three in 0.315; therefore, there are five decimal places in the product of the two numbers. The product is 0.77805.

Dividing Decimals

When a decimal is divided by a whole number, the decimal point in the quotient should be aligned with the decimal point in the dividend. Divide as you would with whole numbers.

Example: Divide 0.264 by 12

$$
\begin{array}{r}
.022\ \ \\
12\overline{)\,.264} \\
24\ \ \ \ \\
\hline
24\ \\
24\ \\
\hline
0
\end{array}
$$

To divide by a decimal, multiply the divisor by the multiple of 10 that will make the divisor a whole number, then multiply the dividend by the same multiple of 10. Divide as you would with whole numbers.

Example: Divide 2.752 by 0.16

$$.16\overline{)2.752}$$

Multiply the divisor and dividend by 100 to get a new divisor of 16 and dividend of 275.2.

$$
\begin{array}{r}
17.2 \\
16\overline{)275.2} \\
\underline{16} \\
115 \\
\underline{112} \\
32 \\
\underline{32} \\
0
\end{array}
$$

Percentages

Percent means "by the hundredths." A **percentage** can be expressed as a fraction with a denominator of 100. $63\% = \dfrac{63}{100}$

Converting decimals and fractions to percentages and vice versa

Example: To convert a decimal to a percentage, multiply the decimal by 100.

$0.134 \times 100 = 13.4\%$

Example: To convert a percentage to a decimal, divide the percent by 100.

$47\% = \dfrac{47}{100} = 0.47$

To find the percentage (the amount) of a given number (the base), change the percent to a decimal and multiply the decimal times the base.

Example: 35% of $80 = 0.35 \times 80 = 28$

Example: The number of patients admitted to Get Well Hospital for opioid drug overdoses was 24% higher in 2017 than in 2016. If 325 patients were admitted for drug overdoses in 2016, how many were admitted in 2017?

24% of $325 = .24 \times 325 = 78$

$325 + 78 = 403$

There were 78 more patients in 2017 than in 2016, making a total of 403 admitted for drug overdoses in 2017.

To determine the base when the percent and amount are known, change the percent to a decimal and divide the amount by the result. (Note that "is" can be interpreted as = and "of" as multiplication.)

Example: 32 is 20% of what number?

$32 = 0.20 \times B$ (B represents the base, which is the unknown number, and 32 is the amount)

$\frac{32}{.20} = B$

$160 = B$

32 is 20% of 160.

To determine what percent a given amount is of a base, divide the amount by the base and change the resulting decimal to a percent.

Example: What percent of 60 is 15?

$15 = P \times 60$ (P is the percent, 60 is the base, and 15 is the amount.)

$\frac{15}{60} = \frac{1}{4} = 0.25 = 25\%$

Example: If a nurse with a salary of $40,000 receives a $2,000 bonus, what percent of his salary is his bonus? (That is, what percent of $40,000 is $2,000?)

$2,000 = P \times 40,000$

$\frac{2,000}{40,000} = \frac{1}{20} = 0.05$ or 5%

To find a percentage increase or percentage decrease in a word problem, write a fraction with the amount of increase or decrease as the numerator and the original amount as the denominator. Then change the fraction to a percentage.

Example: A patient's prescription was decreased from 2 grams to 1.5 grams. What is the percent of decrease of the new prescription?

The amount of decrease was 0.5 grams. What percent of 2 grams is 0.5 grams?

$0.5 = P \times 2$

$\frac{0.5}{2} = 0.25 = 25\%$

The dosage was decreased by 25%.

To determine discount in word problems, change the percentage to a fraction or decimal, multiply by the original cost, and deduct this amount from the original cost.

For word problems dealing with commission or taxes, multiply the total value of the goods or services by the percentage of tax or commission.

Ratios

A **ratio** is the comparison of two numerical quantities by division.

Example: A box contains 3 red balls and 2 blue balls. The ratio of blue to red balls in the box is 2 to 3, or $\frac{2}{3}$.

Proportions

A **proportion** is a statement that two ratios are equivalent.

Example: The ratio of 4 to x is equivalent to the ratio of 5 to 10.

$$\frac{4}{x} = \frac{5}{10}$$

TIP

If $\frac{A}{B} = \frac{C}{D}$, you can cross-multiply to get $AD = BC$.

Direct Proportions

In a **direct proportion**, one quantity increases (↑) or decreases (↓) as the other increases or decreases. In other words, the direction of the changes is the same for both factors. (x increases as y increases, or x decreases as y decreases.)

Example: One orange sells for 15 cents. How much will six oranges cost?

$$\frac{1 \text{ orange}}{15¢} = \frac{6 \text{ oranges}}{y¢}$$

Cross-multiply: $1y = 6 \times 15$

$$y = 90¢$$

The total cost increases as the number of oranges sold increases.

Example: Six oranges cost 90 cents. How much would one orange cost?

$$\frac{6 \text{ oranges}}{90¢} = \frac{1 \text{ orange}}{y¢}$$

Cross-multiply: $6y = 90¢$

$$y = 15¢ \quad \text{(Divide both sides by 6.)}$$

The cost decreases as the number of oranges purchased decreases.

Inverse Proportions

In an **inverse proportion**, one quantity increases (↑) as the other decreases (↓), and vice versa. In other words, the direction of the changes is opposite. (As x increases, y decreases; or as x decreases, y increases.)

Example: A 5-pound bag of dog food lasts one week when the dog is given 2 servings per day. How long would this bag last if the dog were to receive 3 servings per day?

$$\frac{3}{2} = \frac{7}{y}$$

$$3y = 14$$

$$y = 4.\overline{6} \text{ or } 4\frac{2}{3}$$

(As the number of meals increases, the number of days the dog food lasts decreases.)

Algebra

Algebra involves the use of letters and symbols as well as numbers. Some of the introductory concepts of algebra are reviewed in this section.

Operations with signed numbers

For operations with signed numbers (+ or −):

Addition

For numbers with the same sign, add and keep the same sign in the answer. For numbers with different signs, subtract and give the answer using the sign of the higher number.

Subtraction

Combine the two signs of the subtrahend, taking the subtraction sign as a negative sign, [− times − = +] [− times + = −]. Then use the rules for addition.

Examples: $-4 - (-2) = -4 + 2 = -2$
$-4 - (+2) = -4 - 2 = -6$

Multiplication

- The product of an odd number of negative numbers is negative.
- The product of an even number of negative numbers is positive.

Examples: $(-3)(-2)(-5) = -30$
$(-4)(-2)(-3)(-5) = 120$

Division

If the two numbers have the same sign, the quotient is positive; if otherwise, the quotient is negative.

Algebraic Expressions

Algebraic expressions consist of a combination of variables and numbers connected by addition and subtraction signs. The parts of algebraic expressions connected by plus and minus signs are called **terms**.

Combining Like terms

Like terms are terms that contain the same variables. These variables have the same exponents.

$2xy^2$ and $5xy^2$ are like terms.

$3xy$ and $4x^2y$ are not like terms. The variable x in the two terms has different exponents.

Only like terms in an algebraic expression can be combined. To combine like terms, add their numerical coefficients.

Examples: $7x - 4x + 2 + 3 = 3x + 5$

$2xy + 7x^2y - 4xy + 6y = 7x^2y - 2xy + 6y$

Order of Operations

When simplifying an algebraic expression:

1. First remove grouping symbols (parentheses, brackets), starting with the innermost grouping symbols. To remove grouping symbols, perform any operations that you can inside the symbols.

2. Perform the operations of multiplication and division, moving from left to right.

3. Perform the operations of addition and subtraction, moving from left to right.

Example:
$$5x - 2\big[(3x - 1) + (4 - 2x)\big]$$
$$= 5x - 2\big[3x - 1 + 4 - 2x\big]$$
$$= 5x - 2\big[x + 3\big]$$
$$= 5x - 2x - 6$$
$$= 3x - 6$$

Evaluating Algebraic Expressions

Find the value of an algebraic expression for given values of the variable by substituting the value of the variables in the expression.

Example: Evaluate the expression $2x^2y + 3xy$ when $x = 2$ and $y = 3$.

$$2x^2y + 3xy = 2(2)^2(3) + 3(2)(3)$$
$$= 2(4)(3) + 3(2)(3)$$
$$= 24 + 18$$
$$= 42$$

Solving Equations with One Variable

An equation is a statement that two quantities are equal. An equation has one unknown if it has only one variable. Equations with one variable can be solved using inverse operations. One or more of the basic operations of addition, subtraction, multiplication, and division are used to solve equations.

Consider the equation $x - 7 = 3$.

7 has been subtracted from the variable; the inverse operation for subtraction is addition. To solve the equation, add 7 to both sides of the equation.

$$x - 7 = 3$$
$$x - 7 + 7 = 3 + 7$$
$$x = 10$$

Equivalent equations can be obtained by adding or subtracting the same number from both sides of the equation, or by multiplying or dividing both sides of the equation by the same number. (Do not divide by zero.)

Example:
$$3x + 5 = 17$$
$$3x + 5 - 5 = 17 - 5$$
$$3x = 12$$
$$\frac{3x}{3} = \frac{12}{3}$$
$$x = 4$$

Note that to solve an equation, it is necessary to get the variable on one side of the equation and the constant on the other side.

Example:
$$5x + 2 = x - 10$$
$$5x + 2 - 2 = x - 10 - 2$$
$$5x = x - 12$$
$$5x - x = x - 12 - x$$
$$4x = -12$$
$$\frac{4x}{4} = \frac{-12}{4}$$
$$x = -3$$

Solving Word Problems

The previously described methods can be used to solve word problems once they are translated into equations. The first step in translating a word problem into an equation is to represent the unknown quantity by a variable. Then write an equation involving the variable that represents information given in the problem.

Example: When 3 times a number is increased by 4, the result is 19.

Let N represent the unknown number.

$3N$ represents 3 times the number.

$3N + 4$ represents 3 times the number increased by 4.

(To increase a number means to add to it.)

Since the result is 19, the desired equation is

$3N + 4 = 19$.

$3N = 15$ (4 was subtracted from both.)

$N = 5$ (Both sides were divided by 3.)

The solution is 5.

Example: A number decreased by $\frac{1}{2}$ of itself equals $\frac{3}{4}$. What decimal is equivalent to the resulting fraction?

Let y represent the unknown number.

$y - \frac{1}{2} y$ represents y decreased by $\frac{1}{2}$ of itself.

The desired equation is

$$y - \frac{1}{2}y = \frac{3}{4}$$

$$\frac{1}{2}y = \frac{3}{4}$$

Multiply both sides of the equation by 4 to get

$$2y = 3$$

$$y = \frac{3}{2} = 1.5$$

The solution is 1.5.

Formulas

An equation in which a variable is expressed in terms of one or more other variables is called a **formula**.

- $I = PRT$ is a formula for finding interest.
  - P represents the principal.
  - R represents the interest rate.
  - T represents the time.

Example: Find the simple interest that would be paid on a $5,000 loan at 8% after five years.

$$I = PRT$$

$$I = 5,000 \times .08 \times 5$$

$$I = \$2,000$$

- $D = RT$ is the formula for finding distance.
  - R is the rate or speed.
  - T is the time.

Example: How long will it take to drive a distance of 330 miles traveling at a rate of 60 mph?

$$D = R \times T$$

$$330 = 60 \times T$$

$$\frac{330}{60} = T$$

$$5\frac{1}{2} = T$$

It will take $5\frac{1}{2}$ hours to drive the 330 miles at a rate of 60 mph.

- $F = \frac{9}{5}C + 32$ is the formula for changing a temperature from Celsius to Fahrenheit.

  o C = Celsius

  o F = Fahrenheit

  Example: If a temperature reading on the Celsius scale is 40 degrees, what is the Fahrenheit reading?

  $$F = \frac{9}{5}(40) + 32$$

  $$F = \frac{360}{5} + 32 = 72 + 32 = 104$$

  The temperature is 104 degrees Fahrenheit.

- $\frac{T}{A} + \frac{T}{B} = 1$ is the formula for a work problem.

  o T is the time working together.

  o A is time for person A working alone.

  o B is the time for a person B working alone.

  Example: Shelley can paint a wall in 60 minutes and Lisa can do it in 30 minutes. How many minutes will it take them to do the job together?

  $$\frac{T}{60} + \frac{T}{30} = 1$$

  $T + 2T = 60$ (multiplying both sides by 60, the lowest common denominator)

  $3T = 60$ (combine like terms)

  $T = 20$ (divide by 3)

  They can do the job together in 20 minutes.

Inequalities

The symbols $<$ and $>$ are used to represent the inequalities "less than" and "greater than." Various statements of inequality are expressed as follows:

1.	$a < b$ means	a is less than b.
	$7 < 12$ means	7 is less than 12.
2.	$a \leq b$ means	a is either less than or equal to b.
	$5 \leq 9$ means	5 is less than or equal to 9.
3.	$a > b$ means	a is greater than b.
	$18 > 14$ means	18 is greater than 14.
4.	$a \geq b$ means	a is either greater than or equal to b.
	$3 \geq 3$ means	3 is greater than or equal to 3.
5.	$a < b \leq c$ means	a is less than b, and b is less than or equal to c.
	$-1 < 3 \leq 5$ means	-1 is less than 3, and 3 is less than or equal to 5.
	$2 \leq x < 5$ means	2 is less than or equal to x, and x is less than 5.

Defined Functions

Certain questions may include a special sign such as * or # that is defined for you. The sign tells you to perform a specific function or operation. This kind of problem tests your ability to learn and apply a new concept.

Example: For all numbers, $a * b = \frac{a}{b} + 2$. What is $6 * 3$?

$$6 * 3 = \frac{6}{3} + 2$$
$$= 2 + 2$$
$$= 4$$

Geometry

English Standard Measurements

The following are some English standard units of measurement.

Length	Capacity or Volume
inches	ounces
feet (1 ft. = 12 in.)	pints (1 pt. = 16 oz.)
yard (1 yd. = 3 ft.)	quart (1 qt. = 2 pts.)
miles (1 mi. = 5,280 ft.)	gallon (1 gal. = 4 qts.)

Weight	
ounces	pounds (1 lb. = 16 oz.)

Area is expressed in square units, and volume is expressed in cubic units (square feet, cubic inches, etc.).

For **literal expressions** (problems with letters instead of numbers), use the same processes as you would for numbers.

Example: How many inches are in y yards and x feet?

$$y \text{ yd.} \times \frac{36 \text{ in.}}{\text{yd.}} = 36y \text{ in.} \quad x \text{ ft.} \times \frac{12 \text{ in.}}{\text{ft.}} = 12x \text{ in.}$$

Metric Measurements

Metric measurements are based on powers of 10. The basic metric units of measure are as follows:

- **Length—Meter**
- **Volume—Liter**
- **Weight—Gram**
- **Temperature—Celsius**

The chart below illustrates the relationship between metric units.

MILLI	CENTI	DECI	UNIT	DEKA	HECTO	KILO
.001	.01	.1	1	10	100	1,000

Example: 1 gram = 1,000 milligrams

2 liters = 2,000 milliliters

1 hectometer = 100 meters

Computations in the metric system involve multiplication and division by powers of 10. Problems involving metric measurements (other than conversions within the metric system) are solved using the same techniques as problems with English measurement units.

Lines, Segments, and Rays

A **line** extends infinitely in opposite directions. A **segment** is two endpoints and the part of a line that lies between them. A **ray** is an endpoint and the part of a line that extends in one direction from that point.

The length of a segment can be measured using the units for length in either the English standard or metric systems.

Parallel and Perpendicular Lines

- **Parallel lines** are two lines on the same plane that do not intersect (have no points in common). When graphed, the slopes of two parallel lines are equal.

- **Perpendicular lines** are two lines that intersect at right angles. When graphed, the slopes of two perpendicular lines have a product of –1.

Angles and Angle Measure

An **angle** is formed by two rays that share a common endpoint. Units of measurement of angles are called **degrees**.

An **acute angle** has a measure that is less than 90°.

A **right angle** has a measure of exactly 90°. (Perpendicular lines form right angles.)

An **obtuse angle** has a measure that is greater than 90° and less than 180°.

Two angles are **complementary** if the sum of their measures is 90°.

Two angles are **supplementary** if the sum of their measures is 180°.

If the exterior sides of a pair of adjacent angles form a straight line, the two adjacent angles are supplementary.

Example: If $AB \perp DC$ (AB is perpendicular to DC), then

∠ABF and ∠FBC are complementary angles.

(The sum of the measures of ∠ABF and ∠FBC = 90°.)

∠EBD and ∠EBC are supplementary angles.

(The sum of ∠EBD and ∠EBC = 180°.)

∠FBC is an acute angle. ∠ABC is a right angle.

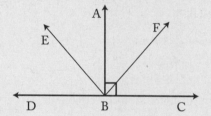

Polygons and Circles

A **polygon** is a simple closed plane figure made up of line segments.

Polygons with three sides are called **triangles**. If the lengths of two sides of a triangle are equal, the triangle is called an **isosceles** triangle. When all three sides of a triangle have the same length, the triangle is called an **equilateral** triangle.

Polygons with four sides are called **quadrilaterals**. A **square** is a quadrilateral with all four sides equal, and with four corners having equal measure of 90 degrees. A **rectangle** is a quadrilateral with four 90-degree corners and opposite sides equal.

A **circle** is a set of all points in a plane that are an equal distance from a given point called the **center**.

In the drawing below, point O is the center of the given circle. Points P, R, and S are points on the circle.

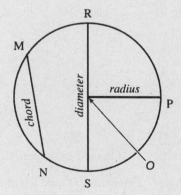

A **chord** of a circle is any segment with its two end points on the circle. $\overline{MN}$ is a chord of the given circle.

A **radius** of a circle is a segment from the center of the circle to any point on the circle. $\overline{OP}$ is a radius of the circle.

A **diameter** of a circle is a chord that passes through the center of a circle. $\overline{RS}$ is a diameter of the given circle.

All radii of a circle have the same length. A diameter of a given circle is always twice the radius of the circle.

> **Example:** If the length of radius $\overline{OP} = 7$ cm. , the diameter $\overline{RS} = 14$ cm.

Perimeter

To find the **perimeter (P)** of a figure, add the lengths of all its sides.

Triangle	$P =$ sum of the three sides, or $P = a + b + c$
Rectangle	$P = 2 \times \text{Length} + 2 \times \text{Width}$, or $P = 2L + 2W$
Square	$P = 4 \times S$, where $S = $ length of each side.
Circle	The circumference (C) is the distance around a circle.
	The circumference of a circle is equal to $\pi \times$ the diameter:
	$C = \pi \times d$

Area

To find the **area (A)** of plane figures:

Square	$A = (\text{side})^2$, or $A = S^2$
Rectangle	$A = \text{length} \times \text{width}$, or $A = L \times W$
Triangle	$A = \frac{1}{2} \text{ Base} \times \text{Height}$, or $A = \frac{1}{2} bh$
Circle	$A = \pi \times (\text{radius})^2$, or $A = \pi r^2$

Choose any side of the triangle to be the base; the height is determined as shown below.

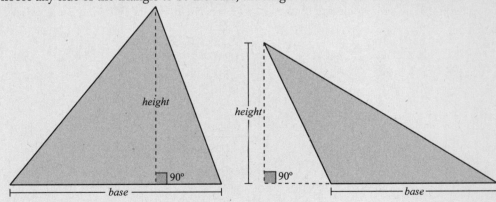

To find the **areas of other polygons**, divide the polygon into nonoverlapping triangles and/or quadrilaterals (squares, rectangles), and then add the areas of the triangles and quadrilaterals.

Nonoverlapping triangles and quadrilaterals may be obtained by drawing diagonals of the polygon. A **diagonal** of a polygon is a line segment joining two nonconsecutive vertices (corners) of a polygon. Segment $\overline{BE}$ is a diagonal of polygon *ABCDE* below.

Example: Given polygon ABCDE with the measurements indicated, draw the diagonal *BE* to divide the polygon into triangle *BAE* and rectangle *BEDC*.

Area of triangle $BAE = \frac{1}{2} \times 10 \times 4 = 20$ sq. in.

Area of rectangle $BEDC = 2 \times 10 = 20$ sq. in.

Since 20 + 20 = 40, the area of polygon *ABCDE* = 40 sq. in.

Similar triangles have the same shape. The angles of one similar triangle are equal to the angles of the other. The ratios of the lengths of corresponding sides of similar triangles are equal.

Example: The two given triangles are similar (measures of corresponding angles are equal). Therefore $\frac{8}{y} = \frac{x}{5}$. (Note that the side of length *x* in the triangle on the left is

opposite the 50° angle. The side across from the 50° angle in the second triangle, of length 5, corresponds to the side of length *x*. Similarly, the side of length 8 in the first triangle corresponds to the side of length *y* in the second.)

A **right triangle** is a triangle with a right angle. The side of the triangle that is opposite the right angle is called the **hypotenuse**.

Pythagorean theorem: The square of the hypotenuse of a right triangle is equal to the sum of the squares of the other two sides.

$$c^2 = a^2 + b^2$$

Example: Find the hypotenuse of the right triangle given below.

The two sides of the triangle are 5 and 12. The hypotenuse, c, can be found with the use of the Pythagorean theorem.

$$c^2 = 5^2 + 12^2$$
$$c^2 = 25 + 144$$
$$c^2 = 169 \quad \text{(To find } c, \text{ take the square root of 169.)}$$
$$c = 13$$

Angles in Triangles

The sum of the measures of the three **interior angles** of a triangle is 180°. If the measures of two angles of a triangle are given, the measure of the third angle can be found by subtracting the sum of the measures of the two known angles from 180°.

Example: If $m\angle A = 40°$ and $m\angle B = 60°$, then
$$m\angle C = 180° - (m\angle A + m\angle B)$$
$$= 180° - (40° + 60°)$$
$$= 180° - (100°)$$
$$= 80°$$

An **exterior angle** of a triangle is formed by a side of a triangle and by the extension of another side of the triangle.

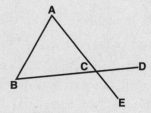

$\angle ACD$ is an exterior angle of $\triangle ABC$.

$\angle BCE$ is also an exterior angle of $\triangle ABC$.

Every triangle has six exterior angles.

- The measure of an exterior angle of a triangle is greater than either of the measures of the remote interior angles. Angles A and B are the remote interior angles for the exterior angle ACD.

- An exterior angle of a triangle equals the sum of the remote interior angles ($m\angle ACD = m\angle A + m\angle B$).

- $m\angle ACD + m\angle ACB = 180°$.

Angles in Circles

The total degree measure of a circle is 360°.

- A **central angle** of a circle is an angle in which the vertex is the center of the circle.
- Angle ∠*AOB* is a central angle in the circle below.
- An **arc** of a circle consists of two points A and B, where the sides of a central angle intersect the circle, and all points of the circle that lie in the interior of the central angle. The measure of an arc is the measure of the central angle that forms the arc (m $\overset{\frown}{AB}$ = m∠*AOB*).

  The **minor arc** $\overset{\frown}{AB}$ is indicated in the given circle. A minor arc measures less than 180°.

- A **major arc** of a circle consists of points *A* and *B* and all points on the circle that lie in the exterior of the central angle. A major arc measures greater than 180° and less than 360°.

  The major arc $\overset{\frown}{AB}$ is indicated in the circle below.

- An **inscribed angle** of a circle is an angle with its vertex on the circle and its rays intersecting the circle in two points different from the vertex. The measure of an inscribed angle equals one-half the measure of its intercepted arc.

  ∠*ACB* is an inscribed angle of the given circle. The measure of ∠*ACB* is one half the measure of the central angle, ∠*AOB*.

MATHEMATICS ANSWER SHEET

Test 1

1. Ⓐ Ⓑ Ⓒ Ⓓ	5. Ⓐ Ⓑ Ⓒ Ⓓ	9. Ⓐ Ⓑ Ⓒ Ⓓ	13. Ⓐ Ⓑ Ⓒ Ⓓ	17. Ⓐ Ⓑ Ⓒ Ⓓ
2. Ⓐ Ⓑ Ⓒ Ⓓ	6. Ⓐ Ⓑ Ⓒ Ⓓ	10. Ⓐ Ⓑ Ⓒ Ⓓ	14. Ⓐ Ⓑ Ⓒ Ⓓ	18. Ⓐ Ⓑ Ⓒ Ⓓ
3. Ⓐ Ⓑ Ⓒ Ⓓ	7. Ⓐ Ⓑ Ⓒ Ⓓ	11. Ⓐ Ⓑ Ⓒ Ⓓ	15. Ⓐ Ⓑ Ⓒ Ⓓ	19. Ⓐ Ⓑ Ⓒ Ⓓ
4. Ⓐ Ⓑ Ⓒ Ⓓ	8. Ⓐ Ⓑ Ⓒ Ⓓ	12. Ⓐ Ⓑ Ⓒ Ⓓ	16. Ⓐ Ⓑ Ⓒ Ⓓ	20. Ⓐ Ⓑ Ⓒ Ⓓ

Test 2

1. Ⓐ Ⓑ Ⓒ Ⓓ	5. Ⓐ Ⓑ Ⓒ Ⓓ	9. Ⓐ Ⓑ Ⓒ Ⓓ	13. Ⓐ Ⓑ Ⓒ Ⓓ	17. Ⓐ Ⓑ Ⓒ Ⓓ
2. Ⓐ Ⓑ Ⓒ Ⓓ	6. Ⓐ Ⓑ Ⓒ Ⓓ	10. Ⓐ Ⓑ Ⓒ Ⓓ	14. Ⓐ Ⓑ Ⓒ Ⓓ	18. Ⓐ Ⓑ Ⓒ Ⓓ
3. Ⓐ Ⓑ Ⓒ Ⓓ	7. Ⓐ Ⓑ Ⓒ Ⓓ	11. Ⓐ Ⓑ Ⓒ Ⓓ	15. Ⓐ Ⓑ Ⓒ Ⓓ	19. Ⓐ Ⓑ Ⓒ Ⓓ
4. Ⓐ Ⓑ Ⓒ Ⓓ	8. Ⓐ Ⓑ Ⓒ Ⓓ	12. Ⓐ Ⓑ Ⓒ Ⓓ	16. Ⓐ Ⓑ Ⓒ Ⓓ	20. Ⓐ Ⓑ Ⓒ Ⓓ

Test 3

1. Ⓐ Ⓑ Ⓒ Ⓓ	5. Ⓐ Ⓑ Ⓒ Ⓓ	9. Ⓐ Ⓑ Ⓒ Ⓓ	13. Ⓐ Ⓑ Ⓒ Ⓓ	17. Ⓐ Ⓑ Ⓒ Ⓓ
2. Ⓐ Ⓑ Ⓒ Ⓓ	6. Ⓐ Ⓑ Ⓒ Ⓓ	10. Ⓐ Ⓑ Ⓒ Ⓓ	14. Ⓐ Ⓑ Ⓒ Ⓓ	18. Ⓐ Ⓑ Ⓒ Ⓓ
3. Ⓐ Ⓑ Ⓒ Ⓓ	7. Ⓐ Ⓑ Ⓒ Ⓓ	11. Ⓐ Ⓑ Ⓒ Ⓓ	15. Ⓐ Ⓑ Ⓒ Ⓓ	19. Ⓐ Ⓑ Ⓒ Ⓓ
4. Ⓐ Ⓑ Ⓒ Ⓓ	8. Ⓐ Ⓑ Ⓒ Ⓓ	12. Ⓐ Ⓑ Ⓒ Ⓓ	16. Ⓐ Ⓑ Ⓒ Ⓓ	20. Ⓐ Ⓑ Ⓒ Ⓓ

Test 4

1. Ⓐ Ⓑ Ⓒ Ⓓ	8. Ⓐ Ⓑ Ⓒ Ⓓ	14. Ⓐ Ⓑ Ⓒ Ⓓ	20. Ⓐ Ⓑ Ⓒ Ⓓ	26. Ⓐ Ⓑ Ⓒ Ⓓ
2. Ⓐ Ⓑ Ⓒ Ⓓ	9. Ⓐ Ⓑ Ⓒ Ⓓ	15. Ⓐ Ⓑ Ⓒ Ⓓ	21. Ⓐ Ⓑ Ⓒ Ⓓ	27. Ⓐ Ⓑ Ⓒ Ⓓ
3. Ⓐ Ⓑ Ⓒ Ⓓ	10. Ⓐ Ⓑ Ⓒ Ⓓ	16. Ⓐ Ⓑ Ⓒ Ⓓ	22. Ⓐ Ⓑ Ⓒ Ⓓ	28. Ⓐ Ⓑ Ⓒ Ⓓ
4. Ⓐ Ⓑ Ⓒ Ⓓ	11. Ⓐ Ⓑ Ⓒ Ⓓ	17. Ⓐ Ⓑ Ⓒ Ⓓ	23. Ⓐ Ⓑ Ⓒ Ⓓ	29. Ⓐ Ⓑ Ⓒ Ⓓ
5. Ⓐ Ⓑ Ⓒ Ⓓ	12. Ⓐ Ⓑ Ⓒ Ⓓ	18. Ⓐ Ⓑ Ⓒ Ⓓ	24. Ⓐ Ⓑ Ⓒ Ⓓ	30. Ⓐ Ⓑ Ⓒ Ⓓ
6. Ⓐ Ⓑ Ⓒ Ⓓ	13. Ⓐ Ⓑ Ⓒ Ⓓ	19. Ⓐ Ⓑ Ⓒ Ⓓ	25. Ⓐ Ⓑ Ⓒ Ⓓ	31. Ⓐ Ⓑ Ⓒ Ⓓ
7. Ⓐ Ⓑ Ⓒ Ⓓ				

answer sheet

TEST 1

20 Questions • 15 Minutes

Directions: Each problem on this test requires logical reasoning and thinking, in addition to simple computations, to find the solution. Read each problem carefully and choose the correct answer from the four choices that follow. Fill in the corresponding space on your answer sheet.

1. Find the interest on $25,800 for 144 days at 6 percent per annum. Base your calculations on a 360-day year.
   A. $619.20
   B. $619.02
   C. $691.02
   D. $691.20

   SHOW YOUR WORK HERE

2. Arthur can shovel snow from a sidewalk in 60 minutes, and Jack can do it in 30 minutes. How many minutes will it take them to do the job together?
   A. 90
   B. 15
   C. 30
   D. 20

3. The visitors' section of a courtroom seats 105 people. The court is in session 6 hours per day. On one particular day, 485 people visited the court and were given seats. What is the average length of time spent by each visitor in the court? Assume that as soon as a person leaves his seat, it is immediately filled and that at no time during the day is one of the 105 seats vacant. Express your answer in hours and minutes.
   A. 1 hour, 20 minutes
   B. 1 hour, 18 minutes
   C. 1 hour, 30 minutes
   D. 2 hours

SHOW YOUR WORK HERE

4. If copy paper costs $14.50 per ream and a 5% discount is allowed for cash, how many reams can be purchased for $690 cash? Do not round off cents in your calculations.

   A. 49 reams

   B. 60 reams

   C. 50 reams

   D. 53 reams

5. How many hours are there between 8:30 a.m. today and 3:15 a.m. tomorrow?

   A. $17\frac{3}{4}$ hours

   B. $18\frac{3}{4}$ hours

   C. $18\frac{2}{3}$ hours

   D. $18\frac{1}{2}$ hours

6. How many days are there from September 19 to December 25 (*inclusive*)?

   A. 98 days

   B. 96 days

   C. 89 days

   D. 90 days

7. A clerk is requested to file 800 cards. If he can file cards at the rate of 80 cards per hour, what is the number of cards remaining to be filed after 7 hours of work?

   A. 40

   B. 240

   C. 140

   D. 260

8. If your monthly electricity bill increases from $80 to $90, the percentage of increase is

   A. 10%

   B. $11\frac{1}{9}$ %

   C. $12\frac{1}{2}$ %

   D. $14\frac{1}{7}$ %

SHOW YOUR WORK HERE

9. Fifteen nurses who work the morning shift at Get Well Hospital are responsible for 135 patients. The average number of patients served by each nurse is

   A. 120.

   B. 10.

   C. 9.

   D. 140.

10. If a nursing exam contained 80 questions and you answered 72 of them correctly, what percentage of the questions did you answer correctly?

   A. 90%

   B. 72%

   C. 8%

   D. 28%

11. If a patient is required to get 45 minutes of exercise each day, how many hours of exercise does he get in a week?

   A. 315 hours

   B. 5.25 hours

   C. 52 hours

   D. 6.4 hours

12. If a hospital has 120 nurses on duty during the afternoon shift and one half as many on duty for the night shift, what is the total number of nurses on duty for the two shifts?

    A. 60
    B. 180
    C. 90
    D. 120.5

13. If an inspector issued 182 summonses in the course of 7 hours, his hourly average of summonses issued was

    A. 23 summonses.
    B. 26 summonses.
    C. 25 summonses.
    D. 28 summonses.

14. Last week, 23 of the 76 patients admitted to Emergency Hospital had been in accidents. How many of the admitted patients had **not** been in accidents?

    A. 23
    B. 99
    C. 53
    D. 76

15. A truck going at a rate of 40 miles per hour will reach a town 80 miles away in how many hours?

    A. 1 hour
    B. 3 hours
    C. 2 hours
    D. 4 hours

16. If a barrel has a capacity of 100 gallons, how many gallons will it contain when it is two-fifths full?

    A. 20 gallons
    B. 60 gallons
    C. 40 gallons
    D. 80 gallons

SHOW YOUR WORK HERE

17. If a monthly salary of $3,000 is subject to a 20 percent tax, the net salary is

   A. $2,000.

   B. $2,400.

   C. $2,500.

   D. $2,600.

18. If $1,000 is the cost of repairing 100 square yards of pavement, the cost of repairing 1 square yard is

   A. $10.

   B. $150.

   C. $100.

   D. $300.

19. If an employee's base pay is $3,000 per month, and it is increased by a monthly bonus of $350 and a seniority increment of $250 this month, her total salary for the month is

   A. $3,600.

   B. $3,500.

   C. $3,000.

   D. $3,700.

20. If an annual salary of $21,600 is increased by a bonus of $7,200 and by a service increment of $1,200, the total pay rate is

   A. $29,600.

   B. $39,600.

   C. $26,900.

   D. $30,000.

SHOW YOUR WORK HERE

STOP

IF YOU FINISH BEFORE TIME IS CALLED, YOU MAY CHECK YOUR WORK ON THIS SECTION ONLY. DO NOT TURN TO ANY OTHER SECTION IN THE TEST.

TEST 2

20 Questions • 15 Minutes

Directions: Each problem on this test requires logical reasoning and thinking, in addition to simple computations, to find the solution. Read each problem carefully and choose the correct answer from the four choices that follow. Fill in the corresponding space on your answer sheet.

SHOW YOUR WORK HERE

1. An emergency medical technician (EMT) was standing 40 feet behind his vehicle when a second emergency medical vehicle arrived and parked 90 feet from the first vehicle. If the EMT is standing between the two vehicles, how much closer is he to the first vehicle than to the second?
   A. 30 feet
   B. 50 feet
   C. 10 feet
   D. 70 feet

2. If an IV bag has a capacity of 1,260 milliliters, how many milliliters does it contain when it's two-thirds full?
   A. 809 mL
   B. 750 mL
   C. 630 mL
   D. 840 mL

3. If an employee's salary is $2,500 a month and there are 23 working days in the month, he earns approximately how much for each day he works that month?
   A. $108.70
   B. $150
   C. $112.50
   D. $186.70

4. A nursing home assistant earns $360 a week and has deductions of $18 for her retirement fund, $15 for medical insurance, $21 for social security, and $72 for with-holding taxes. How much is her take-home pay?

A. $488.

B. $296.

C. $234.

D. $288.

SHOW YOUR WORK HERE

5. A company uses 40 thirty-five-cent stamps, 25 fifty-cent stamps, and 320 seventy-one-cent stamps each day. The total cost of stamps used by the company in a five-day period is

A. $1,268.50.

B. $253.70.

C. $25,370.

D. $126,850.

6. A city department issued 12,000 applications in 2017. The number of applications that the department issued in 2015 was 25 percent greater than the number it issued in 2017. If the department issued 10 percent fewer applications in 2013 than it did in 2015, the number it issued in 2013 was

A. 16,500.

B. 13,500.

C. 9,900.

D. 8,100.

7. A secretary can add 40 columns of figures in an hour by using a calculator and 20 columns of figures an hour without using a calculator. The total number of hours it would take him to add 200 columns if he does three fifths of the work by machine and the rest without the machine is

A. 6.

B. 7.

C. 8.

D. 9.

8. In 2015, a medical office bought 500 dozen rubber gloves at a price of $2.60 per dozen. In 2018, 25 percent fewer gloves were bought than in 2015, but the price per dozen was 20 percent higher than the price in 2015. The total cost of the gloves bought in 2018 was

  A. $1,560.

  B. $1,170.

  C. $975.

  D. $1,040.

9. A nurse is assigned to check the accuracy of the entries on 490 forms. He checks 40 forms per hour. After working 1 hour on this task, he is joined by another nurse, who checks these forms at the rate of 35 per hour. The total number of hours required to do the entire assignment is

  A. 5.

  B. 6.

  C. 7.

  D. 8.

10. Assume there is a total of 420 employees in a medical care building. Thirty percent of the employees are nurses and one seventh are doctors. The difference between the number of nurses and the doctors is

  A. 60.

  B. 66.

  C. 186.

  D. 360.

SHOW YOUR WORK HERE

11. Assume that a copying machine produces copies of a bulletin at a cost of 12 cents per copy. The machine produces 120 copies of the bulletin per minute. If the cost of producing a certain number of copies was $36, how many minutes did it take the machine to produce this number of copies?

   A. 10 minutes
   B. 6 minutes
   C. 2.5 minutes
   D. 1.2 minutes

12. The average number of medical records filed per day by a filing clerk during a five-day week was 720. She filed 610 records the first day, 720 records the second day, 740 records the third day, and 755 records the fourth day. The number of records she filed the fifth day was

   A. 748.
   B. 165.
   C. 775.
   D. 565.

13. A city department employs 1,400 people, of whom 35 percent are clerks and one eighth are stenographers. The number of employees in the department who are neither clerks nor stenographers is

   A. 640.
   B. 665.
   C. 735.
   D. 750.

14. Two nurses were assigned to take blood pressure readings at a health fair. They took the blood pressure of 190 people. If Nurse A took 40 more blood pressures than Nurse B, then the number of blood pressures taken by Nurse A was

   A. 75.
   B. 110.
   C. 115.
   D. 150.

SHOW YOUR WORK HERE

15. A stock clerk had on hand the following items:

500 pads, worth $0.04 each

130 pencils, worth $0.03 each

50 dozen rubber bands, worth $0.02 a dozen

If, from this stock, he issued 125 pads, 45 pencils, and 48 rubber bands, the value of the remaining stock would be

A. $6.43.

B. $8.95.

C. $17.63.

D. $18.47.

16. Joe can paint a fence in 3 hours and his friend can paint the fence in 4 hours. How long will it take them to do the job if they work together?

A. 7 hours

B. $\frac{15}{7}$ hours

C. $1\frac{5}{7}$ hours

D. 2 hours

SHOW YOUR WORK HERE

17. A department head hired a total of 60 temporary employees to handle a seasonal increase in the department's workload.

    The following lists the number of temporary employees hired, their rates of pay, and the duration of their employment:

    One third of the total were hired as clerks, each at the rate of $29,750 per year, for two months.

    Thirty percent of the total were hired as office machine operators (OMOs), each at the rate of $31,500 per year, for four months.

    Twenty-two stenographers (stenos) were hired, each at the rate of $42,000 per year, for three months.

    The total amount paid to these temporary employees was approximately

    A. $585,400.

    B. $519,200.

    C. $173,800.

    D. $103,250.

18. Assume that there are 2,300 employees in a city agency. Also assume that 5 percent of these employees are accountants; that 80 percent of the accountants have college degrees; and that one half of the accountants who have college degrees have five years of experience. Then the number of employees in the agency who are accountants with college degrees and five years of experience is

    A. 46.

    B. 51.

    C. 460.

    D. 920.

19. If a monthly salary of $3,000 is subject to a $425 tax deduction, the net salary is

SHOW YOUR WORK HERE

  A. $2,557.

  B. $2,755.

  C. $2,575.

  D. $2,555.

20. A sanitation worker who reports 45 minutes early for 8:00 a.m. duty will report at

  A. 7:00 a.m.

  B. 7:30 a.m.

  C. 6:15 a.m.

  D. 7:15 a.m.

STOP

IF YOU FINISH BEFORE TIME IS CALLED, YOU MAY CHECK YOUR WORK ON THIS SECTION ONLY. DO NOT TURN TO ANY OTHER SECTION IN THE TEST.

TEST 3

20 Questions • 15 Minutes

Directions: Each problem on this test requires logical reasoning and thinking, in addition to simple computations, to find the solution. Read each problem carefully and choose the correct answer from the four choices that follow. Fill in the corresponding space on your answer sheet.

1. If the average cost of sweeping a square foot of a small town's street is $0.75, the cost of sweeping 100 square feet is

    A. $7.50.

    B. $750.

    C. $75.

    D. $70.

2. After her car broke down on the way to a conference, a nurse had the car towed home 90 miles away. If the car was towed at a rate of 36 miles per hour, how many hours did it take to tow her car home?

    A. 0.4 hours

    B. 54 hours

    C. 2.5 hours

    D. 25 hours

3. A man is standing between a bank and a drugstore. He is 60 feet away from the bank, and the drugstore is 100 feet away from the bank. How many feet nearer is the man to the bank than the drugstore is to the bank?

    A. 60 feet

    B. 40 feet

    C. 50 feet

    D. 20 feet

SHOW YOUR WORK HERE

4. A clerk divided his 35-hour work week as follows:

   One-fifth of his time in sorting mail; one-half of his time in filing letters; and one-seventh of his time in reception work.

   The rest of his time was devoted to messenger work. The percentage of time spent on messenger work by the clerk during the week was nearly

   A. 6%.

   B. 10%.

   C. 14%.

   D. 16%.

5. A city department has a computer unit and rents five computers at a yearly rental of $1,400 per machine. In addition, the cost to the department for the maintenance and repair of each of these machines is $100 per year. Five computer operators, each receiving an annual salary of $40,000, and a supervisor, who receives $47,000 a year, have been assigned to the unit. This unit performs the work previously performed by 10 employees whose combined salary was $324,000 per year. On the basis of these facts, the savings that will result from the operation of this unit for five years will be about

   A. $69,500.

   B. $647,500.

   C. $350,000.

   D. $650,000.

6. Joe can do a certain job in eight days. After working alone for four days, he is joined by Mary, and together they finish the work in two more days. How long would it take Mary alone?

   A. 5 days

   B. 6 days

   C. 7 days

   D. 8 days

SHOW YOUR WORK HERE

7. Eighty dozen pairs of rubber gloves were purchased for a medical facility. If the gloves are used at a rate of 32 pairs per day, what is the maximum number of days the gloves will last?

   A. Two and a half days

   B. Forty-eight days

   C. Thirty days

   D. 360 days

SHOW YOUR WORK HERE

8. At a certain health-care facility, the average cost of providing care for 3 patients for five days is $7,200. What is the average cost of providing care for 24 patients for five days?

   A. $43,200

   B. $36,000

   C. $34,560

   D. $57,600

9. Typist A can do a job in 3 hours. Typist B can do the same job in 5 hours. How long would it take both, working together, to do the job?

   A. 5 hours

   B. $3\frac{1}{2}$ hours

   C. $1\frac{7}{8}$ hours

   D. $1\frac{5}{8}$ hours

10. After gaining 50 percent of his original capital, an investor had capital of $18,000. Find the original capital.

   A. $12,200

   B. $13,100

   C. $12,000

   D. $12,025

11. To work off 60 calories, Brenda needs to walk on the treadmill for 15 minutes. How long will it take her to work off 100 calories?

    A. 25 minutes

    B. 55 minutes

    C. 40 minutes

    D. 45 minutes

12. A student worked thirty days at a part-time job. He paid two-fifths of his earnings for room and board and had $810 left. What was his daily wage?

    A. $45

    B. $50

    C. $55

    D. $62.50

13. A dealer bought motorcycles for $40,000. He sold them for $62,500, making $500 on each motorcycle. How many motorcycles were there?

    A. 40

    B. 38

    C. 43

    D. 44

14. An organization had one-fourth of its capital invested in goods. Two-thirds of the remaining capital was invested in land. The rest was cash in the amount of $1,224. What was the capital of the firm?

    A. $4,986

    B. $4,698

    C. $4,896

    D. $4,869

15. A and B together earn $2,100. If B is paid one-fourth more than A, how many dollars should B receive?

    A. $1,166.66

    B. $1,162.66

    C. $1,617.66

    D. $1,167.66

SHOW YOUR WORK HERE

16. If a boat is purchased for $21,500 and sold for $23,650, what is the percentage of gain?

    A. 8%

    B. 15%

    C. 20%

    D. 10%

17. A person owned five-sixths of a piece of property and sold three-fourths of her share for $1,800. What was the value of the whole property?

    A. $2,808

    B. $2,880

    C. $2,088

    D. $2,880.80

18. A lot costing $21,250 leases for $1,900 per year. The taxes and other expenses are $300 per year. Find the percent net annual income on the investment.

    A. $7\frac{1}{2}$ percent

    B. 6 percent

    C. 4 percent

    D. 10 percent

19. B owned 75 shares of stock in a building association worth $50 each. The association declared a dividend of 8 percent, payable in stock. How many shares did he own then?

    A. 81 shares

    B. 80 shares

    C. 90 shares

    D. 85 shares

SHOW YOUR WORK HERE

20. It requires four men three days to take an inventory; the weekly wages of each is as follows:

A—$750, B—$630, C—$520, D—$490.

Calculate the cost of taking the inventory, assuming that there are five full working days in a week.

A. $478

B. $794

C. $1,434

D. $7,170

SHOW YOUR WORK HERE

STOP

> IF YOU FINISH BEFORE TIME IS CALLED, YOU MAY CHECK YOUR WORK ON THIS SECTION ONLY. DO NOT TURN TO ANY OTHER SECTION IN THE TEST.

TEST 4

31 Questions • 22 Minutes

Directions: Solve the following problems and choose the correct answer from the four choices provided. Fill in the corresponding space on your answer sheet.

1. In simplest form, $-11 - (-2)$ is

    SHOW YOUR WORK HERE

    A. 7

    B. 9

    C. -11

    D. -9

2. Find the average of 6.47, 5.89, 3.42, 0.65, and 7.09.

    A. 5.812

    B. 4.704

    C. 3.920

    D. 4.705

3. $\dfrac{456.3}{0.89}$ equals

    A. $513\dfrac{13}{89}$

    B. 512.70

    C. 513.89

    D. 512.59

4. Add 5 hours, 13 minutes; 3 hours, 49 minutes; and 24 minutes. The sum is

    A. 9 hours, 26 minutes.

    B. 8 hours, 16 minutes.

    C. 9 hours, 76 minutes.

    D. 8 hours, 6 minutes.

5. Two numbers are in the ratio of 18:47. If the smaller number is 126, the larger number is

    A. 376.

    B. 144.

    C. 235.

    D. 329.

6. Change 0.3125 to a fraction.

   A. $\frac{3}{64}$

   B. $\frac{1}{16}$

   C. $\frac{1}{64}$

   D. $\frac{5}{16}$

7. Divide $\frac{7}{8}$ by $\frac{7}{8}$.

   A. 1

   B. 0

   C. $\frac{7}{8}$

   D. $\frac{49}{64}$

8. In the series 5, 8, 13, 20, the next number should be

   A. 23.

   B. 26.

   C. 29.

   D. 32.

9. What is the interest on $300 at 6 percent for ten days? (Assume year = 360 days.)

   A. $0.50

   B. $1.50

   C. $2.50

   D. $5.50

10. If the scale on a map indicates that 1 and one-half inches equal 500 miles, then 5 inches on the map will represent approximately

    A. 1,800 miles.

    B. 1,700 miles.

    C. 1,300 miles.

    D. 700 miles.

SHOW YOUR WORK HERE

11. $\frac{1}{2}$ percent equals

    SHOW YOUR WORK HERE

    A. 0.002.

    B. 0.020.

    C. 0.005.

    D. 0.050.

12. If 20 percent of an employee's bonus was $260, what was her entire bonus?

    A. $2,300

    B. $2,600

    C. $1,600

    D. $1,300

13. If a kilogram equals about 35 ounces, the number of grams in 1 ounce is approximately

    A. 29.

    B. 30.

    C. 31.

    D. 32.

14. An IV pump delivers medication at a constant rate of 24 milligrams per hour. How long does it take to deliver 90 milligrams?

    A. 3 hours, 15 minutes

    B. 3 hours, 45 minutes

    C. 3 hours, 75 minutes

    D. 4 hours, 15 minutes

15. If sound travels at the rate of 1,100 feet per second, in one-half minute it will travel about

    A. 6 miles.

    B. 8 miles.

    C. 10 miles.

    D. 3 miles.

16. If a kilometer is about five-eighths of a mile, 2 miles is about

    A. 1.6 kilometers.

    B. 3.2 kilometers.

    C. 2.4 kilometers.

    D. 3.75 kilometers.

17. A lecture hall that is 25 feet wide and 75 feet long has a perimeter equal to
    A. 1,750 feet.
    B. 200 yards.
    C. $66\frac{2}{3}$ yards.
    D. 1,875 feet.

18. After deducting a discount of $16\frac{2}{3}$ %, the price of a blouse was $35. The list price was
    A. $37.50.
    B. $38.
    C. $41.75.
    D. $42.

19. The number of decimal places in the product of 0.4266 and 0.3333 is
    A. 8.
    B. 4.
    C. 14.
    D. None of the above.

20. What is the cost of 5,500 bandages at $50 per thousand?
    A. $385
    B. $550
    C. $275
    D. $285

21. 572 divided by 0.52 is
    A. 1,100.
    B. 110.
    C. 11.10.
    D. 11,000.

22. 200 percent of 800 equals
    A. 2,500.
    B. 16.
    C. 1,600.
    D. 4.

23. A seventh-grade baseball team won ten games and lost five. Their average (number of wins per game played) is

 A. 0.667.

 B. 0.500.

 C. 0.333.

 D. 0.200.

24. The number of cubic feet of soil needed for a flower box 3 feet long, 8 inches wide, and 1 foot deep is

 A. 24.

 B. 12.

 C. $4\frac{2}{3}$.

 D. 2.

25. At $1,250 per hundred, 228 watches will cost

 A. $2,850.

 B. $36,000.

 C. $2,880.

 D. $360.

26. The area of the shaded portion of the rectangle below is

 A. 54 square inches.

 B. 90 square inches.

 C. 45 square inches.

 D. 36 square inches.

SHOW YOUR WORK HERE

27. On February 12, 1989, the age of a boy who was born on March 15, 1979, was

   A. 10 years, 10 months, and 3 days.

   B. 9 years, 9 months, and 27 days.

   C. 10 years, 1 month, and 3 days.

   D. 9 years, 10 months, and 28 days.

SHOW YOUR WORK HERE

Questions 28–31 are based on the following graph.

INTELLIGENCE QUOTIENTS (IQs)

28. The number of pupils having an IQ above 145 is

   A. 0.

   B. 5.

   C. 10.

   D. 20.

29. The number of pupils having an IQ of 75 is about

   A. 130.

   B. 100.

   C. 120.

   D. 110.

30. The number of pupils having an IQ of 80
    is identical to the number of pupils having
    an IQ of

    A. 100.
    B. 68.
    C. 110.
    D. 128.

31. The IQ that has the greatest frequency is

    A. 100.
    B. 95.
    C. 105.
    D. 160.

SHOW YOUR WORK HERE

STOP

IF YOU FINISH BEFORE TIME IS CALLED, YOU MAY
CHECK YOUR WORK ON THIS SECTION ONLY. DO NOT
TURN TO ANY OTHER SECTION IN THE TEST.

ANSWER KEYS AND EXPLANATIONS

Test 1

1. A	**5.** B	**9.** C	**13.** B	**17.** B
2. D	**6.** A	**10.** A	**14.** C	**18.** A
3. B	**7.** B	**11.** B	**15.** C	**19.** A
4. C	**8.** C	**12.** B	**16.** C	**20.** D

1. **The correct answer is A.**

   Interest = Principal × Rate × Time
   Note: 6% = 0.06
   144 days $= \dfrac{144}{360}$ year
   $I = P \times R \times T$
   $= \$25,800 \times 0.06 \times \dfrac{144}{360}$
   $= \dfrac{\$222,912}{360}$
   $= \$619.20$

2. **The correct answer is D.** Let n = number of minutes in which they can do the job together. Arthur can do $\dfrac{1}{60}$ of the job in 1 minute, so in n minutes he can do $\dfrac{n}{60}$ of the job. Jack can do $\dfrac{1}{30}$ of the job in 1 minute and $\dfrac{n}{30}$ of the job in n minutes. Together, in n minutes they can do the complete job.

   $\dfrac{n}{60} + \dfrac{n}{30} = 1$

   $n + 2n = 60$ (multiplying both sides by 60, the lowest common denominator)

   $3n = 60$ (combine like terms)

   $n = 20$ (divide by 3)

   They can do the job together in 20 minutes.

3. **The correct answer is B.**

   Total seats = 105

   Total time = 6 hours

   Total people involved = 485

   105 seats × 6 hours = 630 seating hours

   To find the average seating time, divide hours by people seated:

   630 ÷ 485 = 1.3 hours

   Now change the 0.3 hours to minutes:

   (1 hour = 60 minutes)

   0.3 hour $\times \dfrac{60 \text{ minutes}}{1 \text{ hour}} = 18$ minutes

   The amount is 1 hour, 18 minutes.

4. **The correct answer is C.**

   Paper per ream = $14.50

   Discount = 5%, or 0.05

   Total cash = $690.00

   First, find the discount on the paper per ream when paying cash.

   $14.50 × 0.05 = $0.725

   The price per ream is
   $14.50 − $0.725 = $13.775.

   Given $690 to spend, divide to find how much paper can be purchased.

   $690.00 ÷ $13.775/ream = 50

   50 reams for $688.75

5. **The correct answer is B.** Use simple logic to solve this problem.

From	To	
8:30 a.m. →	8:30 p.m.	= 12 hours
8:30 p.m. →	3:30 a.m.	= 7 hours

Total = 19 hours, but this is 15 minutes too much.

Note: Change one of the hours to minutes (1 hour = 60 minutes).

$$\begin{array}{r} 18 \text{ hours } 60 \text{ minutes} \\ -15 \text{ minutes} \\ \hline 18 \text{ hours } 45 \text{ minutes} \end{array}$$

45 minutes = $\frac{45}{60}$ hours, or $\frac{3}{4}$ hours

$18\frac{3}{4}$ is the total number of hours.

6. **The correct answer is A.** Again, use logic.

Month	Number of days/month	
September	from 19 to 30	12 days
October	31 days	31 days
November	30 days	30 days
December	from 1 to 25	25 days
		98 days

Note: Remember that September 19 and December 25 are included.

Total = 98 days inclusive

7. **The correct answer is B.**

Total to be filed = 800 cards

Rate cards can be filed = 80 cards per hour

How many cards were filed in the first 7 hours?

7 × 80 = 560 cards were filed

Subtract to find the remaining cards to be filed.

800 − 560 = 240

240 cards remain unfiled.

8. **The correct answer is C.** From $80 to $90, there is a $10 increase; the percent of increase is found by dividing the amount of increase by the original amount:

$10 ÷ 80 = 0.125$, or $12\frac{1}{2}\%$

Note: $0.125 = 12.5\%$, or $12\frac{1}{2}\%$

Percent of increase = $12\frac{1}{2}\%$

9. **The correct answer is C.** To find the *average* number of patients served by each nurse, divide 135 patients by 15 nurses to get 9 patients per nurse.

10. **The correct answer is A.** To find the percent of correct answers on the test, divide the number of correct answers by the total number of items on the test.

$$\frac{72}{80} = .90$$

Change .90 to a percent.

.90 = 90%

90% of the test items were correct.

11. **The correct answer is B.** To find the number of hours of exercise the patient gets in a week, multiply.

45 min. × 7 days = 315 minutes

Convert the minutes to hours by dividing by 60, since there are 60 minutes in an hour.

$$\frac{315}{60} = 5.25 \text{ hours per week}$$

12. **The correct answer is B.** To find the number of nurses on duty for the two shifts, determine the number of nurses who worked on the night shift by finding one half of the number who worked the afternoon shift.

$$120 \times \frac{1}{2} = 60$$

Add the number who worked the afternoon shift to the number who worked the night shift.

$$120 + 60 = 180$$

180 nurses worked on the two shifts.

13. **The correct answer is B.**

Total summonses in 7 hours = 182

To find the *average* number of summonses per hour, divide:

182 summonses ÷ 7 hours = 26

Average = 26 summonses/hour

14. **The correct answer is C.** To find the number of admitted patients who weren't in accidents, subtract the number of patients who were in accidents from the total number of patients.

$$76 - 23 = 53$$

53 of the admitted patients had not been in accidents.

15. **The correct answer is C.** If it takes the truck 1 hour to go 40 miles, it will take 2 hours to go 80 miles.

$$2 \text{ hours } \times 40 \frac{\text{miles}}{\text{hours}} = 80 \text{ miles}$$

16. **The correct answer is C.** If the total capacity is 100 gallons, then

$$\frac{2}{5} \text{ of } 100 = \frac{2}{5} \times 100$$

$$= \frac{200}{5}$$

$$= 40 \text{ gallons}$$

17. **The correct answer is B.**

Total salary = $3,000

Tax = 20%, or .20

Find the amount of 20% tax by multiplying:
$3,000 × .20 = $600

Subtract the tax from the salary to find the net:

$$\$3,000 - \$600 = \$2,400$$
$$2,400 = \text{net pay}$$

18. **The correct answer is A.**

Total cost = $1,000

Total square yards = 100

Find the cost per square yard by dividing:

$1,000 ÷ 100 square yards = $10

$10/square yard

19. **The correct answer is A.**

Base pay	**$3,000**
Bonus	+ 350
Serv. Increment	+ 250
Total pay	$3,600

20. **The correct answer is D.**

Annual salary	**$21,600**
Bonus	+ 7,200
Increment	+ 1,200
Total pay	$30,000

Test 2

1. C	5. A	9. C	13. C	17. B
2. D	6. B	10. B	14. C	18. A
3. A	7. B	11. C	15. D	19. C
4. C	8. B	12. C	16. C	20. D

1. **The correct answer is C.**

The second vehicle is 90 feet – 40 feet = 50 feet from the EMT. The first vehicle is 40 feet from the EMT. The first vehicle is 50 feet – 40 feet = 10 feet closer than the second vehicle.

2. **The correct answer is D.** To find the number of milliliters the IV bag contains when it's two-thirds full, multiply

$$1{,}260 \text{ milliliters} \times \frac{2}{3} = 840 \text{ milliliters}$$

There are 840 milliliters in the IV bag when it's two-thirds full.

3. **The correct answer is A.**

Salary per month = $2,500

Days worked = 23

To find the earnings per day, divide:

$$\frac{\$2{,}500}{\text{month}} \div \frac{23 \text{ days}}{\text{month}} = \frac{\$108.70}{\text{days}}$$

or

$$\frac{\$2{,}500}{\text{month}} \div \frac{23 \text{ days}}{\text{month}}$$

$$= \frac{\$2{,}500}{\text{month}} \times \frac{\text{month}}{23 \text{ days}}$$

$$= \frac{\$2{,}500}{23 \text{ days}} = \frac{\$108.70}{\text{day}}$$

4. **The correct answer is C.** To find the take-home pay of the nursing home assistant, subtract the total amount of her deductions from her weekly salary.

Total deductions	= $18 + $15 + $21 + $72 = $126
Weekly salary	= 360
Salary – deductions	= $360 – $126
	= $234
Take-home pay	= $234

5. **The correct answer is A.**

Stamps per day	Cost per day
$\frac{40}{\text{day}} \times \$0.35$	= $14.00
$\frac{25}{\text{day}} \times \$0.50$	= $12.50
$\frac{320}{\text{day}} \times \$0.71$	= $227.20
Total cost/day	$253.70

For five days, 5 × $253.70 = $1,268.50

Total cost = $1,268.50

6. **The correct answer is B.**

Number of applications issued in 2017 = 12,000

In 2015, 25 percent more were issued, or 0.25 × 12,000 = 3,000 more in 2015.

So there were 3,000 + 12,000 = 15,000 issued in 2015.

In 2013, 10 percent fewer were issued than in 2015, or 0.10 × 15,000 = 1,500 fewer were issued in 2013.

The number issued in 2013 is

$15,000 - 1,500 = 13,500$.

7. **The correct answer is B.** If three fifths of the 200 are done by calculator, then:

$$\frac{3}{5} \times 200 = \frac{600}{5} = 120.$$

120 columns will be done by the machine. To find the number done by hand, subtract:

$200 - 120 = 80$.

80 will be done by hand

To find the time it takes to do the 120 columns by machine and the 80 columns by hand, divide:

120 columns ÷ 40 columns per hour = 3 hours by machine

80 columns ÷ 20 columns per hour = 4 hours by hand

Total time = 7 hours

8. **The correct answer is B.** To find the total cost of the rubber gloves bought in 2018, first determine the amount of the 20% price increase for a dozen gloves in 2018.

$.20 \times \$2.60 = 0.52$

Add the cost in 2015 to the amount of the increase to get the cost of the gloves in 2018.

$\$2.60 + 0.52 = \$3.12$

In 2018, a dozen gloves cost $3.12.

The number of gloves purchased in 2018 was 25 percent less than the number purchased in 2015.

To find how many dozens of gloves were purchased in 2018, find 25 percent of 500 dozen and subtract the result from 500 dozen.

500 dozen − .25 × 500 dozen
= 500 dozen − 125 dozen = 375 dozen

375 dozen gloves were purchased in 2018.

Multiply the price per dozen $3.12 × 375 dozen = $1,170.00.

The total cost of the gloves bought in 2018 was $1,170.00.

9. **The correct answer is C.** During the first hour, 40 forms were checked, leaving 450 to be checked:

$490 - 40 = 450$

The two nurses working together can check 75 forms per hour.

Now find the time it takes to do the 450 forms. Do this by dividing:

450 forms ÷ 75 forms/hour = 6 hours

It takes 6 hours to do the 450 and 1 hour for the first 40 forms:

6 hours + 1 hour = 7 hours to do the job

A total of 7 hours is needed.

10. **The correct answer is B.**

Total employed = 420

If 30 percent are nurses,

$420 \times 0.30 = 126$ nurses

$\frac{1}{7}$ are doctors:

$420 \times \frac{1}{7} = 60$ doctors

The difference is $126 - 60 = 66$.

11. **The correct answer is C.**

Cost = $0.12 per copy

Time = 120 copies per minute

To find the number of copies produced, divide:

$36 ÷ $0.12 = 300 copies

To find the number of minutes, divide:

300 copies ÷ 120 copies/minute = 2.5 minutes

12. The correct answer is C. If the average number of medical records filed for five days was 720, then 5 days × 720 records/day = 3,600 records for the five-day period.

For four days:

610 + 720 + 740 + 755 = 2,825 medical records were filed

Subtract:

3,600 − 2,825 = 775 need to be filed the fifth day to get an average of 720 for the five-day period.

13. The correct answer is C.

Total employees = 1,400

35% clerks = 1,400 × .35 = 490 clerks

$\frac{1}{8}$ stenos = $1,400 \times \frac{1}{8} = 175$ stenos

Together (490 + 175 = 665), there are 665 clerks and stenographers. To find how many employees are neither, subtract:

1,400 − 665 = 735

Answer = 735 other employees

14. The correct answer is C. If Nurse A takes 40 more blood pressure readings than Nurse B, let x represent the number of blood pressure readings taken by Nurse B. Then $x + 40 =$ the number of blood pressure readings taken by Nurse A. Add the number taken by Nurse A to the number taken by Nurse B to get the total number of blood pressure readings taken.

$$x + x + 40 = 190$$
$$2x + 40 = 190$$
$$2x = 150$$

$x = 75$, the number of blood pressure readings taken by Nurse B

$x + 40 = 75 + 40 = 115$, the number of blood pressure readings taken by Nurse A

15. The correct answer is D.

Stock on hand and cost per item:

		Cost
500 pads × $0.04/pad	=	$20.00
130 pencils × $0.03/pencil	=	$3.90
50 dozen rubber bands × $0.02/dozen	=	$1.00
value of stock on hand	=	$24.90

If we issue the items below,

125 pads × $0.04	=	$5.00
45 pencils × $0.03	=	$1.35
48 rubber bands or 4 dozen × $0.02	=	$0.08
		$6.43

To find the value of the remaining stock, subtract:

$24.90 − $6.43 = $18.47

Value = $18.47

16. The correct answer is C. Let t be the amount of time, in hours, for both to do the job. If Joe does $\frac{t}{3}$ part of the job, and here's the classic set up for the work problem, his friend does $\frac{t}{4}$ part of the job, then $\frac{t}{3} + \frac{t}{4} = 1$ (the whole job).

$$4t + 3t = 12 \text{ (multiply lowest common denominator by 12)}$$
$$7t = 12 \text{ (combine like terms)}$$
$$t = \frac{12}{7} \text{ (divide by 7)}$$
$$t = 1\frac{5}{7} \text{ hours}$$

17. **The correct answer is B.**

    Total employees = 60

    $\frac{1}{3} \times 60 = 20$ clerks

    30% × 60, or .30 × 60 = 18 OMOs

    60 − 38 = 22 stenos

    To find their *rate per month*, divide their annual salaries by 12, because there are 12 months in a year:

    clerks: $\frac{\$29,750}{12} = \$2,479.17$ per month

    OMOs: $\frac{\$31,500}{12} = \$2,625.00$ per month

    stenos: $\frac{\$42,000}{12} = \$3,500.00$ per month

    Now find the salary for all employees for the time they worked:

    If 20 clerks worked two months, total pay equals:

    20 × 2 × $2,479.17 = $99,166.80

    If 18 OMOs worked four months, total pay equals:

    18 × 4 × $2,625.00 = $189,000.00

    If 22 stenos worked three months, total pay equals:

    22 × 3 × $3,500 = $231,000.00

    Total salaries = $99,166.80 + $189,000.00 + $231,000.00 = $519,166.80. This amount can be rounded up to $519,200.

18. **The correct answer is A.**

    5 percent of 2,300 are accountants:

    0.05 × 2,300 = 115

    80 percent of the 115 accountants have college degrees:

    0.80 × 115 = 92

    One half of the 92 have five years of experience:

    $\frac{1}{2} \times 92 = 46$

    46 employees have all three qualifications.

19. **The correct answer is C.** $3,000 is subject to $425 tax. The net can be found by subtracting:

    $3,000 − $425 = $2,575

20. **The correct answer is D.** A sanitation worker who reports 45 minutes early for 8:00 a.m. duty reports at 7:15 a.m.

    Note: 1 hour = 60 minutes

    8 hours = 7 hours, 60 minutes

    $$\begin{array}{r} 7 \text{ hours } 60 \text{ minutes} \\ - \quad 45 \text{ minutes} \\ \hline 7 \text{ hours } 15 \text{ minutes} \end{array}$$

    7 hours and 15 minutes = 7:15 a.m.

Test 3

1. C	5. C	9. C	13. D	17. B
2. C	6. D	10. C	14. C	18. A
3. B	7. C	11. A	15. A	19. A
4. D	8. D	12. A	16. D	20. C

1. **The correct answer is C.** If it costs $0.75 to sweep 1 square foot, to find the cost for 100 square feet, multiply 100 square feet × $0.75 per square foot = $75.

   Total cost = $75

2. **The correct answer is C.** To determine how many hours it will take to tow the car 90 miles at a rate of 36 mph, divide

   90 ÷ 36 = 2.5

   It will take 2.5 hours to tow the car 90 miles.

3. **The correct answer is B.** To determine how many feet nearer the man is to the bank than the drugstore is to the bank, use the following diagram:

   The total distance from the bank to the drugstore is 100 feet. Subtract to find the difference between the man's distance from the bank and the drugstore's distance from the bank.

   100 feet − 60 feet = 40 feet

   The man is 40 feet nearer to the bank than the drugstore is to the bank.

4. **The correct answer is D.** A clerk works 35 hours per week. $\frac{1}{5}$ of his time is used to sort mail:

   $\frac{1}{5} \times 35 = 7$ hours

   $\frac{1}{2}$ of his time is used to file letters:

   $\frac{1}{2} \times 35 = 17\frac{1}{2}$ hours

   $\frac{1}{7}$ of his time is used for reception work:

   $\frac{1}{7} \times 35 = 5$ hours

   Total = $29\frac{1}{2}$ hours

   $29\frac{1}{2}$ hours were used for the above. To find the time left for messenger work, subtract

   $35 - 29\frac{1}{2} = 5\frac{1}{2}$ hours

   Now to find what percent of 35 is $5\frac{1}{2}$, divide:

   $5.5 \div 35 = 0.16$ or 16%

   Note: $5\frac{1}{2} = 5.5$

   16% remains for messenger work.

5. **The correct answer is C.**

Item

5 computers $1,400/year	5 × 1,400	$7,000
Maintenance, repairs $100/computer	5 × 100	$500
5 operators' annual salaries $40,000	5 × $40,000	$200,000
Supervisor's annual salary $47,000	1 × $47,000	$47,000
Total cost		$254,500

If 10 employees were paid a total of $324,000, find the savings by subtracting:

$$\$324{,}000 - \$254{,}500 = \$69{,}500, \text{ one year's savings}$$

To find the savings for five years, multiply:

$$\$69{,}500 \times 5 = \$347{,}500$$

This amount *rounds up* to (or, is nearest to) $350,000.

6. **The correct answer is D.** If Joe can do the job alone in eight days, then he can do $\frac{1}{8}$ in one day and $\frac{6}{8}$, or $\frac{3}{4}$, in six days.

Let n be the number of days it would take Mary to do the job alone. Then:

$\frac{1}{n}$ is the part of the job she can do in one day, and $\frac{2}{n}$ is the part of the job she can do in the two days she works with Joe.

Now, the sum of parts done by Joe and Mary equals one whole job:

$\frac{3}{4} + \frac{2}{n} = 1$

$3n + 8 = 4n$ (multiply by the lowest common denominator, $4n$)

$8 = 4n - 3n$ (subtract $3n$ from both sides of the equation)

$8 = n$ (subtract like terms)

$n = 8$

Mary alone could do the job in eight days.

7. **The correct answer is C.**

Eighty dozen = 80 × 12 = 960

960 pairs of gloves were purchased.

To find the maximum number of days the gloves will last, divide:

960 ÷ 32 = 30

If the gloves are being used at a rate of 32 pairs per day, they will last thirty days.

8. **The correct answer is D.** To determine the cost of caring for 24 patients for five days, find the cost of caring for 1 patient for five days by dividing.

$7,200 ÷ 3 = $ 2,400

To get the cost for caring for 24 patients, multiply.

24 × $2,400 = $57,600

The cost for caring for 24 patients is $57,600.

9. **The correct answer is C.** A can do one third of the job in 1 hour. B can do one fifth of the job in 1 hour. Together they can do $\frac{1}{3} + \frac{1}{5}$ of the job in 1 hour. Let t be the time in hours it takes for both to do the job. Together, they can do $\frac{1}{t}$ of the job in 1 hour. Thus:

$$\frac{1}{3} + \frac{1}{5} = \frac{1}{t}$$

$5t + 3t = 15$ (multiply by the lowest common denominator, $15t$ or $3 \times 5 \times t$)

$8t = 15$ (add like terms)

$t = \frac{15}{8}$ (divide both sides by 8 hours)

$t = 1\frac{7}{8}$

10. **The correct answer is C.** Let x be the unknown original capital and $0.50x$ be 50 percent of the unknown capital.

$$x + .50x = \$18,000$$
$$1.50x = \$18,000 \quad \text{(add like terms)}$$
$$\frac{150x}{1.50} = \frac{\$18,000}{1.50} \quad \text{(divide both sides by 1.50)}$$
$$x = \$12,000$$

$12,000 is the original amount of the capital.

11. **The correct answer is A.** Let x represent the amount of time it takes to work off 100 calories.

The ratio of the amount of time it takes to work off 60 calories equals the ratio of the amount of time it takes to work off 100 calories:

$$\frac{15 \text{ minutes}}{60 \text{ calories}} = \frac{x \text{ minutes}}{100 \text{ calories}}$$
$$60x = 15 \times 100$$
$$60x = 1,500$$
$$x = 25 \text{ minutes}$$

It will take 25 minutes on the treadmill to work off 100 calories.

12. **The correct answer is A.** If two-fifths of his salary was used, then three-fifths was left; three-fifths of his salary is $810. Now, since his salary is unknown, let x represent it:

$$\frac{3}{5} \times x = \$810$$
$$x = \$810 \div \frac{3}{5} \left(\text{divide both sides by } \frac{3}{5} \right)$$
$$x = \$810 \times \frac{5}{3} \text{ (invert and multiply)}$$
$$x = \$1,350$$

His salary is $1,350 for 30 days of work. To find the *daily wage*, divide the salary by 30:

$1,350 ÷ 30 days = $45/day

Daily wage = $45

13. **The correct answer is D.** To find the number of motorcycles purchased, first subtract their original purchase price from the selling price:

$62,000 − $40,000 = $22,000 profit

Since the profit was $22,000, and the profit on each motorcycle was $500, divide to find the number of motorcycles sold:

$22,000 profit ÷ $500 profit/motorcycle = 44 motorcycles sold.

14. **The correct answer is C.**

$\frac{1}{4}$ in *goods* (given)

$\frac{2}{3} \times \frac{3}{4} = \frac{1}{2}$ in *land* (because $\frac{3}{4}$ is the remainder after the goods are invested)

$\frac{1}{4}$ is left in *cash*, because if $\frac{1}{4}$ is in goods, and $\frac{1}{2}$ is in land, then $\frac{3}{4}$ is invested, leaving $\frac{1}{4}$ for cash.

If $\frac{1}{4}$ of the capital is cash valued at $1,224, then to find total capital, multiply $1,224 × 4.

Total capital = $4,896

15. **The correct answer is A.** Let *A* equal the amount A earned, and *B* equal the amount B earned.

Together, they earned $A + B = $2,100$.

If B is paid $\frac{1}{4}$ more than A, then A's salary plus $\frac{1}{4}$ of A's salary is equal to B's salary.

Express this as follows:

$$A + B = \$2,100$$

$$B = A + \frac{1}{4}A$$

$$B = 1\frac{1}{4}A$$

$$A + 1\frac{1}{4}A = 2,100$$

$$2\frac{1}{4}A = 2,100$$

$$A = 933\frac{1}{3}$$

A earns $933.33

B earns $933.33 \times 1\frac{1}{4} = 1,166.66$

B earns $1,166.66

16. **The correct answer is D.** The boat costs $21,500 and was sold for $23,650. Subtract:

$23,650 − $21,500 = $2,150

$2,150 was gained. To find the percent gained, divide the amount gained by the original amount:

$2,150 ÷ $21,500 = 0.10, or 10%

Percent gained = 10%

17. **The correct answer is B.**

$\frac{5}{6} \times \frac{3}{4} = \frac{5}{8}$ of the property costs $1,800

Then, letting *y* represent the value of the property,

$$\frac{5}{8} \times y = \$1,800$$

$$y = \$1,800 \div \frac{5}{8} \quad \left(\text{divide both sides by } \frac{5}{8}\right)$$

$$y = \$1,800 \times \frac{8}{5} \quad (\text{invert and multiply})$$

Therefore, $2,880 is the price of the whole property.

18. **The correct answer is A.**

A lot costs $21,250.

$1,900	is received for lease
− 300	is deducted for expenses
$1,600	is net income

To find what percent $1,600 is of the cost of the lot, divide:

$$1,600 \div 21,250 = 0.075, \text{ or } 7\frac{1}{2}\%$$

$7\frac{1}{2}\% =$ percent of cost

19. **The correct answer is A.**

Total shares currently owned = 75

Values per share = $50

To find the value of the stock, multiply

75 × $50 = $3,750

To find 8%, multiply the stock value by 0.08:

$3,750 × 0.08 = $300 (dividend)

Given $300, divide by $50 to see how many additional shares of stock can be purchased:

$300 ÷ 50 = 6 shares

Therefore, he now owns 75 + 6 = 81 shares.

20. **The correct answer is C.** First, find the wages each man is paid for 1 day. To do so, divide their wages by 5 days:

		wages/day	wages/ 3 days
A	$\dfrac{\$750}{5} =$	$150 × 3 =	$450
B	$\dfrac{\$630}{5} =$	$126 × 3 =	$378
C	$\dfrac{\$520}{5} =$	$104 × 3 =	$312
D	$\dfrac{\$490}{5} =$	$98 × 3 =	$294

Total salaries for 3 days = $1,434

Test 4

1. D	**8.** C	**14.** B	**20.** C	**26.** A
2. B	**9.** A	**15.** A	**21.** A	**27.** D
3. B	**10.** B	**16.** B	**22.** C	**28.** A
4. A	**11.** C	**17.** C	**23.** A	**29.** C
5. D	**12.** D	**18.** D	**24.** D	**30.** C
6. D	**13.** A	**19.** A	**25.** A	**31.** A
7. A				

1. The correct answer is D.

$-11 - (-2)$
$= -11 + 2$
$= -9$

2. The correct answer is B.

$6.47 + 5.89 + 3.42 + 0.65 + 7.09 = 23.52$

To find the average, divide the sum by 5 (the number of terms involved)

$23.52 \div 5 = 4.704$

Average = 4.704

3. The correct answer is B.

```
           512.696...
        _____
.89.)456.30.000
       445
       113
        89
       240
       178
       620
       534
       860
       801
       590
       534
        56
```

512.696 rounds up to 512.70.

4. The correct answer is A.

```
   5 hours, 13 minutes
   3 hours, 49 minutes
+            24 minutes
_____
   8 hours, 86 minutes
```

Since there are 60 minutes in 1 hour, then 86 minutes = 60 minutes + 26 minutes or 1 hour and 26 minutes.

So 8 hours and 86 minutes = 9 hours and 26 minutes.

5. The correct answer is D.

$$\frac{18}{47} = \frac{126}{x}$$

$18x = 47(126)$ (cross-multiply)
$18x = 5{,}922$
$x = 329$ (divide by 18)

6. The correct answer is D.

$$0.3125 = \frac{3{,}125}{10{,}000} = \frac{5}{16}$$

7. The correct answer is A.

$$\frac{7}{8} \div \frac{7}{8}$$

$= \frac{7}{8} \times \frac{8}{7}$ (invert the second term and multiply)

$= 1$

8. **The correct answer is C.** 5, 8, 13, 20. To each number, add the next odd number to determine the next number in the series.

		Odd	
Series		Number	
5	+	3	= 8
8	+	5	= 13
13	+	7	= 20
20	+	9	= 29

29 will be the next number.

9. **The correct answer is A.**

   Interest = Principal × Rate × Time

   $$= \$300 \times 0.06 \times \frac{10}{360}$$

   $$= \frac{\$180}{360} = \frac{\$1}{2}$$

   $$= \$0.50$$

10. **The correct answer is B.** First, find the number of $1\frac{1}{2}$ inch units there are in 5 inches. Do this by dividing:

    $$5 \div 1\frac{1}{2}$$

    $$= 5 \div \frac{3}{2} \quad \left(\text{change } 1\frac{1}{2} \text{ to } \frac{3}{2}\right)$$

    $$= 5 \times \frac{2}{3} \quad \text{(invert and multiply)}$$

    $$= \frac{10}{3}$$

    Now find the total miles by multiplying:

    $$500 \times \frac{10}{3} = 1,666.67$$

    Five inches represents approximately 1,700 miles.

11. **The correct answer is C.** $\frac{1}{2}\% = 0.5\%$, or

    $$\frac{0.5}{100} = 0.005$$

12. **The correct answer is D.** $260 is 20% of the bonus. Write this in equation form. Let the bonus be x.

    $$\$260 = .20x$$

    $$\frac{260}{.20} = \frac{.20x}{.20} \quad \text{(divide by 0.20)}$$

    $$\$1,300 = x$$

    Her entire bonus was $1,300.

13. **The correct answer is A.**

    1 kilogram = 35 ounces

    Find how many grams there are in 1 ounce.

    Note: 1 kilogram = 1,000 grams

    1,000 grams = 35 ounces

    $$1 \text{ ounce} \times \frac{1,000 \text{ grams}}{35 \text{ ounces}} = \frac{1,000 \text{ grams}}{35}$$

    $$= 28.6, \text{ or } 29 \text{ grams}$$
    $$\text{in 1 ounce}$$

14. **The correct answer is B.** To find the amount of time it takes to deliver the 90 milligrams at a rate of 24 milligrams per hour, divide:

    amount of time = 90 milligrams ÷

    24 milligrams per hour = 3.75 hours

    3.75 hours = $3\frac{3}{4}$ hours =

    3 hours and 45 minutes

15. **The correct answer is A.** First, find the number of seconds there are in one-half minute:

    $$\frac{1}{2} \times 60 \text{ sec/min} = 30 \text{ seconds}$$

    Since sound travels 1,100 feet per second, it will travel:

    30 sec. × 1,100 ft. = 33,000 ft.

    Change the 33,000 feet to miles
    (1 mile = 5,280 feet)

$$33,000 \text{ feet} \times \frac{1 \text{ mile}}{5,280 \text{ feet}} = \frac{33,000}{5,280}$$
$$= 6.25$$

Round off: 6.25 miles = about 6 miles

16. **The correct answer is B.**

1 kilometer = $\frac{5}{8}$ mile

x kilometers = 2 miles

$$\frac{1 \text{ kilometer}}{\frac{5}{8} \text{ mile}} = \frac{x}{2}$$

$$\frac{5}{8}x = 2$$
$$5x = 16$$
$$x = 3.2$$

2 miles = about 3.2 kilometers

17. **The correct answer is C.** The perimeter of a rectangle (the hall is shaped like a rectangle) is:

$$Perimeter = 2 \; length + 2 \; width$$
$$= 2(75) + 2(25)$$
$$= 150 + 50$$
$$= 200 \text{ feet}$$

The perimeter is 200 feet.

Now change 200 feet to yards (3 feet = 1 yard).

$$200 \text{ feet} \times \frac{1 \text{ yard}}{3 \text{ feet}} = 66\frac{2}{3} \text{ yards}$$

18. **The correct answer is D.** Let the price of a blouse be x. Then:

$$x - \left(16\frac{2}{3}\%\right)x = 35$$

$\frac{2}{3} = 0.67$, so $16\frac{2}{3}\% = 16.67\% = 0.1667$

$x - 0.1667x = \$35$ (change the percent to a decimal)

$0.8333x = \$35$ (combine like terms)

$x = \$42$ (divide by 0.8333)

The list price was \$42.

19. **The correct answer is A.** To find the number of decimal places in the product of two numbers, find the sum of the number of digits to the right of the decimal of each number.

0.4266 has 4 digits to the right.
0.3333 has 4 digits to the right.

There should be 8 digits in the product.

20. **The correct answer is C.** 5.5 thousand × \$50/thousand = \$275

21. **The correct answer is A.**

$$\begin{array}{r} 1100. \\ .52.\overline{)572.00.} \\ \underline{52} \\ 52 \\ \underline{52} \\ 0 \end{array}$$

Answer: 1,100

22. **The correct answer is C.**

200 percent of 800

2.00 × 800 = 1,600

23. **The correct answer is A.** The total games played was 15. To find their average, divide games won by total played:

10 ÷ 15 = 0.667

Their average is 0.667.

24. **The correct answer is D.** To find the soil needed, first change the 8 inches to feet, so all units will be the same.

$$8 \text{ inches} \times \frac{1 \text{ foot}}{12 \text{ inches}} = \frac{2}{3} \text{ feet}$$

Now multiply all units.

$$3 \text{ feet} \times \frac{2}{3} \text{ feet} \times 1 \text{ foot} = 2 \text{ cubic feet}$$

2 cubic feet of soil will be needed to fill the box.

25. **The correct answer is A.** Find the price for one watch by dividing:

    $1,250 (per hundred) ÷ 100 = $12.50 (price of one watch)

    To find the cost of 228 watches, multiply the number of watches by the price per watch.

    228 watches × $12.50 per watch = $2,850

    The cost of 228 watches will be $2,850.

26. **The correct answer is A.** Find the area of the small rectangle and subtract its area from the large rectangle to determine the shaded area.

    Large rectangle

    $A = length \times width$
    $= 6 \times 15$
    $= 90$ square inches

    Small rectangle

    $A = length \times width$
    $= 4 \times 9$
    $= 36$ square inches

    $90 - 36 = 54$ square inches

    The area of the shaded area is 54 square inches.

27. **The correct answer is D.**

From	To	Time
March 15, 1979	March 15, 1988	9 years
March 15, 1988	Jan. 15, 1989	10 months
Jan. 15, 1989	Feb. 12, 1989	28 days

    His age will be 9 years, 10 months, 28 days.

28. **The correct answer is A.** The line on the graph does not extend to the right of 145 on the horizontal axis. So zero students have an IQ above 145.

29. **The correct answer is C.** Locate 75 on the base and trace the vertical grid line up to the graph. The point on the graph directly above 75 is to the right of 120.

30. **The correct answer is C.** There are 100 pupils with an IQ of 80. Looking across the chart, we see that there are also 100 pupils with an IQ of 110.

31. **The correct answer is A.** The highest point on the graph points to an IQ of 100.

FINAL MATHEMATICS EXAMINATION
ANSWER SHEET

1. Ⓐ Ⓑ Ⓒ Ⓓ   10. Ⓐ Ⓑ Ⓒ Ⓓ   19. Ⓐ Ⓑ Ⓒ Ⓓ   27. Ⓐ Ⓑ Ⓒ Ⓓ   35. Ⓐ Ⓑ Ⓒ Ⓓ

2. Ⓐ Ⓑ Ⓒ Ⓓ   11. Ⓐ Ⓑ Ⓒ Ⓓ   20. Ⓐ Ⓑ Ⓒ Ⓓ   28. Ⓐ Ⓑ Ⓒ Ⓓ   36. Ⓐ Ⓑ Ⓒ Ⓓ

3. Ⓐ Ⓑ Ⓒ Ⓓ   12. Ⓐ Ⓑ Ⓒ Ⓓ   21. Ⓐ Ⓑ Ⓒ Ⓓ   29. Ⓐ Ⓑ Ⓒ Ⓓ   37. Ⓐ Ⓑ Ⓒ Ⓓ

4. Ⓐ Ⓑ Ⓒ Ⓓ   13. Ⓐ Ⓑ Ⓒ Ⓓ   22. Ⓐ Ⓑ Ⓒ Ⓓ   30. Ⓐ Ⓑ Ⓒ Ⓓ   38. Ⓐ Ⓑ Ⓒ Ⓓ

5. Ⓐ Ⓑ Ⓒ Ⓓ   14. Ⓐ Ⓑ Ⓒ Ⓓ   23. Ⓐ Ⓑ Ⓒ Ⓓ   31. Ⓐ Ⓑ Ⓒ Ⓓ   39. Ⓐ Ⓑ Ⓒ Ⓓ

6. Ⓐ Ⓑ Ⓒ Ⓓ   15. Ⓐ Ⓑ Ⓒ Ⓓ   24. Ⓐ Ⓑ Ⓒ Ⓓ   32. Ⓐ Ⓑ Ⓒ Ⓓ   40. Ⓐ Ⓑ Ⓒ Ⓓ

7. Ⓐ Ⓑ Ⓒ Ⓓ   16. Ⓐ Ⓑ Ⓒ Ⓓ   25. Ⓐ Ⓑ Ⓒ Ⓓ   33. Ⓐ Ⓑ Ⓒ Ⓓ   41. Ⓐ Ⓑ Ⓒ Ⓓ

8. Ⓐ Ⓑ Ⓒ Ⓓ   17. Ⓐ Ⓑ Ⓒ Ⓓ   26. Ⓐ Ⓑ Ⓒ Ⓓ   34. Ⓐ Ⓑ Ⓒ Ⓓ   42. Ⓐ Ⓑ Ⓒ Ⓓ

9. Ⓐ Ⓑ Ⓒ Ⓓ   18. Ⓐ Ⓑ Ⓒ Ⓓ

answer sheet

FINAL MATHEMATICS EXAMINATION

42 Questions • 40 Minutes

Directions: This part requires logical reasoning and thinking, in addition to simple computations to find the solution to each question. Read each question carefully and choose the correct answer from the four choices provided.

---

1. Jane Doe borrowed $225,000 for five years at $13\frac{1}{2}$ percent. The annual interest charge was

   A. $1,667.

   B. $6,000.

   C. $30,375.

   D. $39,375.

2. A junior salesman gets a commission of 14 percent on his sales. If he wants his commission to amount to $140, he will have to sell merchandise totaling

   A. $1,960.

   B. $10.

   C. $1,000.

   D. $100.

3. On a list price of $200, the difference between a single discount of 25 percent and successive discounts of 20 percent and 5 percent is

   A. $0.

   B. $48.

   C. $8.

   D. $2.

SHOW YOUR WORK HERE

SHOW YOUR WORK HERE

4. *A* worked five days on overhauling an old car. *B* worked four days more to finish the job. After the sale of the car, the net profit was $243. They wanted to divide the profit based on the time spent by each. *A*'s share of the profit was

   A. $108.

   B. $135.

   C. $127.

   D. $143.

5. If cloth costs $42\frac{1}{2}$ cents per yard, how many yards can be purchased for $76.50?

   A. 220

   B. 180

   C. 190

   D. 230

6. A fashionable dress shop offers a 20 percent discount on selected items. For a dress marked at $280, what is the discount price?

   A. $224.00

   B. $232.00

   C. $248.00

   D. $261.00

7. If *A* takes six days to do a task and *B* takes three days to do the same task, working together they should do the same task in

   A. $2\frac{2}{3}$ days.

   B. 2 days.

   C. $2\frac{1}{3}$ days.

   D. $2\frac{1}{2}$ days.

8. The area of a mirror 40 inches long and 20 inches wide is approximately

   A. 8.5 square feet.

   B. 5.6 square feet.

   C. 8.0 square feet.

   D. 2.5 square feet.

9. $\frac{2}{3}$ plus $\frac{1}{8}$ equals

   A. $\frac{37}{72}$

   B. $\frac{82}{72}$

   C. $\frac{3}{11}$

   D. $\frac{19}{24}$

10. A student has received two grades of 90 and two grades of 80 in an English course. Assuming the grades are weighted equally, what is the student's average for the course?

   A. 90

   B. 87

   C. 85

   D. 84

11. If a man has only quarters and dimes totaling $2.00, the number of quarters CANNOT be

   A. 2.

   B. 4.

   C. 6.

   D. 3.

12. The number that increased by one sixth of itself yields 182 is

   A. 156.

   B. 176.

   C. 148.

   D. 160.

13. $0.16\frac{3}{4}$ written as a percent is

   A. $16\frac{3}{4}$ percent.

   B. $16.\frac{3}{4}$ percent.

   C. $0.016\frac{3}{4}$ percent.

   D. $0.0016\frac{3}{4}$ percent.

14. If 4 ounces of protein provide 448 calories, how much protein is needed to provide 392 calories?

   A. 2.8 ounces

   B. 3.5 ounces

   C. 4.57 ounces

   D. 56 ounces

SHOW YOUR WORK HERE

15. $1,296.53 minus $264.87 is

   A. $1,232.76.

   B. $1,032.76.

   C. $1,031.66.

   D. $1,132.53.

16. $12\frac{1}{2}$ minus $6\frac{1}{4}$ is

   A. $5\frac{3}{4}$.

   B. $6\frac{1}{4}$.

   C. $6\frac{1}{2}$.

   D. $5\frac{1}{4}$.

17. Men's handkerchiefs cost $1.29 for three. The cost per dozen handkerchiefs is

   A. $7.74.

   B. $3.87.

   C. $14.48.

   D. $5.16.

18. Add: $\frac{1}{4}, \frac{7}{12}, \frac{3}{8}, \frac{1}{2}$, and $\frac{5}{6}$.

   A. $2\frac{1}{2}$

   B. $2\frac{13}{24}$

   C. $2\frac{3}{4}$

   D. $2\frac{15}{24}$

19. A floor is 25 feet wide by 36 feet long. To cover this floor with carpet will require

   A. 100 square yards.

   B. 300 square yards.

   C. 900 square yards.

   D. 25 square yards.

20. 72 divided by 0.0009 is

   A. 0.125.

   B. 800.

   C. 80,000.

   D. 80.

21. 345 safety pins at $4.15 per hundred will cost

   A. $0.1432.

   B. $1.4320.

   C. $14.32.

   D. $143.20.

22. The number that decreased by one fifth of itself yields 132 is

   A. 165.

   B. 198.

   C. 98.

   D. 88.

23. 285 is 5 percent of

   A. 1,700.

   B. 7,350.

   C. 1,750.

   D. 5,700.

24. A store sold jackets for $65 each. The jackets cost the store $50 each. The percent increase of selling price over cost is

   A. 40 percent.

   B. $33\frac{1}{2}$ percent.

   C. $33\frac{1}{3}$ percent.

   D. 30 percent.

25. The denominator of a fraction is 20 more than the numerator. What is the numerator if the fraction is equivalent to $\frac{3}{5}$?

   A. 12

   B. 30

   C. −50

   D. 10

SHOW YOUR WORK HERE

26. Which statement below is true about the inequality of $2 < x \leq 7$?

A. $x < 2$

B. $x = 2$

C. x is greater than 7

D. $x > 2$

27. $\frac{x}{5} - 4 = 11$. Find the value of x.

A. 75

B. 3

C. 35

D. 59

28. A punch recipe for a half gallon (64 ounces) of punch requires one pint (16 ounces) of grape juice. How many quarts (1 quart = 32 ounces) of grape juice are required for $2\frac{1}{2}$ gallons of the punch?

A. 5 quarts

B. 10 quarts

C. $1\frac{1}{4}$ quarts

D. $2\frac{1}{2}$ quarts

29. Mrs. Bowler got up at 7:00 a.m. last Wednesday morning and went to bed at 11:00 p.m. Wednesday night. During the time that she was up, she spent $\frac{1}{2}$ of her time at work, $\frac{1}{8}$ of her time bowling with friends, and $\frac{1}{4}$ of her time with her family.

How much time did she have left for other activities?

A. 2 hours

B. 4 hours

C. 1 hour

D. 8 hours

SHOW YOUR WORK HERE

30. If 24 percent of the students who enrolled in an algebra class of 50 students dropped the course before the semester ended, how many students remained in the class?

    A. 27
    B. 76
    C. 12
    D. 38

31. How many $\frac{3}{4}$–gram tablets are needed for a dosage of $4\frac{1}{2}$ grams?

    A. 3.75
    B. 1.5
    C. 6
    D. 3

32. $3.6 - 1.2(0.8 - 0.3) + 8 \div 0.4 =$

    A. 23
    B. 20.5
    C. 50
    D. 3.2

33. Find 0.2 percent of 400.

    A. 80
    B. 800
    C. 0.8
    D. 2,000

34. An 8-ounce bottle of fruit juice provides 200 calories. What percent of the 200 calories is provided by 3 ounces of the fruit juice?

    A. 12.5 percent
    B. 22.5 percent
    C. 37.5 percent
    D. 75 percent

SHOW YOUR WORK HERE

35. Find the length of the hypotenuse in the triangle below.

   A. 7
   B. 5
   C. 25
   D. 6

36. What is the width of a rectangle with an area of 63 square feet and a length of 9 feet?

   A. 22.5 feet
   B. 7 feet
   C. 567 feet
   D. 144 feet

37. If the triangles below are similar, find the length of side x.

   A. 21
   B. 11
   C. 13
   D. $3\frac{6}{7}$

38. If two lines are parallel, which of the following statements is true?

    A. The two lines have equal slopes.

    B. The two lines have one point in common.

    C. The product of the slopes of the lines is −1.

    D. The two lines form right angles.

SHOW YOUR WORK HERE

39. If the area of a square is 144 m², what is the length of a side of the square?

    A. 12m

    B. 12m²

    C. 72m

    D. 72m²

40. Find the area of the figure below. The lengths shown are in meters.

    A. 40m

    B. 46m

    C. 80m²

    D. 96m²

Questions 41 and 42 are based on the
following circle.

41. What percent of the circle does the central
angle of 60° represent? (Give answer to the
nearest percent.)

A. 6 percent

B. 60 percent

C. 17 percent

D. 25 percent

42. If $\frac{1}{12}$ of a family's weekly budget is spent
on entertainment and $\frac{1}{8}$ of the budget is
spent on gasoline, which central angle
represents the total spent on entertainment
and gasoline?

A. 20°

B. 45°

C. 90°

D. 75°

ANSWER KEYS AND EXPLANATIONS

Final Mathematics Examination

1. C	10. C	19. A	27. A	35. B
2. C	11. D	20. C	28. D	36. B
3. D	12. A	21. C	29. A	37. D
4. B	13. A	22. A	30. D	38. A
5. B	14. B	23. D	31. C	39. A
6. A	15. C	24. D	32. A	40. C
7. B	16. B	25. B	33. C	41. C
8. B	17. D	26. D	34. C	42. D
9. D	18. B			

1. **The correct answer is C.**

   $I = P \times R \times T$

   $\quad = \$225{,}000 \times 0.135 \times 1 \text{ year}$

   $\quad = \$30{,}375$

2. **The correct answer is C.**

   14% of x = \$140 (Let x be the total sales.)

   $0.14 \times x = \$140$

   $\qquad x = \$1{,}000$ (divide by 0.14)

3. **The correct answer is D.**

   25% of \$200 = 0.25 × \$200 = \$50

   Next, find the 20% discount on \$200:

   $0.20 \times \$200 = \$40$

   The list price discounted 20% is

   $\$200 - \$40 = \$160$

   Now take 5% of \$160:

   $0.05 \times \$160 = \$8$

   The discount is \$48 when taken at 20% and 5% successively.

   $\$50 - \$48 = \$2$

4. **The correct answer is B.**

   The job took nine days to complete.

   A worked five days: he completed $\dfrac{5}{9}$ of the work.

   B worked four days: he completed $\dfrac{4}{9}$ of the work.

   If the net profit was \$243, then A received

   $\dfrac{5}{9} \times \$243 = \$135$

5. **The correct answer is B.**

   $\$76.50 \div 42\dfrac{1}{2} \, \cancel{c}/\text{yard}$

   $\left(42\dfrac{1}{2}\,\cancel{c} = \$0.425 \right)$

   $= \$76.50 \div \$0.425 \, / \text{ yard}$

   $= 180 \text{ yards}$

6. **The correct answer is A.**

   Discount = 20%

   Sale price = 80%

   $0.80 \times \$280.00 = \$224.00$

7. **The correct answer is B.** $\frac{n}{6} + \frac{n}{3} = 1$

$n + 2n = 6$ (multiply by 6)

$\quad 3n = 6$ (combine like terms)

$\quad\quad n = 2$ (divide by 3)

8. **The correct answer is B.**

Area of a rectangle is

$A = length \times width$

$\quad = 40 \text{ inches} \times 20 \text{ inches}$

$\quad = 800 \text{ square inches}$

Note: 1 square foot = 144 square inches

$\frac{800 \text{ square inches}}{144 \text{ square inches}} = 5.6 \text{ square feet}$

9. **The correct answer is D.**

$\frac{2}{3} \times \frac{8}{8} = \frac{16}{24}$ (lowest common

$+\frac{1}{8} \times \frac{3}{3} = \frac{3}{24}$ denominator is 24)

$\quad\quad\quad = \frac{19}{24}$

10. **The correct answer is C.** To arrive at the average, add all numbers and divide by total number of grades.

$\quad 80$

$\quad 80$

$\quad 90$

$\underline{+90}$

$340 \div 4 = 85$

11. **The correct answer is D.** The number of quarters must be even; otherwise, adding dimes will not give $2.00 *exactly*. So the answer cannot be 3 (choice D).

$3 \times 25\text{¢} = 75\text{¢}$ or 0.75

$\$2.00 - 0.75 = \$1.25$

$1.25 cannot be changed to all dimes.

12. **The correct answer is A.** Let the *number* be x. A *number* increased by $\frac{1}{6}$ of itself is 182. To put this in equation form:

$x + \frac{1}{6}x = 182$

$6x + x = 1,092$ (multiple each term by 6)

$\quad 7x = 1,092$ (combine like terms)

$\quad\quad x = 156$ (divide by 7)

13. **The correct answer is A.**

$0.16\frac{3}{4} = 16\frac{3}{4} \text{ percent}$

When changing decimals to percents, move the decimal to the right two places.

14. **The correct answer is B.** Let p represent the amount of protein needed for 392 calories. Use a proportion

$\frac{4 \text{ ounces}}{448 \text{ calories}} = \frac{p \text{ ounces}}{392 \text{ calories}}$

$\quad 448p = 4 \times 392$

$\quad 448p = 1,568$

$\quad\quad p = 3.5 \text{ ounces of protein}$

3.5 ounces of protein are needed for 392 calories.

15. **The correct answer is C.**

$\$1,296.53$

$\underline{-246.87}$

$\$1,031.66$

16. **The correct answer is B.**

$12\frac{1}{2} = 12\frac{2}{4}$

$-6\frac{1}{4} = -6\frac{1}{4}$

$\quad\quad\quad 6\frac{1}{4}$

Note: $\frac{1}{2} \times \frac{2}{2} = \frac{2}{4}$

17. The correct answer is D. Price per dozen can be found by multiplying the $1.29 by 4. (There are 4 groups of 3 in a dozen.)

$$1.29 \times 4 = \$5.16$$

18. The correct answer is B.

$$\frac{1}{4} + \frac{7}{12} + \frac{3}{8} + \frac{1}{2} + \frac{5}{6} = \frac{6}{24} + \frac{14}{24} + \frac{9}{24} + \frac{12}{24} + \frac{20}{24}$$

Note: The lowest common denominator is 24. Each fraction needs to be rewritten to an equivalent fraction, so the denominator will be 24.

$$\frac{6 + 14 + 9 + 12 + 20}{24} = \frac{61}{24}$$

Divide:

$$24\overline{)61} = 2\frac{13}{24}$$
$$\underline{48}$$
$$13$$

19. The correct answer is A.

25 feet × 36 feet = 900 square feet

Now change 900 square feet to square yards.

Note: 9 square feet = 1 square yard

$$900 \text{ square feet} \times \frac{1 \text{ square yard}}{9 \text{ square feet}}$$

$$= 100 \text{ square yards}$$

20. The correct answer is C.

$$72.0000 \div 0.0009$$

$$= 720,000 \div 9$$

$$= 80,000$$

21. The correct answer is C.

One safety pin costs:

$$\$4.15 \div 100 = \$.0415$$

So 345 safety pins cost:

$$345 \times 0.0415 = \$14.32$$

22. The correct answer is A. A number, x, that decreased by $\frac{1}{5}$ of itself equals 132, can be expressed as:

$$x - \frac{1x}{5} = 132$$
$$5x - x = 660 \quad \text{(multiply each term by 5)}$$
$$4x = 660 \quad \text{(combine like terms)}$$
$$x = 165 \quad \text{(divide by 4)}$$

23. The correct answer is D. $285 = 0.05y$ (y is the unknown value)

$$5,700 = y \text{ (divide by 0.05)}$$

24. The correct answer is D. $65 − $50 = $15 is the increase, but to find the percent increase, we divide the increase by the original amount:

$$\$15 \div \$50 = 0.30, \text{ or } 30\%$$

25. The correct answer is B.

Let x represent the numerator of the fraction, then the denominator will be $x + 20$.

Since the fraction is equivalent to $\frac{3}{5}$, we get

$$\frac{x}{x + 20} = \frac{3}{5}$$
$$5x = 3(x + 20)$$
$$5x = 3x + 60$$
$$2x = 60$$
$$x = 30$$

26. The correct answer is D. $2 < x \leq 7$ means that x is greater than 2 and it is less than or equal to 7.

27. The correct answer is A.

$$\frac{x}{5} - 4 = 11$$
$$\frac{x}{5} - 4 + 4 = 11 + 4$$
$$\frac{x}{5} = 15$$
$$5 \times \frac{x}{5} = 5 \times 15$$
$$x = 75$$

28. The correct answer is D. Note that one gallon of punch contains 128 ounces (one-half gallon contains 64 ounces; hence, $2\frac{1}{2}$ gallons equals 320 ounces). A direct proportion can be used to solve the problem.

Let x = the number of ounces of grape juice needed.

$$\frac{16 \text{ ounces grape}}{64 \text{ ounces punch}} = \frac{x}{320 \text{ ounces punch}}$$

$$\frac{1}{4} = \frac{x}{320}$$

$$4x = 320$$

$$x = 80 \text{ ounces grape juice}$$

Since the answer is to be given in quarts, change 80 ounces to quarts by dividing 80 by 32. (There are 32 ounces in a quart.)

$80 \div 32 = 2.5$; thus, 2.5, or $2\frac{1}{2}$ quarts of grape juice are needed to make $2\frac{1}{2}$ gallons of punch.

29. The correct answer is A. There are 16 hours from 7:00 a.m. until 11:00 p.m. Hence, Mrs. Bowler was up 16 hours.

Let x = the time Mrs. Bowler had left for other activities, then

$$\frac{1}{2}(16) + \frac{1}{8}(16) + \frac{1}{4}(16) + x = 16$$

$$8 + 2 + 4 + x = 16$$

$$14 + x = 16$$

$$x = 2$$

30. The correct answer is D.

24 percent of the 50 students dropped the class.

24 percent of $50 = 0.24 \times 50 = 12$

Since 12 students dropped, $50 - 12$, or 38 students remained in the class.

31. The correct answer is C. Divide $4\frac{1}{2}$ by $\frac{3}{4}$. (First change $4\frac{1}{2}$ to $\frac{9}{2}$.)

$$4\frac{1}{2} \div \frac{3}{4} = \frac{9}{2} \times \frac{4}{3} = \frac{36}{6} = 6$$

32. The correct answer is A.

$3.6 - 1.2(0.8 - 0.3) + 8 \div 0.4$

$= 3.6 - 1.2(0.5) + 8 \div 4$

$= 3.6 - 0.6 + 8 \div 0.4$

$= 3.6 - 0.6 + 20$

$= 3 + 20$

$= 23$

(*Note:* Operations must be performed in the correct order. (Parentheses first, then multiplication and division before addition and subtraction.)

33. The correct answer is C. Change 0.2 percent to a decimal and multiply by 400.

$0.002 \times 400 = 0.800$, or 0.8

34. The correct answer is C. Find the number of calories provided by 3 ounces of fruit juice.

$$\frac{8}{200} = \frac{3}{c}$$

$$8c = 600$$

$$c = 75$$

75 calories are provided by 3 ounces of fruit juice.

Now determine what percent 75 is of 200.

$$200n = 75$$

$$n = .375 = 37.5\%$$

Three ounces of the fruit juice provide 37.5% of the 200 calories in 8 ounces.

35. The correct answer is B.

Use the Pythagorean theorem.

$$c^2 = a^2 + b^2$$
$$c^2 = 3^2 + 4^2$$
$$c^2 = 9 + 16$$
$$c^2 = 25$$
$$c = \sqrt{25}$$
$$c = 5$$

36. The correct answer is B. The formula for the area of a rectangle is $A = LW$. We know the area of the rectangle is 63 square feet and the length is 9 feet. Thus,

$$63 = 9W$$
$$\frac{63}{9} = \frac{9W}{9}$$
$$7 = W$$

37. The correct answer is D. The corresponding sides of similar triangles are proportional. Therefore,

$$\frac{3}{7} = \frac{x}{9}$$
$$7x = 27$$
$$x = 3\frac{6}{7}$$

38. The correct answer is A. Parallel lines have equal slopes; they do not intersect.

39. The correct answer is A. The area of a square is found by squaring a side of the square.

If $A = 144\text{m}^2$

$144\text{m}^2 = s^2$ where s is a side of the square

$$\sqrt{144\text{m}^2} = s$$
$$12\text{m} = s$$

40. The correct answer is C. Divide the figure into nonoverlapping rectangles. Find the area of each rectangle. Add the areas of the rectangles to get the total area of the figure.

$$A = 48\text{m}^2 + 20\text{m}^2 + 12\text{m}^2 = 80\text{m}^2$$

41. The correct answer is C. The entire circle contains 360°. The central angle of 60° represents $\frac{60}{360} = \frac{1}{6}$.

Change $\frac{1}{6}$ to a percent by dividing the denominator into the numerator. Thus, $\frac{1}{6} = 16\frac{2}{3}\%$. We get 17 when we express $16\frac{2}{3}$ to the nearest whole percent.

42. The correct answer is D. The weekly budget is represented by the entire circle; $\frac{1}{12}$ of the circle represents $\frac{1}{12} \times 360 = 30°$, which is the measure of the central angle for the amount spent on entertainment. $\frac{1}{8}$ of the circle represents $\frac{1}{8} \times 360 = 45°$, which is the measure of the central angle for the amount spent on gasoline. A central angle that represents the total spent on entertainment and gasoline is $30° + 45° = 75°$.

(Alternatively, $\frac{1}{8} + \frac{1}{12} = \frac{5}{24}$ and $\frac{5}{24} \times 360° = 75°$.)

Science

OVERVIEW

Unit 6 provides a review of important life science and physical science information to help you prepare for the registered nursing school entrance exam. This unit includes relevant concepts and principles related to general biology, chemistry, and physics, as well as practice tests that simulate the testing experience. Emphasis is on the descriptions of the activities and characteristics of life with respect to humans.

CHARACTERISTICS OF ORGANISMS

The modern classification of organisms divides all living species into one of six kingdoms. There is some debate as to how many kingdoms there are, and some taxonomists classify species into only five kingdoms. In the United States, it is currently accepted practice to classify species into six kingdoms.

1. **Eubacteria:** The kingdom Eubacteria consists of prokaryotic organisms. Prokaryotes are cells that do not have a nucleus or any membrane-bound organelles. Eubacteria are single-cell organisms that reproduce asexually. While most bacteria are heterotrophic (they obtain energy from an outside food source), these organisms can also be autotrophic (self-feeders) or decomposers that feed off dead matter (saprotrophic).

2. **Archaeabacteria:** The kingdom Archaeabacteria also consists of single-celled prokaryotes. These organisms are bacteria that can live under very extreme conditions such as extreme temperatures, acidity, alkalinity, or salinity. Some archaeabacteria can live under extremely low oxygen conditions.

3. **Protista:** The kingdom Protista consists of unicellular and multicellular eukaryotic organisms. Eukaryotic cells are those with a nucleus and compartmentalized, membrane-bound organelles. There are three informal groups of Protista: protozoa (amoeba, flagellates, ciliates), algae, and slime and water molds. Organisms in the kingdom Protista can be autotrophs, saprotrophs, or heterotrophs.

4. **Fungi:** Members of the kingdom Fungi are unicellular or multicellular heterotrophs. This kingdom includes mushrooms, yeasts, and molds. Multicellular fungi are composed of a mass of slender filaments called mycelium, and yeasts are a type of unicellular fungi. Fungi do not perform photosynthesis because they lack chlorophyll. Some fungi are parasitic and pathogenic. Fungi are generally saprotrophic.

5. **Plantae:** Members of the kingdom Plantae are eukaryotic, multicellular organisms that consist of a cell wall made of cellulose. The kingdom Plantae includes flowering plants, conifers, ferns, and mosses. They are all photosynthetic green plants that contain chlorophyll. These species are autotrophs and nonmotile. Plants are the primary producers for all living land organisms, and they are an essential source of oxygen on Earth.

6. **Animalia:** The kingdom Animalia consists of eukaryotic multicellular heterotrophs. Heterotrophs are consumers that must ingest food as an energy source. They can be herbivores, carnivores, omnivores, or decomposers. Species belonging to the kingdom Animalia include all vertebrates and invertebrates. These species commonly exhibit tissue differentiation and complex organ systems, and they are motile. Parasitic organisms are sometimes included in the kingdom Animalia.

Regardless of the kingdom into which a species is classified, all living organisms share certain common characteristics. These characteristics are sometimes used to describe life. In particular, all living organisms are composed of cells, respond to stimuli (external or internal), reproduce, exhibit growth and development, obtain and metabolize food as an energy source, possess nucleic acids, and are able to adapt to their environments.

Organisms can be interdependent. Two species can exist in an indirect relationship in which they adapt to occupy the same habitat without interacting with each other. Other species can exist in a direct relationship in which one or both species benefit from the relationship (symbiosis), or one species is threatened by the other (predation). In addition, organisms can have an effect on their environment, or an environment may have an effect on the organisms that live within it.

NOTE

The science part of the Registered Nursing Exam tests knowledge of concepts rather than critical thinking ability.

BASIC PRINCIPLES OF LIFE SCIENCES

All substances, whether inorganic or organic, are composed of matter. We'll begin with the makeup of all living organisms: the cell.

The Cell

All living organisms are composed of cells. Cells are the basic unit of life. There are two types of cells that define an organism: prokaryotic and eukaryotic. **Prokaryotic cells** are cells that lack a nuclear membrane and defined organelles. These cells make up organisms such as bacteria and archaea. **Eukaryotic cells** are more complex. The genetic material (DNA) of eukaryotic cells is contained within a nuclear membrane, separating it from the cytoplasm. Within the cytoplasm are clearly defined membrane-bound organelles. Some types of eukaryotic cells, such as red blood cells, lack a clearly defined nucleus when they are fully mature. Immature red blood cells have a nucleus, but lose it for functional reasons when they are fully developed. All vertebrates, including humans, are composed of eukaryotic cells.

There are several differences between plant and animal cells. Organelles that are found in animal cells, but not in plant cells, include lysosomes, centrioles, and flagella (although these are found in some plant sperm cells). Organelles that are found in plant cells, but not in animal cells, include chloroplasts, central vacuole and tonoplasts, cell wall, and plasmodesmata.

Cell Division

All eukaryotic cells divide in order to reproduce. Typical non-sex cells divide through the process of **mitosis**. Mitosis is the division of the cell's nuclear material, and it is divided into five stages: prophase, prometaphase, metaphase, anaphase, and telophase. DNA replicates in a cell during the cell cycle phase known as interphase. Interphase occurs before the process of mitosis. Mitosis conserves numbers of chromosomes equally, allocating replicated chromosomes to each of the new daughter nuclei. One round of mitosis of a diploid cell (two copies of each chromosome) produces two new daughter cells that are also diploid. In some cases, mitosis may occur without cell division, resulting in a multinucleate cell.

Sex cells in eukaryotic organisms undergo a variation of cell division called **meiosis**. Meiosis results in four nonidentical daughter cells that each have only one set of chromosomes. Meiosis occurs only in the gonads (ovaries and testes). Cells that undergo meiosis are called **gametes** and include ovum and sperm cells.

Cellular Organelles

Cellular functions are accomplished by one or more parts, or **organelles**, in each cell.

- **Cell membrane:** The cell, or plasma, membrane is a phospholipid bilayer impregnated with proteins. It is differentially permeable and functions in regulating the passage of materials into and out of the cell. Mechanisms by which material can pass through the plasma membrane include osmosis, diffusion, and active transport. Cells constantly interact with their environment through osmosis and diffusion. **Diffusion** is the passive movement of a substance from an area of higher concentration to an area of lower concentration. **Osmosis** is another mechanism of passive transport in which a solvent (usually water) will travel from an area of higher concentration to an area of lower concentration. Mechanisms of active transport include a sodium-potassium ion pump, endocytosis, phagocytosis, pinocytosis, and exocytosis. The outside surface of the plasma membrane of animal cells is covered with tiny microvilli, projections that increase the surface area of the cell.

- **Cell wall:** The cell wall is the outer layer of plant cells that maintains the cell's shape and protects the cell from mechanical and physical damage. The cell wall is composed of cellulose, other polysaccharides, and proteins.

- **Central vacuole:** The central vacuole is an organelle found in plant cells, but not in animal cells. Its functions include storage, the breakdown of waste products, and the hydrolysis of macromolecules. The enlargement of the central vacuole is a major mechanism in plant growth.

- **Centrosome:** The centrosome is the region of the cell where microtubules initiate. Each animal cell contains a pair of centrioles within the centrosome. **Centrioles** are tiny, barrel-shaped organelles that provide a framework for functional structure construction, such as centrosomes and cilia. Centrioles occur in pairs and move toward the poles of the cell nucleus during cell division.

- **Contractile vacuole:** Contractile vacuoles are membranous sacs that maintain a proper concentration of water inside the cell. They function to drain excess water from the cytoplasm and remove it from the cell. Contractile vacuoles are found in many protists and some animal cells.

- **Cytoskeleton:** The cytoskeleton reinforces and maintains a cell's shape. It also functions in cell movement. The components of the cytoskeleton are microfilaments, intermediate filaments, and microtubules.

- **Endoplasmic reticulum:** The endoplasmic reticulum (ER) is a network of membranous sacs and tubules. The ER is active in membrane synthesis and functions as an intracellular transport system for many proteins and substances. The ER extends throughout the cytoplasm.

  There are two types of endoplasmic reticulum: the rough ER and the smooth ER. The rough ER is studded with ribosomes that produce many secretory proteins in the cell. The rough ER is also involved in membrane synthesis. The smooth ER is involved in processes including the synthesis of lipids, cellular metabolism of carbohydrates, and the detoxification of drugs and poisons.

- **Flagella/Cilia:** Flagella and cilia are slender projections from the cell that aid in cell movement. Flagella are longer than cilia and are composed of membrane-enclosed microtubules. Cilia are small hair-like structures that also have an internal arrangement of microtubules.

- **Golgi apparatus:** The Golgi apparatus functions in the synthesis, modification, sorting, and secretion of cell products. Products of the ER are modified and stored in the Golgi and then sent to other destinations. The Golgi apparatus consists of flattened membranous sacs called cisternae. These are responsible for carbohydrate synthesis, phosphorylation of proteins, and synthesis of other non-protein macromolecules.

- **Lysosome:** The lysosomes are digestive organelles in which macromolecules are hydrolyzed. In addition, phagocytic vacuoles, also called food vacuoles, are membranous sacs used by some types of cells to engulf and digest food material. Other vacuoles, called autophagic vacuoles, function to engulf, digest, and recycle worn-out cytoplasmic organelles.

- **Mitochondria:** Mitochondria are important organelles in the cell in which cellular respiration occurs. Macromolecules such as carbohydrates, fats, and proteins are oxidized, resulting in the release of ATP, a form of usable energy that all cells require.

- **Nucleus:** The nucleus is the genetic control center of the cell. The cell nucleus is enclosed within a porous, double membrane called the nuclear envelope. The nucleus contains all the cell's DNA. DNA and protein form a complex of genetic material called chromatin, which condenses and forms chromosomes during cell division. The nucleolus is a nonmembraneous organelle within the nucleus that is involved in the production of ribosomal RNA (rRNA) and ribosomes.

  Transcription, the biosynthesis of RNA from a DNA template, occurs within the cell's nucleus. The messenger RNA (mRNA) then moves to the ribosomes in the cytosol, or the intracellular fluid, where the mRNA acts as a template for protein synthesis in the process of translation.

- **Peroxisome:** A peroxisome is an organelle with specialized metabolic functions that produce hydrogen peroxide as a by-product.

- **Plasmodesmata (plasmodesma, singular):** Plasmodesmata are found only in plant cells. They are the channels through cell walls that connect the cytoplasm of adjacent cells.

- **Plastid:** Plastids, found only in plant cells, are involved in the synthesis and storage of food. Chloroplasts are green organelles that give plants their green color and in which photosynthesis takes place. Chloroplasts convert the energy from sunlight into chemical energy, which is stored in a plant cell in the form of glucose. The other common plastid types are chromoplasts, gerontoplasts (pigmented plastids), and leucoplasts (nonpigmented plastids). Chromoplasts and leucoplasts function in storage and other processes such as starch collection.

- **Ribosomes:** Ribosomes are small nonmembranous organelles that synthesize proteins from mRNA. They may be found free in the cytoplasm or bound to the endoplasmic reticulum.

Cells are grouped together to form tissues. Well-developed tissues are specialized for certain functions. Furthermore, different tissues work together to form organs, and organs are grouped together by function to form a system. Throughout the body, organ systems have highly specialized functions, but in many cases the function of one system is dependent on the function of one or more other systems. Most organisms, from the round and segmented worm to vertebrates, are characterized by the organization of their systems.

The Cell Cycle

Cell growth occurs in a regular pattern called the **cell cycle**. The cell cycle is divided into the mitotic (M) phase and the interphase, which is divided into the G1, S, and G2 phases.

1. **M phase:** Mitosis occurs during the M phase of the cell cycle. Mitosis is the division of the cell nucleus, followed immediately by division of the cytoplasm in a process known as cytokinesis. There are five phases of mitosis that are involved in division of the nucleus. Chromatin fibers become denser during prophase. The nuclear envelope fragments and microtubules that form spindles invade the nuclear area during prometaphase. Metaphase is the longest phase of mitosis, in which the chromosomes line up along the center of the cell, midway between the poles of the mitotic spindle. Anaphase is the shortest phase of mitosis during which the chromatid pairs separate and each chromosome moves to opposite poles of the cell. During telophase, two daughter cells begin to form, two nuclear envelopes form, and the original nucleus is now divided into two. The cytoplasm divides during cytokinesis, and the result is two new cells.

2. **G1 and G2 phase:** The cell grows during both the G1 and the G2 portions of interphase. The G1 phase is known as the first "gap," and the G2 phase is called the second "gap."

3. **S phase:** The S phase, or the synthesis phase, is the phase in which the DNA of the cell is replicated, resulting in duplication of each chromosome.

Reproduction

All living organisms undergo either sexual or asexual reproduction. Reproduction maintains the continuity of a species or population.

Asexual Reproduction

Asexual reproduction occurs through mitosis and does not involve a union of reproductive cells (gametes). There are several mechanisms of asexual reproduction.

- **Sporulation:** Sporulation is a process that involves the production of asexual reproductive cells called spores. These spores develop into mature individuals that are identical.

- **Binary fission:** Binary fission involves the division of an organism (usually a unicellular organism) into two organisms. In the case of unicellular eukaryotes, binary fission usually involves mitosis.

- **Multiple fission or fragmentation:** Fragmentation is seen in organisms such as filamentous algae. It involves the breaking of an organism into smaller units. Each of these fragments can then develop into an identical member of the same species.

- **Budding:** Budding involves the production of an outgrowth or miniature organism that eventually breaks away from the parent, forming a new identical individual.

Sexual Reproduction

Sexual reproduction involves the process of meiosis followed by fertilization. Thus, there is a union between the nuclei of a male reproductive cell and a female reproductive cell. Sexual reproduction allows for variation between parents and offspring, whereas asexual reproduction produces offspring that are identical to the parent. There are three general mechanisms of sexual reproduction.

1. **Isogamy:** Isogamy is a mechanism of sexual reproduction involving the fusion of gametes of identical size and structure. This type of reproduction is most common in lower plant species.

2. **Heterogamy:** Heterogamy is a mechanism of sexual reproduction involving the fusion of gametes that differ in size and/or structure. Ansiogamy is a type of heterogamy that involves motile gametes that differ only in size. Oogamy is a type of heterogamy that involves gametes that differ in size and structure.

   Human sexual reproduction is a form of oogamy. The spermatozoa produced by males differs in size and structure from the ovum produced by females. In humans and most other mammals, gametes are produced in gonads or sex organs. The male gonads are the testes, and the female gonads are the ovaries. Gonads in humans and other higher-order animal species also have an endocrine function. Gonads produce hormones that function in the development of secondary sex characteristics and reproductive cycles (female menstruation cycle).

3. **Conjugation:** Conjugation is a mechanism of sexual reproduction that involves the temporary union of cells to allow for the exchange or transmission of DNA or nuclei.

Meiosis

The production of gametes (sex cells) or spores involves the process of meiosis. Gametes are haploid cells, meaning that they have half the number of chromosomes of a zygote, or fertilized ovum. Meiosis has several stages that occur in two rounds (meiosis I and meiosis II). Round 1 consists of interphase, prophase, prometaphase, metaphase I, anaphase I, and telophase I. Round 2 consists of interphase II, metaphase II, anaphase II, telophase II, and cytokinesis. During the first round (interphase through telophase I), two diploid cells are formed. The cell undergoes DNA replication during interphase, just as it would in the process of mitosis. During the second round (interphase II through cytokinesis), four haploid cells are formed. The process of meiosis is similar to mitosis, except that a single replication of chromosomes is followed by two consecutive cell divisions (meiosis I and meiosis II).

Once the two gametes, such as a sperm and an ovum, are united, the zygote forms, and there is a diploid number of chromosomes. This process is called fertilization. The zygote typically develops mitotically into an embryo; thus, the developing embryo has cells that contain a diploid number of chromosomes (except for any developing gametes). Because of meiosis and the union of two gametes (syngamy), the individual developing from the zygote receives half of its chromosomes (DNA) from each parent. In this way, the number of chromosomes in a species remains constant.

Growth and Development

The growth and development of an organism allows for the characteristic size range of a species to be maintained. Also, through the development and growth of offspring, differentiation of tissue and organs is accomplished. In a multicellular organism, growth most often involves an increase in the number of cells. It may also occur through an increase in the size of the cells or an increase in both the number and size of the cells.

Embryogenesis is the process by which an embryo forms and develops, eventually becoming a fetus. In higher-order animals such as humans, the basic pattern of development is as follows:

1. **Cleavage:** The zygote undergoes cleavage that results in the formation of a cluster of cells called a morula.

2. **Blastocyst or a Blastula:** The morula develops into a blastula or blastocyst. The blastocyst is a hollow ball of cells with a cavity known as a blastocoel.

3. **Gastrula:** The blastocyst develops into a two-layered gastrula. The gastrula has a cavity known as a gastrocoel or archenteron. The outer, or germ, layer of the gastrula is called the **ectoderm**, and the inner layer is called the **endoderm**. A third germ layer called the **mesoderm** develops between the ectoderm and the endoderm.

Each of these three germ layers gives rise to specific tissues and body structures. The nervous system, including some sensory organs such as the eyes and the outer skin, develops from the ectoderm layer. The musculoskeletal system, muscles of the viscera, mesenteries, and the circulatory system develop from the mesoderm. The lungs, liver, pancreas, thyroid, parathyroid, thymus glands, and the lining of the digestive tract all develop from the endoderm layer.

In addition to these three primary germ layers, some animals develop extraembryonic membranes. There are four basic extraembryonic membranes: the yolk sac, amnion, chorion, and allantois. The yolk sac provides nutrition to the embryo. The amnion forms a fluid-like sac filled with amniotic fluid that protects the developing embryo. The allantois is the membrane involved in gas exchange to and from the developing embryo. The outermost fetal membrane, the chorion, is formed from the secretion of ectoderm.

The complete development of a human takes about 38 weeks. During the first two months, the developing baby is referred to as an embryo. From the third month until the ninth month, the baby is then referred to as a fetus.

Nutrition

The nutritional processes of ingesting and utilizing food as an energy source are exhibited by all organisms. Food is defined "as any substance that can be used by an organism as an energy source that helps to promote growth and maintenance of the body."

Most food sources ingested by humans are organic (carbon-based substances). In plants, the process of converting inorganic materials into an organic food source is carried out through the process of photosynthesis. Sunlight provides energy for the process of photosynthesis, and green plants have chloroplasts that are the major site of photosynthesis. Chloroplasts are found mainly in the mesophyll, the tissue in the interior of the leaf. Light energy absorbed by chlorophyll drives the synthesis of inorganic compounds into organic molecules. During photosynthesis, light energy drives a reaction between carbon dioxide and water in the leaf tissue. The resulting products are the sugar glucose ($C_6H_{12}O_6$) and oxygen. Carbon dioxide enters the leaf and oxygen exits the leaf through microscopic pores called stomata. All organisms (with the exception of some algae and prokaryotes) depend either directly or indirectly on photosynthesis for food.

Organisms such as green plants that are able to manufacture food and energy within their bodies from inorganic materials in the environment are called autotrophs. Organisms that receive an organic food source from their environment are called heterotrophs. In addition to what they eat, heterotrophs can be classified into three categories based on how they eat or obtain nutrition.

1. **Saprotrophs:** Saprotrophs digest food externally and absorb the digested food into the body. Most bacteria and fungi are saprotrophs.

2. **Parasites:** Parasites are dependent on a host for survival and are harmful to the host on or in which they live.

3. **Phagotrophs:** Humans and most animals are phagotrophs. Phagotrophs ingest solid food into a digestive cavity. The digestive cavity may be as simple as a food vacuole in primitive organisms. Other simple organisms, such as coelenterates and flatworms, have a gastrovascular cavity with a mouth opening at one end. More complex organisms such as humans and other animals have a complete digestive tract. The human digestive system has a mouth opening for ingesting food and an anal opening for expelling food waste.

Food that has been ingested by an organism must be changed into a usable and absorbable state. The digestive system alters ingested food so that the body can absorb the necessary nutrients. The undigested and nutritionally expended food remains are expelled as waste. In humans and most animals, this occurs in the digestive tract. In lower organisms, this will occur in the food vacuole or gastrovascular cavity.

Once food has been digested, nutrients and molecules from the food are distributed to cells throughout the body. In humans, it is the circulatory system that distributes food products to the cells. Within the cells, the process of metabolism converts these molecules obtained from food into energy for the cell.

There are three classes of organic macromolecules found in foods that are essential to life: proteins, carbohydrates, and lipids.

1. **Proteins:** Proteins are made up of long chains of amino acids. Twenty different types of amino acids form long polypeptide chains that can be folded into a three-dimensional structure. The final folded structure is a protein. Structural proteins are made up of long filaments (collagen). Structural proteins are found in hair, skin, and connective tissue. Globular proteins are larger proteins such as hemoglobin, enzymes, and antibodies. Most proteins are globular.

2. **Carbohydrates:** Carbohydrates consist of carbon, hydrogen, and oxygen atoms. All sugars are carbohydrates. A sugar molecule is called a **saccharide**. A saccharide can contain one, two, or many sugar molecules. **Monosaccharides** are simple sugars such as glucose and fructose. **Disaccharides** contain two sugars. These include sucrose, lactose, and maltose. **Polysaccharides** have many sugars. Examples of polysaccharides include glycogen (the form in which animals store glucose), starch (the form in which plants store glucose), and cellulose (a structural polysaccharide that forms cell walls in plants). Saccharides serve as an energy source for cells. This energy can be used immediately or stored as glycogen for later use.

3. **Lipids:** Lipids are organic compounds that, like carbohydrates, contain carbon, hydrogen, and oxygen. Lipids are important for maintaining the structure of cell membranes, and they are a source of insulation and a means of storing energy in the body. Lipids include fats, oils, waxes, phospholipids, and steroids. A fat molecule contains one glycerol molecule and three fatty acid chains; thus, the term triglyceride is also used to refer to fats. The human body stores both health beneficial lipids called high-density lipids, or

HDLs, and health harmful lipids called low-density lipids, or LDLs. Too many lipids can lead to clogged arteries, which cause coronary diseases such as arteriosclerosis and atherosclerosis. These conditions can lead to heart attacks and stroke. Both LDL and HDL are referred to as cholesterols. Cholesterol is a unique organic lipid made up of hydrocarbon rings that is necessary to build and maintain cell membranes and give the cell an elastic quality. Cholesterol also functions to produce steroid hormones in the body.

Metabolism

Metabolism occurs in cells and is the sum of the chemical reactions that take place within a cell. Macromolecules such as carbohydrates, lipids, and proteins are metabolized in the cell to provide energy for cell maintenance and function. The steps of cellular respiration in human and animal cells are glycolysis, the Krebs cycle (or citric acid cycle), and oxidative phosphorylation. Respiration breaks down fuel in the form of glucose and generates ATP, the usable form of energy in the cell.

- **Glycolysis:** Glycolysis takes place in the cytosol in the absence of oxygen and involves the splitting of a glucose molecule (through the process of oxidation) into two molecules of pyruvate (the ionized form of pyruvic acid). The initial glycolysis reaction involves the breakdown of two ATP molecules into adenosine diphosphate (ADP). However, the overall glycolysis reaction produces four ATP molecules, so there is a net gain of two ATP molecules in the overall reaction. The overall reaction also produces two NADH molecules, also a form of usable energy in the cell. Therefore, the overall yield of one round of glycolysis in which glucose is oxidized in the cell is two pyruvate, two ATP, and two NADH molecules. No CO_2 is released during glycolysis because the reaction takes place in the absence of oxygen.

- **Krebs Cycle:** After the completion of glycolysis, pyruvate is transported to the mitochondria. In the mitochondria, each pyruvate is first converted into acetyl coenzyme A. Pyruvate's COOH group is removed, and CO_2 is released from the reaction. The remaining fragment of pyruvate is oxidized and several more reaction steps take place involving NAD^+ and coenzyme A, resulting in acetyl CoA. During the Krebs cycle, eight reaction steps are catalyzed by different enzymes. The result is the release of two ATP molecules, six NADH molecules, and two FADH molecules, all of which provide usable energy to the cell.

TIP

Remember that the Krebs cycle is also called the citric acid cycle. You might find either term on the exam

The Krebs Cycle (Citric Acid Cycle)

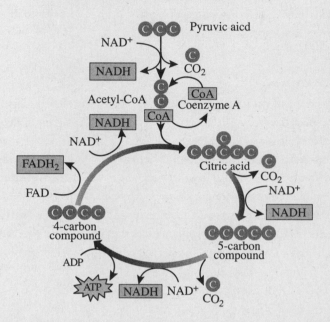

- **Oxidative phosphorylation:** The process of oxidative phosphorylation is comprised of two stages: electron transport and chemiosmosis. The electron transport chain is a collection of molecules embedded in the inner membrane of the mitochondrion. Most components of the electron transport chain are protein complexes. Electron transport through these complexes creates an H^+ ion gradient across the cell membrane. The two sources of H^+ for the electron transport chain are NADH and $FADH^2$. No ATP is made during this process, but the purpose of the electron transport chain is to enable the mitochondrion to couple the electron transport with the process of chemiosmosis. Oxygen is the final electron acceptor of the electron transport chain. The energy stored in the H^+ gradient across the membrane couples the redox reaction of the chain to ATP synthesis. Protons (H^+) from the electron transport chain flow through the membrane by way of a large enzyme complex called ATP synthase. There are three catalytic sites in the enzyme complex that join ADP with inorganic phosphate to form ATP. Oxidative phosphorylation results in the production of 32 to 34 ATP molecules.

The total yield of ATP molecules during cellular respiration is 36 to 38 ATP molecules. Energy conversion via cellular respiration is a remarkably efficient process.

During the process of cellular respiration, aerobic oxidation requires free molecular oxygen. Oxygen is made available to the cells by means of the human respiratory system or, in other animals, by the respiratory organs. Oxygen is inhaled and absorbed from the air into the lungs. It is transported throughout the body by the circulatory system. In humans, oxygen is transported through the blood by hemoglobin and red blood cells. Once glucose is oxidized, CO_2 is produced. The resulting CO_2 is removed from cells by the circulatory system and is expelled from the body through expiration of air from the lungs (respiratory system). Liquid waste formed as a result of metabolism is collected, concentrated, and eliminated through the excretory (urinary) system.

When food is ingested, the production of other necessary compounds such as proteins and secretory products also occurs in the cell. Any solid indigestible waste from food is eliminated from the digestive system through the excretory system.

Enzymes

All cellular functions depend on specific proteins, and in particular, they depend upon enzymes. Enzymes are highly specialized proteins that serve as biological catalysts to help speed up certain biological reactions. Enzymes are able to change the rate of a chemical reaction without themselves being changed or consumed during the reaction. A **substrate** is a particular substance acted upon by an enzyme. A substrate fits into a region of the enzyme called the **active site**, which is typically a pocket or groove on the enzyme's surface. Enzymes are specific because their active sites will fit only a specific substrate molecule. Once the substrate fits into the enzyme's active site, the reaction is catalyzed and product is formed. The enzyme releases the product and emerges unchanged from the reaction, so it can bind to another of the same type of substrate molecule.

Nucleic Acids

Nucleic acids are macromolecules found in every cell. There are two types of nucleic acids: DNA (deoxyribonucleic acid) and RNA (ribonucleic acid). All living organisms possess one or both types of nucleic acids. DNA functions as the source of genetic information for an individual. DNA exists as two long chains of individual molecules called nucleotides. The long strands of DNA nucleotides are twisted into a double helix structure in which one nucleotide forms a base pair with another. These base pairs are held together by hydrogen bonds. Each nucleotide consists of a sugar called deoxyribose, a phosphate group, and a purine or pyrimidine base. There are two purine bases, guanine and adenine, and two pyrimidine bases, cytosine and thymine. The purine guanine (G) forms base pairs only with the pyrimidine cytosine (C) and the purine adenine (A) forms base pairs only with the pyrimidine thymine (T). All eukaryotic cells contain DNA within their nucleus, and prokaryotic cells contain DNA attached to the inside of the cell membrane.

DNA can function in several processes, including cellular metabolism, reproduction (heredity), and the production of another nucleic acid called RNA. RNA is synthesized from a DNA template during the process of transcription. RNA is also composed of nucleotides. However, RNA exists mostly as a single strand of nucleotide molecules, and it is generally smaller in size than DNA. The nucleotides of RNA are slightly different than those of DNA in that the pyrimidine base uracil (U) replaces thymine. Uracil pairs with adenine. Guanine pairs with cytosine.

There are three types of RNA, all of which play a role in protein synthesis. **Messenger RNA** (mRNA) is the template for amino acid synthesis. These amino acid chains, or polypeptide chains, synthesized by an mRNA template, are modified and folded into a protein structure. The information in the mRNA that leads to the synthesis of a protein comes from the original DNA template that was transcribed into RNA. The segments of DNA that code for specific proteins are called genes.

Transfer RNA (tRNA) matches each specific amino acid to its codon on an mRNA strand. The codon is a three-nucleotide sequence that is specific for only one of the 26 amino acids. Thus, tRNA molecules are able to pick up a specific amino acid and deliver it to a specific amino acid codon. This ensures that all amino acids are placed in the correct sequence for a particular protein.

Ribosomal RNA (rRNA) is the third type of RNA and the key component of ribosomes. Ribosomes are present in the cytoplasm of the cell and are the site of protein synthesis.

Heredity

Heredity is defined as the transmission of traits from one generation to the next. The transmission of these traits can be explained in terms of several concepts, including gene theory, Mendel's law, meiosis, and chromosomes.

Gene Theory

Gregor Mendel deduced the fundamental principles of modern genetics by breeding garden peas. The pea plants he studied produced a large number of offspring and came in many distinguishable varieties. A heritable feature that varies among individuals in a population is called a character, and each variable of a character is called a trait. Mendel was able to strictly control the breeding of the pea plants and worked with his plants until he had true breeding varieties that produced offspring identical to the parent. Mendel was then able to create hybrid offspring by mating two different true breeds of a pea plant variety. The cross fertilization of two species is called hybridization, or a cross.

Mendel's Laws

Mendel performed many experiments in which he tracked the inheritance patterns of specific traits in plants. The results of his experiments led him to formulate several ideas about inheritance.

- **The law of segregation:** Mendel's law of segregation, based on his observations during his studies of inheritance patterns of plants, states that for a specific inheritable trait, there are two alleles (versions of the same gene) that separate during gamete formation and end up in two separate gametes during meiosis. For each trait, an individual inherits one allele from each parent. An individual with two identical alleles for a gene is said to be homozygous for that allele, and an individual with two different alleles for a gene is said to be heterozygous for that gene. If the two alleles for one gene are different, one allele determines the physical trait expressed by the gene and is called the dominant allele. The other allele has no noticeable effect on the appearance of the individual and is called the recessive allele.

- **The law of independent assortment:** Mendel's law of independent assortment states that each pair of alleles for a specific gene segregates independently of the alleles for a different gene. This law was revealed by the tracking of two traits at one time.

Punnett Squares

Since Mendel's laws of segregation and independent assortment reflect the rules of probability, the distribution of hereditary traits among offspring can be predicted using a tool called the **Punnett square**. In order to construct a Punnett square, the genotypes of each parent must be known. The genotype of an individual identifies each allele for a specific gene. Individuals can either be homozygous for the dominant trait, homozygous for the recessive trait, or heterozygous for both traits. The Punnett square predicts the percentage of each type of offspring based on the genotypes of the parents. For example, if two heterozygous individuals mate, 50% of the offspring will be heterozygous, 25% will be homozygous for the dominant trait, and 25% will be homozygous for the recessive trait.

MATERNAL	PATERNAL	
	A	a
A	AA	Aa
a	Aa	aa

AA = 25% heterozygous (two dominates)

Aa = 50% heterozygous (one dominate and one recessive)

aa = 25% homozygous (two recessives)

Meiosis and Chromosomes

During meiosis, four haploid gamete cells are produced. Each of these cells contains one copy of each gene packaged into chromosomes. When two gametes are joined during fertilization, the offspring receives one copy of each allele from each of its parents. In this way, a population experiences genetic variation during sexual reproduction that is not seen in asexual reproduction.

DNA in most species is divided into separate segments and packaged into chromosomes. Genes occupy specific loci, or positions, on a chromosome, and it is the chromosomes that undergo segregation and independent assortment. Therefore, it is the behavior of chromosomes during meiosis and fertilization that accounts for inheritance patterns.

Many species have a pair of sex chromosomes, designated by the symbols X and Y. These sex chromosomes are responsible for determining the sex of an individual. In humans, individuals with one X chromosome and one Y chromosome are male, and those with two X chromosomes are female. All ova contain a single copy of the X chromosome, and sperm can contain either an X or a Y chromosome. Thus, the sex of an individual is determined by whether the sperm that fertilizes the ovum is carrying an X or a Y chromosome.

CHEMISTRY

The Periodic Table and Bonding

The periodic table of elements shows all of the chemical elements discovered up to this point. The numbers provided for each element on the periodic table are indicative of the elements' properties.

Periodic Table

Group

	Alkali metals		Alkaline earth metals		Lanthanides		Actinides		Transition metals
	Poor metals		Metalloids		Nonmetals		Halogens		Noble gases

State at standard tempurature and pressure

Atomic number in red: gas

Atomic number in blue: liquid

Atomic number in black: solid

solid border: at least one isotope is older than the Earth (Primordial elements)

dashed border: at least one isotope naturally arise from decay of other chemical elements and no isotopes are older than the earth

dotted border: only artificially made isotopes (synthetic elements)

no border: undiscovered

Table courtesy of Wikimedia Commons (**https://commons.wikimedia.org/wiki/Periodic_table_of_elements**)

Note: It is recommended that you reference a full-color version of the periodic table either online or at your local library. The periodic table provided is simplistic in nature and for reference only.

The letter representing an element is its **chemical symbol**. For carbon, the chemical symbol is C. The **atomic number** uniquely identifies an element and, in a neutral atom, is equivalent to the number of electrons in the atom. For carbon, the atomic number is 6. The **mass number** is equivalent to the sum of proton and neutron masses. Since electrons are significantly smaller than protons and neutrons, they are not included in the calculation of the mass number. An **ion** is an atom that has gained or lost electrons, while an **isotope** has a different number of neutrons in its nucleus than usual. For a given isotope, the half-life can be calculated my multiplying $ln(2)$, or 0.693, by the number of atoms and dividing by the number of decays. Put more simply, based on first order kinetics, the half-life is equivalent to $ln(2)$, or 0.693, divided by the rate **constant**.

On the periodic table, columns are called **groups**, and rows are called **periods**. With a focus on the main groups (namely, all but the transition metals), elements within the same group have the same number of **valence electrons**, the outer electrons that are involved in chemical bonding. When atoms bond, they generally aim to generate an **octet** (8) of valence electrons. This is often done by sharing electrons between nonmetals (**covalent bonding**), transferring electrons from a nonmetal to a metal (**ionic bonding**), and sharing delocalized electrons among metals (**metallic bonding**). **Alloys** are metals made by combining two or more metallic elements, particularly to allow for greater resistance to corrosion. Bronze, for example, is an alloy of copper and tin.

On the periodic table, a number of periodic trends can be observed. From left to right across the periodic table, and up a group, ionization energy and electron affinity increase. **Ionization energy** is the energy needed to remove an electron from an atom, while **electron affinity** is the affinity an atom has to take on additional electrons. **Atomic radius** decreases from left to right across the periodic table because nuclear charge increases without adding additional energy levels; atomic radius increases moving down a group due to increased numbers of energy levels. **Metallic character** increases from the top right to the bottom left of the periodic table, while **nonmetallic character** increases in the opposite direction. **Electronegativity** is a measure of the tendency of an atom to attract a bonding pair of electrons. In general, electronegativity increases from left to right across the periodic table, and from bottom to top of the periodic table. Fluorine is the most electronegative element.

A compound made of nonmetals only is a **molecular compound**, while a compound made of a metal and a nonmetal is an **ionic salt**. In a molecular compound, like ozone (O_3), there are only covalent bonds. In an ionic salt, the negatively charged ion that donates electrons is called an **anion**, while the positively charged ion that receives electrons is called a **cation**. Within a compound of any type, the **molecular mass** of a compound is the sum of masses of its elements, and the **percent composition** of a particular element can be determined by dividing the mass contributed by that element alone by the total molecular mass of the compound. The **law of multiple proportions** states that when two elements combine with one another to form multiple compounds, the masses of an element that combine with a fixed mass of another do so in a ratio of small whole numbers. The **law of definite composition** states that a particular compound is always composed of the same proportions of elements by mass.

A molecule is **polar** if it exhibits a separation of charge, while a molecule is **nonpolar** if it is symmetrical or shows a uniform charge distribution. Some bonds are stronger than others. A bond with a significant electronegativity difference between the two involved atoms is more polar than a bond with a smaller electronegativity difference between the two involved atoms. Bond length and bond strength are related. As bond length increases, bond strength decreases, and vice versa.

Despite its name, **hydrogen bonds** are intermolecular forces rather than true bonds. Hydrogen bonds occur between hydrogen atoms on one molecule (or part of a molecule) and electronegative atoms (like N or O) on another molecule (or part of a molecule). Hydrogen bonds are important in holding together amino acid structures together in proteins and complementary nucleotide base pairs in nucleic acids (like DNA).

Reactivity

A particular substance can have **physical** or **chemical** properties. Physical properties are properties of a substance that can be observed without changing its composition, while **chemical properties** involve reactivity and changing the identity of the compound. Color of a substance, for example, is a physical property, while corrosiveness is a chemical property.

Fractional distillation is a technique, often used in organic chemistry, that separates components of a liquid mixture based on the physical properties of its components, namely their boiling points. When a liquid mixture is heated, the component with the lowest boiling point vaporizes first and is re-condensed back into liquid in a separate container. The component with the next highest boiling point is vaporized next, re-condensed, and collected, and so on until all components are separated.

Chemical reactions can be classified in a number of ways. **Synthesis** reactions involve two or more compounds combining to form one compound, while **decomposition** reactions involve one compound breaking apart into two or more compounds. **Single displacement** reactions occur when an element reacts with a compound and takes the place of another element in that compound, while **double displacement** reactions occur when two ionic compounds react and exchange cations and anions. In **acid-base** reactions, acids and bases react to form a more neutral product solution. In **reduction-oxidation (redox)** reactions, one molecule gains electrons and is **reduced**, while another molecule loses electrons and is **oxidized**.

To determine if a redox reaction has taken place, the **oxidation numbers** of the involved elements must be determined. The oxidation number of a free element is always zero, and the oxidation number of a monatomic ion always equals the charge of the ion. The oxidation number of H is +1, but it is -1 in when combined with less electronegative elements, and for other main-group metals, the oxidation number is generally equivalent to its group number. The sum of oxidation numbers in a neutral compound is zero.

In any chemical reaction, specific numbers of molecules react. The molecules that go into a reaction are called **reactants**, and the resulting output molecules are called **products**. Within compounds, **subscripts** denote the numbers of atoms, while **coefficients** indicate relative numbers of compounds that react in a given chemical reaction. In particular, the coefficients represent the numbers of moles of involved compounds; one **mole** of a particular compound is equivalent to 6.022×10^{23} molecules of that compound. If two (or more) reactants are mixed in quantities that do not match up with the coefficient ratio indicated in the chemical reaction, one reactant will be used up first. The reactant that is used up first is the **limiting reagent**, while the one that is leftover is the **excess reagent**.

Some chemical reactions are **reversible**; that is, they can proceed in both the forward and backward directions. The balanced dynamic of a reversible reaction is referred to as **equilibrium**. **LeChatelier's principle** describes how reversible reactions adjust to maintain equilibrium. For example, if extra compound on the right side of a reversible equation is added to a system, the equilibrium will shift to the left to compensate for the excess. If the temperature of an equilibrium is decreased, for instance, the equilibrium will shift in the direction that produces heat. A reaction that produces heat is **exothermic**, while a reaction that takes in heat is **endothermic**.

The change in heat of a system can be described by the equation $\Delta Q = mc\Delta T$, where Q represents heat flow, m represents mass, c represents the **specific heat capacity**, and ΔT represents the temperature change of the system. The specific heat of a substance is the heat needed to raise the temperature of a gram of a substance by 1°C. If the mass of a substance and its specific heat capacity in a process are known, along with the difference between the final and initial temperatures of the system, the change in heat for the process can be calculated.

Gas-forming reactions make up a special class of chemical reactions. For example, when a strong acid reacts with a carbonate or bicarbonate, a salt, carbon dioxide, and water are produced. The reaction of a strong acid with a sulfide evolves H_2S gas, while the reaction of a strong acid with a sulfite or bisulfite evolves SO_2 gas. Finally, the reaction of a strong base with an ammonium compound evolves ammonia. Hydrogen gas is evolved along with an ionic salt when a strong acid reacts with solid metal. This is a redox reaction because the acid oxidizes the metal.

Reactivity in molecular compounds is often determined by **functional groups**, groups of atoms that are bonded in very specific ways. Examples of functional groups include hydroxides (ROH), esters ($R_1C=OOR_2$), ketones ($R_1C=OR_2$), and aldehydes (RC=OH). A benzene ring is an **aromatic** functional group; the term *aromatic* describes a planar, unsaturated ring of atoms often stabilized by **conjugated** (alternating) double bonds.

Ideal Gases and Solutions

The four fundamental states of matter are solid, liquid, gas, and plasma.

Gas is a state of matter that has no fixed volume or fixed shape. Gases can be analyzed using the **ideal gas law**. In order to apply this law, several assumptions must be made in order to treat a gas as an ideal gas. An ideal gas by definition consists of many identical molecules that have a **point-mass**; that is, the volume they occupy is negligible but they have mass. Additional, ideal gas molecules move in random motion, and collisions between molecules are **perfectly elastic**; that is, energy transfer is perfect and complete, with no losses.

The ideal gas law summarizes the behavior of an ideal gas, describing the relationship of pressure (P), volume (V), number of moles (n), and temperature (T). R represents the ideal gas constant, which can have different values based on units. Widely used values include 8.31 J/mol-K and 0.0821 L-atm/mol-K. If all but one of the variables in the ideal gas law are known, the last remaining variable can be calculated.

There are a number of simpler laws that can be derived from the ideal gas law. **Avogadro's law** states that the volume of a gas is directly proportional to the number of moles. **Boyle's law** states that the volume of a gas is inversely proportional to its pressure. **Charles' law** states that the volume of a gas is directly proportional to its temperature. These simpler laws can be applied when all conditions remain the same except for the two involved in each law.

Solutions also have their own sets of rules. A **solution** is, by definition, a liquid mixture in which the **solute** (minor component) is dissolved within the **solvent** (major component). Solutions involving water as the solute are **aqueous**. A solution in which the amount of dissolved solute is lower than the capacity the solvent can handle is described as **unsaturated**. A solution in which the amount of dissolved solute is equivalent to the capacity the solvent can handle is described as **saturated**. A solution in which the amount of dissolved solute is higher than the capacity the solvent can handle is described as **supersaturated**.

Biochemistry

The four classes of biomolecules are carbohydrates, lipids, nucleic acids, and proteins. These biological molecules provide the building blocks of life, making up cells and the important molecules within cells.

Carbohydrates serve as the major energy source for most cells, and they are critical in the synthesis of lipids and proteins. The three key elements that make up carbohydrates are carbon, hydrogen, and oxygen, which are actually the three elements that comprise nearly 99% of the human body. Carbohydrates have the general empirical formula of $(CH_2O)_n$. In general, carbohydrates consist of a set of carbons arranged in a linear or ring structure, with a number of hydroxyl (-OH), keto (-[C=O]-), or aldehyde (-[CH=O)] groups attached to them. **Monosaccharides** are simple sugars and represent the monomer of carbohydrates, linked together via **glycosidic bonds**. Carbohydrates distinctively end in the suffix *-ose*.

Glucose is a well-known example of a monosaccharide, a hexose, and has the chemical formula $C_6H_{12}O_6$. Note that this formula corresponds with the empirical formula noted in the previous paragraph. While glucose can take on a number of three-dimensional forms called **stereoisomers**, the one that exists in nature is called D-glucose. Glucose is critical to the function of cells because it is the major input carbohydrate for cellular respiration, the process by which cells aerobically use oxygen to produce significant quantities of ATP, or cellular energy.

Lipids cover a wide expanse of molecules that include waxes, oils, phospholipids, triglycerides, and fatty acids. In general, they are important for energy storage, cell signaling, and cell membrane structure, as well as hormone regulation. Many lipids can be acquired from one's diet, but some lipids can only be made in the cell. Lipids are formed via fatty acid synthesis, the elongation of hydrocarbon chains that end with a carboxylic acid termination group. A **saturated** fatty acid consists of a hydrocarbon chain consisting entirely of single bonds, while an **unsaturated** fatty acid has at least one double bond that causes a "kink" in the chain. During fatty acid synthesis, NADPH is used as an energy source to polymerize fatty acid chains. The hydrocarbon chains within lipids represent nonpolar regions, while carbonyl and charged portions of lipids represent polar regions.

The three main classes of lipids are triglycerides, steroids, and phospholipids. **Triglycerides** consist of a glycerol head group with three attached fatty acids. **Steroids** tend to be hydrophobic and insoluble in water. Examples of steroids are cholesterol and testosterone. **Phospholipids** consist of a polar head group and a number of fatty acid tails. These tend to have both hydrophobic and hydrophilic parts, and these are the lipids found in membranes. The central portion of a membrane bilayer is hydrophobic due to the presence of the hydrophobic tails interacting with one another, while the head groups that face water and the surrounding solution are hydrophilic. An **ester bond** is the bond between a head group and a fatty acid in a lipid.

DNA and RNA represent nucleic acids, which store genetic information. The monomer of a nucleic acid is the **nucleotide**, which consists of three parts: a nitrogenase base, a pentose sugar, and a phosphate group. Nucleotides are connected via phosphodiester bonds, which can again form via condensation reactions.

DNA and RNA have a number of similarities and differences. Deoxyribonucleic acid (DNA) and ribonucleic acid (RNA) are named for their pentose sugars, which are deoxyribose and ribose, respectively. DNA and RNA both consist of nucleotides, and nearly the same ones—the nucleotides of DNA are adenine (A), cytosine (C), guanine (G), and thymine (T), while those of RNA are adenine (A), cytosine (C), guanine (G), and uracil (U). DNA takes on the structure of a double helix and is consequently double-stranded. The two strands of DNA are held together by hydrogen bonds between bases; the sugar and phosphate groups make up the backbone of each strand, with the bases centrally holding the strands together. Within DNA, C and G pair up, and A and T pair up. That means that in DNA, for every C in one strand, there is a G in the opposite strand. The same goes for A and T, and vice versa for each. RNA, on the other hand, is single-stranded, but if RNA pairs up with DNA or another nucleic acid, the same pairings happen, with U in place of T.

Among the nitrogenous bases in nucleic acids, the five can be categorized as purines or pyrimidines. Purines have two rings in their structure, while pyrimidines only have one ring in their structure. Purines and pyrimidines always pair up with one another, keeping the stands of DNA (or in some cases, RNA) consistently far apart.

Proteins have a vast array of functions. Proteins play both structural and functional roles in the cell. Hemoglobin, for example, is found in the blood and binds oxygen, allowing for its circulation and subsequent use throughout the body. Actin and myosin are key players in muscle contraction. Antibodies are produced by the immune system to target antigens. Many proteins are **enzymes**, which catalyze chemical reactions by lowering the **activation energy** required to get the reaction started, converting **substrates** to **products**. Enzymes are almost exclusively proteins, though ribozyme is a ribonucleic acid that acts as an enzyme to catalyze specific reactions.

The monomer of a protein is the **amino acid**. An amino acid consists of a central carbon surrounded by four main functional groups: a simple hydrogen atom, a carboxylic acid group (-COOH), an amino group ($-NH_2$), and a variable R group. There are twenty naturally occurring amino acids that have unique R groups. R groups can be polar or nonpolar, charged or uncharged, small or large—this variety allows for a wide array of different kinds of proteins to be formed. The type of bond that forms between amino acids is called the **peptide bond**, forming between the carboxyl group of one amino acid and the amino group of the next amino acid. Proteins fold by a variety of mechanisms, but the way proteins fold is extremely important to their function. Much of protein folding is directed by the **hydrophobic effect**, which indicates that hydrophobic molecules tend to interact with each other rather than with water. As a result, many of the hydrophobic amino acids in a protein will tend toward the inside of the protein, avoiding contact as much as possible with the surrounding solution. On the other hand, hydrophilic amino acids are more likely to be found on the external surface of a protein because they favorably interact with water.

Proteins can be finicky with regard to the types of conditions in which they can survive. **Buffers** can help to resist changes in the pH of solutions to ensure that proteins are maintained at favorable, functional pH levels. Dramatic pH increases or decreases can result in the unfolding of a protein and the loss of its function; this is called **denaturation**. Denaturation can also result from changes in temperature, particularly a dramatic increase in temperature. Hot temperatures can weaken the intramolecular forces holding proteins together, which could then result in the unfolding of the protein and the loss of function. Other chemicals can destroy protein function by influencing the way they fold or by chemically changing the functional groups found within the structure of the proteins.

Catalysts speed up chemical reactions by lowering activation energy input required to make the reactions happen, and protein catalysts are called **enzymes**, which have specific inputs (**substrates**) and outputs (**products**).

Acids and Bases

Buffers regulate **pH**, an indication of the hydrogen ion concentration in a solution. An acidic solution has a high concentration of hydrogen ions, while a basic solution has a low concentration of hydrogen ions. Acids have pHs below 7, while bases have pHs above 7. A strong acid or base dissociates 100% into its ions, while a weak acid or base does not dissociate 100%. To calculate the pH of a particular solution, one simply uses the equation pH = $-\log[H^+]$.

Acids and bases can be further broken down into subcategories. The first subcategory is Arrhenius acids and bases. An Arrhenius acid is a molecule that donates an H^+ when dissolved in water, or a proton donor. An example is HCl. An Arrhenius base is a molecule that donates an OH^- when dissolved in water. An example is NaOH. The Arrhenius definitions of acids and bases are rather widely used, but they apply only to solutions in water. The second subcategory is Bronsted-Lowry acids and bases. Bronsted-Lowry acids are also proton donors, but the key difference here is that the solution does not have to be water. Bronsted-Lowry base are proton acceptors, extending the definition beyond molecules that contribute hydroxides to the solution. If ammonia (NH_3) mixes with nitric acid (HNO_3) to form ammonium (NH_4^+) and nitrate (NO_3^-) in solution, ammonia is the Bronsted-Lowry base and nitric acid is the Bronsted-Lowry acid. That also means that ammonium is the **conjugate acid** to ammonia, and that nitrate is the **conjugate** base to nitric acid. Finally, the last subcategory is Lewis acids and bases. Lewis acids are simply electron pair acceptors, while Lewis bases are electron pair donors. These are most relevant in organic chemistry. For example, in a halogenation reaction, a chloride ion might act as a Lewis base if it attacks the boron in boron trihydride (BH_3) to form a complex, making BH_3 the Lewis acid.

Acid-base titrations can be used to quantify the concentration of an unknown acid or base by neutralizing it with a standard base or acid solution of known concentration. To track progress along the way, a pH indicator is used. Once an appropriate amount of the standard is added to reach a neutral pH, the number of moles of the standard added can be calculated based on the volume added and the concentration of the standard. This number of moles can then be divided by the volume of the unknown solution to determine its concentration.

PHYSICS

Motion of Objects

There are two main types of motion: **linear** (in a straight line) and **circular**. The properties that can influence motion can be **scalar**, meaning only one number is involved, or **vector**, which have multiple influences. Mass, for example, is scalar.

Energy, Force, and Work

Kinetic energy is the energy of motion—there cannot be motion without energy. **Potential energy** is energy waiting to turn into kinetic energy, like a coiled spring. If the spring is released, its potential energy becomes kinetic energy as the spring expands.

There are many influences on motion. Anything that causes an object's motion to change (e.g., speeding it up, slowing it down, changing direction, etc.) is **force**. A commonly discussed force in physics is **gravity**, which attracts a body toward the center of any object with mass. In most cases, a body, such as a planet, needs a lot of mass in order to have a noticeable effect. There is also **work**, a scalar property that is the change in energy of an object resulting from a force. The two concepts are related but different; force *causes* work.

An object's **speed** (scalar) is the distance covered by an object in a set time. Similarly, **velocity** is an object's speed and its direction, making it a vector quantity. **Acceleration** is the rate at which velocity changes over time, so it is also a vector. If the rate decreases, acceleration is negative. Force influences acceleration, speed, and velocity; the stronger the force acting on an object, typically the greater its velocity and acceleration. If you know the distance a mass travels and its velocity, you can calculate acceleration using the following formula:

$$a = \frac{\text{distance/time}}{\text{time}} = \frac{\text{distance}}{\text{time}^2}$$

Force can be calculated using the formula $F = MA$.

Pay attention to units. Force is measured in Newtons (N), or the force required to accelerate a Mass of 1kg to 1m/s. Acceleration units are m/s². **Standard gravitational acceleration**, also known as **standard gravity** (g_n), is a constant value defined by 9.806 m/s₂. Standard gravity is the same regardless of the mass of an object *in a vacuum*, so a 100-pound brick accelerates toward the earth at the same rate as a half-pound golf ball. Outside a vacuum, forces such as friction or resistance (see below) will act on a falling object. Under those circumstances, the size or shape of a falling object may make a big impact.

Momentum is any object with mass in motion, so if an object in motion has mass, then it also has momentum. Momentum is related to mass and velocity; the more mass and velocity an object has, the more momentum it has, and the more force required to counteract that momentum and stop its motion. A related term is **inertia**, which means "resistance to changes in motion." Inertia forces objects in motion to try to keep moving.

Other forces counteract motion. **Wind resistance**, or **drag**, is the force of air acting against an object. As an object passes through air, air pushes against it, countering forward motion. Similarly, **friction** is the force that results when one object passes over (or through) another object or substance. The rubbing of the two objects creates resistance, which impedes motion. For example, a child's slide is made of smooth metal to reduce friction, allowing for faster sliding. Friction would prevent movement down the slide if the same slide were made of thick wool. When one object moves over another, there is pressure; the ratio of the force needed to move one of the objects over the other to that pressure is called the **coefficient of friction**.

Motion isn't always in a straight line. **Centripetal force** is the net force that acts on an object moving in a curved or circular path that is directed toward the center of the circular path. The opposite is **centrifugal force**, the apparent force which pulls outward on an object moving on a curve, trying to force it to go straight despite the curve. Without a seatbelt, centrifugal force would fling riders of a spinning amusement park ride out into space. **Rotational force**, or **torque**, rotates an object around an axis.

Electricity is the energy that results from charged particles. Like any energy, it can be used to do work. Outside of solution, electrons are the main charge carriers (in solution, charges are carried by ions. Recall that electrons are negatively charged particles (protons have a positive charge). Also remember that opposite charges attract each other, so, for example, electrons will attract protons, but repel other electrons.

These charged particles, generating electrical energy, will all move at light speed in a particular direction; the path they follow is called a **circuit**. The charged particles begin at a **source** (e.g., a battery in a cell phone). The source has a negatively charged end called the **cathode**, and a positive end called the **anode**. The cathode attracts positively charged particles (protons) and is the source of the electrons in a circuit. It's counterintuitive, but even though the main moving particles in a circuit are the electrons, the direction of a current is defined as the direction a positive charge would actually move in the circuit. So current flow is measured in the direction of the anode to the cathode.

An interesting source for electricity is static electricity, a charge imbalance on the surface of a material. The static charge will stay put in the material until it is discharged when the charge is neutralized by contact with another charge; e.g., when a person scuffing a carpet touches a metal doorknob. Light can also be used to generate electricity; certain materials, when struck by light, force electrons to move through a circuit instead of just moving in place (heating up).

From the source, electricity moves through a **conductor** (wires in the cell phone) to the **load** (functions of the cell phone). Water is an excellent conductor, which is why electricity is dangerous near water. The load is a component of the circuit that consumes power. A **switch** or breaker is something that interrupts a circuit; it is usually a small component that will connect or break the conductor, turning the circuit on or off. A switch is like a drawbridge across a wire. Anything that impedes electrical current is an **insulator**, like the rubber sheathing around many wires.

The rate at which the electricity flows (charge/time) is called the **current**, which is measured in amperes (A) and symbolized by I or i. Think of current as the volume of electricity moving through a circuit. Voltage, measured in volts and symbolized by V or E, is the measure of potential energy of charged objects. Another key aspect of circuits is **resistance** (opposite is **conductance**), symbolized by R, which is electrical friction, or opposition to an electrical current. Resistance is measured in ohms (Ω).

Resistance can be caused by the material through which a circuit passes, or by the volume of material; a rubber wire will have much more resistance than a highly conductive copper wire. Resistance also increases with length of the conductor, but decreases with width (cross sectional area).

In a circuit, resistance (R), current (I), or voltage (V) can all be calculated using

Ohm's law: $I = \dfrac{V}{R}$.

You should be familiar with a circuit diagram, or a schematic drawing of a circuit:

Resistors are any component that adds resistance to a circuit. A **series circuit** has resistors arranged in a row, or chain, one after the other (e.g., a string of holiday lights). In a series circuit, **total resistance** (**equivalent resistance** in a series circuit) is the sum of the resistance provided by each resistor or $R_{eq} = R_1 + R_2 + \ldots\ldots + R_N$.

The other major circuit type is a **parallel circuit**, where each resistor is on a separate branch of the circuit. In parallel circuits, $R_{eq} = (1/ R_1) + (1/ R_2) + \ldots + (1/ R_n)$.

Optics

Properties of Light

Light is a type of energy that exists either as a wave or a particle. A light particle is called a **photon**, but light also exists as an electromagnetic **wave**. A light wave is like an unbroken stream of light. Light also has **intensity**, which is the rate at which a light wave delivers energy to a fixed area.

When light bounces off an object back toward the observer, as in a mirror, it is called a **reflection**. Cameras have an internal mirror, but the eyepiece rights the image for you. Light that hits a reflective surface will bounce back at exactly the same angle. If you look in a mirror, the light from that person is heading toward the mirror. If you could watch from inside the mirror, you could see your own face exactly as it appears. However, what you really see is exactly the same light, but coming at you from a reverse direction. That is why mirror images are reversed. A reflective surface must be smooth, or else it will scatter the light into many directions, diffusing the image rather than forming a reflection. When the light does not scatter or reflect, it is absorbed. A black cloth will absorb more light than a white cloth will.

Light passes through transparent materials, such as windows. Sometimes, the light goes through directly with no changes. **Refraction** occurs when light bends as it is passing through a material. Water is refractory; objects under water are slightly offset from their real position. **Lenses**, or curved pieces of transparent material, also bend or focus light. **Convex** lenses are curved outward and bend light inward; **concave** lenses are curved inward and reflect light outward. Magnifying lenses (and the surface of water) are convex.

The Electromagnetic (EM) Spectrum

Why are some types of light different from others? If you could look at light from the side, it would look like a row of uniform hills. Light as a wave acts like a wave and oscillates up and down in an endlessly repeating pattern. The distance between the peaks, which is always the same in a given light wave, is called the **wavelength**, depicted by the Greek letter lambda (λ), and is measured in nanometers (nm). The number of peaks in a fixed time is the **frequency**.

The wavelength and frequency of a light wave determine its nature. The complete collection of all wavelengths of electromagnetic radiation are the **electromagnetic** or **EM spectrum**. Humans can see light only from 390 nm to 700 nm; this is called the **visible spectrum**. The visible spectrum is also known as white light, since humans see all colors of light simultaneously, not each color separately. Different colored objects absorb some colors of light but reflect the others; this is why we see objects as different colors. A **prism** can separate white light into its component colors. Frequencies lower than the visible spectrum are ultraviolet light; infrared frequencies are higher.

A form of energy that often accompanies light (and vice versa) is heat, or thermal energy caused by the movement of atoms. As molecular movement increases, thermal energy increases in whatever is heating up, or cooling down as movement decreases. **Heat** (that you feel) or **heat transfer**, is the transfer of thermal energy from an area of greater thermal energy to an area of less. A hot pie left to cool is transferring thermal energy into the air around it; in other words, the air feels warm around the pie. Heat and thermal energy are similar. In **combustion**, fuel and oxygen have a rapid reaction that produces a lot of heat and light-fire.

Temperature is the unit of measurement of thermal energy. There are a variety of temperature scales, most based on the difference between the freezing and boiling points of water. The Celsius scale sets the freezing point of water at 0° and the boiling point at 100°. Fahrenheit sets the freezing point of water at 32° and the boiling point at 212°; 0° Fahrenheit is based on the freezing point of a brine solution. In the Kelvin scale (used mostly by scientists), 0 K is **absolute zero**, the point at which all molecular motion stops and there is no thermal energy at all. Since temperature is a unit of measurement, a higher temperature is measuring more thermal energy. Instruments such as thermometers are measuring temperature, but not thermal energy itself.

A related concept is **specific heat** (denoted by c), which is the energy required to raise a specified mass of a material 1°C. Specific heat is an inherent property of a material, not a type of radiation.

Specific heat can be calculated based on the added heat (Q) with the formula $Q = cM\Delta T$, where c is specific heat, M is the mass being heated, and ΔT is the change in temperature.

Heat is transferred by three different methods. In **conduction**, the molecules of an object with more thermal energy collide directly with the molecules in another object, making that object warmer. A metal spoon in a hot liquid is an example.

In **convection,** thermal energy moves upward, forcing molecules to move farther apart and decrease in density as they do so. Heat rises for this reason; when you see birds circling on updrafts, they are riding convection currents. As the hotter molecules move upward, the cooler, denser molecules move downward, until eventually, all the molecules in the affected area are the same temperature. At that point of even temperature, the sample is in **thermal equilibrium**.

Radiation is heat transfer through electromagnetic waves. Radiation can occur without any intermediate material or particles; there is no need for direct contact as in conduction or convection. For example, the sun's light and heat come straight to Earth with nothing in between.

Insulation blocks or limits heat transfer through a material or barrier that does not easily conduct heat, such as a mitten. The mitten prevents heat transfer from the wearer's hand to the environment.

Volume is the amount of space occupied by an object or sample of material. How to determine the volume of a sample will depend on its shape. Liquids and gases have no fixed shape; they have the same volume as the container they occupy. Solids don't have to fill a container, but their volume is still shape dependent. For example, the volume of a cube is side × side × side, or length $(l)^3$.

A square rock, for example, that is 2 m high × 2 m wide × 2 m deep has a volume of 8 cm³. The volume of a sphere is $\frac{4}{3}\pi r^3$, where r is the radius of the sphere.

Objects expand as their thermal energy increases, so most substances increase in volume as their temperature increases. A notable exception is water, which expands into ice as it cools.

Volume can also be relative to other properties, such as mass or other substances. For example, when an object is completely submerged in a fluid, the object and the fluid can't both occupy exactly the same space at the same time, so an equal volume of fluid must be displaced to make room for the submerged object. However, when an object is buoyant, or floats, unless it is floating exactly on the liquid's surface it will displace some of the liquid but not an amount equal to the volume of the buoyant object.

Archimedes' principle, which states that an object is buoyed by a force equal to the weight of the fluid that the object displaces. So from $F = MA$, F and A are equal, so M, mass, must be equal as well. If an object sinks, then its mass is greater than the mass of the water being displaced. The full equation for calculating the mass of displaced fluid is

$$W = pVg$$

where p is the density of the liquid being displaced (1g/mL, if its water), V is the volume of displaced liquid, and g is gravitational acceleration.

In practice, if you know the mass of the displacing object, you won't need this formula, thanks to Archimedes' principle.

Related to volume is **pressure**, or force exerted per unit area. Everything has pressure. All around us is air pressure, or the pressure of air on a surface. Air pressure decreases with altitude, so it is highest at sea level. The atmosphere thins as altitude increases, so there are fewer molecules of air to exert any force. A **barometer** is an instrument that measures the air pressure on a container of mercury; higher pressure causes the mercury level to rise, and lower pressure causes it to fall. The standard **atmospheric pressure** at sea level is 14.7 psi (pounds per square inch), or 29.2 inches of mercury. When calculating air pressure, air can be treated as fluid using the formula.

Changes in air pressure are associated with changes in the weather. Highs, or high-pressure areas, are generally clear and nice; storms are created by low-pressure systems. Air moving down a pressure gradient is a local source of wind. Water pressure is exerted opposite that of air pressure. At sea level, the pressure is at its lowest; in the ocean, the pressure increases with depth as there is more water above an object, pressing down with greater force.

Pressure also applies to moving gases or fluids, and it is connected to both the force with which the fluid is being forced through an area as well as the volume of that area. Water being pumped with equal velocity will be under greater pressure when forced through a narrow pipe as opposed to a very wide pipe.

Pressure, especially pressure gradients, can have serious consequences. Pressure differences can be beneficial; for example, an airplane can fly because the pressure above the wing is lower than the pressure below. However, a very large difference in air pressure, such as the extremely low pressure inside a tornado, can destroy structures as air pressure forcefully equalizes. When there is no air pressure at all, a vacuum exists. Gases or fluids under high pressure will move into areas of low pressure; a big enough change can result in considerable destruction. The hulls of ships and submarines must be very strong to resist water pressure pushing inwards. Certain shapes, such as spheres, tend to be more pressure resistant as they disperse the force around the curve.

SCIENCE GLOSSARY

A

absolute zero
The lowest known temperature possible, where all molecular motion nearly ceases.
Fahrenheit Scale—approximately -460°F (actual -459.67°F)
Celsius Scale—approximately -273°C (actual -273.15°C)
Kelvin Scale 0°K

absorption
The movement of water and/or dissolved substances into a cell, tissue, or organism.

acceleration
A change in the speed of an object. If the object speeds up, it is called *positive acceleration*. If the object slows down, it is called *negative acceleration*.

acid
A compound with a pH less than 7, which means that it releases hydrogen ions when dissolved in water. An acid changes blue litmus paper to red and tastes sour.

acquired immunity
Immunity that is not natural or congenital; obtained after birth.

active immunity
Immunity brought about by activity of certain cells of the body as a result of being exposed to an antigen.

active transport
An energy-requiring process by means of which materials are moved across a cell membrane.

adsorption
The gathering of molecules of a substance on a surface.

aerobe
Any organism living in the presence of and utilizing free, molecular oxygen (that is, oxygen not in chemical combination) in its oxidative processes.

alchemy
The science of transforming less valuable metals into gold or silver, and the philosophy behind this idea. The theories of the alchemists of the Middle Ages were false, but their experiments laid the foundation for modern chemistry.

alkali
A compound, when dissolved in water, with a pH greater than 7. An alkaline substance changes red litmus paper to blue, and it can combine with hydrogen ions of acids. *See* BASE.

alkaline
A substance having the properties of an ALKALI.

allantois

One of four extraembryonic membranes attached to the body of the embryo or fetus of a land-dwelling vertebrate. In humans, it is modified to form part of the placenta and umbilicus.

amino acid

An organic molecule containing an amino group (NH_2) and a carboxyl group (COOH) bonded to the same carbon atom; the "building blocks" of proteins. There are 20 amino acids that are used in metabolic processes.

amnion

The innermost of four extraembryonic membranes attached to the body of the embryo or fetus of a land-dwelling vertebrate. It forms a fluid-filled sac around the body that provides an aqueous environment (amniotic fluid) and cushions the embryo from shocks.

ampere

A measurement of electric current, abbreviated *amp*. It was named after French scientist ANDRÉ-MARIE AMPÈRE.

Ampère, André-Marie

A French scientist (1775–1836) whose work and theory laid the foundation for the André-Marie science of electrodynamics. His name lives on in the electrical measurement AMPERE.

amphipods

A crustacean group that includes sand fleas.

anaerobe

Any organism not requiring free, molecular oxygen (O_2) for its cellular oxidative processes. Some anaerobes are *obligate* and cannot survive in the presence of oxygen; others are *facultative* and can survive with or without oxygen.

anatomy

The study of the structure of living things. Usually refers to the structure of the human body.

anemone

A sea animal (a coelenterate) that resembles the flower of the same name.

antibiotic

A substance derived from lower organisms that can be used to prevent growth of certain pathogens, thus combating infection.

antibody

A specific type of protein molecule that is manufactured in the tissues, blood, or lymph in response to the presence of viruses or foreign cells. Each variety of antibody will attach to the surface of only one type of invader, enabling it to be recognized and marked for destruction by the immune system.

antigens

Protein molecules on the surface of viruses or foreign cells that provoke the manufacture of matching antibodies, enabling invaders to be recognized as such so they can be destroyed.

apolipoprotein

(apo E) A gene that codes for a protein that facilitates the transport of cholesterol and influences human longevity.

ATP

(adenosine triphosphate) The energy-transport compound of a cell which is produced in the mitochondria.

atrium

One of the two anterior chambers of the heart of vertebrates.

attenuated

The state of being weakened, as in the case of pathogens used to induce active immunity.

auricle

The projecting outer portion, or pinna, of the ear.

autotroph

An organism, such as a green plant, capable of manufacturing its food from inorganic environmental materials.

B

bacteria

Unicellular, microscopic, prokaryotic organisms, mostly saprotrophic or parasitic.

base

A compound, when dissolved in water, with a pH greater than 7 that can react with an acid to accept a hydrogen ion and form a salt. *See* ALKALI.

biochemistry

The study of the chemical makeup of organisms. This science is a branch of both chemistry and biology.

biology

The study of living things; a major science.

biome

A type of community recognized by certain characteristics of plants and climate, such as the plains of the Midwest United States, tropical rainforests, and arctic tundra.

bond

The force of attraction that holds 2 atoms together in a molecule. There are two major types of chemical bonds: COVALENT BONDS and IONIC BONDS.

botany

The study of plant life. Botany is a branch of BIOLOGY.

Brahe, Tycho

A Danish astronomer (1546–1601) who made a systematic study of the movement of celestial bodies. He is often referred to simply as *Tycho*.

C

carbohydrate

A food substance made up of carbon, hydrogen, and oxygen.

carbon

An important chemical element that forms the basic skeleton of all ORGANIC compounds. Atoms of other elements are bonded to the carbon skeleton to form the many different varieties of organic compounds.

carbon dioxide (CO_2)

A compound made up of 1 atom of carbon (C) and 2 atoms of oxygen (O). It exists in the form of a gas and is one of the principal waste byproducts resulting from CELLULAR RESPIRATION.

carcinogen

A cancer-causing substance that may be physical, chemical, biological, or radiological.

catalyst

A chemical substance that lowers the energy necessary for a chemical reaction to take place and makes the reaction proceed more rapidly. ENZYMES act as catalysts in living organisms. Catalysts do not become part of the end-product. They can be reused many times.

celestial

An adjective referring to the sky.

cell

The basic structural and functional unit of organisms.

cellular respiration

The oxidation of glucose into carbon dioxide and water (or into other products, in the case of anaerobic respiration), leading to the release of energy.

Celsius

A system of measurement of temperature, often referred to as *centigrade*. On the Celsius scale, the freezing point for water is 0 degrees and the boiling point is 100 degrees.

centriole

A cellular organelle characteristic of animal cells, but not plant cells, that migrates to the poles during mitosis; spindle fibers and astral rays arise from it.

centromere

The portion of the chromosome that holds the chromatids together and to which spindle fibers attach.

chelicerae

The pincer-like claw appendages in front of the mouth of arachnids and certain arthropods, such as spiders.

chemistry

The science that studies the composition and transformation of matter; a major science.

chlamydiae

Small intracellular obligate parasites closely related to the *Rickettsiae*.

chlorophylls
The green pigments of plants, produced in the presence of light and essential for photosynthesis.

chromosomes
Small cellular bodies containing tightly bound and packaged DNA that are formed during MITOSIS and MEIOSIS from loosely packaged DNA (chromatin). The hereditary determinants called GENES are coded on chromosomes.

colloid
A type of mixture intermediate between a SOLUTION and a SUSPENSION, consisting of liquid plus particles that are too small to settle out of the mixture and too large to dissolve. Colloids can exist in the form of a gel and pass through membranes either slowly or not at all.

commensalism
A symbiotic relationship in which one member is benefited, and the other member is neither benefited nor harmed.

compound
The combination of two or more elements into a single unit.

condensation
The transition of water vapor to liquid water due to a lowering of temperature.

conduction
The transfer of heat from one object or physical medium to another by direct contact.

conservation of energy
The principle that energy changes its form but cannot be created or destroyed.

conservation of matter
The principle that matter can change its form but cannot be created or destroyed.

constellation
A particular grouping of stars.

copepod
A small aquatic crustacean.

Copernicus, Nicholas
A Polish astronomer (1473–1543) who proposed the theory that the earth moves through space. It was generally believed up to that time that the earth was the immobile center of the universe.

cosmic year
The time it takes the sun to go around its galaxy. Also known as a *galactic year*.

covalent bond
A type of chemical bond created by the sharing of electrons between 2 atoms to achieve the maximum number of electrons in the outer electron orbit of each atom. Covalent bonds are the strongest type of chemical bonds.

crop rotation
An agricultural method by which crops in an area are changed each year, helping to maintain the fertility of the soil.

crustaceans

A group of aquatic animals with a hard outside covering. They are often included with MOLLUSKS in the group of "shellfish."

crystal

A form of solid in which the constituent atoms or molecules are arranged in a very regular, repeating pattern.

cytoplasm

In a prokaryotic cell, the entire contents of the cell contained within the plasma membrane. In a eukaryotic cell, the region of the cell lying within the plasma membrane but exterior to the nucleus.

D

Dalton, John

An English chemist and physicist (1766–1844) who introduced the theory that matter is composed of atoms.

Darwin, Charles

An English naturalist (1809–1883) who developed a THEORY OF EVOLUTION.

deforestation

The process by which land is cleared of forests. Excessive removal of forests for agriculture, development, mining, timber, and other human interests. If deforested areas remain barren, it can result in many negative ecological and environmental consequences, such as soil erosion and flooding.

density

Mass per unit volume, often expressed as grams per milliliter.

dictyosome

The *Golgi apparatus* of plant cells, which serves as a collecting and packaging center for secretions.

diffusion

The spontaneous movement of dissolved molecules from an area where they are in high concentration to an area where they are in lower concentration. This process requires no energy and, in living organisms, often takes place across semipermeable membranes.

distillation

The purification of a liquid substance by heating it until it vaporizes and then cooling it to cause it to condense into liquid again. Useful for separating and purifying liquids with different boiling points.

DNA

Deoxyribonucleic acid; a large, helical, double-stranded molecule in which the chromosomes code hereditary information.

dorso-ventral

An adjective referring to a back-to-front plane.

Down Syndrome

A genetic disorder of humans caused by the presence of an extra, third copy of chromosome 21. Individuals with Down Syndrome are intellectually disabled and possess characteristic physical features.

E

eclipse

The obscuring of a celestial body that takes place when one celestial object moves in front of another. When the moon comes between the earth and the sun, it casts a shadow, or *umbra*, on part of the earth. This is known as a *solar* eclipse, since during this time the sun cannot be seen on that part of the earth. When the earth comes between the sun and the moon, it casts a shadow on the moon. Since the moon cannot be seen during this time, this is called a *lunar* eclipse.

Einstein, Albert

A German physicist (1879–1955) who lived the last years of his life in the United States. His theories changed the field of PHYSICS. He, more than any other scientist, was responsible for nuclear fission.

electron

A negatively charged particle in the atom that moves in an orbit around the NUCLEUS of the atom.

electronics

The study of the motion or movement of free electrons and ions to power countless communication and entertainment devices.

electrophoresis

A biochemical technique used to separate organic molecules such as PROTEINS or NUCLEIC ACIDS out of a mixture. In the most commonly used version of the technique, a sample of the mixture is placed at one end of a slab-shaped gel immersed in a buffer solution. An electric current is passed through the chamber containing the gel, and molecules travel through the gel at different distances according to their size and electrical charge. Each type of molecule accumulates in its own distinct zone or band in the gel.

element

One of more than 118 known basic substances. These substances and their combinations make up all matter, as far as is known. A pure chemical substance composed of a single type of atom, distinguished by having the same number of protons and electrons.

embryology

The study of the development of organisms from the time of conception until birth.

energy

The capacity to do work.

enthalpy

The heat content of the reactants and products in a chemical reaction.

entropy

The concept that closed systems move to a state of maximum disorder unless energy enters from the surroundings.

enzyme

An organic CATALYST; specific types of proteins produced by cells that govern or otherwise affect all biological reactions. *Exoenzymes* act outside the cells that produce them, and *endoenzymes* act within the cells that produce them. Enzymes are sensitive to the pH and temperature of their environment, and deviations from the optimal pH and temperature for an enzyme will lessen its activity. The maintenance of optimal internal environments for enzymes is a major objective of HOMEOSTASIS.

erg

A unit of work or energy.

erythrocytes

Red blood cells.

eugenics

A science that deals with the improvement of hereditary qualities of a race or breed.

eukaryote

An organism characterized by cells containing a true or visible nucleus.

evaporation

The process by which liquids change to gases.

evolution, theory of

Usually refers to Darwin's theory that changes occur in populations because natural selection favors the survival of those organisms best fitted for their environment.

exergonic reaction

Downhill reaction, whose products have less energy than the reactant.

experiment

A test to see if an idea is true or false.

F

Fahrenheit

The system of measuring temperature as generally used in the United States was developed by Gabriel Fahrenheit (1686–1736), a German scientist. On the Fahrenheit scale, 32 degrees is the freezing point of water, 212 degrees is the boiling point of water, and 98.6 degrees is the average temperature of the human body. Another widely used temperature measurement is the CELSIUS scale.

Faraday, Michael

An English physicist and chemist (1791–1867) who developed the first dynamo (electric generator) and discovered that a magnet could induce an electric current in a conductor, such as metal.

fertility

The ability to reproduce. *See* REPRODUCTION.

force

That which stops, creates, or changes the velocity of motion.

friction

The resistance created to the movement of an object when it rubs against or collides with other objects.

fungi

A group of organisms, typically saprotrophic (or parasitic), many of which have a MYCELIUM. A few fungi, such as yeasts, do not have a mycelial body. *See* SAPROTROPH.

G

galaxy

A massive grouping of stars, often orbiting a central black hole. Astronomers estimate there are over 100 billion galaxies in the visible universe.

Galileo

An Italian astronomer and physicist (1564–1642) who made many contributions to science. He discovered that objects of different weights and shapes fall to the ground at the same rate of speed, attracted by GRAVITY. He was a strong believer in COPERNICUS' theory that the earth moved in space, and he was persecuted for this belief.

gene

A hereditary determinant consisting of a segment of a DNA molecule that contains the coded information necessary for assembling a specific type of protein molecule. Each gene occupies a fixed locus on a specific CHROMOSOME, enabling the transmission of hereditary determinants from one generation to the next.

genetic code

The sequence of NUCLEOTIDE bases in a molecule of DNA or RNA that, when translated by a RIBOSOME, specifies the sequence of AMINO ACIDS in a PROTEIN molecule.

genetic disorder

A metabolic disorder caused by inheritance of a damaged gene, a damaged chromosome, or an incorrect number of chromosomes. *See* DOWN SYNDROME, HEMOPHILIA, PHENYLKETONURIA, and SICKLE CELL ANEMIA.

genetics

The study of HEREDITY, or the manner in which hereditary traits are passed on from one generation to the next.

genome

The genetic makeup of an individual; the genotype.

geology

The study of the formation, structure, and history of the earth.

geriatrics

The science of the diseases of aged persons.

glycolysis

The anaerobic decomposition of a glucose into 2 molecules of pyruric acid, with the production of 2 net molecules of ATP.

Golgi

An organelle in animal and plant cells within which proteins from the endoplasmic reticulum are processed, modified, and secreted.

gravitation

The tendency of objects in space to move toward each other.

gravity

A fundamental force in nature. The force of attraction between two bodies where the strength of the force is proportional to the bodies' masses and distance between them.

greenhouse effect

The warming effect of the earth caused by an accumulation of carbon dioxide and other gases, such as methane, which are expelled from vehicles and industrial operations into the atmosphere. Heat is trapped under the layer of greenhouse gases and is attributed to causing global warming and climate change.

H

habitat

The immediate surroundings or environment in which a particular species may live.

half-life

The length of time required for the degradation to another substance of half the molecules in an amount of radioactive substance. The half-lives of radioactive ISOTOPES of elements can be used to date material containing radioactive substances. An example is the carbon-14 dating of living material.

Harvey, William

An English physician and anatomist (1578–1657) who discovered how the blood moves through the body.

heat

A measurable form of energy.

heat shock proteins

A protein that prevents the denaturation of other proteins when the temperature rises to abnormally high levels.

hemoglobin

A type of protein molecule that is bright red in color and binds reversibly to oxygen. It is carried within ERYTHROCYTES, enabling them to transport oxygen.

hemophilia
A GENETIC DISORDER caused by inheritance of a defective gene for one of the proteins that act as blood-clotting factors. The blood of affected persons fails to clot normally if an injury occurs, creating the danger that they might bleed to death from even minor wounds.

heredity
The transmission of traits from generation to generation.

homeostasis
The maintenance of internal balance by a living organism.

hormone
A chemical regulator of many bodily activities. A hormone is produced by an endocrine gland.

hydridoma
Recombinant (mixed) cells produced by the fusion of plasma cells and cancer cells.

hydrogen
The element with the smallest atom, consisting of one (1) proton and one (1) electron. It exists as a gas and is common in nature. Hydrogen is important to living organisms because it is a constituent of water and most organic compounds.

hypha
A mycelial thread; one of the "strands" making up a MYCELIUM, which is a fungus body.

hypothesis
An unproven explanation of something that has happened or might happen.

I

immunity
Resistance to a particular disease or condition. *See* ACQUIRED IMMUNITY, ACTIVE IMMUNITY, NATURAL IMMUNITY, and PASSIVE IMMUNITY.

immunization
The process of making one immune, usually by giving antigens to induce active immunity via the production of antibodies specific to that antigen.

immunoglobulins
Antibodies.

indicator
A substance whose color is sensitive to the hydrogen-ion concentration of the solution to which it is added.

inorganic
An adjective meaning "not organic" and generally applied to any atom other than carbon, or to a molecule not containing carbon. *See* ORGANIC.

insecticides
Natural or synthetic chemical compounds used to control insects.

interferon

An antiviral agent secreted by cells under attack from viruses.

interstellar

An adjective meaning "between stars."

ion

An atom or radical that has acquired a positive charge by giving up or losing electron(s), or a negative charge by gaining electron(s).

ionic bond

A type of chemical bond created when one atom gives up all its electrons to another atom to achieve the maximum number of electrons in the outer orbit of each atom. Ionic compounds will separate in water to yield IONS in a process called *dissociation*.

isotopes

Atoms that belong to the same chemical element, having the same number of protons and electrons, differing only in the number of neutrons and therefore atomic mass.

K

Kepler, Johannes

A German astronomer (1571–1630) who made important discoveries about the orbits of planets.

kinetic energy

Energy that is in motion. The energy of a boulder tumbling down a mountainside is an example of kinetic energy. *See* POTENTIAL ENERGY.

Koch, Robert

A German doctor (1843–1910) who studied bacteria. He and LOUIS PASTEUR are considered the founders of the science of bacteriology.

Krebs cycle

The aerobic breakdown of glucose, forming carbon dioxide, water, and ATP.

L

Lamarck, Chevalier de

A French naturalist (1744–1829) who developed a theory of evolution. *See* CHARLES DARWIN.

Lavoisier, Antoine

A French chemist (1743–1794) who made important discoveries concerning combustion, the conservation of matter, and the role of oxygen in respiration.

leukocytes

White blood cells that defend the body against bacteria, infectious diseases, and foreign bodies.

lever system

An assemblage of parts for moving weight with the least amount of applied force. A lever system consists of a rigid rod (*lever*) applied to the weight, a point of balance (*fulcrum*) for the lever, and mechanical force applied to the lever. These parts can be arranged in different ways to accommodate different amounts of weight, but a common principle of all lever systems is that the greatest amount of lifting force is achieved when the point at which the force is applied is farthest from the fulcrum.

light year
The distance light travels in one year. 9.46 trillion kilometers; 5.88 trillion miles.

Linnaeus, Carolus
A Swedish botanist (1707–1778) best known for developing a system of nomenclature for animals and plants.

lipopoly-saccharide
A polymer of simple sugars linked with fragments of lipid molecules.

litmus
An indicator used to test for pH, or hydrogen-ion concentration. Litmus is red in acid solutions and blue in basic solutions.

litmus paper
A special paper containing LITMUS, used by chemists to test for acid and alkali.

lunar
An adjective referring to the moon. A lunar eclipse is an eclipse of the moon.

lymph
A colorless fluid that has passed from the bloodstream through capillary walls into the intercellular spaces; lymph is collected by lymph ducts and returned to the bloodstream.

lysosomes
Cellular organelles that contain powerful hydrolytic enzymes.

M

mandible
The lower jaw bone of vertebrates; the mouth part of arthropods that resembles a jaw and functions in biting.

marine
An adjective meaning "of or relating to the sea."

mechanics
The study of the effects of force on moving or motionless bodies; a branch of PHYSICS.

meiosis
A type of cellular division that results in gametes (sex cells) or gametic nuclei. It consists of two divisions resulting in four daughter cells, and the number of chromosomes in each daughter is reduced by half (haploid).

membrane

A thin sheet forming a semipermeable boundary, as in (1) a thin layer of soft tissue; (2) the outer boundary of a cell (*see* PLASMA MEMBRANE); or (3) the enclosing boundary of an intracellular structure (for example, the nucleus).

Mendel, Gregor Johann

An Austrian monk and botanist (1822–1884) who made important discoveries concerning HEREDITY.

metabolism

The sum total of the cellular chemical processes that allow a cell to survive.

meteorology

A science that studies the weather and the atmosphere.

microscope

An instrument that produces a magnified image of an object. Light microscopes use a set of glass lenses to focus and magnify rays of light that either pass through or bounce off the object. Electron microscopes use magnetic lenses and beams of electrons to produce more sharply focused and highly magnified images than can be produced with a light microscope.

mineral

An INORGANIC substance that occurs naturally in rocks or soil. Minerals such as calcium, sodium, potassium, and zinc are used by living organisms in various metabolic processes. Calcium carbonate (limestone) is an example.

mitochondrion

The cellular organelle of EUKARYOTES in which cellular oxidation (*cellular respiration*) generates energy in the form of ATP.

mitosis

A type of cellular division that results in exact duplicates of the parent cell, as in asexual reproduction or growth. It consists of one division resulting in two daughter cells, and the number of chromosomes in each daughter is the same as in the parent (diploid).

molecule

A collection of atoms arranged in a specific manner; the smallest unit into which a compound can be divided, yet still retain its physical and chemical properties.

mollusks

Animals of the phylum *Mollusca*, characterized by a *mantle*, a *radula*, and a *muscular foot*. Some mollusks are aquatic, like the octopus, clam, and oyster. Others are terrestrial, like the snail and slug.

mutation

A stable and abrupt change in a gene, and thus in the trait the gene determines, that is transmitted from generation to generation.

mutualism

A symbiotic relationship of mutual benefit to its partners.

mycelium

A mass of fungal threads or hyphae, composing the fungus body.

N

natural immunity

Immunity or resistance to disease with which a person is born.

nebula

An intersteller gas cloud mostly composed of ionized hydrogen and helium atoms, primarily responsible for star formation.

nephron

A functional unit of the kidney, consisting of Bowman's capsule with its glomerulus, and the associated ducts and convoluted tubules, with their capillaries.

neutron

A small particle that is part of the atom and has no electrical charge. *See* ELECTRON and PROTON.

Newton, Isaac

An English mathematician and natural philosopher (1642–1727) who made major discoveries in astronomy and PHYSICS. His most important works were his study of GRAVITATION and OPTICS.

nonpolar compound

A substance in which the electromagnetic charge of each molecule is balanced so that there is no positively or negatively charged end to the molecule. Oils and fats are examples. *See* POLAR COMPOUND and SOLUBLE.

norepinephrine

A biogenic amine derivative of tyrosine that serves as a neurotransmitter in the central nervous system and the peripheral nervous system.

nuclear

An adjective referring to the NUCLEUS of an atom or cell.

nuclear fission

The splitting of an atom in order to produce energy and different atomic weight elements.

nuclear fusion

The joining together of lightweight atoms resulting in the release of energy.

nucleic acid

DNA and RNA; the nucleic acids code and transcribe information about heredity.

nucleolus

A separate area within the NUCLEUS in which RNA is synthesized.

nucleotide

The "building unit" of NUCLEIC ACIDS, consisting of a sugar (ribose or deoxyribose), a phosphate, and a base (a purine or a pyrimidine).

nucleus

The center core of an object, as (1) the center of an atom, containing protons and neutrons; or (2) the regulatory center of a cell of an organism.

O

observatory

A specially constructed building containing one or more telescopes for observation of the heavens.

ohm

A unit for measuring electrical resistance.

oncogene

A gene that has the potential to cause a normal cell to become cancerous.

optics

The study of light and its effects; a branch of PHYSICS.

orbit

The path of an object or particle around a body, such as the moon circling the earth, and an electron around an atomic nucleus.

organ

A structure consisting of several different types of TISSUE combined into a single unit. A single organ can perform one or more major functions and is usually linked with other organs to form a *system*.

organelle

An intracellular structure that performs a major function for the cell; the cellular equivalent of an organ.

organic

Characteristic of, pertaining to, or derived from organisms; an adjective referring to living things or organisms.

organism

A living thing, such as a human, a plant, or an animal.

osmosis

The movement of a solvent (such as water) through a semipermeable membrane.

oxidation

Any chemical reaction that results in a molecule losing an electron, losing a hydrogen atom, or gaining an oxygen atom.

oxide

A compound made of oxygen and another element.

P

parasitism

A symbiotic relationship in which one organism (*parasite*) lives on and at the expense of another (*host*).

passive immunity

(usually temporary) Imparted without the person's body acting in its immunity build-up; the immunity is imparted by the administration of foreign antibodies.

Pasteur, Louis

A French chemist (1822–1895) who made major discoveries in chemistry and biology, especially in the control of many diseases. He and ROBERT KOCH were the founders of the science of bacteriology.

pasteurization

The heating of milk, or some other liquid, to a certain temperature for a definite period of time to destroy certain pathogens without changing the flavor or quality of the beverage.

peptide bond

A chemical bond that joins two amino acids by connecting the carboxyl group of one amino acid and the amino group of the other.

peptidoglycan

A polymer of amino acids and sugars arranged in a mesh-like structure to form bacteria cell walls.

pH

A symbol used in expression of acidity or alkalinity. It denotes the negative logarithm of the concentration of hydrogen ions in gram atoms or moles per liter.

phagotroph

A heterotrophic organism that obtains its nutrients by ingesting solid organic matter; often refers to organisms that feed on other organisms by engulfing them to allow digestion and absorption to take place within the body.

phenylketonuria (PKU)

A GENETIC DISORDER caused by inheritance of a damaged gene for the enzyme that converts excess molecules of the AMINO ACID phenylalanine to the AMINO ACID tyrosine. High levels of phenylalanine and phenylketones, molecules intermediate between phenylalanine and tyrosine, accumulate in the blood of the affected person unless dietary intake of phenylalanine is severely restricted. Untreated PKU in infants results in severe brain damage and mental retardation.

physics

The study of matter and energy and their interactions.

phytogeographic map

A visual reference, illustration, or imagery of vegetarian and plant distribution in a given area.

Planck, Max
A German physicist (1858–1947) who did notable work in thermodynamics; the "father of quantum physics."

planet
A large body that moves around the sun or another star. Earth, Venus, Jupiter, Mars, Mercury, and Saturn are examples of planets.

plankton
A group of sea life—both plant and animal—that drifts with tides and currents.

plasma
The liquid portion of the blood in which proteins and other substances are dissolved. Also, a fourth state of matter.

plasma membrane
The cell membrane; the living covering of the cell.

plasmid
An extrachromosomal ring of DNA especially of bacteria that replicates autonomously .

plastids
Cellular organelles that are found in plant cells and may contain pigments. The types of plastids are (1) *chloroplasts,* which contain the chlorophyll and carotenoid pigments and which are green; (2) *chromoplasts,* which contain carotenoid pigments and range in color from yellow to brown; and (3) *gerodontoplasts,* which develop from chloroplasts in plants that are aging; (4) *leucoplasts,* which are colorless.

polar compound
A substance (for example, water) in which the electromagnetic charge of each molecule is unevenly distributed so that the molecule is positively charged on one end and negatively charged on the other end. *See* NONPOLAR COMPOUND and SOLUBLE.

polymerase chain reaction (PCR)
An *in-vitro* technique for the rapid reproduction of many copies of DNA segments.

potential energy
Energy that is available for use. The energy of a boulder balanced on a mountainside is an example of potential energy. It becomes KINETIC ENERGY when the boulder begins to roll.

precipitation
The settling out of particles suspended in liquid. Precipitation can be the result of a chemical reaction in which dissolved reactants form an insoluble product. Material that settles out of a suspension is a *precipitate.*

Priestley, Joseph
The English chemist (1738–1804) who discovered oxygen, though the element was named, and its importance first recognized, by ANTOINE LAVOISIER.

primeval
An adjective meaning "the first" or "early."

prokaryote

An organism characterized by cells not containing a true or definite NUCLEUS surrounded by a nuclear membrane.

protein

A complex organic compound consisting of AMINO ACIDS in polymeric form.

proton

A positively charged particle found in the nucleus of atoms.

protoplasm

An outdated term for the living substance within a cell. Current terminology divides cellular content into CYTOPLASM and *nucleoplasm* (material within the nuclear membrane).

protoplast

The entire cellular contents, surrounded by and including the cell membrane. The cell wall and/or capsule are not a part of the protoplast.

R

radical

An atom or compound that contains an unpaired electron.

radio astronomy

The study of radio waves received from outside the earth's atmosphere.

reduction

Any chemical reaction that results in a molecule gaining an electron, gaining a hydrogen atom, or losing an oxygen atom.

regeneration

The ability of an organism to regrow parts of itself after an injury.

replication

The process by which DNA duplicates itself for distribution to daughter nuclei during mitosis and/or meiosis.

reproduction

The process by which organisms create offspring of their own species.

respiration

In cells, the oxidation of food for the release of energy; in aerobes, the intake of oxygen and the release of carbon dioxide.

restriction fragment

A piece of DNA produced by breaking a large piece of DNA at specific points with restriction enzymes extracted from bacteria.

retrovirus

An RNA virus that produces new DNA from its RNA, as catalyzed by the enzyme reverse transcriptase. Example, human immunodeficiency virus (HIV).

RFLP

(restriction fragment length polymorphism) Differences in the lengths of RESTRICTION FRAGMENTS seen when DNA from different individuals is exposed to the same set of restriction enzymes. Using RFLPs to determine the identity of a person with DNA obtained from blood or other bodily materials is often referred to as "DNA fingerprinting." RFLPs can also be used to diagnose the presence of genetic disorders resulting from damaged genes.

ribosome

An intracellular structure consisting of RNA and protein whose function is to provide a site for the TRANSLATION phase of protein synthesis.

RNA

(ribonucleic acid) A large, helical, single-stranded molecule whose different types perform various tasks in the process of protein synthesis. Responsible for decoding the DNA sequence to construct protein chains.

S

salinity

The amount of dissolved salt in a fluid, typically referring to sodium chloride. However, other salts can be present.

salt

A substance formed when an acid is mixed with a base and composed of ionic bonds.

saprotroph

An organism feeding on dead organic matter, usually digesting the food externally and absorbing the digested material into its body such as fungi.

satellite

A man-made or natural object that orbits around a planet.

serotonin

A biogenic amine derivative of tryptophan that serves as a neurotransmitter in the central nervous system.

serum

The fluid portion of blood plasma after clotting.

sickle cell anemia

A GENETIC DISORDER caused by inheritance of a damaged gene for two of the four PROTEIN subunits of the HEMOGLOBIN molecule. The defective hemoglobin molecules stick to one another, forming clusters that distort the shape of the ERYTHROCYTES, reducing their ability to transport oxygen. Defective erythrocytes can also burst or clog capillaries.

slime mold

Large amoeboid protozoans that form spores similar to those of fungi.

solar

An adjective referring to the sun. A solar eclipse is an eclipse of the sun.

solar system

The sun, planets, moons, asteroids, and comets.

soluble

The ability of a substance to mix completely with a liquid at the molecular level, such that no particles of any kind are visible in the mixture. The substance must be compatible with the liquid; nonpolar substances will not dissolve in polar liquids, nor will the reverse occur. Dissolved substances will often be able to pass through semipermeable membranes. *See* NONPOLAR COMPOUND, POLAR COMPOUND, SOLUTE, and SOLUTION.

solute

The substance dissolved in a fluid to form a solution. *See* SOLUTION, SOLUBLE, and SOLVENT.

solution

A solution is a type of mixture formed when one substance mixes completely with a liquid at the molecular level. For example, when sugar (a POLAR COMPOUND) is mixed with hot water (also a POLAR COMPOUND), the result is a solution. *See* SOLUTE, SOLVENT, and SOLUBLE.

solvent

The fluid in which a solute is dissolved to form a SOLUTION. *See* SOLUBLE.

sonic

An adjective referring to sound.

spawn

(noun) Eggs of certain aquatic and marine animals, such as fish, crabs, shrimp, frogs, and turtles (verb) To lay eggs.

stimulus

Any change in the external or internal environment of a living organism. Many stimuli cause a change in the organism's activity (response). For example, if a person has not eaten for some time, the smell of the food might make his mouth water. The stimulus is the sudden presence of food (detected by smell); the response is secretion of saliva.

sublimation

The transformation of a substance from a solid directly to a gaseous state without passing through a liquid state.

substratum

A layer lying beneath the top layer (geology); the surface of a medium on which microorganisms grow (biology); a material or compound on which enzymes act (biology). Also called the *substrate*.

supersonic

Faster than the speed of sound.

suspension

A type of mixture in which large particles are mixed with a liquid and remain mixed only as long as they are agitated. The particles in a suspension will settle out if not continuously agitated. An example is the suspension of blood cells in the plasma of blood. Particles in suspension will not pass through a semipermeable membrane. *See* COLLOID and SOLUTION.

symbiosis

A relationship between two different species living together. The relationship may be PARASITISM, MUTUALISM, or COMMENSALISM.

synergism

A phenomenon in which the total is greater than the sum of the individual parameters.

T

theory

An explanation of natural events based on hypotheses and confirmed by testing.

thermodynamics

The study of heat and energy flow.

tissue

A group of similar CELLS specialized to perform a single task. When different tissues are combined, they are arranged in sequential layers. *See* ORGAN.

transcription

The formation of messenger RNA from the coded DNA.

transduction

The passage of genetic material from one bacterial cell to another by means of viral parasites called *phages*.

transformation

The passage of genetic material from one bacterium to another through the medium in which they are growing.

translation

The formation of proteins from amino acids by the use of the coded information in the messenger RNA (mRNA) and transfer (tRNA).

translocation

The movement of materials throughout a plant.

U

unicellular

An adjective meaning single-celled. *See* CELL.

universe

All existing matter and space considered as a whole; the cosmos.

V

valence

The number of electrons that can be accepted, given up, or shared by an atom or RADICAL. Positive valence numbers indicate electrons that can be given up to or shared with another atom or radical; negative valence numbers indicate electrons that can be accepted from another atom or radical. The positive and negative valences of reactants must balance for a chemical reaction to occur.

vapor

The gaseous phase of a substance that is usually in a liquid state. Vaporization (*evaporation*) of water or another liquid is accomplished by heating the liquid.

vascular tissue

Tissue used to transport materials in multicellular organisms. In higher animals, blood is vascular tissue; in higher plants, xylem and phloem are vascular tissues.

vector

An organism that carries and transmits pathogens from one animal to another.

velocity

The rate of motion of one object relative to another object.

Vesalius, Andreas

A Flemish anatomist (1514–1564) who studied the body. His discoveries were so important that he is often referred to as "the father of anatomy." *See* ANATOMY.

virus

An obligate intracellular parasite consisting essentially of a nucleic acid surrounded by a protein coat.

vitamin

An organic substance other than an ENZYME that is necessary for the proper maintenance of a metabolic process. A vitamin deficiency will cause metabolic dysfunction and an overall decline in health. Animals, including humans, must get their vitamins from the foods they eat.

volt

The practical unit of measurement of electric potential and electromotive force.

W

water table

The level nearest to the surface of the ground where water is found.

work

The result of energy expenditure. Common examples of work are movement, chemical reactions, and changes from one physical state to another.

Y

yeast

A unicellular nonmycelial fungus. Some yeasts are of commercial importance in the brewing and baking industries.

Z

zoology

The study of animals; a branch of BIOLOGY.

SCIENCE ANSWER SHEET

Test 1: Chemistry and Physics

1. Ⓐ Ⓑ Ⓒ Ⓓ   14. Ⓐ Ⓑ Ⓒ Ⓓ   27. Ⓐ Ⓑ Ⓒ Ⓓ   40. Ⓐ Ⓑ Ⓒ Ⓓ   53. Ⓐ Ⓑ Ⓒ Ⓓ
2. Ⓐ Ⓑ Ⓒ Ⓓ   15. Ⓐ Ⓑ Ⓒ Ⓓ   28. Ⓐ Ⓑ Ⓒ Ⓓ   41. Ⓐ Ⓑ Ⓒ Ⓓ   54. Ⓐ Ⓑ Ⓒ Ⓓ
3. Ⓐ Ⓑ Ⓒ Ⓓ   16. Ⓐ Ⓑ Ⓒ Ⓓ   29. Ⓐ Ⓑ Ⓒ Ⓓ   42. Ⓐ Ⓑ Ⓒ Ⓓ   55. Ⓐ Ⓑ Ⓒ Ⓓ
4. Ⓐ Ⓑ Ⓒ Ⓓ   17. Ⓐ Ⓑ Ⓒ Ⓓ   30. Ⓐ Ⓑ Ⓒ Ⓓ   43. Ⓐ Ⓑ Ⓒ Ⓓ   56. Ⓐ Ⓑ Ⓒ Ⓓ
5. Ⓐ Ⓑ Ⓒ Ⓓ   18. Ⓐ Ⓑ Ⓒ Ⓓ   31. Ⓐ Ⓑ Ⓒ Ⓓ   44. Ⓐ Ⓑ Ⓒ Ⓓ   57. Ⓐ Ⓑ Ⓒ Ⓓ
6. Ⓐ Ⓑ Ⓒ Ⓓ   19. Ⓐ Ⓑ Ⓒ Ⓓ   32. Ⓐ Ⓑ Ⓒ Ⓓ   45. Ⓐ Ⓑ Ⓒ Ⓓ   58. Ⓐ Ⓑ Ⓒ Ⓓ
7. Ⓐ Ⓑ Ⓒ Ⓓ   20. Ⓐ Ⓑ Ⓒ Ⓓ   33. Ⓐ Ⓑ Ⓒ Ⓓ   46. Ⓐ Ⓑ Ⓒ Ⓓ   59. Ⓐ Ⓑ Ⓒ Ⓓ
8. Ⓐ Ⓑ Ⓒ Ⓓ   21. Ⓐ Ⓑ Ⓒ Ⓓ   34. Ⓐ Ⓑ Ⓒ Ⓓ   47. Ⓐ Ⓑ Ⓒ Ⓓ   60. Ⓐ Ⓑ Ⓒ Ⓓ
9. Ⓐ Ⓑ Ⓒ Ⓓ   22. Ⓐ Ⓑ Ⓒ Ⓓ   35. Ⓐ Ⓑ Ⓒ Ⓓ   48. Ⓐ Ⓑ Ⓒ Ⓓ   61. Ⓐ Ⓑ Ⓒ Ⓓ
10. Ⓐ Ⓑ Ⓒ Ⓓ   23. Ⓐ Ⓑ Ⓒ Ⓓ   36. Ⓐ Ⓑ Ⓒ Ⓓ   49. Ⓐ Ⓑ Ⓒ Ⓓ   62. Ⓐ Ⓑ Ⓒ Ⓓ
11. Ⓐ Ⓑ Ⓒ Ⓓ   24. Ⓐ Ⓑ Ⓒ Ⓓ   37. Ⓐ Ⓑ Ⓒ Ⓓ   50. Ⓐ Ⓑ Ⓒ Ⓓ   63. Ⓐ Ⓑ Ⓒ Ⓓ
12. Ⓐ Ⓑ Ⓒ Ⓓ   25. Ⓐ Ⓑ Ⓒ Ⓓ   38. Ⓐ Ⓑ Ⓒ Ⓓ   51. Ⓐ Ⓑ Ⓒ Ⓓ   64. Ⓐ Ⓑ Ⓒ Ⓓ
13. Ⓐ Ⓑ Ⓒ Ⓓ   26. Ⓐ Ⓑ Ⓒ Ⓓ   39. Ⓐ Ⓑ Ⓒ Ⓓ   52. Ⓐ Ⓑ Ⓒ Ⓓ   65. Ⓐ Ⓑ Ⓒ Ⓓ

Test 2: Chemistry and Physics

1. Ⓐ Ⓑ Ⓒ Ⓓ   10. Ⓐ Ⓑ Ⓒ Ⓓ   19. Ⓐ Ⓑ Ⓒ Ⓓ   28. Ⓐ Ⓑ Ⓒ Ⓓ   37. Ⓐ Ⓑ Ⓒ Ⓓ
2. Ⓐ Ⓑ Ⓒ Ⓓ   11. Ⓐ Ⓑ Ⓒ Ⓓ   20. Ⓐ Ⓑ Ⓒ Ⓓ   29. Ⓐ Ⓑ Ⓒ Ⓓ   38. Ⓐ Ⓑ Ⓒ Ⓓ
3. Ⓐ Ⓑ Ⓒ Ⓓ   12. Ⓐ Ⓑ Ⓒ Ⓓ   21. Ⓐ Ⓑ Ⓒ Ⓓ   30. Ⓐ Ⓑ Ⓒ Ⓓ   39. Ⓐ Ⓑ Ⓒ Ⓓ
4. Ⓐ Ⓑ Ⓒ Ⓓ   13. Ⓐ Ⓑ Ⓒ Ⓓ   22. Ⓐ Ⓑ Ⓒ Ⓓ   31. Ⓐ Ⓑ Ⓒ Ⓓ   40. Ⓐ Ⓑ Ⓒ Ⓓ
5. Ⓐ Ⓑ Ⓒ Ⓓ   14. Ⓐ Ⓑ Ⓒ Ⓓ   23. Ⓐ Ⓑ Ⓒ Ⓓ   32. Ⓐ Ⓑ Ⓒ Ⓓ   41. Ⓐ Ⓑ Ⓒ Ⓓ
6. Ⓐ Ⓑ Ⓒ Ⓓ   15. Ⓐ Ⓑ Ⓒ Ⓓ   24. Ⓐ Ⓑ Ⓒ Ⓓ   33. Ⓐ Ⓑ Ⓒ Ⓓ   42. Ⓐ Ⓑ Ⓒ Ⓓ
7. Ⓐ Ⓑ Ⓒ Ⓓ   16. Ⓐ Ⓑ Ⓒ Ⓓ   25. Ⓐ Ⓑ Ⓒ Ⓓ   34. Ⓐ Ⓑ Ⓒ Ⓓ   43. Ⓐ Ⓑ Ⓒ Ⓓ
8. Ⓐ Ⓑ Ⓒ Ⓓ   17. Ⓐ Ⓑ Ⓒ Ⓓ   26. Ⓐ Ⓑ Ⓒ Ⓓ   35. Ⓐ Ⓑ Ⓒ Ⓓ   44. Ⓐ Ⓑ Ⓒ Ⓓ
9. Ⓐ Ⓑ Ⓒ Ⓓ   18. Ⓐ Ⓑ Ⓒ Ⓓ   27. Ⓐ Ⓑ Ⓒ Ⓓ   36. Ⓐ Ⓑ Ⓒ Ⓓ   45. Ⓐ Ⓑ Ⓒ Ⓓ

answer sheet

Test 3: Biology

1. Ⓐ Ⓑ Ⓒ Ⓓ   13. Ⓐ Ⓑ Ⓒ Ⓓ   25. Ⓐ Ⓑ Ⓒ Ⓓ   37. Ⓐ Ⓑ Ⓒ Ⓓ   49. Ⓐ Ⓑ Ⓒ Ⓓ
2. Ⓐ Ⓑ Ⓒ Ⓓ   14. Ⓐ Ⓑ Ⓒ Ⓓ   26. Ⓐ Ⓑ Ⓒ Ⓓ   38. Ⓐ Ⓑ Ⓒ Ⓓ   50. Ⓐ Ⓑ Ⓒ Ⓓ
3. Ⓐ Ⓑ Ⓒ Ⓓ   15. Ⓐ Ⓑ Ⓒ Ⓓ   27. Ⓐ Ⓑ Ⓒ Ⓓ   39. Ⓐ Ⓑ Ⓒ Ⓓ   51. Ⓐ Ⓑ Ⓒ Ⓓ
4. Ⓐ Ⓑ Ⓒ Ⓓ   16. Ⓐ Ⓑ Ⓒ Ⓓ   28. Ⓐ Ⓑ Ⓒ Ⓓ   40. Ⓐ Ⓑ Ⓒ Ⓓ   52. Ⓐ Ⓑ Ⓒ Ⓓ
5. Ⓐ Ⓑ Ⓒ Ⓓ   17. Ⓐ Ⓑ Ⓒ Ⓓ   29. Ⓐ Ⓑ Ⓒ Ⓓ   41. Ⓐ Ⓑ Ⓒ Ⓓ   53. Ⓐ Ⓑ Ⓒ Ⓓ
6. Ⓐ Ⓑ Ⓒ Ⓓ   18. Ⓐ Ⓑ Ⓒ Ⓓ   30. Ⓐ Ⓑ Ⓒ Ⓓ   42. Ⓐ Ⓑ Ⓒ Ⓓ   54. Ⓐ Ⓑ Ⓒ Ⓓ
7. Ⓐ Ⓑ Ⓒ Ⓓ   19. Ⓐ Ⓑ Ⓒ Ⓓ   31. Ⓐ Ⓑ Ⓒ Ⓓ   43. Ⓐ Ⓑ Ⓒ Ⓓ   55. Ⓐ Ⓑ Ⓒ Ⓓ
8. Ⓐ Ⓑ Ⓒ Ⓓ   20. Ⓐ Ⓑ Ⓒ Ⓓ   32. Ⓐ Ⓑ Ⓒ Ⓓ   44. Ⓐ Ⓑ Ⓒ Ⓓ   56. Ⓐ Ⓑ Ⓒ Ⓓ
9. Ⓐ Ⓑ Ⓒ Ⓓ   21. Ⓐ Ⓑ Ⓒ Ⓓ   33. Ⓐ Ⓑ Ⓒ Ⓓ   45. Ⓐ Ⓑ Ⓒ Ⓓ   57. Ⓐ Ⓑ Ⓒ Ⓓ
10. Ⓐ Ⓑ Ⓒ Ⓓ   22. Ⓐ Ⓑ Ⓒ Ⓓ   34. Ⓐ Ⓑ Ⓒ Ⓓ   46. Ⓐ Ⓑ Ⓒ Ⓓ   58. Ⓐ Ⓑ Ⓒ Ⓓ
11. Ⓐ Ⓑ Ⓒ Ⓓ   23. Ⓐ Ⓑ Ⓒ Ⓓ   35. Ⓐ Ⓑ Ⓒ Ⓓ   47. Ⓐ Ⓑ Ⓒ Ⓓ   59. Ⓐ Ⓑ Ⓒ Ⓓ
12. Ⓐ Ⓑ Ⓒ Ⓓ   24. Ⓐ Ⓑ Ⓒ Ⓓ   36. Ⓐ Ⓑ Ⓒ Ⓓ   48. Ⓐ Ⓑ Ⓒ Ⓓ   60. Ⓐ Ⓑ Ⓒ Ⓓ

Test 4: Cells, Structure, and Function

1. Ⓐ Ⓑ Ⓒ Ⓓ   8. Ⓐ Ⓑ Ⓒ Ⓓ   15. Ⓐ Ⓑ Ⓒ Ⓓ   22. Ⓐ Ⓑ Ⓒ Ⓓ   29. Ⓐ Ⓑ Ⓒ Ⓓ
2. Ⓐ Ⓑ Ⓒ Ⓓ   9. Ⓐ Ⓑ Ⓒ Ⓓ   16. Ⓐ Ⓑ Ⓒ Ⓓ   23. Ⓐ Ⓑ Ⓒ Ⓓ   30. Ⓐ Ⓑ Ⓒ Ⓓ
3. Ⓐ Ⓑ Ⓒ Ⓓ   10. Ⓐ Ⓑ Ⓒ Ⓓ   17. Ⓐ Ⓑ Ⓒ Ⓓ   24. Ⓐ Ⓑ Ⓒ Ⓓ   31. Ⓐ Ⓑ Ⓒ Ⓓ
4. Ⓐ Ⓑ Ⓒ Ⓓ   11. Ⓐ Ⓑ Ⓒ Ⓓ   18. Ⓐ Ⓑ Ⓒ Ⓓ   25. Ⓐ Ⓑ Ⓒ Ⓓ   32. Ⓐ Ⓑ Ⓒ Ⓓ
5. Ⓐ Ⓑ Ⓒ Ⓓ   12. Ⓐ Ⓑ Ⓒ Ⓓ   19. Ⓐ Ⓑ Ⓒ Ⓓ   26. Ⓐ Ⓑ Ⓒ Ⓓ   33. Ⓐ Ⓑ Ⓒ Ⓓ
6. Ⓐ Ⓑ Ⓒ Ⓓ   13. Ⓐ Ⓑ Ⓒ Ⓓ   20. Ⓐ Ⓑ Ⓒ Ⓓ   27. Ⓐ Ⓑ Ⓒ Ⓓ   34. Ⓐ Ⓑ Ⓒ Ⓓ
7. Ⓐ Ⓑ Ⓒ Ⓓ   14. Ⓐ Ⓑ Ⓒ Ⓓ   21. Ⓐ Ⓑ Ⓒ Ⓓ   28. Ⓐ Ⓑ Ⓒ Ⓓ

Test 5: Biology

1. Ⓐ Ⓑ Ⓒ Ⓓ   5. Ⓐ Ⓑ Ⓒ Ⓓ   9. Ⓐ Ⓑ Ⓒ Ⓓ   13. Ⓐ Ⓑ Ⓒ Ⓓ   16. Ⓐ Ⓑ Ⓒ Ⓓ
2. Ⓐ Ⓑ Ⓒ Ⓓ   6. Ⓐ Ⓑ Ⓒ Ⓓ   10. Ⓐ Ⓑ Ⓒ Ⓓ   14. Ⓐ Ⓑ Ⓒ Ⓓ   17. Ⓐ Ⓑ Ⓒ Ⓓ
3. Ⓐ Ⓑ Ⓒ Ⓓ   7. Ⓐ Ⓑ Ⓒ Ⓓ   11. Ⓐ Ⓑ Ⓒ Ⓓ   15. Ⓐ Ⓑ Ⓒ Ⓓ   18. Ⓐ Ⓑ Ⓒ Ⓓ
4. Ⓐ Ⓑ Ⓒ Ⓓ   8. Ⓐ Ⓑ Ⓒ Ⓓ   12. Ⓐ Ⓑ Ⓒ Ⓓ

Test 6: Biology

1. Ⓐ Ⓑ Ⓒ Ⓓ　　5. Ⓐ Ⓑ Ⓒ Ⓓ　　9. Ⓐ Ⓑ Ⓒ Ⓓ　　13. Ⓐ Ⓑ Ⓒ Ⓓ　　17. Ⓐ Ⓑ Ⓒ Ⓓ
2. Ⓐ Ⓑ Ⓒ Ⓓ　　6. Ⓐ Ⓑ Ⓒ Ⓓ　　10. Ⓐ Ⓑ Ⓒ Ⓓ　　14. Ⓐ Ⓑ Ⓒ Ⓓ　　18. Ⓐ Ⓑ Ⓒ Ⓓ
3. Ⓐ Ⓑ Ⓒ Ⓓ　　7. Ⓐ Ⓑ Ⓒ Ⓓ　　11. Ⓐ Ⓑ Ⓒ Ⓓ　　15. Ⓐ Ⓑ Ⓒ Ⓓ　　19. Ⓐ Ⓑ Ⓒ Ⓓ
4. Ⓐ Ⓑ Ⓒ Ⓓ　　8. Ⓐ Ⓑ Ⓒ Ⓓ　　12. Ⓐ Ⓑ Ⓒ Ⓓ　　16. Ⓐ Ⓑ Ⓒ Ⓓ　　20. Ⓐ Ⓑ Ⓒ Ⓓ

Test 7: Chemistry

1. Ⓐ Ⓑ Ⓒ Ⓓ　　5. Ⓐ Ⓑ Ⓒ Ⓓ　　9. Ⓐ Ⓑ Ⓒ Ⓓ　　13. Ⓐ Ⓑ Ⓒ Ⓓ　　17. Ⓐ Ⓑ Ⓒ Ⓓ
2. Ⓐ Ⓑ Ⓒ Ⓓ　　6. Ⓐ Ⓑ Ⓒ Ⓓ　　10. Ⓐ Ⓑ Ⓒ Ⓓ　　14. Ⓐ Ⓑ Ⓒ Ⓓ　　18. Ⓐ Ⓑ Ⓒ Ⓓ
3. Ⓐ Ⓑ Ⓒ Ⓓ　　7. Ⓐ Ⓑ Ⓒ Ⓓ　　11. Ⓐ Ⓑ Ⓒ Ⓓ　　15. Ⓐ Ⓑ Ⓒ Ⓓ　　19. Ⓐ Ⓑ Ⓒ Ⓓ
4. Ⓐ Ⓑ Ⓒ Ⓓ　　8. Ⓐ Ⓑ Ⓒ Ⓓ　　12. Ⓐ Ⓑ Ⓒ Ⓓ　　16. Ⓐ Ⓑ Ⓒ Ⓓ　　20. Ⓐ Ⓑ Ⓒ Ⓓ

Test 8: Chemistry and Physical Science

1. Ⓐ Ⓑ Ⓒ Ⓓ　　11. Ⓐ Ⓑ Ⓒ Ⓓ　　21. Ⓐ Ⓑ Ⓒ Ⓓ　　31. Ⓐ Ⓑ Ⓒ Ⓓ　　41. Ⓐ Ⓑ Ⓒ Ⓓ
2. Ⓐ Ⓑ Ⓒ Ⓓ　　12. Ⓐ Ⓑ Ⓒ Ⓓ　　22. Ⓐ Ⓑ Ⓒ Ⓓ　　32. Ⓐ Ⓑ Ⓒ Ⓓ　　42. Ⓐ Ⓑ Ⓒ Ⓓ
3. Ⓐ Ⓑ Ⓒ Ⓓ　　13. Ⓐ Ⓑ Ⓒ Ⓓ　　23. Ⓐ Ⓑ Ⓒ Ⓓ　　33. Ⓐ Ⓑ Ⓒ Ⓓ　　43. Ⓐ Ⓑ Ⓒ Ⓓ
4. Ⓐ Ⓑ Ⓒ Ⓓ　　14. Ⓐ Ⓑ Ⓒ Ⓓ　　24. Ⓐ Ⓑ Ⓒ Ⓓ　　34. Ⓐ Ⓑ Ⓒ Ⓓ　　44. Ⓐ Ⓑ Ⓒ Ⓓ
5. Ⓐ Ⓑ Ⓒ Ⓓ　　15. Ⓐ Ⓑ Ⓒ Ⓓ　　25. Ⓐ Ⓑ Ⓒ Ⓓ　　35. Ⓐ Ⓑ Ⓒ Ⓓ　　45. Ⓐ Ⓑ Ⓒ Ⓓ
6. Ⓐ Ⓑ Ⓒ Ⓓ　　16. Ⓐ Ⓑ Ⓒ Ⓓ　　26. Ⓐ Ⓑ Ⓒ Ⓓ　　36. Ⓐ Ⓑ Ⓒ Ⓓ　　46. Ⓐ Ⓑ Ⓒ Ⓓ
7. Ⓐ Ⓑ Ⓒ Ⓓ　　17. Ⓐ Ⓑ Ⓒ Ⓓ　　27. Ⓐ Ⓑ Ⓒ Ⓓ　　37. Ⓐ Ⓑ Ⓒ Ⓓ　　47. Ⓐ Ⓑ Ⓒ Ⓓ
8. Ⓐ Ⓑ Ⓒ Ⓓ　　18. Ⓐ Ⓑ Ⓒ Ⓓ　　28. Ⓐ Ⓑ Ⓒ Ⓓ　　38. Ⓐ Ⓑ Ⓒ Ⓓ　　48. Ⓐ Ⓑ Ⓒ Ⓓ
9. Ⓐ Ⓑ Ⓒ Ⓓ　　19. Ⓐ Ⓑ Ⓒ Ⓓ　　29. Ⓐ Ⓑ Ⓒ Ⓓ　　39. Ⓐ Ⓑ Ⓒ Ⓓ　　49. Ⓐ Ⓑ Ⓒ Ⓓ
10. Ⓐ Ⓑ Ⓒ Ⓓ　　20. Ⓐ Ⓑ Ⓒ Ⓓ　　30. Ⓐ Ⓑ Ⓒ Ⓓ　　40. Ⓐ Ⓑ Ⓒ Ⓓ　　50. Ⓐ Ⓑ Ⓒ Ⓓ

PERIODIC TABLE

Table courtesy of Wikimedia Commons (**https://commons.wikimedia.org/wiki/Periodic_table_of_elements**)

Note: It is recommended that you reference a full-color version of the periodic table either online or at your local library. The periodic table provided is simplistic in nature and for reference only.

TEST 1: CHEMISTRY AND PHYSICS

65 Questions • 55 Minutes

Directions: Read each question carefully and consider all possible answers. When you have decided which choice is best, blacken the corresponding space on your answer sheet. There is only one best answer for each question.

1. Oxygen gas can be obtained in appreciable quantities by heating all of the following EXCEPT:
   A. H_2O
   B. H_2O_2
   C. HgO
   D. PbO_2

2. All of the reactions between the following pairs will produce hydrogen EXCEPT:
   A. Copper and hydrochloric acid
   B. Iron and sulfuric acid
   C. Magnesium and steam
   D. Sodium and alcohol

3. Choose the correct description, relative to scalar and vector quantities.
   A. Vectors = magnitude and direction
   B. Scalar = direction
   C. Vector = magnitude
   D. Scalar = magnitude and direction

4. Use the formula: $c = Q/M\Delta T$.
   c = specific heat
   Q = number of calories
   M = mass
   T = temperature

   If 3,480 calories of heat are required to raise the temperature of 300 grams of a substance from 50° C to 70° C, the substance would be:

	Substances	Specific Heat
A.	ethyl alcohol	0.581
B.	aluminum	0.214
C.	liquid ammonia	1.125
D.	water	1.0

5. Ozone is a molecular variety of
   A. oxygen.
   B. chlorine.
   C. hydrogen.
   D. sulfur.

6. If a eudiometer tube were filled with 26 mL of hydrogen and 24 mL of oxygen and the mixture exploded, which of the following would remain uncombined?
   A. 2 mL hydrogen
   B. 14 mL hydrogen
   C. 23 mL hydrogen
   D. 11 mL oxygen

7. The gas resulting when hydrochloric acid is added to a mixture of iron filings and sulfur is
   A. H_2S.
   B. SO_2.
   C. SO_3.
   D. H_2.

8. Calculate the time required for 100 mg of I^{131} (dissociation constant, K = 0.086625) to decay to 50 mg. Use the formula
   $$K = \frac{0.693}{t_{\frac{1}{2}}}.$$

   A. 0.5 days
   B. 0.4 days
   C. 64 days
   D. 8 days

9. What is the percentage composition of oxygen in a mole of glucose ($C_6H_{12}O_6$)?

    (C = 12, H = 1, O = 16)

    A. 53

    B. 35

    C. 6

    D. 20

10. In sulfuric acid, the valence number of sulfur is

    A. + 2.

    B. − 2.

    C. − 4.

    D. + 6.

11. The boiling points of the following gases are as follows:

    argon −185.7° C   nitrogen −195.8° C
    helium −268.9° C   oxygen −183° C

    In the fractional distillation of liquid air, the gas that boils off last is

    A. argon.

    B. helium.

    C. nitrogen.

    D. oxygen.

12. The chemical reaction $2Zn + 2HCl = 2ZnCl + H_2$ is an example of

    A. double displacement.

    B. synthesis.

    C. analysis.

    D. single displacement.

13. When carbon dioxide gas is bubbled through water in a test tube, the product is

    A. ozone.

    B. methane.

    C. hydrogen peroxide.

    D. carbonic acid.

14. Of the following electrical devices, a(n) _____ produces the highest voltage.

    A. electric broiler

    B. radio tube

    C. television picture tube

    D. electric steam-iron

15. Which of the following substances will raise the pH of a solution of hydrochloric acid?

    A. NaCl

    B. H_2CO_3

    C. $NaHCO_3$

    D. HNO_3

16. An oxide whose water solution will turn litmus red is

    A. BaO.

    B. Na_2O.

    C. P_2O_3.

    D. CaO.

17. 100 mL of a H_2SO_4 solution is completely neutralized with 50 mL of 1.0 M NaOH.

    What is the molarity of the H_2SO_4 solution? (S = 32, O = 16, Na = 23, H = 1).

    A. 1.0 M

    B. 0.25 M

    C. 0.5 M

    D. None of the above

18. A solution of zinc chloride should NOT be stored in a tank made of aluminum because

    A. aluminum will displace the zinc in the zinc chloride solution.

    B. the zinc will become contaminated.

    C. the chloride ion will react with impurities in the solution.

    D. the two metals will react to produce an undesirable compound.

19. The valence number of sulfur in the ion SO_4^{-2} is
   A. −2.
   B. +2.
   C. +6.
   D. +10.

20. The chemical name for sulfuric acid is
   A. hydrogen sulfate.
   B. hydrogen sulfite.
   C. sulfur trioxide.
   D. hydrogen sulfide.

21. The number of grams (g) of hydrogen formed by the action of 6 g of magnesium (atomic weight = 24) on an appropriate quantity of acid is
   A. 0.5.
   B. 8.
   C. 22.4.
   D. 72.

22. Identify the statement that is NOT characteristic of exergonic reactions.
   A. They are downhill reactions.
   B. They have a negative energy change (−H).
   C. They are uphill reactions.
   D. The products have less energy than the reactants.

23. What is the formula for sodium bisulfate?
   A. $NaBiSO_4$
   B. $NaHSO_4$
   C. NaH_2SO_4
   D. Na_2SO_4

24. The law of multiple proportions was first proposed by
   A. Dalton.
   B. Davy.
   C. Priestley.
   D. Williams.

25. One liter of a certain gas, under standard conditions, weighs 1.16 grams. A possible formula for the gas is
   A. C_2H_2.
   B. CO.
   C. NH_3.
   D. O_2.

26. Which of the following compounds would be classified as a salt?
   A. Na_2CO_3
   B. $Ca(OH)_2$
   C. H_2CO_3
   D. CH_3OH

27. Of the following, which is an aromatic compound?
   A. Benzene
   B. Ethyl alcohol
   C. Iodoform
   D. Methane

28. Of the following, which is a monosaccharide?
   A. Dextrose
   B. Glycogen
   C. Lactose
   D. Sucrose

29. Fats belong to the class of organic compounds represented by the general formula, RCOOR', where R and R' represent hydrocarbon groups; therefore, fats are
   A. ethers.
   B. soaps.
   C. esters.
   D. lipases.

30. Oil and water are immiscible (do not mix) because
   A. oil is polar, and water is polar.
   B. oil is nonpolar, and water is polar.
   C. water is nonpolar, and oil is polar.
   D. water is nonpolar, and oil is nonpolar.

31. The chemical bond that forms between the carboxyl (RCOOH) group of one amino acid and the amino (RC-NH$_2$) of another is a(n)

    A. peptide bond.

    B. coordinate covalent.

    C. ionic bond.

    D. high energy bond.

32. Two atoms have the same atomic number but different atomic weights (masses); therefore, these atoms are

    A. compounds.

    B. isotopes.

    C. neutrons.

    D. different elements.

33. What is the formula for commercial bleach?

    A. CaCl$_2$

    B. CaOCL

    C. Ca(OCl)$_2$

    D. Ca(ClO$_3$)$_2$

34. In forming an ionic bond with an atom of chlorine, a sodium atom will

    A. receive one electron from the chlorine atom.

    B. receive two electrons from the chlorine atom.

    C. give up one electron to the chlorine atom.

    D. give up two electrons to the chlorine atom.

Questions 35–40 are based on the periodic table.

35. Which of the following is an example of a transition element?

    A. Aluminum

    B. Astatine

    C. Nickel

    D. Rubidium

36. Identify those elements that are inert gases (by group number) in the periodic table.

    A. 1

    B. 18

    C. 13

    D. 16

37. The element neon is considered an inert gas because it has _____ electrons in its outermost energy shell.

    A. 8

    B. 7

    C. 4

    D. 2

38. Identify the two atoms with the same number of electrons in their outermost energy level.

    A. Na and K

    B. K and Ca

    C. Na and Mg

    D. Ca and Na

39. By use of the periodic table, it can be determined that the atoms with the greatest affinity would be

    A. Na and Cl.

    B. K and F.

    C. Na and F.

    D. K and Cl.

40. Using the periodic table, determine the valence of a sodium ion.

    A. +1

    B. 0

    C. −1

    D. +12

41. A gas lighter than air is

    A. CH$_4$.

    B. C$_6$H$_6$.

    C. HCl.

    D. N$_2$O.

42. Of the following gases, which is odorless and heavier than air?
    A. CO
    B. CO_2
    C. H_2S
    D. N_2

43. In a volume of air at a pressure of one atmosphere at sea level, the partial pressure of oxygen is equal to
    A. 593 mm of mercury.
    B. 494 mm of mercury.
    C. 380 mm of mercury.
    D. 160 mm of mercury.

44. The complete combustion of carbon disulfide would yield carbon dioxide and
    A. sulfur.
    B. sulfur dioxide.
    C. sulfuric acid.
    D. water.

45. Alcoholic beverages contain
    A. wood alcohol.
    B. isopropyl alcohol.
    C. glyceryl alcohol.
    D. ethyl alcohol.

46. Of the following compounds, which is more difficult to decompose than lithium fluoride?
    A. Lithium bromide
    B. Lithium chloride
    C. Lithium iodide
    D. None of the above

47. Which of the following molecules would be classified as a ketone?

48. Which of the following copper wires would have the greatest resistance to an electrical current?
    A. Length of 1 m and diameter of 4 mm
    B. Length of 2 m and diameter of 8 mm
    C. Length of 1 m and diameter of 8 mm
    D. Length of 2 m and diameter of 2 mm

49. What is the general formula for an organic acid?
    A. RCOOR
    B. ROH
    C. ROR
    D. RCOOH

50. An example of a strong electrolyte is
    A. sugar.
    B. calcium chloride.
    C. glycerin.
    D. boric acid.

51. A lead ball, a wooden ball, and a polystyrene foam ball, all with a mass of 1 kg, are thrown at a wall 16 m away. Each of the balls hit the wall in 2 seconds. Which ball will strike the wall with the greatest force?

   A. Lead ball

   B. Wooden ball

   C. Polystyrene foam ball

   D. All strike with the same force.

52. When copper oxide is heated with charcoal, the reaction that occurs is an example of

   A. reduction.

   B. oxidation.

   C. both oxidation and reduction.

   D. neither oxidation nor reduction.

53. Nonmetal oxides, when dissolved in water, tend to form

   A. acids.

   B. bases.

   C. salts.

   D. hydrides.

54. Choose the correct structural formula for acetylene (C_2H_2).

   A. $HC = CH$

   B. $HC - CH$

   C. $HC \equiv CH$

   D. $HC\ CH$

55. The best reducing agent is

   A. mercury.

   B. hydrogen.

   C. copper.

   D. carbon dioxide.

56. For a solution of H_2SO_4, the equivalency between molarity and normality would be

   (H = I, S = 32, O = 16)

   A. $IM = IN$

   B. $IM = 2\ N$

   C. $IN = 2\ M$

   D. $IM = 0.5\ N$

57. The test for a nitrate results in

   A. a precipitate.

   B. a red flame.

   C. a brown ring.

   D. litmus turning blue.

58. A solution that contains all the solute it can normally dissolve at a given temperature must be

   A. concentrated.

   B. supersaturated.

   C. saturated.

   D. unsaturated.

59. The oxides of barium and sulfur combine to form a(n)

   A. salt.

   B. base.

   C. acid.

   D. anhydride.

60. A pencil is dropped into a glass half filled with water. It looks as if the end that is underwater does not match up with the end that is in the air. This optical illusion is the result of

   A. diffraction of light.

   B. convection of light.

   C. diffusion of light.

   D. refraction of light.

61. The reason concentrated H_2SO_4 is used extensively to prepare other acids is that concentrated sulfuric acid

    A. is highly ionized.

    B. is an excellent dehydrating agent.

    C. has a high specific gravity.

    D. has a high boiling point.

62. In a 0.001 M solution of HCl, the pH is:

    A. 2

    B. −3

    C. 1

    D. 3

63. The portion of an atom directly involved in the ionic bonding is the

    A. protons in the nucleus.

    B. neutrons in the nucleus.

    C. electrons in the outer energy level.

    D. electrons in the innermost energy level.

64. When hydrochloric acid is added to sodium sulfite and the gas that is formed is bubbled through barium hydroxide, the salt formed is

    A. $BaCl_2$.

    B. $BaSO_2$.

    C. NaCl.

    D. NaOH.

65. A tornado passed over a house and destroyed it, primarily because

    A. the air pressure over the roof was lower than the pressure in the attic.

    B. the air pressure over the roof was equal to the pressure in the attic.

    C. the air pressure over the roof was higher than the pressure in the attic.

    D. None of the above

STOP

IF YOU FINISH BEFORE TIME IS CALLED, YOU MAY CHECK YOUR WORK ON THIS SECTION ONLY. DO NOT TURN TO ANY OTHER SECTION IN THE TEST.

TEST 2: CHEMISTRY AND PHYSICS

45 Questions • 45 Minutes

Directions: Read each question carefully and consider all possible answers. When you have decided which choice is best, blacken the corresponding space on your answer sheet. There is only one best answer for each question.

1. Which of the following properties is considered a physical property?
   A. Flammability
   B. Boiling point
   C. Reactivity
   D. Osmolarity

2. Which one of the following substances is a chemical compound?
   A. Blood
   B. Water
   C. Oxygen
   D. Air

3. What are the differentiating factors between potential and kinetic energy?
   A. Properties—physical or chemical
   B. State—solid or liquid
   C. Temperature—high or low
   D. Activity—in motion or in storage

4. How many calories are required to change the temperature of 2 g of H_2O from 20° C to 38° C?
   A. 36 calories
   B. 24 calories
   C. 18 calories
   D. 12 calories

5. A 1,000-ton ship must displace a weight of water equal to
   A. 500 tons.
   B. 1,000 tons.
   C. 1,500 tons.
   D. 2,000 tons.

6. What is the atomic weight of the element in the figure below?

   A. 2
   B. 3
   C. 4
   D. 7

7. Which of the following kinds of radiation is most penetrating?
   A. Alpha
   B. Beta
   C. Gamma
   D. X-rays

8. I^{131} has a half-life of eight days. A 100-milligram sample of this radioactive element would decay to what amount after eight days?
   A. 50 milligrams
   B. 40 milligrams
   C. 30 milligrams
   D. 20 milligrams

9. A direct physiological effect of radiation on human tissues is
   A. impairment of cellular metabolism.
   B. proliferation of white blood cells.
   C. formation of scar tissue.
   D. reduction of body fluids.

10. What is the gram molecular weight of $C_6H_{12}O_6$? (C = 12, H = 1, O = 16)
    A. 29 grams
    B. 174 grams
    C. 180 grams
    D. 696 grams

11. Which one of the following equations is balanced?
    A. $H_2O \rightarrow H_2 \uparrow + O_2 \uparrow$
    B. $Al + H_2SO_4 \rightarrow Al_2(SO_4)_3 + H_2 \uparrow$
    C. $S + O_2 \rightarrow SO_3$
    D. $2HgO \rightarrow 2Hg + O_2 \uparrow$

12. What is the current in a 60-volt circuit where $R_{eq} = 15\Omega$?
    A. 0.25 A
    B. 4 A
    C. 60 A
    D. 900 A

13. Which of the following bodily substances is a catalyst?
    A. Bile
    B. Hemoglobin
    C. Enzyme
    D. Mucus

14. In order to increase the temperature of a gas in a closed unit, it would be necessary to
    A. increase the pressure.
    B. decrease the density.
    C. decrease the volume.
    D. increase the space.

15. Which of the following equations represents an oxidation-reduction reaction?
    A. $2Na + Cl_2 \rightarrow NaCl$
    B. $CO_2 + H_2O \rightarrow H_2CO_3$
    C. $HNO_3 + KOH \rightarrow KNO_3 + H_2O$
    D. $CaO + H_2O \rightarrow Ca(OH)_2$

16. Which of the following instruments can convert light into an electric current?
    A. A radiometer
    B. A dry cell
    C. An electrolysis apparatus
    D. A photoelectric cell

17. When you mix salt with water, what is the water called?
    A. Solute
    B. Solvent
    C. Solution
    D. Ionizer

18. A 10-percent solution of glucose will contain
    A. 1 gram of glucose per 1,000 milliliters of solution.
    B. 1 gram of glucose per 100 milliliters of solution.
    C. 1 gram of glucose per 10 microliters of solution.
    D. 10 grams of glucose per 100 milliliters of solution.

Questions 19–21 refer to the diagrams below.

Each diagram represents one solution: One gram molecular weight of NaOH, one of KOH, and one of HCl, each dissolved in enough H_2O to make 1 liter.

19. What is the weight of NaOH in the solution diagram?

    A. 40

    B. 20

    C. 23

    D. 16

20. These are molar quantities because

    A. their molecular weights are equal to each other.

    B. the volume for each solution is the same.

    C. each solution contains 1 gram molecular weight.

    D. the percentage of solute to solvent is equal in each solution.

21. Identify the products of the chemical reaction between 1 cubic centimeter of KOH and 1 cubic centimeter of HCl.

    A. $K^+ + Cl_2 + 2H + OH$

    B. $KCl + H_2 + O_2$

    C. $K + Cl + HOH$

    D. $KCl + H_2O$

22. CA^{++} (atomic weight 40) is bivalent; hence, 1 gram equivalent weighs

    A. 40 grams.

    B. 30 grams.

    C. 20 grams.

    D. 10 grams.

23. A covalent bond between two amino acid molecules can be created by

    A. inserting a water molecule between them.

    B. removing a water molecule from them.

    C. inserting a carbon atom between them.

    D. removing a carbon atom from one of them.

24. The atomic number of fluorine is 9; this indicates that a fluoride atom contains

    A. nine neutrons in its nucleus.

    B. nine protons in its nucleus and nine electrons in orbit around the nucleus.

    C. a total of nine protons and neutrons.

    D. a total of nine protons and electrons.

25. The basic inorganic raw materials for photosynthesis are

    A. water and oxygen.

    B. water and carbon dioxide.

    C. oxygen and carbon dioxide.

    D. sugar and carbon dioxide.

26. A 2 kg bowling ball is accelerating down the lane at a rate of 7 m/s^2. How much force did the bowler apply to the ball with her throw?

    A. 3.5 N

    B. 14 N

    C. 1400 g/cm^2

    D. It's impossible to calculate because of friction.

27. A ray of light strikes a mirror at a 45°
angle. At what angle does the light reflect
back from the mirror?

    A. 45°

    B. 90°

    C. 180°

    D. 315°

28. Firefighters battling a fire suddenly discover a tear in their hose. This decreases
the effectiveness of the hose by which
mechanism?

    A. The tear increases the area of the hose,
reducing the water pressure.

    B. The water is now forced through a
smaller area, making the pressure too
high to control.

    C. The leaking water reduces the volume
of water in the hose, reducing the
pressure.

    D. All of the above.

**Questions 29 and 30 refer to the following
diagrams.**

I

II

29. A person who turns off the television
does not also cause the refrigerator to stop
because the appliances are

    A. in circuit I; TV in series and
refrigerator in parallel.

    B. in circuit II; TV in parallel and
refrigerator in series.

    C. in circuit II; both the TV and
refrigerator are in parallel circuits.

    D. in circuit I; both TV and refrigerator
are in series.

30. Along a string of lights on a Christmas
tree, if one half goes out, they all go out.
Use the diagram to determine which of
the following illustrates this circuitry.

    A. Both I and II

    B. I

    C. II

    D. Neither I nor II

31. Bronze is an alloy of copper and

    A. iron.

    B. lead.

    C. zinc.

    D. tin.

32. Which is NOT a characteristic of
enzymes?

    A. They are proteins.

    B. They catalyze metabolic reactions.

    C. They act on substances.

    D. They are phospholipids.

33. The symbol for two molecules of hydrogen
is

    A. H_2

    B. $2H$

    C. $2H+$

    D. $2H_2$

34. As electrons from aerobic respiration are moved through the electron transport system (ETS), the final electron acceptor is
    A. hydrogen.
    B. carbon dioxide.
    C. oxygen.
    D. water.

35. The oxidation of 1 gram of CHO produces 4 calories. How much CHO must be oxidized in the body to produce 36 calories? (CHO is a carbohydrate.)
    A. 4 grams
    B. 7 grams
    C. 9 grams
    D. 12 grams

36. Which one of the following equations represents neutralization?
    A. $2Na + Cl_2 \rightarrow 2NaCl$
    B. $CO_2 + H_2O \rightarrow H_2CO_3$
    C. $HNO_3 + KOH \rightarrow KNO_3 + H_2O$
    D. $CaO + H_2O \rightarrow Ca(OH)_2$

37. Which of the following could react chemically with ammonia?

    A. H
    B. Cl⁻
    C. Na
    D. H⁺

38. The lightest element known on Earth is
    A. hydrogen.
    B. helium.
    C. oxygen.
    D. air.

39. Of the following gases in the air, the most plentiful is
    A. argon.
    B. nitrogen.
    C. oxygen.
    D. carbon dioxide.

40. Per liter, compared with a 3-molar aqueous solution, a 3-molal aqueous solution contains
    A. the same amount of solute.
    B. more solute.
    C. less solute.
    D. a variable amount of solute.

41. Of the following, the process that will result in water most nearly chemically pure is
    A. aeration.
    B. chlorination.
    C. distillation.
    D. filtration.

42. For the reaction $H_2(g) + Br_2(g) \rightarrow 2HBr(g)$, the reaction can be driven to the left by
    A. increasing the pressure.
    B. increasing the hydrogen.
    C. increasing hydrogen bromide.
    D. decreasing hydrogen bromide.

43. Which of the following groups contain no ionic compounds?
    A. $HCN, NO, Ca(NO_3)_2$
    B. KOH, CCL_4, SF_6
    C. $NaH, CaF_2, NaNH_2$
    D. $CH_2O, H2S, NH_3$

44. Of the 92 naturally occurring elements, the number found in the human body is closest to

A. 50.

B. 10.

C. 25.

D. 75.

45. Inasmuch as the molecular formula for glucose is $C_6H_{12}O_6$ and the molecular formula for fructose is $C_6H_{12}O_6$, the two substances are

A. hextomers.

B. isomers.

C. heteromers.

D. anomers.

STOP

IF YOU FINISH BEFORE TIME IS CALLED, YOU MAY CHECK YOUR WORK ON THIS SECTION ONLY. DO NOT TURN TO ANY OTHER SECTION IN THE TEST.

TEST 3: BIOLOGY

60 Questions • 50 Minutes

> **Directions:** Read each question carefully and consider all possible answers. When you have decided which choice is best, fill in the corresponding space on your answer sheet. There is only one best answer for each question.

1. Passage of water through the membrane of a cell is called
   - A. assimilation.
   - B. osmosis.
   - C. circulation.
   - D. transpiration.

2. The largest portion of the iron supplied to the body by foods is used by the body for the
   - A. growth of hard bones and teeth.
   - B. manufacture of insulin.
   - C. development of respiratory enzymes.
   - D. formation of hemoglobin.

3. Phenylketonuria is a genetic disorder that involves an inability of
   - A. blood to clot properly.
   - B. one amino acid to be converted to another.
   - C. blood cells to carry a sufficient load of oxygen.
   - D. lung alveoli to stay open.

4. A new drug for treatment of tuberculosis was being tested in a hospital. Patients in group A received doses of the new drug; those in group B were given only sugar pills. Group B represents a(n)
   - A. scientific experiment.
   - B. scientific method.
   - C. experimental error.
   - D. experimental control.

5. Which is most closely associated with the process of transpiration?
   - A. Spiracles of a grasshopper
   - B. Root of a geranium
   - C. Leaf of a maple
   - D. Gills of a fish

6. Which term includes all the others?
   - A. Organ
   - B. Tissue
   - C. System
   - D. Organism

7. When several drops of pasteurized milk were placed in a petri dish containing sterilized nutrient agar, many colonies developed. This experiment shows the milk
   - A. contained some bacteria.
   - B. contained harmful bacteria.
   - C. should have been sterilized.
   - D. was incorrectly stamped "pasteurized."

8. The growth of green plants toward light is related most specifically to the distribution of _____ in the plant.
   - A. minerals
   - B. enzymes
   - C. auxins
   - D. amino acids

9. In humans, the digestion of carbohydrates begins in the
   - A. stomach.
   - B. small intestine.
   - C. mouth.
   - D. liver.

10. To determine whether an unknown black guinea pig is pure or hybrid black, it should be crossed with

   A. a white guinea pig.

   B. a hybrid black guinea pig.

   C. a pure black guinea pig.

   D. another unknown.

11. Photosynthesis is a cellular process that

   A. is an exergonic reaction.

   B. produces simple sugar and O_2.

   C. is initiated by chemical energy.

   D. produces CO_2 and H_2O.

12. The principal way in which forests help to prevent soil erosion is that the

   A. trees provide homes for wildlife.

   B. leaves of the trees manufacture food.

   C. forest floors absorb water.

   D. forest shields the soil from the sun's heat.

13. Which factor in the environment of an organism causes it to react?

   A. A stimulus

   B. A response

   C. A reflex

   D. An impulse

14. A breeder wanted to develop a strain of beef cattle with high-quality meat and the ability to thrive in a hot, dry climate. How can the breeder best accomplish this?

   A. Continued selection among the members of a prize herd

   B. Crossbreeding followed by selection

   C. Inbreeding to bring out desirable hidden traits

   D. Inbreeding followed by selection

15. The inhaling and exhaling of air by the human lungs is mainly an application of

   A. Boyle's Law—the inverse relationship between the pressure and the volume of a gas.

   B. the volume of a gas at standard temperature and pressure (STP).

   C. Charles' Law—the direct relationship between the temperature and the volume of a gas.

   D. the number of O_2 and CO_2 particles per mole.

16. Which plant tissues are mostly concerned with storage?

   A. Phloem and xylem

   B. Phloem and cambium

   C. Palisade cells and epidermis

   D. Pith and spongy cells

17. Movement of a solute across a biological membrane from an area of high concentration to an area of low concentration occurs via

   A. osmosis.

   B. diffusion.

   C. active transport.

   D. inertia.

18. Which reagent should be used in the urine test for diabetes?

   A. Iodine

   B. Nitric acid

   C. Ammonia

   D. Benedict's solution

19. The major benefit of buffer systems is that they

   A. increase pH significantly.

   B. resist significant changes in pH.

   C. decrease pH significantly.

   D. None of the above

20. The Krebs cycle produces
    A. H_2O and NADH.
    B. CO_2 and H_2.
    C. pyruvic acid and lactic acid.
    D. amino acids.

21. The removal for microscopic examination of a small bit of living tissue from a patient is called
    A. a biopsy.
    B. surgery.
    C. a dissection.
    D. therapy.

22. The presence of which substance is most important for all cell activity?
    A. Light
    B. Carbon dioxide
    C. Water
    D. Chlorophyll

23. The end products of digestion that enter the lacteals are
    A. glucose.
    B. amino acids.
    C. minerals.
    D. fatty acids.

24. A student in the laboratory tossed two pennies from a container 100 times and recorded these results: both heads, 25; one head and one tail, 47; both tails, 28. Which cross between plants would result in approximately the same ratio?
    A. Aa × AA
    B. Aa × Aa
    C. AA × aa
    D. Aa × aa

25. In the following equation for photosynthesis, $CO_2 + H_2O \rightarrow C_6H_{12}O_6 + O_2$, the oxygen comes
    A. entirely from CO_2.
    B. from a simple sugar molecule.
    C. partially from CO_2 and H_2O.
    D. entirely from H_2O.

26. Tissue culture has been extensively used as a research method in all of the following fields of biological investigation EXCEPT:
    A. Photosynthesis
    B. Virology
    C. Development of nerve cells
    D. Experimental embryology

27. After each transfer of a culture of bacteria, the wire loop should be
    A. dipped into alcohol.
    B. held in a flame.
    C. dipped into liquid soap.
    D. washed repeatedly in water.

28. Identify the statement that is NOT true of cellular respiration.
    A. It is a downhill process.
    B. It occurs in both plant and animal cells.
    C. It uses CO_2 and H_2O for reactants.
    D. It is an exergonic process.

29. In which one of the following ways does combustion differ from cellular respiration?
    A. More heat is produced.
    B. More energy is wasted.
    C. It is less rapid.
    D. It occurs at a higher temperature.

30. Of the following, an enzyme responsible for the digestion of proteins is
    A. maltase.
    B. trypsin.
    C. ptyalin.
    D. steapsin.

31. Failure of blood to clot readily when exposed to air may be due to a(n)
    A. oversupply of erythrocytes.
    B. deficiency of leucocytes.
    C. overabundance of fibrin.
    D. inadequacy of thrombokinase.

32. Cone cells are most closely associated with the function of
    A. digestion.
    B. absorption.
    C. vision.
    D. secretion.

33. The part of the vertebrate eye that controls the amount of light entering the eye is the
    A. cornea.
    B. ciliary body.
    C. iris.
    D. conjunctiva.

34. Most of the carbon dioxide in the blood is carried in the
    A. liquid portion.
    B. leucocytes.
    C. erythrocytes.
    D. platelets.

35. Increased blood pressure may be brought about by excess secretion of
    A. thyroxin.
    B. insulin.
    C. ACTH.
    D. adrenaline.

36. Of the following, the plant hormone concerned with growth is
    A. auxin.
    B. estrogen.
    C. testosterone.
    D. ATP.

37. Bread mold resembles ferns in that both develop
    A. mycelia.
    B. hyphae.
    C. pinnules.
    D. spores.

38. Sap rises in woody stems because of root pressure and
    A. transpiration pull.
    B. enzyme action.
    C. molecular adhesion.
    D. photosynthesis.

39. Vascular tissues present in the body of a flowering plant are xylem and
    A. cambium.
    B. phloem.
    C. meristem.
    D. lenticels.

40. Stored food for the embryo of a bean seed is found in the
    A. plumule.
    B. hypocotyl.
    C. cotyledons.
    D. testa.

41. Which of the following is NOT a characteristic of cancer cells?
    A. High power for self-affinity
    B. Altered genetic material
    C. Uncontrolled division
    D. Loss of normal functions

42. In the structure of a flower, the stigma is most closely positioned to the
    A. style.
    B. ovary.
    C. sepal.
    D. ovule.

43. The basic structure of cell membranes is a
    A. protein bilayer.
    B. protein-impregnated phospholipid bilayer.
    C. carbohydrate bilayer.
    D. phospholipid bilayer.

44. When catalyzed by sucrase, sucrose decomposes to yield glucose + fructose. The reaction is
    A. fermentation.
    B. hydrolysis.
    C. denaturation.
    D. condensation.

45. Movement of particles across a biological membrane is enhanced by
    A. large particle size.
    B. lipid solubility.
    C. particle charge.
    D. lipophobic properties.

46. Carbohydrates are a combination of carbon, hydrogen, and oxygen in an approximate ratio of
    A. 2:1:2
    B. 3:2:1
    C. 1:2:1
    D. 1:1:1

47. Rod-shaped bacteria are classified as
    A. bacilli.
    B. cocci.
    C. vibrios.
    D. spirilla.

48. A stain used in classifying bacteria is
    A. Gram's.
    B. Wright's.
    C. Loeffler's.
    D. Giemsa.

49. A bacteriophage is a kind of
    A. enzyme.
    B. toxin.
    C. bacterium.
    D. virus.

50. Of the following, the marsupial native to the United States is the
    A. raccoon.
    B. wombat.
    C. opossum.
    D. armadillo.

51. The first fully terrestrial vertebrates were the
    A. amphibians.
    B. reptiles.
    C. birds.
    D. mammals.

52. Enzyme molecules are all of the following EXCEPT:
    A. Lipids
    B. Proteins
    C. Macromolecules
    D. Biological catalysts

53. The size of most eukaryotic cells is
    A. 0.1–1.0 microns.
    B. 10–100 microns.
    C. 1.0–10 microns.
    D. greater than 100 microns.

54. Sickle-cell anemia is a genetic disorder that involves an inability of

  A. erythrocytes to contain a sufficient amount of hemoglobin.

  B. bone marrow to produce a sufficient number of erythrocytes.

  C. bone marrow to produce erythrocytes of normal size.

  D. erythrocytes to carry a sufficient load of oxygen.

55. Of the following, a crustacean that lives on land is the

  A. centipede.

  B. millipede.

  C. sow bug.

  D. tick.

56. Where would you find a leucoplast?

  A. In a liver cell

  B. In white blood cell

  C. In a white potato

  D. In a bacterium

57. Of the following, the hydra is most closely related to

  A. coral.

  B. flatworm.

  C. sponge.

  D. roundworm.

58. The process responsible for the continuous removal of carbon dioxide from the atmosphere is

  A. respiration.

  B. metabolism.

  C. oxidation.

  D. photosynthesis.

59. Cytoplasmic structures that contain powerful hydrolysis enzymes, which could lead to cell destruction in the absence of surrounding membranes, are

  A. lysosomes.

  B. golgi.

  C. ribosomes.

  D. None of the above

60. If the carrying capacity (k-value) represents the maximum number of individuals of a species that a habitat can support, it suggests that the population

  A. is regulated by density-dependent factors.

  B. will ultimately become extinct.

  C. is regulated by density-independent factors.

  D. can increase at an exponential rate, indefinitely.

STOP

IF YOU FINISH BEFORE TIME IS CALLED, YOU MAY CHECK YOUR WORK ON THIS SECTION ONLY. DO NOT TURN TO ANY OTHER SECTION IN THE TEST.

TEST 4: CELLS, STRUCTURE, AND FUNCTION

34 Questions • 30 Minutes

Directions: Read each question carefully and consider all possible answers. When you have decided which choice is best, fill in the corresponding space on your answer sheet. There is only one best answer for each question.

1. Which movement requires carrier proteins but no direct cellular energy?
   A. Diffusion
   B. Osmosis
   C. Dialysis
   D. Facilitated diffusion

2. The polymerase chain reaction (PCR) technique is more efficient than cloning for copying large quantities of a gene because it is performed
   A. without DNA polymerase.
   B. in vitro.
   C. without primers.
   D. in vivo.

3. Which term denotes the movement of glucose molecules from an area of lower concentration to an area of higher concentration?
   A. Osmosis
   B. Diffusion
   C. Dialysis
   D. Active transport

4. You place a cell in a solution of substance x and water. Substance x is always present in the cell, but you do not know the concentration ratio in either case. The cell increases in size. What is the tonicity of the solution in which you placed the cell?
   A. Hypotonic
   B. Isotonic
   C. Hypertonic
   D. None of the above.

5. Substance x passes through a plasma membrane easily. What phrase best describes the probable nature of the substance?
   A. It is hydrophilic and nonpolar.
   B. It is hydrophobic and polar.
   C. It is hydrophilic and polar.
   D. It is hydrophobic and nonpolar.

6. Cells that contain more dissolved salts and sugars than the surrounding solution are called
   A. isotonic.
   B. hypertonic.
   C. hypotonic.
   D. osmosis.

7. Foods containing unsaturated fatty acids are healthier than those with saturated ones because they contain
   A. more hydrogen.
   B. less oxygen.
   C. more nitrogen.
   D. less hydrogen.

8. You are watching an amoeba engulf another organism. This process is an example of
   A. receptor-mediated endocytosis.
   B. facilitated transport.
   C. pinocytosis.
   D. phagocytosis.

9. The concentration of glucose in blood cells is lower than the concentration of glucose in liver cells. During active transport, glucose moves from blood cells into the liver. Which organelle would you expect to find in large numbers in the liver?

   A. Golgi bodies
   B. Endoplasmic reticulum
   C. Ribosomes
   D. Mitochondria

10. If a red blood cell is placed in sea water, it will be in what kind of solution?

   A. Isotonic
   B. Hypotonic
   C. Hypertonic
   D. Facilitated diffusion

11. *Plasmolysis* is a term describing

   A. cytoplasmic movement.
   B. cells that become turgid.
   C. cellular shrinkage, which occurs when cells are immersed in hypertonic solution.
   D. amoeboid movement.

12. The movement of substances from lesser concentration to higher concentration is called

   A. osmosis.
   B. diffusion.
   C. active transport.
   D. pinocytosis.

13. Which structure is present in both eukaryotic and prokaryotic cells?

   A. Membrane-bound nucleus
   B. Mitochondria
   C. Plastids
   D. Cell membrane

14. In photosynthesis, the reactants CO_2 and H_2O, in the presence of sunlight and chlorophyll, combine chemically to produce glucose and O_2. The O_2 comes from

   A. H_2O.
   B. CO_2.
   C. CO_2 and H_2O.
   D. N_2.

15. Which of the following organelles are found only in plants?

   A. Golgi apparatus
   B. Plasmodesmata
   C. Endoplasmic reticulum
   D. Mitochondria

16. Nerve cells transmit impulses by varying the permeability of their membranes primarily to

   A. Na^+ and K^+.
   B. Cl^- and K^+.
   C. Na^+ and Cl^-.
   D. K^+ and Mg^{++}.

17. As you try to mix water and oil in your salad dressing, they do not mix because

   A. water is hydrophilic, and oil is hydrophobic.
   B. water is polar, and oil is nonpolar.
   C. both are hydrophilic.
   D. None of the above

18. Plant cells differ from animal cells in that plant cells

   A. have a glycoprotein covering their plasma membrane.
   B. have a cell wall and animal cells do not.
   C. have mitochondria and animal cells do not.
   D. do not have a nucleus.

19. Which cell type is characterized by the lack of a true nucleus and the absence of membrane-bound organelles?

   A. Animal cell type

   B. Plant cell type

   C. Fungal cell type

   D. Prokaryotic cell

20. The cytoskeleton within the cell is thought to function

   A. in a structural capacity.

   B. in positioning certain enzymes in close proximity for increased efficiency.

   C. as a means of enhancing secretion of metabolites within the cell.

   D. Both A and B

21. Which organelle is associated with hydrolytic enzymes and is sometimes referred to as a "suicide bag"?

   A. Golgi apparatus

   B. Lysosome

   C. Mitochondrion

   D. Ribosome

Questions 22 and 23 refer to the following structural formula.

$$H_2N - \underset{\underset{H}{|}}{\overset{\overset{H}{|}}{C}} - COOH$$

22. This compound is an

   A. amino acid.

   B. aldehyde.

   C. alpha-keto acid.

   D. alcohol.

23. In human digestion, this compound is the end product of

   A. fats.

   B. vitamins.

   C. proteins.

   D. carbohydrates.

24. The virus belongs to which one of the following kingdoms?

   A. Eubacteria

   B. Plantae

   C. Protista

   D. None of the above

25. Pinocytosis is the process of

   A. enclosing a food source or other substance in a membrane and bringing it into a cell.

   B. enclosing a liquid substance in a membrane and bringing it into the cell.

   C. enclosing a manufactured substance in a membrane and secreting it from the cell.

   D. binding a substance and a receptor and bringing it into the cell.

26. The AIDS virus is transported in bodily fluids. The US Surgeon General sends out information about the disease and its transmission. In one section, there is a recommendation that one should use latex (a form of plastic) condoms rather than those made of natural membranes. This recommendation is probably based upon the principal of

   A. diffusion.

   B. facilitated transport.

   C. active transport.

   D. varied selectivity, permeability of membranes.

27. The plasma membrane of the eukaryotic cell determines selectively which substances can enter and leave the cell. Such a membrane is said to be

   A. impermeable.

   B. selectively permeable.

   C. isotonic.

   D. hypotonic.

28. What primarily determines the shape of cells that lack cell walls?

A. Microtubules and microfilaments

B. Nucleus

C. Endoplasmic reticulum (ER)

D. Ribosomes

29. Which pair of organelles is responsible for energy supply to eukaryotic cells?

A. Ribosomes and mitochondria

B. Chloroplasts and mitochondria

C. Nuclei and ribosomes

D. Mitochondria and nuclei

Questions 30 and 31 relate to the following equation and graph of an enzyme-catalyzed cellular reaction.

30. The linear distance between P_1 and P_2 on the graph shown is the initial velocity of the reaction, as expressed by the slope (m) of the line (see the formula shown), which is

A. 60.

B. 10.

C. 40.

D. 6.

31. Choose the correct statement, relative to 10 minutes of reaction time.

A. The enzyme has been denatured.

B. All ES has been converted to [P].

C. All enzyme [E] is occupied with substrate [S].

D. All product has been converted to substrate.

32. You collect some pond water and filter out the different organisms into separate jars. You add no food to the water, but one kind of organism is still alive long after the others have died. That species is best described as being

A. autotrophic.

B. hydrophilic.

C. autonomous.

D. heterotrophic.

33. With which organelle is the synthesis of ATP associated?

A. Ribosome

B. Plastid

C. Mitochondrion

D. Lysosome

34. The plasma membrane is soluble to
    A. lipids.
    B. proteins.
    C. acids.
    D. nucleic acids.

STOP

IF YOU FINISH BEFORE TIME IS CALLED, YOU MAY CHECK YOUR WORK ON THIS SECTION ONLY. DO NOT TURN TO ANY OTHER SECTION IN THE TEST.

TEST 5: BIOLOGY

18 Questions • 15 Minutes

> **Directions:** Read each question carefully and consider all possible answers. When you have decided which choice is best, fill in the corresponding space on your answer sheet. There is only one best answer for each question.

1. The process whereby muscle cells produce lactic acid is called

    A. aerobic respiration.

    B. glycolysis.

    C. fermentation.

    D. electron transport chain.

2. Aerobic respiration can produce up to _____ with a single molecule of glucose.

    A. 2 ATP

    B. 22 ATP

    C. 32 ATP

    D. 38 ATP

$\Delta G = \Delta H - T\Delta S$

In cellular metabolism, the energy available for doing biological work is called free energy (G). It is equal to the molecular energy, enthalpy (H) minus the disorder, entropy (S) times the absolute temperature (T).

3. Choose the correct statement describing reaction I.

    A. The reaction is exergonic.

    B. ΔG is negative.

    C. Glucose and O_2 have less energy than CO_2 and H_2O.

    D. The reaction is endergonic.

4. Choose the correct statement describing reaction II.

    A. ΔG is positive.

    B. CO_2 and H_2O have more energy than glucose and O_2.

    C. The reaction is exergonic.

    D. The reaction is endergonic.

5. In exergonic reactions, the energy is

    A. used.

    B. stored.

    C. released.

    D. lost.

6. Most human enzymes function best in the temperature range of

    A. 5–15°C.

    B. 20–30°C.

    C. 35–40°C.

    D. 45–50°C.

7. Vitamins are important to the human diet because they are incorporated into

    A. enzyme substitutes.

    B. ATP.

    C. co-enzymes.

    D. inhibitors.

8. Stored energy is referred to as

    A. activation energy.

    B. kinetic energy.

    C. potential energy.

    D. electrical energy.

9. Noncyclic-photophosphorylation takes place inside the
   A. stroma.
   B. cytoplasm.
   C. thylakoids.
   D. Golgi bodies.

10. The products of the light reaction of photosynthesis are
    A. carbohydrate + CO_2.
    B. $NADPH_2$ + ATP + O_2.
    C. PGAL + CO_2 + H_2O.
    D. starch + CO_2.

11. The dark reaction of photosynthesis takes place in
    A. thylakoids.
    B. cytoplasm.
    C. stroma.
    D. grana.

12. Aerobic cellular respiration is more important to sustaining life than anaerobic because it produces more
    A. pyruvic acid.
    B. sugar.
    C. energy.
    D. lactic acid.

13. Which organelle is responsible for oxygen production?
    A. Mitochondria
    B. Cilia
    C. Golgi body
    D. Chloroplasts

14. An organic catalyst that enhances the chemical reaction is called a(n)
    A. fat.
    B. lactic acid.
    C. polysaccharide.
    D. enzyme.

15. The first stage of aerobic cellular respiration is
    A. electron transport chain.
    B. Krebs cycle.
    C. glycolysis.
    D. light reaction.

16. Glycolysis occurs in the
    A. nucleus.
    B. mitochondrion.
    C. plasma membrane.
    D. cytoplasm.

17. For the aerobic pathway, electron transport systems are located in the
    A. cytoplasm.
    B. Golgi bodies.
    C. lysosomes.
    D. mitochondrion.

18. Aerobic oxidation of glucose occurs in which two major stages?
    A. Glycolysis and reduction.
    B. Synthesis and the Krebs cycle.
    C. Glycolysis and the Krebs cycle.
    D. Degradation and hydrolysis.

STOP

IF YOU FINISH BEFORE TIME IS CALLED, YOU MAY
CHECK YOUR WORK ON THIS SECTION ONLY. DO NOT
TURN TO ANY OTHER SECTION IN THE TEST.

TEST 6: BIOLOGY

20 Questions • 15 Minutes

> **Directions:** Read each question carefully and consider all possible answers. When you have decided which choice is best, fill in the corresponding space on your answer sheet. There is only one best answer for each question.

1. If body cells of cows contain a total of 40 chromosomes, sperm and egg cells of cows contain how many chromosomes total?
   - A. 10
   - B. 20
   - C. 25
   - D. 40

2. Codominance occurs when
   - A. both the alleles in a heterozygote are expressed phenotypically in an individual.
   - B. expression of two different alleles alternates from one generation to the next.
   - C. a heterozygote expresses an intermediate phenotype.
   - D. offspring exhibit several different phenotypic expressions of a single trait.

3. Mitosis in a single human cell usually results in the formation of
   - A. two diploid cells.
   - B. two haploid cells.
   - C. four diploid cells.
   - D. four haploid cells.

4. Meiosis in a single human cell usually results in the formation of
   - A. two diploid cells.
   - B. two haploid cells.
   - C. four diploid cells.
   - D. four haploid cells.

5. If you reproduce sexually, you produce gametes via
   - A. fertilization.
   - B. mitosis.
   - C. meiosis.
   - D. recombination.

6. An organism that reproduces asexually produces offspring via
   - A. fertilization.
   - B. mitosis.
   - C. meiosis.
   - D. recombination.

7. According to Mendel's Law of Segregation, an organism with the genotype Aa
   - A. produces gametes containing only the A allele.
   - B. produces gametes containing only the a allele.
   - C. half the time produces gametes containing A, and half the time containing a.
   - D. three quarters of the time produces gametes containing A, and one quarter of the time containing a.

8. What type of allele is expressed in the phenotype of only a homozygous individual?
   - A. Incompletely dominant
   - B. Haploid
   - C. Recessive
   - D. Dominant

9. The sex of a human child is determined by the sex chromosome from
   A. the mother.
   B. the father.
   C. both parents.
   D. neither parents.

10. Cell division occurs most rapidly in
    A. heart tissue.
    B. muscle tissue.
    C. nervous tissue.
    D. cancerous tissue.

11. If the sperm cells of a fish have 30 chromosomes, the body cell of the fish has
    A. 80 chromosomes.
    B. 60 chromosomes.
    C. 120 chromosomes.
    D. None of the above

12. A condition resulting from the presence of an extra twenty-first chromosome is
    A. hemophilia.
    B. the Rh-positive condition.
    C. phenylketonuria.
    D. Down syndrome.

13. A woman who is a heterozygous carrier for a sex-linked recessive gene will pass it to
    A. all of her sons.
    B. all of her daughters.
    C. all children.
    D. one-half of her sons and one-half of her daughters.

14. Which of the following is an example of a sex-linked genetic disorder?
    A. Tay-Sachs disease
    B. Cystic fibrosis
    C. Turner's syndrome
    D. Hemophilia

15. In the case of the sex-linked trait red-green color blindness, which one of the following CANNOT occur?
    A. A carrier mother passing the gene on to her son
    B. A carrier mother passing the gene on to her daughter
    C. A color-blind father passing the gene on to his son
    D. A color-blind father passing the gene on to his daughter

16. The genotype for a man who has blue eyes and hemophilia is
    A. $x^b y\, x^h y$
    B. bb hh
    C. bb $x^h y$
    D. Bbh

17. Which blood type would be a universal donor?
    A. A
    B. AB
    C. B
    D. O

18. Males who tend to be abnormally tall, have severe acne, and are poorly coordinated have which of the following sex chromosomes?
    A. XXY
    B. XY
    C. XYY
    D. XYXY

19. The Central Dogma of molecular biology states that information is passed in what sequence?
    A. RNA to proteins to DNA
    B. DNA to RNA to proteins
    C. Proteins to RNA to DNA
    D. RNA to DNA to proteins

20. The end products of the Krebs cycle are
    A. carbon dioxide and water.
    B. urea and bile pigments.
    C. lactic acid and pyruvic acid.
    D. ketones and acetones.

STOP

IF YOU FINISH BEFORE TIME IS CALLED, YOU MAY
CHECK YOUR WORK ON THIS SECTION ONLY. DO NOT
TURN TO ANY OTHER SECTION IN THE TEST.

TEST 7: CHEMISTRY

20 Questions • 15 Minutes

Directions: Read each question carefully and consider all possible answers. When you have decided which choice is best, fill in the corresponding space on your answer sheet. There is only one best answer for each question.

1. A high concentration of H^+ ions is characteristic of
   A. high pH.
   B. strong acid.
   C. alkaline base.
   D. Both A and C

2. Long chains of glucose molecules are involved in the structure of
   A. proteins.
   B. fats.
   C. cholesterol.
   D. polysaccharides.

3. When a solution has a pH of 7, it is
   A. a strong base.
   B. a strong acid.
   C. a weak base.
   D. neutral.

4. Which one of the following is NOT a carbohydrate?
   A. Maltose
   B. Cellulose
   C. Glycogen
   D. Cholesterol

5. An example of an organic compound is
   A. water (H_2O).
   B. ammonia (NH_3).
   C. salt (NaCl).
   D. glucose ($C_6H_{12}O_6$).

6. A covalent bond is believed to be caused by
   A. the transfer of electrons.
   B. the sharing of electrons.
   C. the release of energy.
   D. None of the above

7. An atom has the electron configuration (2-8-8-2). This atom would tend to
   A. gain electrons.
   B. lose two electrons.
   C. be inert.
   D. None of the above

8. Which of the following is a disaccharide?
   A. Glucose
   B. Maltose
   C. Fructose
   D. Chilin

9. Which one of the following is NOT a carbohydrate?
   A. Maltose
   B. Cellulose
   C. Glycogen
   D. Wax

10. The basic building blocks of proteins are
    A. polypeptides.
    B. glucose.
    C. amino acids.
    D. None of the above

11. If the atomic number of magnesium is 12, how many protons will its nucleus contain?
    A. 6
    B. 10
    C. 14
    D. 12

12. Which is an inert element?
    A. Hydrogen
    B. Neon
    C. Oxygen
    D. Nitrogen

13. Atoms are electrically neutral. This means that an atom will contain
    A. more protons than neutrons.
    B. more electrons than protons.
    C. an equal number of protons and electrons.
    D. None of the above

14. Which is true of alkaline solutions?
    A. More H^+ ion than OH ion
    B. Same amount of H^+ ion + OH^- ion
    C. More OH^- ion than H^+ ion
    D. None of the above

15. A common detergent has pH 11.0, so the detergent is
    A. neutral.
    B. acidic.
    C. alkaline.
    D. None of the above

16. The basic building block of carbohydrate is
    A. starch.
    B. chitin.
    C. sucrose.
    D. glucose.

17. The number of different amino acids used to create proteins in humans is
    A. 20.
    B. 26.
    C. 50.
    D. 92.

18. A nucleotide is composed of a
    A. phospholipid, sugar, and base.
    B. phosphate, sugar, and base.
    C. phosphate, protein, and base.
    D. phospholipid, sugar, and protein.

19. Polar bonds form when
    A. electrons are shared unequally between atoms.
    B. more than one pair of electrons is shared.
    C. ions are formed.
    D. an acid and base are combined.

20. Completion of the human genome project gave further proof that genes are
    A. nucleic acid.
    B. phospholipids.
    C. protein.
    D. protein and nucleic acid.

STOP

IF YOU FINISH BEFORE TIME IS CALLED, YOU MAY CHECK YOUR WORK ON THIS SECTION ONLY. DO NOT TURN TO ANY OTHER SECTION IN THE TEST.

TEST 8: CHEMISTRY AND PHYSICAL SCIENCE

50 Questions • 45 Minutes

Directions: Read each question carefully and consider all possible answers. When you have decided which choice is best, fill in the corresponding space on your answer sheet. There is only one best answer for each question.

---

1. The compound that has the greatest polarity is
   A. $CH_3—CH_2—O—CH_2—CH_3$.
   B. $CH_3—CH_2CH_2CH_2—CH_3$.
   C. $CH_3—CH_2—CH_2—CH_2—CH_2—Cl$.
   D. $CH_3—CH_2—CH_2—CH_2—CH_2—OH$.

2. In a film camera, the image from a lens that is imprinted on the film by comparison with the original subject is
   A. right side up and reversed from left to right.
   B. upside down and reversed from left to right.
   C. right side up and not reversed from left to right.
   D. upside down and not reversed from left to right.

3. The sugar with the highest molecular weight of those listed is
   A. fructose.
   B. sucrose.
   C. glucose.
   D. None of the above. All have the same molecular weight.

4. A hydride ion and a hydrogen atom both have
   A. the same number of electrons.
   B. the same charge.
   C. the same number of protons.
   D. equal atomic radii.

5. The general formula for an aldehyde is
   A. RCOOH.
   B. RCOOR.
   C. ROH.
   D. RCHO.

6. The compound that will NOT be acidic when dissolved in water is
   A. HBr.
   B. N_2O_5.
   C. CaO.
   D. NH_4Cl.

7. Atoms that have the same atomic number but different atomic masses
   A. are from different elements.
   B. are isobars.
   C. have different numbers of electrons.
   D. are isotopes.

8. When electrolysis is done with molten NaCl, the substance produced at the anode is
   A. chlorine.
   B. hydrogen.
   C. sodium.
   D. oxygen.

9. The non-electrolyte in the following group is
   A. acetic acid.
   B. calcium chloride.
   C. sodium bromide.
   D. sugar.

10. Rubbing alcohol is
   A. methyl alcohol.
   B. ethyl alcohol.
   C. phenol.
   D. isopropyl alcohol.

11. Which of the following elements is a transition element?
   A. Argon
   B. Copper
   C. Barium
   D. Aluminum

12. When calcium reacts with chlorine to form calcium chloride, it
   A. shares two electrons.
   B. gains two electrons.
   C. loses two electrons.
   D. gains one electron.

13. The compound NaClO is called
   A. sodium perchlorate.
   B. sodium oxychloride.
   C. sodium chlorate.
   D. sodium hypochlorite.

14. Reaction kinetics deals with
   A. equilibrium position.
   B. reaction rates.
   C. molecular reactant size.
   D. None of the above

15. A 1-molar solution of potassium phosphate (K_3PO_4) contains in 1 liter
   A. one mole of potassium ions.
   B. one mole of oxygen atoms.
   C. one mole of phosphorus atoms.
   D. no ions.

16. In the compound propene, $H_2C=CH—CH_3$, the single bond between two carbon atoms is
   A. stronger than the double bond.
   B. shorter than the double bond.
   C. equal to the double bond in bond strength.
   D. longer than the double bond.

Questions 17 and 18 refer to the diagram below.

The boulder at the top of an inclined plane has potential energy, E_p = mgh, and if it rolls down the plane, the energy becomes kinetic, $E_k = \frac{1}{2}mV^2$. Therefore, mgh = $\frac{1}{2}mV^2$.

17. Choose the correct formula for calculating the boulder's velocity when it reaches position 2.
   A. $V = \sqrt{2gh}$
   B. $V = 2gh$
   C. $V = mgh^2$
   D. $V = \sqrt{mg^2h}$

18. The expression mgh = $\frac{1}{2}mV^2$ represents
   A. conservation of momentum.
   B. constancy of velocity.
   C. variability of acceleration.
   D. conservation of energy.

19. For a molecular substance, a gram formula weight
    A. is unrelated to the gram molecular weight.
    B. is always equal to the mass corresponding to its empirical formula.
    C. can always be calculated from its empirical formula alone.
    D. is identical to its gram molecular weight.

20. If gas A has a molecular weight four times that of gas B, the average speed of gas
    A. A is about four times that of gas B.
    B. B is about four times that of gas A.
    C. A is about twice that of gas B.
    D. B is about twice that of gas A.

21. Ice can be melted most effectively by _____ if 1 mole is used.
    A. sucrose
    B. calcium chloride
    C. sodium chloride
    D. methanol

22. Per atom, an element that has an atomic number of 19 contains
    A. 19 electrons and 19 neutrons.
    B. 19 electrons and 19 protons.
    C. 19 protons and 19 neutrons.
    D. a total of 19 protons and neutrons.

23. In a volume of air at one atmosphere pressure at sea level, the partial pressure of nitrogen will be about
    A. 490 mm of mercury.
    B. 760 mm of mercury.
    C. 106 mm of mercury.
    D. 608 mm of mercury.

24. If the stirring of a solution results in precipitation of solute with no change in temperature, the solution must have been
    A. saturated.
    B. concentrated.
    C. dilute.
    D. supersaturated.

25. If the reaction $A + B \rightarrow C + D$ is designated as first order, the rate depends on
    A. the concentration of only one reactant.
    B. the concentration of each reactant.
    C. no specific concentration.
    D. the temperature only.

26. The loss of an alpha particle from the radioactive atom $\frac{228}{88}$ would leave
    A. $\frac{224}{86}$ Rn
    B. $\frac{222}{86}$ Rn
    C. $\frac{224}{88}$ Ra
    D. $\frac{230}{90}$ Th

27. Which of the following is NOT a form of radioactive decay?
    A. Electron capture
    B. Beta emission
    C. Alpha emission
    D. Proton emission

28. The greatest amount of energy would be produced by the burning of 1 gram of
    A. fat.
    B. carbohydrate.
    C. protein.
    D. ribonucleic acid.

29. The number of degrees on the Fahrenheit thermometer between the freezing point and the boiling point of water is
   A. 100.
   B. 180.
   C. 212.
   D. 273.

30. Carbon-14 has a half-life of 5.73×10 years. If a sample contained 1 gram of C-14, the time required to decay to only 0.0625 g would be
   A. 11.46×10 years.
   B. 5.73×10 years.
   C. 22.92×10 years.
   D. None of the above

31. The oxidation number of Mn in the compound K_2MnO_4 is
   A. +7.
   B. +2.
   C. 0.
   D. +6.

32. The element with the highest ionization energy of those following is
   A. Mg.
   B. Sr.
   C. Ca.
   D. Ba.

33. The LEAST electronegative of the following elements is
   A. Cl.
   B. F.
   C. Br.
   D. I.

34. The element with the smallest atomic radius of the following is
   A. Sr.
   B. Mg.
   C. Ba.
   D. Ra.

35. Which of the following salts would be more soluble in 1.0 M acid than in pure water?
   A. KCl
   B. $CaCO_3$
   C. $CaCl_2$
   D. KNO_3

36. Which of the following is NOT an acid/conjugate base pair?
   A. HCN/CN
   B. H_2CO_3/OH^-
   C. H_2SO_4/HSO_4^-
   D. $H_3PO_4/H_2PO_4^-$

37. In a titration of 40.0 ml of 0.20 M NaOH with 0.4 M HCl, what will be the final volume of the solution when the sodium hydroxide is completely neutralized?
   A. 42 ml
   B. 20 ml
   C. 60 ml
   D. 80 ml

38. When dissolved in water to form 0.2 M solutions, which of the following would have the highest pH?
   A. The salt of a strong acid
   B. A weak acid
   C. The ammonium salt of a strong acid
   D. The sodium salt of a weak acid

39. Consider the reaction $N_2(g) + 3H_2(g) \rightarrow 2NH_3(g)$ + heat. Indicate the incorrect statement.
   A. An increase in temperature will shift the equilibrium to the right.
   B. An increase in pressure applied will shift the equilibrium to the right.
   C. The addition of ammonia will shift the equilibrium to the left.
   D. The addition of H_2 will shift the equilibrium to the right.

40. All of the following are colligative properties of solutions EXCEPT:
    A. Vapor pressure
    B. Osmotic pressure
    C. Density
    D. Boiling point elevation

41. Which of the following statements is incorrect?
    A. London dispersion forces are among those binding the units of molecular solids.
    B. Molten ionic compounds are conductors of electricity.
    C. Molecular solids have high melting points.
    D. Molecular solids are non-conductors.

42. One is most likely to feel the effects of static electricity on a
    A. cold, damp day.
    B. cold, dry day.
    C. warm, humid day.
    D. warm, dry day.

43. In a cubic lattice, an atom lying at the corner of a unit cell is shared by how many unit cells?
    A. 2
    B. 4
    C. 8
    D. 12

44. On the basis of the following boiling point data, which of the following liquids would be expected to have the highest vapor pressure at room temperature?

	SUBSTANCE	BOILING POINT
A.	acetone	56.2°C
B.	ethanol	78.5°C
C.	water	100°C
D.	ethylene glycol	198°C

45. $\frac{34}{17}$ Cl has
    A. 17 protons, 17 electrons, and 17 neutrons.
    B. 17 protons, 19 electrons, and 17 neutrons.
    C. 17 protons, 18 electrons, and 17 neutrons.
    D. 34 protons, 34 electrons, and 17 neutrons.

46. Which of the following arrangements gives the correct trend of electronegativity?
    A. $I < Br < Cl < F$
    B. $Sr < Ca < Ra < Mg$
    C. $Al > Si > P > S$
    D. $Na < K < Li < H$

47. The number of unpaired electrons in the outer subshell of a phosphorus atom (atomic number: 15) is
    A. 2.
    B. 0.
    C. 3.
    D. 1.

48. An atom that has five 3p electrons in its ground state is
    A. Si.
    B. P.
    C. Cl.
    D. O.

49. The density of gold (Au) is 19.3g/cm³ and that of iron (Fe) is 7.9g/cm³. A comparison of the volumes (V) of 50-gram samples of each metal would show that
    A. $V_{Au} = V_{Fe}$.
    B. $V_{Au} < V_{Fe}$.
    C. $V_{Au} > V_{Fe}$.
    D. There is no predictable relationship between volumes.

50. Consider three 1-liter flasks at STP. Flask A contains NO gas; Flask B contains NH_3 gas; and Flask C contains N_2 gas. Which flask contains the greatest number of atoms?

   A. Flask A

   B. Flask B

   C. Flask C

   D. All contain the same number of atoms.

STOP

IF YOU FINISH BEFORE TIME IS CALLED, YOU MAY CHECK YOUR WORK ON THIS SECTION ONLY. DO NOT TURN TO ANY OTHER SECTION IN THE TEST.

ANSWER KEYS AND EXPLANATIONS

Test 1: Chemistry and Physics

1. A	14. C	27. A	40. A	53. A
2. A	15. C	28. A	41. A	54. C
3. A	16. C	29. C	42. B	55. B
4. A	17. B	30. B	43. D	56. B
5. A	18. A	31. A	44. B	57. C
6. D	19. C	32. B	45. D	58. C
7. D	20. A	33. C	46. D	59. A
8. D	21. A	34. C	47. C	60. D
9. A	22. C	35. C	48. D	61. D
10. D	23. B	36. B	49. D	62. D
11. D	24. A	37. A	50. B	63. C
12. D	25. A	38. A	51. D	64. B
13. D	26. A	39. B	52. C	65. A

1. **The correct answer is A.** Heating water to a very high temperature (about 2,000°C) will cause only about 2% of the water to dissociate into hydrogen and oxygen— not a very economical or efficient way of obtaining oxygen. Electrolysis will decompose water at a much lower temperature. Hydrogen peroxide and many oxides or metals can be decomposed more easily by heating alone.

2. **The correct answer is A.** All acids contain hydrogen, which may be displaced by certain metals. However, copper ranks below hydrogen in the electromotive or activity series. *Activity* refers to the activity of a metal in displacing hydrogen in acids and in water. Metals ranked below hydrogen in the series do not displace hydrogen from acids.

3. **The correct answer is A.** Scalar quantities have only magnitude; vectors have magnitude and direction.

4. **The correct answer is A.** The problem can be solved by using the formula: $c = Q/$ $M\Delta T$. Inasmuch as Q, M, D, and T are given, no algebraic rearrangement is necessary to solve for c (specific heat).

5. **The correct answer is A.** Ozone is a molecule variety of oxygen in which three oxygen atoms bond to make one molecule of O_3. Ozone is easily formed by the action of electricity or ultraviolet radiation on the normal diatomic form (O_2) of oxygen.

6. **The correct answer is D.** Since there is twice as much hydrogen as there is oxygen in a molecule of water (H_2O), the 26 milliliters of hydrogen could combine with only 13 milliliters of oxygen. This would leave 11 of the 24 milliliters of oxygen uncombined.

7. **The correct answer is D.** Hydrochloric acid reacts with active metals, forming the chloride of that metal and releasing hydrogen.

8. **The correct answer is D.** Inasmuch as 100 milligrams will decay to 50.0 milligrams, the formula $K = \dfrac{0.693}{t_{\frac{1}{2}}}$ should

be algebraically rearranged to solve for $t_{\frac{1}{2}}$ (half-life).

To do this, multiply both sides by $t_{\frac{1}{2}}$ and divide both sides by K.

9. **The correct answer is A.** The percentage composition of oxygen in 1 mole of glucose (180 grams) is calculated as follows

Atomic Mass				No. of Atoms
Carbon 12	×	6	=	72
Hydrogen 1	×	12	=	12
Oxygen 16	×	6	=	96
				180

% Comp. $O_2 = \dfrac{96}{180} \times 100 \approx 53$

10. **The correct answer is D.** Sulfuric acid (H_2SO_4) contains four oxygens, each with a valence of -2; the total negative valence is 8. Each of the two hydrogens has a valence of $+1$; the total hydrogen valence equals $+2$. Therefore, sulfur would need a valence of $+6$ to equalize the positive and negative valences in the molecule.

11. **The correct answer is D.** Fractional distillation can be used to separate the components of a mixture; the mixture is heated to boiling and the temperature is constantly raised. The component with the lowest boiling point vaporizes first; the component with the highest boiling point will vaporize last. Liquid oxygen has a boiling point of $-183°C$, which is higher than the boiling point of the other components; therefore, oxygen will boil off last.

12. **The correct answer is D.** Only one substance (HCl) is dissociated; therefore, the reaction is a single displacement.

13. **The correct answer is D.** Free carbon dioxide and water will combine to produce carbonic acid (H_2CO_3). Different reactants would be needed to produce ozone (O_3), methane (CH_4), or hydrogen peroxide (H_2O_2).

14. **The correct answer is C.** In a cathode ray tube, such as those found in television sets (i.e., picture tube), a cathode (negative terminal) and an anode (positive terminal) are present. There is no material between the two through which electricity (electrons) can flow from one terminal to another: in other words, a vacuum exists in the tube. A heated cathode generates electrons, which become excited by heat and can acquire enough energy to leave the cathode. Once they do, they are attracted to the anode because of the difference in charges (electrons have a negative charge) and flow across the gap toward the anode. In other appliances, the material through which the electricity flows may produce some resistance; in a picture tube, the electrons are flowing across a space in a vacuum and encounter no resistance.

15. **The correct answer is C.** $NaHCO_3$ will combine with HCl (hydrochloric acid) to form NaCl and H_2CO_3. H_2CO_3 is a weaker acid than HCl; therefore, the net effect of replacing HCl molecules with H_2CO_3 molecules is to raise the pH of the solution. In causing this reaction, $NaHCO_3$ is acting as a buffer. NaCl is a salt that will have no effect on the pH of an HCl solution. The other two compounds are acids that would lower the pH of the solution further if added.

16. **The correct answer is C.** Litmus turns red in acid solution. When phosphorus trioxide dissolves in water, phosphorus acid is formed. The other compounds named form alkaline solutions.

17. **The correct answer is B.** The 50 mL of a 1.0 M NaOH solution required to neutralize an unknown amount of H_2SO_4 contains 0.05 moles of NaOH. Since each mole of H_2SO_4 has two protons that are neutralized in the reaction, the number of moles of H_2SO_4 in the 100 mL solution is

0.05 divided by 2 = 0.025 moles of H_2SO_4. Since molarity is the number of moles per 1,000 mL and we have 0.025 moles H_2SO_4 per 100 mL, multiply 0.025 moles times 10, which equals 0.25 moles per liter, or 0.25 M.

18. **The correct answer is A.** Zinc is ranked above the others but below aluminum in the activity series of metals. The higher the metal is ranked, the more energetic it is in its displacement ability. Therefore, aluminum could displace zinc in the zinc chloride solution, forming aluminum chloride. For this reason, zinc chloride should not be stored in a tank made of aluminum because aluminum will displace the zinc in the zinc chloride.

19. **The correct answer is C.** The four oxygen ions would have a total *valence* of −8 (each oxygen, −2); if the valence of the SO_4 ion is −2, the remaining valence of 6 would be matched to a positive valence. Therefore, sulfur must have a valence of +6.

20. **The correct answer is A.** Sulfuric acid is composed of two hydrogen ions and one sulfate ion. The chemical formula is H_2SO_4; thus, its chemical name is hydrogen sulfate.

21. **The correct answer is A.** Magnesium has an atomic weight of 24; hydrogen's atomic weight is approximately 1. As is true with many metals, magnesium can react with an acid, such as hydrochloric acid, to produce hydrogen ($Mg + 2HCl \rightarrow MgCl_2 + H_2$). The amount of hydrogen produced can be calculated by using the following equation:

$$\frac{\text{amount Mg}}{\text{atomic weight}} = \frac{\text{amount } H_2}{\text{atomic weight}}$$

Substituting in the equation, we get the following:

$$\frac{6 \text{ grams}}{24} = \frac{x \text{ grams}}{2} = 0.5 \text{ grams}$$

In working out problems in which one must determine the amount of a substance derived from a given reaction, the chemical equation must be balanced, and molecular weight must be used. Thus, for diatomic gases, use twice the atomic weight.

22. **The correct answer is C.** Exergonic reactions are downhill reactions.

23. **The correct answer is B.** Sodium bisulfate differs from sodium sulfate in having hydrogen as a part of the molecule. Since the sulfate ion has a valence of −2, and hydrogen and sodium each have a valence of +1, then one sodium and one hydrogen must be in combination with the sulfate ion ($NaHSO_4$).

24. **The correct answer is A.** John Dalton discovered the facts concerning chemical combinations and suggested that materials are composed of atoms. He first proposed the law of multiple proportions in 1804. The law states that in a series of compounds formed by the same two or more elements, given a definite weight for one element, the different weights of the second element are in the ratio of small whole numbers to the weight of the first. For example, in sulfur dioxide (SO_2), the weight of oxygen is 32 (atomic weight = 16); in sulfur trioxide (SO_3), the weight of oxygen is 48. Therefore, the ratio is 2:3.

25. **The correct answer is A.** One mole (gram molecular weight) of a gas occupies 22.4 liters under standard conditions. Since 1 liter of the gas in question is $\frac{1}{22.4}$ of 1 mole, it is $\frac{1}{22.4}$ of its gram molecular weight. Knowing this, the molecular weight of the gas can be determined. We can set up the equation as follows:

$$\frac{x \text{ unknown gram mol. wt.}}{22.4 \text{ liters}} = \frac{1.16 \text{ grams}}{1 \text{ liters}}$$

Solving the equation, we get 26 as 1 gram molecular weight. C_2H_2 (ethane) fits this weight ($C = 12 \times 2$, $H = 1 \times 2$).

26. **The correct answer is A.** A salt is an ionic compound that yields ions other than hydrogen ions (H^+) or hydroxide ions (OH^-) when it dissociates. Na_2CO_3 will yield neither when it dissociates into $2\ Na^+ + CO_3(2^-)$. $Ca(OH)_2$ will yield hydroxide ions when it dissociates, and H_2CO_3 will yield hydrogen ions. CH_3OH is a covalent compound and will not dissociate.

27. **The correct answer is A.** Aromatic compounds are so named because of their odors; they occur in ring structure (molecular structure) and include such compounds as benzene, toluene, and xylene.

28. **The correct answer is A.** Dextrose is a monosaccharide, in that its molecule is composed of one "sugar unit" and cannot be hydrolyzed into simpler sugars. Lactose and sucrose are disaccharides, each yielding two monosaccharides by hydrolysis. Glycogen is a polysaccharide composed of a large number of monosaccharide units.

29. **The correct answer is C.** Fats are glyceryl esters that, when hydrolyzed, yield glycerol and fatty acids. The cleavage of the ester linkage upon hydrolysis can be achieved by saponification, acids, superheated steam, or lipase, which is an enzyme that hydrolyzes fats. This may be represented as follows: $RCOOR' + H_2O \rightarrow RCOOH + R'OH$.

30. **The correct answer is B.** As a rule, polar liquids dissolve in polar liquids and nonpolar liquids dissolve in nonpolar liquids. Water is polar, and oil is nonpolar. Therefore, oil and water are immiscible.

31. **The correct answer is A.** The bond formed between the carboxyl (RCOOH) and the amino ($R - (NH_2)$) of two amino acids is a peptide bond, and the resulting compound is a dipeptide.

32. **The correct answer is B.** The atomic number represents the number of protons within the nucleus of an atom. Since an atom is electrically neutral, the atomic number also equals the number of electrons of the atom. The atomic weight (mass number) represents the total number of nuclear particles (protons plus neutrons). All atoms of the same element have the same number of protons and, thus, the same atomic number. If the number of neutrons differ, the mass number is different; these atoms, then, are isotopes.

33. **The correct answer is C.** Calcium hypochlorite ($Ca(OCl)_2$) is effective as a bleach due to the oxidizing activity of hypochlorous acid (HClO), which is produced from calcium hypochloride, and from which chlorine gas can also be liberated.

34. **The correct answer is C.** An ionic bond will form between two atoms if the loss of electrons from one to the other will result in both atoms having a completely filled outer electron orbit. A sodium atom has 11 electrons—two in its first electron orbit, eight in its second electron orbit, and one in its outer electron orbit. The loss of one electron from the sodium atom will eliminate its outer electron orbit, making the next orbit in toward the nucleus the new outer orbit with a full complement of eight electrons. A chlorine atom has 17 electrons—two in its first electron orbit, eight in its second, and seven in its outer electron orbit. The acceptance of one electron by the chlorine atom will fill its outer electron orbit with the full complement of eight electrons.

35. **The correct answer is C.** Transition elements are characterized by their $4s$ electron shell being completely filled, but the $3d$

shell is not completely filled. Also known as transition metals, these elements are found between Groups 2 (metals) and 13 (nonmetals) in the periodic table. Nickel is classified as a transition metal.

36. **The correct answer is B.** The periodic table places elements according to similarities in properties due to the number and arrangement of electrons in the atom. Group 18 is the inert gases. Metals and nonmetals are included in the remaining groups.

37. **The correct answer is A.** Inert gases, such as neon, have a complete octet (eight electrons) in the outer shell of electrons.

38. **The correct answer is A.** Sodium (Na) and potassium (K) are both in group IA, with one electron in the outer energy level. Sodium and potassium have three and four energy levels, respectively.

39. **The correct answer is B.** Reactivity of elements in group IA increases from top to bottom because valence electrons are progressively further from the positive charges in the nucleus of atoms. Reactivity of elements in group VIIA increases from bottom to top because valence electrons are progressively closer to the positive charges of the nucleus.

40. **The correct answer is A.** Sodium (Na) is a metal in group IA, with 1.0 electron in its outermost shell. Its most stable configuration is achieved by donating 1.0 electron, resulting in a +1 valence.

41. **The correct answer is A.** Air is a mixture of gases; the gases present in greatest quantity are nitrogen and oxygen. The quantity of nitrogen in the air is almost four times that of oxygen. Of the compounds listed, methane (CH_4), with a molecular weight of 16, is lighter than air.

42. **The correct answer is B.** Carbon dioxide (CO_2) is an odorless gas in relatively low concentrations. High concentrations of carbon dioxide have an acidic odor.

43. **The correct answer is D.** The pressure of a gas is measured by the distance in millimeters (mm) that it will lift a column of mercury in a barometer. The pressure of air is 760 mm of mercury at sea level. Air is a mixture of gases, and the pressure of each gas in such a mixture, referred to as its partial pressure, is equal to its concentration in the mixture. Oxygen constitutes 21% of air; therefore, its partial pressure at sea level would be 21% of 760 mm of mercury of pressure, or 160 mm of mercury.

44. **The correct answer is B.** Carbon disulfide is highly flammable; its complete combustion yields carbon dioxide and sulfur dioxide.

$$CS_2 + 3O_2 \rightarrow CO_2 + 2SO_2$$

45. **The correct answer is D.** The ethyl alcohol of alcoholic beverages is produced by fermentation of monosaccharides; usually, yeast is used to supply the enzymes needed, and the fermentation process supplies the energy needed by the yeast.

$$C_6H_{12}O_6 \rightarrow 2\ C_2H_5OH + 2CO_2$$

46. **The correct answer is D.** Because fluorine is extremely active, it does not occur freely in nature but combines naturally with all elements except the inert gases, forming very stable compounds. Because it is a vigorous oxidizing agent, it cannot be oxidized by other oxidizing agents. For these reasons, fluorides are more difficult to decompose than are compounds of the other halogens.

47. **The correct answer is C.** A *ketone* is an organic molecule that contains a carbon atom double-bonded to an oxygen atom located between 2 other carbon atoms

$-C-C-C-$. The compound shown in choice A is an aldehyde because it contains a terminal CHO $-C\mathrel{\substack{H\\=}}O$ group. The compound shown in choice B is an alcohol because it contains an OH group bonded to a carbon. The compound shown in choice D is both an alcohol and an aldehyde.

48. **The correct answer is D.** The resistance of a metal wire is directly proportional to its length and inversely proportional to its cross-sectional area. The longest wire with the smallest diameter will therefore have the greatest resistance.

49. **The correct answer is D.** An *organic* acid is characterized by the presence of a carboxyl group (—COOH), or $-C\mathrel{\substack{O\\OH}}$. R represents a hydrocarbon group or a radical derived from a hydrocarbon.

50. **The correct answer is B.** An electrolyte is a substance that forms an electrically conducting solution when dissolved in water. This is caused by the dissociation of the compound into ions, or ionization. The greater the ionization, the stronger the electrolyte. Calcium chloride ionizes to a much greater degree than the others and is a strong electrolyte.

51. **The correct answer is D.** Force is a function of mass, distance, and acceleration. Since all these factors are equal in this example, all of the balls strike the wall with the same force. The force is calculated as 1 kg × 16 m/(2 sec)^2 = 4 newtons.

52. **The correct answer is C.** Charcoal is an amorphous form of carbon, and carbon can react with oxides of many metals and other substances to form CO, CO_2, and the carbides of the metals. Thus, the oxides would be reduced by the removal of oxygen, and carbon would be oxidized to carbon monoxide or carbon dioxide; therefore, oxidation and reduction would occur.

53. **The correct answer is A.** Nonmetal oxides, such as oxides of sulfur, carbon, and nitrogen, can react with water to form acids. The equations below are examples:
$$CO_2 + H_2O \rightarrow H_2CO_3$$
$$SO_2 + H_2O \rightarrow H_2SO_3$$

54. **The correct answer is C.** Triple bonds, sharing six electrons between two carbon atoms, provide each with a complete octet.

55. **The correct answer is B.** Although hydrogen is relatively inert at ordinary temperatures, it can combine with free oxygen, with oxygen that is in chemical combination, with some metallic elements, and with many nonmetallic elements. The addition of hydrogen reduces a substance.

56. **The correct answer is B.** A 1-molar solution of H_2SO_4 is prepared by dissolving 98 g into water and adjusting the volume to 1 liter. However, H_2SO_4 has two titratable or reactive protons per mole, and the normality is equal to two.

57. **The correct answer is C.** The nitrate test involves the use of a sulfate, such as iron sulfate, and sulfuric acid. The nitrate and sulfate ions react, forming nitric oxide. Nitric oxide then combines with the ferrous ion to form a ferrous-nitrogen-oxygen complex, which produces a brown color.

58. **The correct answer is C.** A saturated solution is one that is in equilibrium; a condition of equilibrium exists between the solvent and the solute, and no more of the solute can dissolve.

59. **The correct answer is A.** Oxides of barium and sulfur can combine to produce barium sulfate, a salt.
$$BaO + SO_3 \rightarrow BaSO_4$$

60. **The correct answer is D.** The optical illusion described is the result of refraction, the abrupt bending of a ray of light when it passes at an angle from a medium of one density to a medium of a different density. Air and water have very different densities, resulting in the refraction of light. Diffraction (choice A) is the separation of light into bands of different wavelengths, as in a rainbow. Convection (choice B) does not apply to light; it is the transfer of heat by circulation of air or water. Diffusion (choice C) is the scattering of light, such as the effect produced when light passes through frosted glass.

61. **The correct answer is D.** Sulfuric acid has a high boiling point: 317° C. Because of this, it is not very volatile and can be used to prepare more volatile acids, such as hydrochloric and nitric acids.

$$NaCl + H_2SO_4 \rightarrow NaHSO_4 + HCl$$

62. **The correct answer is D.** The pH of a solution is a measure of the negative logarithm of the hydrogen ion concentration (e.g., pH = $-\log[H^+]$). The H+ in question is 1×10^{-3}. Therefore, the pH = +3.

63. **The correct answer is C.** The electrons in the outer energy level comprise the portion of an atom directly involved in ionic bonding. The outer energy level will either gain or lose electrons in order to achieve a complete octet (eight electrons).

64. **The correct answer is B.** Hydrochloric acid can react with sodium hydrogen sulfite to produce sodium chloride, water, and sulfur dioxide. Sulfur dioxide can react with barium hydroxide to form barium sulfite and water.

65. **The correct answer is A.** The circular winds that form a tornado create an area of extremely low pressure in the center. When rotating areas of low pressure move over most structures that have areas of higher air pressure, the structure explodes outward, as air is forced down a pressure gradient.

Test 2: Chemistry and Physics

1. B	10. C	19. A	28. C	36. C
2. B	11. D	20. C	29. C	37. D
3. D	12. B	21. D	30. B	38. A
4. A	13. C	22. C	31. D	39. B
5. B	14. A	23. B	32. D	40. C
6. D	15. A	24. B	33. D	41. C
7. C	16. D	25. B	34. C	42. C
8. A	17. B	26. B	35. C	43. D
9. A	18. D	27. A	36. C	44. C
				45. B

1. **The correct answer is B.** Physical properties are those that do not involve any change in the nature or chemical composition of the substance. Heating a substance to the temperature at which it boils (its boiling point) will change its physical state but will not alter its chemical state.

2. **The correct answer is B.** Water is a compound formed by oxygen and hydrogen in chemical combination. Blood and air are mixtures, and oxygen is an element.

3. **The correct answer is D.** Potential energy is, in effect, energy in storage that can be released when conditions are conducive. Kinetic energy is energy of activity; it is released as the activity occurs.

4. **The correct answer is A.** One calorie (kilocalorie) will raise 1 kilogram (1 grams) of water 1 degree Celsius. It would take 18 calories to raise 1,000 grams of water 18 degrees ($38° - 20°$), or 36 calories to raise 2 grams of water 18 degrees Celsius.

5. **The correct answer is B.** Archimedes' Principle indicates that an object will displace its weight in water. Thus, a 1,000-ton ship would displace 1,000 tons of water.

6. **The correct answer is D.** The atomic weight (or mass number of an atom) equals the total of the number of protons and neutrons in the nucleus of the atom, or the total number of particles in the nucleus. In the drawing shown, there are 3 P and 4 N in the nucleus. The atomic weight is 7.

7. **The correct answer is C.** Nearly every unstable nucleus of an atom gives off one or more of the three kinds of radiation: alpha, beta, and gamma. Alpha and beta radiation are particle emission. Gamma rays and X-rays are more penetrating than alpha and beta radiation. Gamma rays are shortwave energy rays similar to X-rays, but stronger and more penetrating.

8. **The correct answer is A.** The half-life period can be defined as the time needed for half of a given amount of a substance to undergo spontaneous decomposition. This varies with different radioactive elements. There would be 50 milligrams left of a 100-milligram sample of material with a half-life of eight days after the eight days pass.

9. **The correct answer is A.** Radiation can cause *mutations* or genetic change. Any change in the genetic code would alter or destroy the trait associated with that particular gene. This could involve changes in enzymes produced and other factors associated with cellular metabolism.

10. **The correct answer is C.** Gram molecular weight may be defined as the weight of the molecule expressed in grams. The molecular weight of glucose ($C_6H_{12}O_6$) is 180, as the following indicates:

The weight of the six atoms of carbon equals 72 (6×12);

twelve hydrogens weigh 12 (12×1);

the weight of the six oxygens equals 96 (6×16).

The total is 180.

Thus, the gram molecular weight of glucose is 180 grams.

11. **The correct answer is D.** Equation D is balanced because the amount of each substance is equal on both sides of the equation. There are two mercury atoms and two oxygen atoms on each side.

12. **The correct answer is B.** You can use Ohm's law to calculate the current I. So if $V = I/R$, where $V = 60V$ and $R = 15\Omega$, then $I = 60V/15\Omega$, or 4 A. Choices A and D are incorrect due to improper constructions of Ohm's law (either dividing R/V or multiplying RV). Choice C is incorrect because voltage and current are not the same thing.

13. **The correct answer is C.** Enzymes are called organic catalysts, in that they are produced by the organisms and catalyze reactions that occur within that organism. The other substances named do not function as catalysts.

14. **The correct answer is A.** Gases are affected by temperature and pressure. If the gas is in a closed system, it cannot change its volume if temperature or pressure changes. Therefore, in a closed system, increasing the pressure would increase the temperature.

15. **The correct answer is A.** For every oxidation, there must be a reduction. Oxidation can involve the removal of electrons, the removal of hydrogen, or the addition of oxygen; reduction, the opposite. In equation A, metallic sodium loses an electron to become a positively charged ion; chlorine gains an electron to become a negatively charged chloride ion. Thus, sodium is oxidized and chlorine is reduced.

16. **The correct answer is D.** A photoelectric cell works on the principle that light can be used to produce electric currents in some metals. When light energy strikes the metal (usually cesium) in the photoelectric cell, it is converted into electric energy. The cesium emits electrons. The greater the amount of light striking the metal, the more electric energy produced.

17. **The correct answer is B.** The liquid part of the solution is called a solvent.

18. **The correct answer is D.** The concentration of a solution, on a percentage basis, contains a specific amount of solute in grams per 100 milliliters of solution. Thus, a 10-percent solution would have 10 grams of solute per 100 milliliters of solution.

19. **The correct answer is A.** A 1-molar solution is the amount of (NaOH) per liter as defined by its gram molecular weight, which can be calculated by adding the weights of the individual chemical elements.

20. **The correct answer is C.** A molar solution contains 1 gram molecular weight (the molecular weight of the molecule expressed in grams), or 1 mole per liter of solution. Therefore, each is a 1-molar solution.

21. **The correct answer is D.** Potassium hydroxide (KOH) and hydrochloric acid (HCl) react to form potassium chloride (KCl) and water. This is a double displacement.

$$KOH + HCl \rightarrow K^+ Cl^- + H_2O$$

22. **The correct answer is C.** An equivalent weight of an element is that weight of the element that combines with or displaces 1 atomic weight of hydrogen. Since calcium has a valence of +2 while hydrogen has a valence of +1, one half of the atomic weight of calcium will displace 1 atomic weight of hydrogen. Calcium has an atomic weight of 40; therefore, its equivalent weight is 20 or, expressed as grams, 20 grams. The following equation can apply: equivalent weight = [atomic weight/valence].

23. **The correct answer is B.** Two amino acid molecules can be bonded together by removing a hydrogen atom from the amino group (NH_2) of 1 amino acid molecule and removing a hydroxyl ion ($OH-$) from the carboxyl group (COOH) of the other. The result is a molecule of water removed from the two amino acids and a covalent bond between the nitrogen atom in the amino group of one amino acid and the carbon atom in the carboxyl group of the other. This type of reaction is called dehydration synthesis and results in the production of water within cells that is called metabolic water. Creation of a bond between two amino acids can be illustrated as follows (R represents any of the 20 different side chains that can be included in amino acids):

Removing this water molecule will create a bond between the nitrogen and carbon.

24. **The correct answer is B.** The atomic number indicates the number of protons (positively charged particles) within the nucleus of an atom. Since an atom is electrically neutral, the number of protons is equal to the number of electrons (negatively charged particles) of the atom. Thus, the atomic number can indicate the number of electrons as well as the number of protons.

25. **The correct answer is B.** Carbon dioxide and water, in the presence of light and the chlorophylls, yield glucose and oxygen. The water is absorbed by the root system of green plants and translocated through xylem to the leaves and other parts, which are the photosynthetic organs. Carbon dioxide enters the plants through epidermal stomates.

26. **The correct answer is B.** This is an application of $F = MA$, or $F = 2kg/7ms^2$, or 14N. Choice A results from using the force equation incorrectly and dividing by mass instead of multiplying. In choice C, there is no reason to convert into grams, but if you did you would need to take units into account. Since 1,400 g is the same as 14kg, so this answer would only be correct if it were 1,400 g/m^2. For choice D, it is true that friction from contact with the lane and air resistance are acting on the ball, but these are forces of their own and would need to be calculated separately. Regardless of these other forces, you know the mass and acceleration of the ball.

27. **The correct answer is A.** Light reflects at the exact angle as the angle with which the light first hits the mirror. Choice B (90°) is the total angle between the angle of strike and the angle of departure; if the light ray hits from about at 45° relative to the mirror, it will bounce downwards at 45°, but 45° also relative to the mirror, not the strike angle. When light strikes the mirror head on at 90°, it reflects directly backwards at 180°.

28. **The correct answer is C.** The water that spills out of the tear is now no longer moving through the hose, decreasing the pressure of water at the nozzle where the firefighters need it. A tear will not increase the area of the hose at all, but it will cause the hose to lose water (choice A). If the tear is very small, the water may emerge from the leak at high pressure, but the bigger problem is that the water is emerging from the wrong place, reducing the volume where it is needed.

29. **The correct answer is C.** Parallel circuits enable electrical currents to take separate paths through individual resistors as shown in circuit II.

30. **The correct answer is B.** All circuits in a series circuit, as shown in circuit I, must travel through all resistors.

31. **The correct answer is D.** Bronze is an alloy of copper and tin. An alloy is made by mixing two or more metals while in molten condition and then allowing the mixture to cool and solidify. The metals remain completely dissolved in one another after solidification, forming a homogenous substance with properties different from any of the constituent metals in their pure forms. For example, bronze is both harder and more resistant to corrosion than pure copper.

32. **The correct answer is D.** Enzymes are proteins that catalyze reactions of substances known as substrates.

33. **The correct answer is D.** Hydrogen in molecular form is composed of two atoms; the formula for one molecule of hydrogen is H_2. Therefore, two molecules of hydrogen is $2H_2$.

34. **The correct answer is C.** As oxygen accepts electrons from the ETS, it acquires a $^-2$ valence, which attracts $2H^+$ to form HOH.

35. **The correct answer is C.** If 1 gram of carbohydrate produces 4 calories, 9 grams are required to produce 36 calories. 36 calories ÷ 4 calories/gram = 9 grams.

36. **The correct answer is C.** Nitric acid reacts with the base potassium hydroxide to form potassium nitrate and water. For each hydrogen ion of the acid, there is a hydroxyl ion of the base to combine with it to form water. Therefore, neutralization occurs.

37. **The correct answer is D.** The H^+ has no electrons, which enables it to use 2 unshared electrons from N to form a coordinate covalent bond.

38. **The correct answer is A.** Hydrogen is the lightest element known, having an atomic weight of 1.008. The atom contains one proton, no neutrons, and one electron.

39. **The correct answer is B.** Nitrogen composes nearly four-fifths of the air; oxygen nearly one-fifth. The remainder of air consists of other gases.

40. **The correct answer is C.** A molar solution contains 1 mole of solute per liter of solution. Therefore, 1 mole of solute is combined with less than 1 kilogram (1 liter) of water. In a 1-molal solution, which contains 1 mole of solute per kilogram of water, the total volume for a solution of 1 mole exceeds 1 liter. Therefore, 1 liter of a 1-molal solution contains less than 1 mole.

41. **The correct answer is C.** Distillation involves evaporation, or changing the water from a liquid to a gaseous state (usually by heating), and collecting and condensing the gaseous water back to a liquid. The water, because it is in a gaseous state, is separated from any impurities since they cannot evaporate with the water.

42. **The correct answer is C.** The total number of moles of reactants and products are equal; therefore, a change of pressure has

no effect on the equilibrium. Increasing hydrogen or reducing hydrogen bromide drives the reaction to the right. Only increasing hydrogen bromide shifts the equilibrium to the left.

43. **The correct answer is D.** Ionic compounds form readily between nonmetals and metals. The only set that has no such combination is CH_2O, H_2S, and NH_3.

44. **The correct answer is C.** The human body is composed primarily of oxygen, carbon, hydrogen, and nitrogen, which comprise approximately 96% of the body's mass. There are about 21 other elements found in the human body for a total of 25.

45. **The correct answer is B.** Glucose and fructose are isomers because they are composed of identical numbers of carbon, hydrogen, and oxygen atoms, with different structural arrangements and different functional groups. The carbon-oxygen bonding in glucose and fructose form aldehydes and ketones, respectively.

Test 3: Biology

1. B	13. A	25. D	37. D	49. D
2. D	14. B	26. A	38. A	50. C
3. B	15. A	27. B	39. B	51. B
4. D	16. D	28. C	40. C	52. A
5. C	17. B	29. D	41. A	53. B
6. D	18. D	30. B	42. A	54. D
7. A	19. B	31. D	43. B	55. C
8. C	20. B	32. C	44. B	56. C
9. C	21. A	33. C	45. B	57. A
10. A	22. C	34. A	46. C	58. D
11. B	23. D	35. D	47. A	59. A
12. C	24. B	36. A	48. A	60. A

1. **The correct answer is B.** Although other mechanisms may be involved in passage of materials through a cell membrane, the passage of some materials, especially water, occurs by diffusion; diffusion occurs from regions of higher concentration of the substance to regions of lower concentration. Diffusion through a membrane, such as the cell membrane, is known as osmosis.

2. **The correct answer is D.** Iron is a part of the hemoglobin molecule, and, as such, is essential for its formation. Hemoglobin is the oxygen-carrying pigment found in red corpuscles.

3. **The correct answer is B.** Phenylketonuria (PKU) is a genetic disorder characterized by the inability of the affected person to convert excess molecules of the amino acid phenylalanine to molecules of the amino acid tyrosine. It is caused by inheriting a defect in the gene for the enzyme that catalyzes the conversion.

4. **The correct answer is D.** A control is used with experiments for comparison. The control is treated in the same manner as is the experimental group except for one variable. In this case, the variable would be the administering of the drug or sugar pills.

Thus, any differences between the groups in experimental results could be attributed to this one variable.

5. **The correct answer is C.** Transpiration is the loss of water in a gaseous state, through epidermal stomata, from the aerial parts of a plant. Most transpiration occurs through the leaf epidermis. Stomata are not found in root epidermis.

6. **The correct answer is D.** An organism is a living thing or individual. An organism consists of "systems," which are made up of organs. Organs consist of tissues, especially in the case of higher organisms. This statement would not apply to lower organisms that have not reached the system level of phylogenetic development.

7. **The correct answer is A.** Milk is not sterile; it contains numerous bacteria. Pasteurization does not sterilize milk but does destroy certain harmful bacteria that can be carried in milk.

8. **The correct answer is C.** Auxins are growth hormones found in plants; in stems, auxins stimulate growth. If a plant is unevenly illuminated, auxins are more concentrated on the side of the stem that

is more poorly illuminated, stimulating growth on that side. This will cause the stem to bend toward the light.

9. **The correct answer is C.** In humans, carbohydrate digestion begins in the mouth with the enzyme ptyalin, produced by the salivary glands.

10. **The correct answer is A.** Black is dominant over white in this case; therefore, the white guinea pig carries only white genes and is homozygous, or pure recessive. When such a test cross is made, the offspring will indicate the genotype of the black guinea pig. If the black guinea pig is hybrid, or heterozygous black (carrying one white gene), black and white offspring will result in a theoretical ratio of 1:1; if the black guinea pig is pure, or homozygous black, all offspring will be black because of dominance, although all of the offspring will be hybrid because they carry a white gene.

11. **The correct answer is B.** Photosynthesis is an endergonic reaction that uses CO_2 + H_2O to produce simple sugar and O_2. It is driven by radiant energy from sunlight.

12. **The correct answer is C.** The roots of plants help to hold the soil in place and prevent soil erosion; the ground can absorb water. Eroded lands do not absorb water readily. Water may run off, carrying with it some of the topsoil. This condition reduces the quality of the land. Where plants are present, the run-off is reduced or diminished, and the ground absorbs water.

13. **The correct answer is A.** A stimulus is anything that can cause a reaction or response by the organism. The reaction may be involuntary, such as batting the eye when an object approaches, or voluntary, such as moving from an area of discomfort.

14. **The correct answer is B.** Crossbreeding between strains with the desired traits, followed by selection of the offspring for future breeding and establishing the herd, is the best way to accomplish the breeder's goal. Inbreeding is just as likely to bring out undesirable hidden traits.

15. **The correct answer is A.** The inhaling and exhaling of air by the human lungs demonstrate Boyle's Law. Inhaling results from the expansion of the chest cavity (increase in volume and decrease in air pressure), and exhaling results from compression of the chest cavity (decrease in volume and increase in air pressure). These changes are accomplished by movement of the ribs and diaphragm.

16. **The correct answer is D.** Pith typically consists of parenchyma cells, which store starch in typical green plants. Spongy cells, characteristic of dicot leaves, also store starch, but temporarily.

17. **The correct answer is B.** Diffusion is the process by which solutes move from an area of high concentration to an area of low concentration. Osmosis is the movement of water down a concentration gradient. Movement of solute against a concentration gradient requires active transport processes and energy.

18. **The correct answer is D.** A symptom of diabetes is sugar (glucose) in the urine. Benedict's solution is a reagent used to test for the presence of reducing sugars such as glucose.

19. **The correct answer is B.** Buffer systems resist significant changes in pH. When a strong acid or a strong base is added to a buffer system, it produces a weak acid and a salt or a weak base and water, respectively. In each case, the pH would change only slightly.

20. The correct answer is B. Each turn of the Krebs cycle generates 2 moles of CO_2 and four pairs of H_2.

21. The correct answer is A. The removal of a small bit of living tissue from a patient for microscopic examination is called a biopsy, a useful diagnostic tool—especially for diseases of a cancerous nature.

22. The correct answer is C. Water constitutes about 75–85% of the typical living cell. No activities associated with life can occur without water.

23. The correct answer is D. Fats are emulsified, or broken down into small droplets, by bile secreted from the liver into the small intestine. The enzyme lipase then digests the fat droplets into fatty acids and glycerin. These products are not absorbed through capillary walls directly into the bloodstream, but enter the small lymph vessels, or lacteals, located in the villi of the intestine.

24. The correct answer is B. The results of the penny toss approximate a 1:2:1 ratio, which is the same ratio that is obtained from a monohybrid cross:

$$Aa \times Aa \rightarrow 1AA:2Aa:1aa$$

25. The correct answer is D. In the light phase of photosynthesis, H_2O is dissociated into $H_2 + O_2$. The O_2 comes entirely from the water molecules. The resulting H_2 is then used to reduce CO_2 to simple sugar.

26. The correct answer is A. Tissue culture is the technique of growing tissues or cells in solutions of water and nutrients. This technique is especially useful in studying growth, differentiation, and morphology.

27. The correct answer is B. Incineration is an effective method of sterilization; holding a loop in a flame sterilizes the loop, preventing contamination of surfaces on work areas, etc., and the possible spread of infectious bacteria.

28. The correct answer is C. Cellular respiration oxidizes digested food molecules and produces CO_2 and H_2O as end products. It is a downhill reaction and occurs in both plant and animal cells.

29. The correct answer is D. Combustion, or burning, is a rapid reaction giving off much heat and light in a short period of time. The energy is expended more rapidly; thus, the reaction occurs at a higher temperature since the temperature of the combustible material must be raised to a combustion point. Cellular respiration occurs more slowly, at lower temperatures, and is controlled by enzymes. If cellular respiration occurred at combustion temperatures, cells would be destroyed.

30. The correct answer is B. Trypsin, an enzyme found in pancreatic juice, digests proteins, peptones, and proteoses to peptides. The digestion of peptides to amino acids also occurs in the small intestine under the control of the enzyme erepsin. Some protein digestion (to peptones and proteoses) occurs in the stomach, under the control of the enzyme pepsin. Ptyalin and maltase act on carbohydrates; steapsin on fats.

31. The correct answer is D. Thrombocytes disintegrate when ruptured, as when blood flows from an injured blood vessel, releasing thrombokinase (thromboplastin), which acts to convert prothrombin to thrombin. Thrombin acts on fibrinogen in the plasma, converting it to insoluble fibrin, the material that forms the clot. Inadequacy of thrombokinase would prevent the first step of clotting, the formation of thrombin from prothrombin.

32. **The correct answer is C.** Cone cells are photoreceptor cells found in the retina of the eye. They are responsible for color vision. Cone cells are functional only in bright light; therefore, color is not perceived in dim light.

33. **The correct answer is C.** The iris is a circular muscle that regulates the diameter of the pupil, the aperture that allows light to enter the posterior chamber of the eye where the light-sensitive retina is located. The cornea allows light to enter the eye but does not regulate the amount of light entering. The ciliary body is a muscle that changes either the position or shape of the lens to focus the light coming through the pupil. The conjunctiva is a thin, protective layer of epithelium that covers the exposed surface of the eyeball.

34. **The correct answer is A.** Most of the carbon dioxide is transported in the blood plasma in the form of sodium bicarbonate ($NaHCO_3$). Erythrocytes, leucocytes, and platelets (thrombocytes) are blood cells suspended in the plasma.

35. **The correct answer is D.** Adrenalin, a hormone secreted by the adrenal glands, causes increases in blood pressure, heart rate, breathing, blood glucose levels, etc., preparing the body for heightened situations.

36. **The correct answer is A.** Auxins are plant growth hormones; testosterone and estrogen are animal sex hormones. ATP (adenosine triphosphate) is an energy-transport compound found in cells.

37. **The correct answer is D.** Bread mold is a fungus, while ferns are vascular plants. Both bread mold and ferns, however, produce spores as asexual reproductive cells. A mycelium is a mass of fungal hyphae and is not a part of the fern-plant body. Pinnules are the "leaflets" of a fern frond and are not part of a fungus.

38. **The correct answer is A.** Transpiration is the loss of gaseous water from a plant through epidermal stomata of the aerial parts of the plant, especially the leaves. Water forms a continuous column in the xylem tissue. The pull of water effected by transpiration is a factor in the rise of sap (water plus dissolved materials). The process is much the same as drinking liquid through a straw.

39. **The correct answer is B.** Xylem and phloem serve the purpose of transporting materials in vascular tissues. Upward translocation of plant sap is accomplished mainly through vessels (in angiosperms) and tracheids of xylem. Downward translocation is accomplished through the sieve tubes of phloem.

40. **The correct answer is C.** The cotyledons of dicotyledonous plants (such as beans) store food for use by the plant embryo as it develops into a seedling that can carry on photosynthesis. The plumule is composed of the embryonic or first leaves of the embryo; the hypocotyl is the lower embryonic stem; and the testa is the seed coat.

41. **The correct answer is A.** Normal cells have a high power of self-affinity (tendency to adhere to their own kind). Cancer cells lose this ability, as demonstrated by the spreading of cancer from one organ to another (malignancy).

42. **The correct answer is A.** The stigma is the top portion of the pistil on which pollen lands in pollination. The style (choice A) is the neck-like portion of the pistil, located between the stigma and the ovary (choice B), the basal part. Ovules (choice D) are potential seeds.

43. **The correct answer is B.** Intensive research has demonstrated that the basic structure of cell membranes is a mosaic of proteins in an outer and inner layer of phospholipids.

44. **The correct answer is B.** The enzyme sucrase adds a molecule of water (hydrolysis) to the band that binds the monosaccharides forming sucrose to decompose the disaccharide to simple sugars.

45. **The correct answer is B.** Small, uncharged lipid soluble molecules cross biological membranes more readily than other species. Water-soluble molecules cross if they are sufficiently small.

46. **The correct answer is C.** The generic formula for carbohydrates is $(CH_2O)^n$ = 1C:2H:1O (1:2:1).

47. **The correct answer is A.** There are three morphological types, or shapes, of bacteria: spherical-shaped bacteria are called cocci; rod-shaped bacteria are called bacilli; curved or spiral-shaped bacteria are usually known as spirilla.

48. **The correct answer is A.** Bacteria are classified as gram positive or gram negative; this classification depends on their ability to retain crystal violet, the primary stain of the gram stain. Those bacteria that cannot be decolorized with ethanol, but retain crystal violet, are classified as gram positive. Those that can be decolorized are gram negative. The difference is due to the chemical composition of the cell wall.

49. **The correct answer is D.** A bacteriophage is a kind of virus that attacks and destroys the bacterial cell. The viruses can pass their DNA into the bacterial cells and cause the cells to manufacture vital DNA and viral protein.

50. **The correct answer is C.** A marsupial is a viviparous mammal that gives birth to immature embryos; the development of the young is completed in the female's pouch, located on her ventral side. Nourishment for the embryo is from the mammary glands, the nipples of which are located in the pouch.

51. **The correct answer is B.** Reptiles are the first vertebrates in evolutionary development that spend the early or developmental part of their lives, as well as adult stages, on land. They do not possess gills for breathing in water as do the larval stages of amphibians.

52. **The correct answer is A.** Enzymes are macromolecular proteins that serve as biological catalysts that lower activation energy requirements in cellular reactions.

53. **The correct answer is B.** Most eukaryotic cells are in the range of 10 microns to 100 microns.

54. **The correct answer is D.** Sickle-cell anemia is caused by inheriting the defective form of a gene that codes for part of the protein portion of the hemoglobin molecule. The number of erythrocytes produced and the amount of hemoglobin in each erythrocyte are normal, but the altered structure of the hemoglobin molecules causes them to stick together in a manner that distorts erythrocytes into an abnormal crescent shape, making them less able to carry oxygen. Other types of anemia are due to insufficient hemoglobin within erythrocytes, too few erythrocytes, or erythrocytes that are abnormally small.

55. **The correct answer is C.** All named are members of the phylum Arthropoda, but only the sow bug is a crustacean. The characteristics of the class Crustacea are two pairs of antennae, three pairs of mouth parts, and a three-part body. Most crustaceans are aquatic, gilled animals, but a few live on land. The sow bug is one of these.

56. **The correct answer is C.** Leucoplasts are cellular plastids that store starches and are found only in plant cells.

57. **The correct answer is A.** The hydra and corals are coelenterates, diploblastic animals characterized by a gastrovascular cavity.

58. **The correct answer is D.** Photosynthesis is the process characteristic of green plants by which carbon dioxide and water react to produce glucose and oxygen. The carbon dioxide used in the process enters the tissue from the air, passing in through stomata of the epidermis; oxygen produced by the reaction passes through the stomata into the air. This process occurs only in the presence of light, and therefore, continuous carbon dioxide removal occurs only in the presence of light.

59. **The correct answer is A.** Lysosomes store powerful hydrolysis enzymes.

60. **The correct answer is A.** All environments have limited amounts of food and space, allowing animal populations to increase up to these limits, and regulating the populations by the number of individuals per unit of space (density-dependent).

Test 4: Cells, Structure, and Function

1. D	8. D	15. B	22. A	29. B
2. B	9. D	16. A	23. C	30. B
3. D	10. C	17. B	24. D	31. C
4. A	11. C	18. B	25. B	32. A
5. D	12. C	19. D	26. D	33. C
6. B	13. D	20. D	27. B	34. A
7. D	14. A	21. B	28. A	

1. **The correct answer is D.** In facilitated diffusion, large molecules and ions diffuse through channels within membrane proteins. The process requires no input of energy on the part of the cell, since materials move down a concentration gradient. Facilitated diffusion occurs more rapidly when the temperature is higher, and when the concentration gradient is steeper.

2. **The correct answer is B.** The polymerase chain reaction (PCR) is an in vitro technique.

3. **The correct answer is D.** In active transport, the transport proteins move a solute against its concentration gradient. Active transport does not proceed spontaneously. It requires an energy (ATP) input.

4. **The correct answer is A.** A cell immersed in a solution with a lower concentration of dissolved materials (solutes) is in a hypotonic environment. The concentration of water is higher outside of the cell than inside. Under these conditions, water diffuses into the cell.

5. **The correct answer is D.** Substance x is hydrophobic and nonpolar, so it can easily pass through the membrane due to the phospholipid structure of the membrane.

6. **The correct answer is B.** A cell is hypertonic when it has higher solute concentration and less water concentration compared to the outside solution, which has more water and less solute (hypotonic), so the water will diffuse inside the cell.

7. **The correct answer is D.** Oxidation is the loss of electrons or the loss of hydrogen from a substance. Therefore, the carbon-carbon double bonds of unsaturated fats are oxidized more easily than the simple bonds of saturated fats.

8. **The correct answer is D.** Macromolecules and fluid cross cellular membranes by bulk transport, in which the transported materials are contained within vesicles and do not mix with other materials of the cytoplasm. There are two forms of bulk transport: endocytosis and exocytosis. Endocytosis of a solid is known as phagocytosis.

9. **The correct answer is D.** In active transport, energy (ATP) is needed. Mitochondria are the organelles primarily involved in ATP synthesis.

10. **The correct answer is C.** Red blood cells have 0.9% salt solution, whereas sea water has more solute than red blood cells, so it is a hypertonic solution compared to red blood cells.

11. **The correct answer is C.** If any cell is placed in a hypertonic solution, the cell loses its water, dehydrates, and dies because the cell is hypotonic (more water) in comparison to outside solutions.

12. **The correct answer is C.** The movement of materials against a concentration gradient needs energy. (See the explanation for question 3.)

13. **The correct answer is D.** Every living organism is covered by a cell membrane.

14. **The correct answer is A.** In the presence of sunlight, CO_2 and H_2O combine chemically to produce glucose and O_2 (which comes from H_2O.)

15. **The correct answer is B.** Plasmodesmata are found only in plants.

16. **The correct answer is A.** The reverse outside-inside concentration and membrane crossing of Na^+ and K^+ are the major ions responsible for resting potentials and action potentials.

17. **The correct answer is B.** Water is a polar molecule, whereas oil is a nonpolar molecule. Water molecules have a slightly negative charge in one side and a slightly positive charge in the other side, but lipid molecules do not have any charges.

18. **The correct answer is B.** All plant cells have an outer rigid covering called a cell wall made up of polysaccharide cellulose; animal cells have cell membranes, not cell walls.

19. **The correct answer is D.** Prokaryote cells (e.g., bacteria and blue-green algae) do not have a membrane-bound nucleus, but they have naked DNA in their cytoplasm.

20. **The correct answer is D.** The cytoskeleton is a web of fibrous protein that extends throughout the cell. It alters the shape of a cell, moves the whole cell from one place to another, and pushes or pulls organelles.

21. **The correct answer is B.** Lysosomes are essentially membrane bags that enclose hydrolytic enzymes, which are involved in breaking down proteins, polysaccharides, and lipids. If the lysosomes break open, the cell itself will be destroyed, because the enzymes they carry are capable of hydrolyzing all the major types of molecules found in a living cell.

22. **The correct answer is A.** Note the $-COOH$ group, which makes the compound an acid, with the $-NH_2$ (amino group) in the alpha position.

23. **The correct answer is C.** Proteins are composed of chains of amino acids linked by peptide bonds, with primary, secondary, and tertiary structure.

24. **The correct answer is D.** A virus is not a living cell; it is a submicroscopic, noncellular particle composed of a nucleic acid core and a protein coat, reproducing only within a host. Therefore, it does not belong to any living kingdom.

25. **The correct answer is B.** There are two forms of endocytosis, depending on the kind of material brought into the cell. Endocytosis of fluid is known as pinocytosis.

26. **The correct answer is D.** All cells can exist as distinct entities because of the cell membrane, which regulates the passage of materials into and out of the cell. A latex membrane does not allow the HIV virus to pass through the membrane, preventing HIV infection.

27. **The correct answer is B.** Membranes control the types of molecules that can pass in and out of the cell and organelles. Cell membranes are permeable to certain molecules and impermeable to others—a phenomenon known as selective permeability.

28. **The correct answer is A.** Three different types of filaments have been identified as major participants in the cytoskeleton: microtubules, microfilaments, and intermediate filaments. They maintain the

shape of the cell, enable it to move, anchor its organelles, and direct its traffic.

29. **The correct answer is B.** Both mitochondria and chloroplasts are energy-producing organelles. Mitochondria release the energy from food as a form of ATP, and the chloroplasts pick up the solar energy and convert it to chemical energy (ATP).

30. **The correct answer is B.** The slope (m) is 10.

31. **The correct answer is C.** In enzyme-catalyzed reactions, substrate molecules generally outnumber enzyme molecules, which allow the enzyme to become saturated and the reaction to proceed at maximum velocity.

32. **The correct answer is A.** Autotrophic organisms, such as plants, all algae, and some bacteria, are able to synthesize their own organic food by using CO_2, H_2O, and sunlight.

33. **The correct answer is C.** The mitochondrion is the powerhouse of the cell. It produces maximum amounts of chemical energy (ATP) for sustaining life.

34. **The correct answer is A.** Membranes are composed of a phospholipid bilayer of molecules interspersed with protein molecules. Any kind of nonpolar molecule, such as lipids or some other organic solvents (ether, acetone, etc.), can easily pass through the lipid layer of membrane.

Test 5: Biology

1. C	5. C	9. C	13. D	17. D
2. D	6. C	10. B	14. D	18. C
3. D	7. C	11. C	15. C	
4. C	8. C	12. C	16. D	

1. **The correct answer is C.** This is the process by which a glucose molecule is changed to two molecules of pyruvic acid with the liberation of a small amount of energy. In the absence of oxygen, pyruvic acid can be converted to ethanol or to one of several organic acids, of which lactic is the most common. This process is called fermentation.

2. **The correct answer is D.** In the first stage, aerobic respiration (glycolysis) produces 2 ATP. In the second stage (Krebs cycle), it produces 2 ATP. During the final stage (electron transport chain), it produces 32–34 ATP, depending upon whether or not oxygen is present. Therefore, up to 38 ATP can be produced per glucose molecule.

3. **The correct answer is D.** Reaction I is an uphill process that takes in radiant energy from the sun and converts it to chemical energy to combine CO_2 and H_2O to produce $C_6H_{12}O_6$ and O_2—which have additional energy.

4. **The correct answer is C.** The reaction in II is downhill, with energy being released from $C_6H_{12}O_6$, generating CO_2 and H_2O with less energy.

5. **The correct answer is C.** The reactants of some reactions have more energy than the products. Many such reactions release energy that cells can use, which is what happens during aerobic respiration.

6. **The correct answer is C.** Each type of enzyme functions best within a certain temperature range. The chemical reaction rates decrease sharply when the temperature becomes too high. Humans usually die when their internal body temperature reaches 44°C (112°F) because it destroys the shape of the enzyme and thereby stops the metabolism.

7. **The correct answer is C.** The enzyme helpers called co-enzymes are complex organic molecules, many of which are derived from vitamins. These co-enzymes can pick up hydrogen atoms that are liberated during glucose breakdown.

8. **The correct answer is C.** The stored form of energy is called potential energy. An example is the glucose molecule; when it breaks down, it releases a large quantity of chemical energy to do work.

9. **The correct answer is C.** All the pigments are present inside the thylakoids; therefore, the chlorophyll molecules and other pigments pick up the solar energy, convert it to chemical energy as a form of ATP and NADPH, and release oxygen during the non-cyclic light reaction.

10. **The correct answer is B.** During non-cyclic light reactions, energy from the sun drives the formation of ATP (which carries energy) and NADPH (which carries hydrogen and electrons). Oxygen is a byproduct of photosynthesis.

11. **The correct answer is C.** The light independent reactions are the "synthesis" part of photosynthesis. ATP molecules deliver the required energy for the reaction. NADPH

molecules deliver the required hydrogen and electrons, and carbon dioxide diffuses inside the stroma. It then forms the energy-rich molecule glucose (the process is called dark reaction).

12. **The correct answer is C.** Aerobic cellular respiration is more important to sustaining life because it produces 36 ATP compared to anaerobic, which only releases 2 ATP.

13. **The correct answer is D.** The organelle chloroplast is responsible for photosynthesis, which produces O_2 and the energy-rich molecule carbohydrate.

14. **The correct answer is D.** All enzymes are protein molecules, and protein is one of the organic molecules necessary for sustaining life.

15. **The correct answer is C.** Glycolysis is the first stage of cellular respiration in which glucose is broken down step by step to form 2 pyruvic acid inside the cytoplasm.

16. **The correct answer is D.** The first stage of respiration, the breaking down of the glucose molecules, always takes place inside the cytoplasm because all the enzymes are there for the reaction.

17. **The correct answer is D.** Electron transport systems and neighboring channel proteins are the machinery embedded in the inner membrane that divides a mitochondrion into two compartments.

18. **The correct answer is C.** In the first stage of aerobic oxidation, glucose is oxidized to pyruvic acid; this is known as glycolysis. The two pyruvates resulting from glycolysis of a molecule of glucose enter into the Krebs cycle (citric acid cycle) and are oxidized to carbon dioxide and water.

Test 6: Biology

1. B	5. C	9. B	13. D	17. D
2. A	6. B	10. D	14. D	18. C
3. A	7. C	11. B	15. C	19. B
4. D	8. D	12. D	16. C	20. A

1. **The correct answer is B.** The adult bodies of most plants and animals consist of diploid (2n) rather than haploid (n) cells. A gamete (male sperm and female egg) is always a haploid cell, which means it has one set of chromosomes formed by meiosis of germ cells (2n). So if the germ cell is 40, the gamete will be 20.

2. **The correct answer is A.** When two alternative alleles are fully apparent in a hybrid, with both phenotypes showing in the organism, we say that the hybrids exhibit codominance. Blood typing of humans provides an excellent example of codominance. The AB blood type inherits an A allele and a B allele. Neither allele is dominant over the other; therefore, codominance causes a new blood type, AB.

3. **The correct answer is A.** The blood cells of humans divide by mitosis. In mitosis, the diploid number of chromosomes is maintained, and the resulting daughter cells are identical to the parent cell.

4. **The correct answer is D.** Meiosis is the nuclear division that reduces the number of chromosomes in the resulting cells by half. Meiosis is necessary for the production of gametes or sex cells and results in four nonidentical haploid cells (sperms and eggs).

5. **The correct answer is C.** The first part of sexual reproduction is meiosis, where the germ cells divide and produce four haploid gametes.

6. **The correct answer is B.** Asexual reproduction occurs without sex and transfers the genes of just one parent to each offspring; it produces offspring that are genetically identical to one another and to their single parent by the process of mitosis.

7. **The correct answer is C.** The first pattern of inheritance discovered by Mendel was the Law of Segregation. This law describes how the two copies of each gene segregate (separate) during meiosis so that just one copy ends up in each gamete (sperm and egg).

8. **The correct answer is D.** The dominant allele will always show the dominant characteristic in their phenotype.

9. **The correct answer is B.** The sex chromosome of a mother is always XX and the father XY. The sex of the child depends on whether he or she gets X or Y from the father. If the child gets X from the father and X from the mother, the child will be a female. If the child gets Y from the father and X from the mother, the child will be a male.

10. **The correct answer is D.** In normal cells, the cell division is controlled by two sets of genes: one set stimulates, and the other set suppresses. In cancer, defective genes may overstimulate cell division or fail to halt cell division.

11. **The correct answer is B.** Sperm cells are haploid (N), which are formed by meiosis of germ cells (2N); therefore, if the haploid is 30, then germ cells should be 60.

12. **The correct answer is D.** A person with Down syndrome has three copies in chromosome 21 rather than two copies. The extra chromosome affects practically every part of the body.

13. **The correct answer is D.** If we do the Punnett square for a woman who is a heterozygous carrier for a sex-linked recessive gene and married to a normal man, half of her sons and half of her daughters will receive this gene.
    X^{C}X—girl with recessive gene
    X^{C}Y—boy with recessive gene
    XY—normal boy
    XX—normal girl

14. **The correct answer is D.** Hemophilia is a sex-linked disorder because the defective gene is present in the Y sex chromosome.

15. **The correct answer is C.** The sex-linked trait is present in the X chromosome; therefore, the father cannot pass the gene to his son because the son always receives the Y chromosome, not the X chromosome, from his father.

16. **The correct answer is C.** The blue gene is the autosomal recessive trait, whereas hemophilia is the sex-linked recessive trait. To get the blue eyes, the person should have two blue-eyes recessive genes. If the person is male, he needs only one recessive gene for hemophilia.

17. **The correct answer is D.** Blood type O is a universal donor because it has neither A nor B polysaccharides (antigen) for antibodies to attack.

18. **The correct answer is C.** Non-disjunction of sex chromosomes (XY) in a man produces four types of abnormal sperms. When these abnormal sperm (YY) fertilize normal X carrying chromosomes, they produce abnormal genotypes (XYY). Males that inherit an extra Y chromosome tend to be unusually tall (above 6 feet), have severe facial acne, and are poorly coordinated.

19. **The correct answer is B.** Genetic information is encoded in the particular order of nucleotide bases, which follow one another in DNA. RNA molecules function in the processes by which the genetic information in DNA is used to build proteins.

20. **The correct answer is A.** Carbon dioxide and water are the end products of the Krebs cycle, which is the second phase of aerobic cellular oxidation of glucose for the release of energy.

Test 7: Chemistry

1. B	5. D	9. D	13. C	17. A
2. D	6. B	10. C	14. C	18. B
3. D	7. B	11. D	15. C	19. A
4. D	8. B	12. B	16. D	20. A

1. **The correct answer is B.** Acidic solutions contain hydrogen (H⁺) ions, while basic (or alkaline) solution contain a basic ion, such as the hydroxyl ion (OH⁻).

2. **The correct answer is D.** Carbohydrates consist of molecules made up of C, H, and O in a ratio of 1:2:1 (e.g., glucose is $C_6H_{12}O_6$). Polysaccharides are chains of three or more simple sugars (e.g., glucose).

3. **The correct answer is D.** Whether a watery solution is acidic or alkaline depends on its concentration of hydrogen ions (H⁺) in relation to hydroxyl ions (OH⁻). The ratio is expressed as the solution pH (the letters stand for potential of hydrogen). The pH scale ranges from 0 (most acidic) to 14 (most alkaline). Pure water is neutral with a pH of 7 because it has equal amounts of hydrogen and hydroxyl ions.

4. **The correct answer is D.** Carbohydrates consist of molecules made up of C, H, and O in a ratio of 1:2:1, whereas cholesterol is a lipid (steroid) formed of four carbon rings.

5. **The correct answer is D.** Organic molecules are molecules that contain carbon; they are found in living things.

6. **The correct answer is B.** Covalence is the mutual attraction between two atoms that share a pair of electrons. It is the strongest type of chemical bond.
$$H^+ = H^+ \rightarrow H^2$$

7. **The correct answer is B.** For many atoms, the simplest way to attain a completely filled outer energy level is either to gain or to lose 1 or 2 electrons.

8. **The correct answer is B.** Disaccharides are double sugars and are formed by linking two simple sugars. For example, glucose and fructose form sucrose, a disaccharide (table sugar).

9. **The correct answer is D.** Wax is made of glycerol and fatty acids. It is nonpolar and insoluble in water. It is a lipid molecule.

10. **The correct answer is C.** Proteins are made up of units called amino acids. Amino acids join together by a covalent bond and form polypeptide chains (the primary structure of proteins).

11. **The correct answer is D.** The nucleus of an atom consists of protons and neutrons. A proton is a subatomic particle with a positive electric charge. The number of protons in the nucleus of an atom is equal to an element's atomic number.

12. **The correct answer is B.** The chemical activity of an atom is how it reacts with other atoms. Atoms are governed by the number of electrons in their outermost shell. Helium, neon, and other atoms with no electron vacancies in their outermost shell are inert; they tend not to enter into chemical reactions. Hydrogen, oxygen, and other atoms with electron vacancies in their outermost shell tend to interact with other atoms.

13. **The correct answer is C.** Regardless of the element, atoms have just as many electrons as protons. This means that they carry no

net charge, overall. A proton is always positively charged, and an electron is negatively charged.

14. **The correct answer is C.** Basic or alkaline solutions have fewer H^+ than OH^- ions; their pH is above 7.

15. **The correct answer is C.** Alkaline solutions always have a higher pH and more OH^- ions.

16. **The correct answer is D.** Glucose is a 6-carbon simple sugar and serves as a precursor of many complex compounds and as a building block for larger carbohydrates.

17. **The correct answer is A.** There are 20 different amino acids used to create proteins in humans. The basic building block of protein is the amino acid. Each amino acid is a small organic compound with an amino group, a carboxyl group (an acid), a hydrogen atom, and one or more atoms, called its R group. Examples of amino acids are tryptophane, alanine, glycine, aspartic acid, lysine, and proline.

18. **The correct answer is B.** The small organic compounds called nucleotides have three components: a 5-carbon sugar, a phosphate group, and a nitrogen-containing base. Nucleotides are the basic building blocks of DNA and RNA.

19. **The correct answer is A.** In polar covalent bonds, atoms of different elements, which have a different number of protons, do not exert the same pull in shared electrons. The more attractive atom ends up with a slight negative charge; the atom is electronegative. Its effect is balanced out by the other atoms, resulting in a slight positive charge. In simple words, a polar covalent bond has no net charge—but the charge is distributed unevenly between the bond's two ends.

20. **The correct answer is A.** Genes are composed of segments of nucleotide bases of DNA molecules.

Test 8: Chemistry and Physical Science

1. D	11. B	21. B	31. D	41. C
2. B	12. C	22. B	32. A	42. B
3. B	13. D	23. D	33. D	43. C
4. C	14. B	24. D	34. B	44. A
5. D	15. C	25. A	35. B	45. A
6. C	16. D	26. A	36. B	46. A
7. D	17. A	27. D	37. C	47. D
8. A	18. D	28. A	38. D	48. C
9. D	19. D	29. B	39. A	49. B
10. D	20. D	30. C	40. C	50. B

1. **The correct answer is D.** Polarity is determined by differences in electronegativities between atoms involved in a bond. The difference in electronegativities between hydrogen and oxygen on a scale devised by Linus Pauling is 1.4, and between carbon and oxygen, it is 1.0. Carbon and hydrogen differ by only 0.4 and consequently form nonpolar bonds.

2. **The correct answer is B.** A camera lens is convex; light passing through such a lens is bent toward the center of the lens. Light reflected near the object and passing through the thinner outer edges of a convex lens bends more than light passing through the thicker areas, and light passing through the exact center of the lens does not bend at all. Because light reflected from an object is focused through such a lens and bent, rather than passing in a straight line, as it would if passing through plain glass, the image formed is reversed and is smaller than the original object.

3. **The correct answer is B.** Sucrose is a disaccharide that has nearly twice the molar mass of the other two sugars, which are monosaccharides.

4. **The correct answer is C.** A hydrogen atom must accept an electron in order to form a hydride ion. No other changes occur.

The hydride therefore has a single negative charge, whereas the hydrogen atom is neutral. An extra negative charge with no change in positive charge expands the radius.

5. **The correct answer is D.** The functional group contains carbonyl plus a hydrogen linked to the carbon (—C—H). The other connection of the carbonyl group is to another carbon atom. The groups COOH, —OH, and —COOR are found in carboxylic acids, alcohols, and esters, respectively.

6. **The correct answer is C.** Calcium oxide (CaO) is the only compound in the four that is a metal oxide. Metal oxides form hydroxides (bases) when dissolved in water, but nonmetal oxides form acids.

7. **The correct answer is D.** The statement given is the definition of an isotope, a form of an atom of an element that differs from other atoms of the same element by the number of neutrons.

8. **The correct answer is A.** Oxidation, the loss of electrons, occurs at the anode. Molten sodium chloride has only sodium (Na^+) and chloride (Cl^-) ions, the latter of which each have a single electron to donate to achieve neutrality. Loss of one electron

each yields chlorine atoms, which stabilize by forming diatomic molecules of chlorine gas.

9. **The correct answer is D.** Sugar is the only molecular compound of this group. The others readily dissociate as ions in polar solvents, such as water.

10. **The correct answer is D.** Isopropyl alcohol has a low enough molecular weight to make it volatile and thus capable of giving a noticeable cooling effect during evaporation. It is unsuitable for internal consumption, but it is relatively inexpensive. There are disadvantages for the use of any of the others as rubbing alcohol. Methyl alcohol is toxic, phenol causes skin burns, and ethyl alcohol is too valuable for internal consumption and other commercial purposes.

11. **The correct answer is B.** Argon, barium, and aluminum are in groups VIIIA, IIA, and IIIA, respectively. Copper is the only element that is in the transition area of the periodic table (group IB).

12. **The correct answer is C.** Calcium and the other metals of the group IIA ionize by losing two electrons. It achieves the stable electron structure of argon, with eight electrons in the outer shell.

13. **The correct answer is D.** In the series for the oxyhalogen ions (e.g., ClO_4^-, ClO_3^-, ClO^-), the one with the least amount of oxygen is designated hypochlorite.

14. **The correct answer is B.** Chemical kinetics is the study of reaction rates and how these change with variation of conditions along with the various molecular events that transpire during the overall reaction.

15. **The correct answer is C.** There is one phosphorus in the formula, but there are three potassiums and four oxygens. The number of atoms or ions present per

formula unit equals the corresponding number of moles of each type in one molecule of the compound (the amount present in a liter of a 1-molar solution). In solution, potassium phosphate would separate as potassium ions and phosphate ions.

16. **The correct answer is D.** Single bonds between carbon atoms are longer but weaker than double bonds between carbon atoms.

17. **The correct answer is A.** After the common multiplier (M) was removed from $mgh = \frac{1}{2}mV^2$, the equation was multiplied by 2 to eliminate the $\frac{1}{2}$, and the square root of both sides was extracted.

18. **The correct answer is D.** Total potential energy was connected to kinetic energy.

19. **The correct answer is D.** For a molecular compound, the gram formula weight is the same as the gram molecular weight. The empirical formula represents the smallest ratio of the different atoms possible in the compound. The molecular formula may be a multiple of the empirical formulas (e.g., twice).

20. **The correct answer is D.** The ratio of the rates of effusion of two gases (proportional to the speeds of the gas molecules) is inversely proportional to the square roots of their molecular weights; consequently, rate of effusion of A/rate of effusion of $B = \sqrt{\frac{1}{4}} = \frac{1}{2}$.

21. **The correct answer is B.** The greater the concentration of soluble particles, the greater the lowering of the freezing point of the solvent. A mole of calcium chloride contains 1 mole of calcium ions and 2 moles of chloride ions. A mole of sodium chloride contains only 2 moles of ions, and

sucrose and methanol have only 1 mole of particles each per liter of 1-molar solution.

22. **The correct answer is B.** If the atomic mass of an isotope is unknown, the number of neutrons cannot be determined. However, if the atomic number is known, the number of protons is known. In an atom, there is no charge, so the number of electrons must equal the number of protons and the atomic number.

23. **The correct answer is D.** Nitrogen makes up about 80% of the air and therefore contributes about 80% of the total atmospheric pressure—0.80×760 mm = 608 mm.

24. **The correct answer is D.** A supersaturated solution contains more dissolved solute than is normal at a given temperature. A disturbance will cause the solution to adjust to the normal concentration with the concurrent expulsion of the excess solute. A saturated solution will remain stable.

25. **The correct answer is A.** A first-order reaction has a rate that is proportional to the concentration of only one reactant.

26. **The correct answer is A.** The loss of an alpha particle reduces the number of positive charges by 2 and the atomic mass by 4.

27. **The correct answer is D.** Positron (with the mass of an electron) emission can occur, but protons are never expelled from the nucleus during radioactive decay.

28. **The correct answer is A.** Fat yields the highest amount of energy per gram of any of the foods consumed.

29. **The correct answer is B.** On the Fahrenheit scale, the boiling point of water is 212°; the freezing point is 32°. Subtracting 32° from 212° results in a difference of 180°, the number of degrees between the boiling and the freezing points of water.

30. **The correct answer is C.** One gram of carbon-14 must go through 4 half-lives to be reduced to 0.0625 grams. $4 \times 5.73 \times 10$ years equal 22.92×10 years.

31. **The correct answer is D.** Since the oxidation number of a compound is 0, the total positive values must equal the total negative values. Consequently, four times the value for oxygen (-2) must equal the positive values due to potassium ($+1$ each) and manganese (Mn).
1 (Oxidation number of Mn) +
2 (Oxidation number of K) +
4 (Oxidation number of 0) = 0
Oxidation number of Mn + 2(+1) + 4(−2) = 0
Oxidation number of Mn = +8 − 2 = +6

32. **The correct answer is A.** Within a group, the element with the lowest atomic number has the highest ionization energy.

33. **The correct answer is D.** Within a group of nonmetals such as the halogens, the one with the highest atomic number has the least electronegative value.

34. **The correct answer is B.** The atomic radii of a group of metals increase as the atomic number increases. Therefore, the element with the lowest atomic number has the smallest atomic radius.

35. **The correct answer is B.** The salt that would yield a weak acid when mixed with acid would dissolve most readily. Calcium carbonate yields carbonic acid (H_2CO_3) when it is acidified. The other salts yield hydrochloric acid (HC1), nitric acid (HNO_3), or phosphoric acid (H_3PO_4), which are all strong acids.

36. **The correct answer is B.** The conjugate base is obtained when the acid loses a hydrogen ion. Therefore, the conjugate base of carbonic acid, H_2CO_3, is the hydrogen carbonate ion (HCO_3^-).

37. **The correct answer is C.** The number of moles of HCl required for the titration must equal the number of moles of NaOH (40 ml × 0.2 m = 8 moles). Therefore, 20 ml of 0.4 ml Cl is required. After titration, the total volume of the mixture is 40 + 20 = 60 ml.

38. **The correct answer is D.** The salt of a weak acid would hydrolyze in solution to remove hydrogen ions from water and leave an excess of hydroxide ions. $H_2O + A \rightarrow HA + OH$. The salt of a strong acid would hydrolyze by removing hydroxide ions from water.

$$NH_4 + H_2O \rightarrow NH_4OH + H^+.$$

39. **The correct answer is A.** Heat is produced by the reaction, and, according to Le Chatalier's Principle, the system will adjust to maintain equilibrium. Heating would force the reaction to the left. A pressure increase shifts the reaction in the direction of smaller volumes (right), and addition of more reactant (N_2 or H_2) also pushes the reaction to the right.

40. **The correct answer is C.** Colligative properties are based on the number of particles. Vapor pressure, osmotic pressure, boiling point elevation, and freezing point lowering all are colligative properties. Density is not.

41. **The correct answer is C.** Molecular solids are held together by rather weak London forces, which increase with molecular weight. The melting points of molecular substances are relatively low since there are no strong forces, such as ionic forces, to overcome.

42. **The correct answer is B.** Static electricity is a non-moving electrical charge that accumulates on the surface of an object. A substance that contains an equal number of protons (positively charged particles) and electrons (negatively charged particles) is electrically neutral. If electrons are gained or lost, the substance becomes charged. When one object loses electrons and becomes positively charged, another must gain electrons and become negatively charged. If electrons are not in motion, the electricity is static. However, warm, moist air is a good conductor of electricity; moisture collects on the surfaces of objects and conducts electrons away from the surface, preventing the object from becoming charged. Cold air acts as a good insulator, preventing the movement of electrons away from the object. Therefore, static electricity can best be felt on a cold, dry day, when the electrons can accumulate on an object or surface.

43. **The correct answer is C.** An atom lying at the corner of a unit cell will touch four corners of cubes below and four corners of cubes above.

44. **The correct answer is A.** A higher boiling point for a liquid is seen when more energy is needed to separate the gaseous molecules from the liquid. It shows that for the same amount of energy, a higher boiling liquid would expel fewer molecules as vapor at any temperature, resulting in a lower vapor pressure. The lowest boiling substance vaporizes most easily and therefore would have the highest vapor pressure at a specific temperature.

45. **The correct answer is A.** The mass number of an isotope is the sum of the protons and neutrons in an atom. 17 protons and 17 neutrons are necessary to give a mass number of 34. The number of electrons equals the number of protons in an atom.

46. **The correct answer is A.** Electronegativity decreases within a group in the periodic table as the atomic number increases. The

example shown is the progression from fluorine to iodine.

47. **The correct answer is D.** Phosphorus has 15 electrons, all of which are paired except one.

48. **The correct answer is C.** Chlorine is in the third period and has seven electrons in its outermost shell. Two electrons are in an S orbital, leaving five electrons for the P orbitals.

49. **The correct answer is B.** Density is defined as mass per unit volume $\left(d = \dfrac{m}{v}\right)$. The mathematical relationship shows that when equal masses of two substances of different densities are compared, the one with greater density occupies less space (volume).

50. **The correct answer is B.** Since all three gases are in equal size flasks with the same temperature and pressure, the total number of moles (hence, the total number of molecules) is equal in each case. However, a molecule of NH_3 contains 4 atoms, a molecule of NO contains 2 atoms, and a molecule of N_2 contains 2 atoms.

FINAL SCIENCE EXAMINATION ANSWER SHEET

1. Ⓐ Ⓑ Ⓒ Ⓓ   16. Ⓐ Ⓑ Ⓒ Ⓓ   31. Ⓐ Ⓑ Ⓒ Ⓓ   46. Ⓐ Ⓑ Ⓒ Ⓓ   61. Ⓐ Ⓑ Ⓒ Ⓓ

2. Ⓐ Ⓑ Ⓒ Ⓓ   17. Ⓐ Ⓑ Ⓒ Ⓓ   32. Ⓐ Ⓑ Ⓒ Ⓓ   47. Ⓐ Ⓑ Ⓒ Ⓓ   62. Ⓐ Ⓑ Ⓒ Ⓓ

3. Ⓐ Ⓑ Ⓒ Ⓓ   18. Ⓐ Ⓑ Ⓒ Ⓓ   33. Ⓐ Ⓑ Ⓒ Ⓓ   48. Ⓐ Ⓑ Ⓒ Ⓓ   63. Ⓐ Ⓑ Ⓒ Ⓓ

4. Ⓐ Ⓑ Ⓒ Ⓓ   19. Ⓐ Ⓑ Ⓒ Ⓓ   34. Ⓐ Ⓑ Ⓒ Ⓓ   49. Ⓐ Ⓑ Ⓒ Ⓓ   64. Ⓐ Ⓑ Ⓒ Ⓓ

5. Ⓐ Ⓑ Ⓒ Ⓓ   20. Ⓐ Ⓑ Ⓒ Ⓓ   35. Ⓐ Ⓑ Ⓒ Ⓓ   50. Ⓐ Ⓑ Ⓒ Ⓓ   65. Ⓐ Ⓑ Ⓒ Ⓓ

6. Ⓐ Ⓑ Ⓒ Ⓓ   21. Ⓐ Ⓑ Ⓒ Ⓓ   36. Ⓐ Ⓑ Ⓒ Ⓓ   51. Ⓐ Ⓑ Ⓒ Ⓓ   66. Ⓐ Ⓑ Ⓒ Ⓓ

7. Ⓐ Ⓑ Ⓒ Ⓓ   22. Ⓐ Ⓑ Ⓒ Ⓓ   37. Ⓐ Ⓑ Ⓒ Ⓓ   52. Ⓐ Ⓑ Ⓒ Ⓓ   67. Ⓐ Ⓑ Ⓒ Ⓓ

8. Ⓐ Ⓑ Ⓒ Ⓓ   23. Ⓐ Ⓑ Ⓒ Ⓓ   38. Ⓐ Ⓑ Ⓒ Ⓓ   53. Ⓐ Ⓑ Ⓒ Ⓓ   68. Ⓐ Ⓑ Ⓒ Ⓓ

9. Ⓐ Ⓑ Ⓒ Ⓓ   24. Ⓐ Ⓑ Ⓒ Ⓓ   39. Ⓐ Ⓑ Ⓒ Ⓓ   54. Ⓐ Ⓑ Ⓒ Ⓓ   69. Ⓐ Ⓑ Ⓒ Ⓓ

10. Ⓐ Ⓑ Ⓒ Ⓓ   25. Ⓐ Ⓑ Ⓒ Ⓓ   40. Ⓐ Ⓑ Ⓒ Ⓓ   55. Ⓐ Ⓑ Ⓒ Ⓓ   70. Ⓐ Ⓑ Ⓒ Ⓓ

11. Ⓐ Ⓑ Ⓒ Ⓓ   26. Ⓐ Ⓑ Ⓒ Ⓓ   41. Ⓐ Ⓑ Ⓒ Ⓓ   56. Ⓐ Ⓑ Ⓒ Ⓓ   71. Ⓐ Ⓑ Ⓒ Ⓓ

12. Ⓐ Ⓑ Ⓒ Ⓓ   27. Ⓐ Ⓑ Ⓒ Ⓓ   42. Ⓐ Ⓑ Ⓒ Ⓓ   57. Ⓐ Ⓑ Ⓒ Ⓓ   72. Ⓐ Ⓑ Ⓒ Ⓓ

13. Ⓐ Ⓑ Ⓒ Ⓓ   28. Ⓐ Ⓑ Ⓒ Ⓓ   43. Ⓐ Ⓑ Ⓒ Ⓓ   58. Ⓐ Ⓑ Ⓒ Ⓓ   73. Ⓐ Ⓑ Ⓒ Ⓓ

14. Ⓐ Ⓑ Ⓒ Ⓓ   29. Ⓐ Ⓑ Ⓒ Ⓓ   44. Ⓐ Ⓑ Ⓒ Ⓓ   59. Ⓐ Ⓑ Ⓒ Ⓓ   74. Ⓐ Ⓑ Ⓒ Ⓓ

15. Ⓐ Ⓑ Ⓒ Ⓓ   30. Ⓐ Ⓑ Ⓒ Ⓓ   45. Ⓐ Ⓑ Ⓒ Ⓓ   60. Ⓐ Ⓑ Ⓒ Ⓓ   75. Ⓐ Ⓑ Ⓒ Ⓓ

answer sheet

FINAL SCIENCE EXAMINATION

75 Questions • 75 Minutes

Directions: After carefully reading each test item, select the best answer. Fill in the corresponding space on your answer sheet.

1. Of the following human traits, the one under both genetic and hormonal control is
   A. hemophilia.
   B. color blindness.
   C. baldness.
   D. blood type.

2. If a sexually reproducing animal has a diploid number of 12, how many chromosomes would a mature sperm have?
   A. 3
   B. 24
   C. 4
   D. 6

3. The tissue to which gland cells belong is
   A. connective.
   B. epithelial.
   C. secretory.
   D. nerve.

4. Of the following, which is closest to the speed of sound in air at sea level?
   A. $\frac{1}{5}$ mile per second
   B. $\frac{1}{2}$ mile per second
   C. 1 mile per second
   D. 5 miles per second

5. The general formula for the acetylene series of hydrocarbons is
   A. C_nH_{2n+2}.
   B. C_nH_{2n}.
   C. C_nH_{2n-2}.
   D. None of the above

6. How many molecules of ATP are required to activate a molecule of glucose in glycolysis?
   A. 2
   B. 6
   C. 3
   D. None

7. The vitamin that helps clotting of the blood is
   A. C.
   B. D.
   C. E.
   D. K.

8. Each nucleotide in a DNA molecule contains
   A. a sugar.
   B. a nitrogen base.
   C. a phosphate group.
   D. All of the above

9. The wavelength (nm) of the visible portion of the electromagnetic spectrum is in the range of
   A. 350–700.
   B. 800–1,000.
   C. 200–350.
   D. 550–900.

10. A person is more buoyant when swimming in salt water than in fresh water because

    A. the person keeps his or her head out of salt water.

    B. salt water has greater tensile strength.

    C. salt coats the person's body with a floating membrane.

    D. salt water is denser than an equal volume of fresh water.

11. Two parameters (e.g., the volume and the temperature of a gas) are directly proportional if a constant value can be calculated from their

    A. product.

    B. ratio.

    C. sum.

    D. difference.

12. Cellular proteins are synthesized by

    A. ribosomes.

    B. mitochondria.

    C. lysosomes.

    D. golgi.

13. All of the following mechanisms affect the amount of glucose in the blood EXCEPT:

    A. Adrenaline secretion

    B. Insulin secretion

    C. Level of oxygen intake

    D. Level of physical activity

14. The most active mixing of many digestive juices occurs in the

    A. stomach.

    B. duodenum.

    C. ileum.

    D. jejunum.

15. A *cold-blooded* animal is one that

    A. has a body temperature colder than that of other types of animals.

    B. uses heat from its blood to warm other tissues of the body, lowering the blood temperature.

    C. depends on external heat sources to regulate its body temperature.

    D. is incapable of regulating its body temperature.

16. The basic mechanism of hereditary transmission is

    A. sexual reproduction.

    B. polyploidy.

    C. separation, rearrangement, and distribution of chromosomes.

    D. the mitotic mechanism.

17. If sound waves have the following pattern, what is the frequency?

    A. 4 hertz

    B. 8 hertz

    C. 12 hertz

    D. 16 hertz

18. Of the following, the highest bactericidal activity of light occurs at a wavelength in angstrom units of

    A. 2,536.

    B. 3,256.

    C. 5,236.

    D. 6,532.

19. In the diagram below, the refraction of the light rays indicates that the lens is

Light rays

A. thicker in the center than the edges.

B. thinner at the center than the edges.

C. uniform in thickness.

D. consistent in dimensions.

20. Which of the following compounds is an ether?

A. CH_2CHO

B. CH_3-O-CH_3

C. CH_3-COOH

D. CH_3-CH_2OH

21. Which of the following statements about wavelengths is true?

A. Visible wavelengths vary in lengths.

B. The wavelength of green is the longest.

C. Radio waves are electromagnetic waves shorter than infrared.

D. Infrared rays are shorter than red light rays.

22. An object appears white, or colorless, when it

A. absorbs the light reaching it.

B. transmits only blue light.

C. rejects all colors.

D. reflects all colors at the same time.

23. Another name for animal starch is

A. cellulose.

B. lecithin.

C. glycogen.

D. chitin.

24. Of the following, a human blood disease that has been definitely shown to be due to a hereditary factor or factors is

A. pernicious anemia.

B. sickle cell anemia.

C. polycythemia.

D. leukemia.

25. All of the following elements are major constituents of a cell EXCEPT:

A. Carbon.

B. Potassium.

C. Hydrogen.

D. Phosphorus.

26. If a machine listed for 1,800 watts is plugged into a 110-volt system, approximately how many amps will it use?

A. 6.6

B. 13.0

C. 16.0

D. 19.8

27. The selection of algae as a possible nutritional supplement for humans is based primarily on their ability to carry on

A. fermentation.

B. digestion.

C. photosynthesis.

D. oxidation.

28. A nurse administered a medication at 10^{-4} molar concentrated to a patient. The doctor instructed that the dosage be reduced by one-half strength, which was

A. $10^{-2}M$

B. $5 \times 10^{-5}M$

C. $10^{-8}M$

D. $10^{-3}M$

29. In eukaryotic cells, the phase of division that produces two daughter cells is
    A. G_1.
    B. mitosis.
    C. G_2.
    D. cytokinesis.

30. Efficiency (mechanical and biological) is a relationship between input, output, and total available energy for work. Which of the following is the correct formula for efficiency?
    A. $E = \dfrac{Input}{Output} \times 100$
    B. $E = \dfrac{Input \times Output}{100}$
    C. $E = \dfrac{Output - Input}{100}$
    D. $E = \dfrac{Output}{Input} \times 100$

31. When a molecule of glucose in humans is degraded, the percent of its energy capable of generating ATP is nearest to
    A. 100.
    B. 50.
    C. 25.
    D. 80.

32. Velocity, defined as the rate of displacement of an object, is
    A. scalar.
    B. inertia.
    C. vector.
    D. centripetal.

33. The fundamental principle expressed by the Einstein equation ($E = mc^2$) on mass-energy equivalency is that
    A. small mass = much energy.
    B. small mass = little energy.
    C. little energy = great mass.
    D. All of the above

34. Exophthalmic goiter is caused by
    A. hypoactivity of the thyroid.
    B. hyperactivity of the thyroid.
    C. deficiency of vitamin A.
    D. radioactive iodine.

35. If other factors are compatible, a person who can most safely receive blood from any donor belongs to this basic blood group.
    A. O
    B. A
    C. B
    D. AB

36. The Schick test indicates whether or not a person is probably immune to
    A. tuberculosis.
    B. diptheria.
    C. poliomyelitis.
    D. scarlet fever.

37. Evaporation of water is likely to be greatest on days of
    A. high humidity.
    B. low humidity.
    C. little or no wind.
    D. low pressure.

38. The generic formula for alkane, aliphatic hydrocarbons is $C_N H_{2N+2}$, from which the formula for propane is derived, is what?
    A. $C_2 H_4$
    B. $C_3 H_8$
    C. NaNO
    D. $C_3 H_4$

39. The percentage of oxygen by weight in $Al_2(SO_4)_3$ (atomic weights: Al = 27, S = 32, O = 16) is approximately
    A. 19.
    B. 21.
    C. 56.
    D. 92.

40. In backcrossing, a hybrid is always mated with
    A. its own parent.
    B. another hybrid.
    C. a pure dominant.
    D. a pure recessive.

41. The diameter of a light microscope on low power is 2 mm. The number of 50Φ wide paramecia (side-by-side) that stretches across the entire field is
    A. 400.
    B. 500.
    C. 40.
    D. 4.

42. Of the following, a structure found in mammals but NOT in reptiles is the
    A. lung.
    B. brain.
    C. diaphragm.
    D. ventricle.

43. If the osmotic pressure of human blood is determined by the number of dissolved particles, and a 0.315 molar glucose solution is isotonic to blood, the concentration of isotonic sodium chloride (NaCl) would be
    A. 0.630 M.
    B. 0.3 M.
    C. 0.157 M.
    D. 0.2 M.

44. The resistance of matter to changes in motion is
    A. elasticity.
    B. inertia.
    C. momentum.
    D. inflexible.

45. Some substances are transported across cell membranes by proteins known as
    A. ligases.
    B. permeases.
    C. hydrolases.
    D. monomers.

46. Which sequence correctly illustrates a food chain?
    A. algae → insect larvae → fish → human
    B. algae → fish → insect larvae → human
    C. insect larvae → algae → fish → human
    D. fish → insect larvae → algae → human

47. Grasses are usually pollinated by
    A. wind.
    B. water.
    C. birds.
    D. insects.

48. Among vertebrates, the embryonic ectoderm gives rise to which of the following?
    A. Nervous system
    B. Digestive system
    C. Skeletal system
    D. Respiratory system

49. Generally, life depends directly or indirectly for food, energy, and oxygen upon
    A. parasitic organisms.
    B. green plants.
    C. fungi.
    D. animals.

50. Pathogenic bacteria responsible for food poisoning are becoming resistant to the antibiotic Ciprofloxacin. This phenomenon illustrates that the populations are
    A. photosynthesizing nutrients.
    B. encapsulating practices.
    C. evolving.
    D. dominating amino acids.

51. The weight in grams of 22.4 liters of nitrogen (atomic weight = 14) is
    A. 3
    B. 7
    C. 14
    D. 28

52. In the production of sounds, the greater the number of vibrations per second, the
    A. greater the volume.
    B. higher the tone.
    C. lower the volume.
    D. lower the tone.

53. A segment of a DNA molecule transcribes a base sequence, AGAUAU, on an mRNA codon. Which of the following is the compatible sequence on the tRNA anticodon?
    A. UUAGCG
    B. UCUAUA
    C. AAUAUA
    D. CGCAAA

54. Which of the following species will combine with a chloride ion to produce ammonium chloride?
    A. NH_3
    B. K^+
    C. NH_4^+
    D. Al^{+++}

55. The newest vaccine for a human cancer controls the HPV-16 virus of the
    A. cervix.
    B. lungs.
    C. colon.
    D. breasts.

56. Which one of the following graphs represents Boyle's Law?

    A.

    B.

    C.

    D.

57. Which of the following minerals is restored to the soil by plants of the pea and bean family?
    A. Sulfates
    B. Nitrates
    C. Carbonates
    D. Phosphates

58. In humans, any hereditary defect caused by a gene on the Y chromosome would occur
    A. in males.
    B. in females.
    C. only if the gene were recessive.
    D. about equally in males and females.

59. There is no oxidation-reduction in a reaction that involves
    A. single replacement.
    B. double replacement.
    C. simple decomposition.
    D. direct combination of elements.

60. A cross between two black guinea pigs yields 3 black and 1 white offspring. The white allele in the parents was
    A. dominant.
    B. recessive.
    C. sex-linked.
    D. absent.

61. The cellular organelle in which respiratory reactions for the release of energy occurs is a

A. centrosome.

B. chromosome.

C. chromoplast.

D. mitochondrion.

62. Members of a population that are reproductively isolated from other populations form a

A. race.

B. species.

C. community.

D. genus.

63. The most efficient cellular respiratory process, in terms of energy-yield per molecule of glucose, is

A. aerobic respiration.

B. anaerobic respiration.

C. fermentation.

D. phosphorylation.

64. Which of the following is/are NOT a requirement(s) for photosynthesis?

A. Oxygen

B. Carbon dioxide and water

C. Sunlight

D. Chlorophyll

65. A cellular organelle found in typical plant cells but not in typical animal cells is the

A. chloroplast.

B. ribosome.

C. mitochondrion.

D. centrosome.

66. In the absence of oxygen, plants and microbes convert pyruvic acid into

A. alcohol and CO_2.

B. lactic acid.

C. CO_2 and H_2O.

D. amino acids.

67. Every cell contains

A. a cell membrane and cytoplasm.

B. a cell wall and cytoplasm.

C. a nucleus and cell wall.

D. plastids and pigments.

68. Digestion in humans is

A. extracellular.

B. intracellular.

C. vacuolar.

D. intercellular.

69. An example of an obligate intracellular parasitic microorganism is a

A. tapeworm.

B. virus.

C. bacterium.

D. spirochaete.

Questions 70–72 refer to the following graph and equation.

70. At time zero, the percentage of substance that is [A] [B] is approximately

A. 100.

B. 0.

C. 50.

D. 25.

71. The comparative affinity of the reactants and products is

A. [C] [D] > [A] [B].

B. [A] [B] = [C] [D].

C. [A] [B] > [C] [D].

D. None of the above

72. Choose the INCORRECT statement, relative to the reaction at equilibrium.

    A. Concentration of reactants and products remains constant.

    B. Reaction is shifted to the right.

    C. Forward and reverse reactions occur at equal rates.

    D. Reaction is shifted to the left.

73. The second law of thermodynamics (entropy) states that systems (ranging from a single organism to the entire universe) become increasingly disordered or random with time. Early scientists erroneously believed that the human body, by maintaining its structural and functional integrity, violated this law.

    It is currently understood that the human body conforms to the second law of thermodynamics because it is a(an)

    A. closed system.

    B. assembly of organic molecules.

    C. open system.

    D. composite of inorganic and organic molecules.

74. Data from the human genome project have shown that the total number of genes in humans is close to

    A. 30

    B. 1,000,000

    C. 3,000

    D. 30,000

75. The smallest chromosome in the human genome is

    A. 1

    B. 51

    C. 21

    D. Y

STOP

IF YOU FINISH BEFORE TIME IS CALLED, YOU MAY CHECK YOUR WORK ON THIS SECTION ONLY. DO NOT TURN TO ANY OTHER SECTION IN THE TEST.

ANSWER KEY AND EXPLANATIONS

Final Science Examination

1. C	16. C	31. B	46. A	61. D
2. D	17. A	32. C	47. A	62. B
3. B	18. A	33. A	48. A	63. A
4. A	19. B	34. B	49. B	64. A
5. C	20. B	35. D	50. C	65. A
6. A	21. A	36. B	51. D	66. A
7. D	22. D	37. B	52. B	67. A
8. D	23. C	38. B	53. B	68. A
9. A	24. B	39. C	54. C	69. B
10. D	25. B	40. A	55. A	70. A
11. B	26. C	41. C	56. B	71. A
12. A	27. C	42. C	57. B	72. D
13. C	28. B	43. C	58. A	73. C
14. B	29. D	44. B	59. B	74. D
15. C	30. D	45. B	60. B	75. C

1. **The correct answer is C.** All conditions are under genetic control; however, hereditary baldness is also under hormonal control. Baldness is expressed as a dominant characteristic in males but recessive in females because of the hormones present. Thus, a male and female may inherit the same genes for baldness, but the expression of the genes will depend on the sex hormones.

2. **The correct answer is D.** Diploid cells in the testes undergo meiosis to reduce the chromosome number by one half to the haploid condition.

3. **The correct answer is B.** There are only four basic kinds of tissues: epithelial, connective, muscle, and nerve. Gland cells are among the epithelial tissues that cover the internal and external surfaces of various parts of the body.

4. **The correct answer is A.** The speed of sound in air varies slightly with temperature, increasing slightly as temperature increases. For convenience, the speed of sound in air is referred to as 1,100 feet per second. This is an approximate value that can be used despite various conditions. 1,100 feet is approximately one fifth of a mile (1 mile = 5,280 feet).

5. **The correct answer is C.** A member of the acetylene series is unsaturated, with a triple bond between two carbons. The formula for acetylene, for example, is H–C $\equiv$ C–H; because of the triple bond between 2 carbons, the number of hydrogens is reduced by 2. Thus, the general formula is $C_{n2}H_{2n-2}$.

6. **The correct answer is A.** A molecule of glucose uses 2 molecules of ATP to supply activation energy to initiate the glycolytic pathway.

7. **The correct answer is D.** Prothrombin is produced in insufficient quantities if there is a deficiency of vitamin K; prothrombin produces thrombin, which acts as an enzyme to convert fibrinogen to fibrin, the mesh that traps blood cells, forming

the clot. Thus, if vitamin K is deficient, prothrombin is deficient, and clotting is delayed or does not occur.

8. **The correct answer is D.** Each nucleotide of a DNA molecule contains a molecule of deoxyribose sugar, a nitrogen base, and a phosphate group, which is attached to the 3' carbon of 1 sugar molecule and the 5' carbon of a second sugar.

9. **The correct answer is A.** The wavelength of energy in the electromagnetic spectrum ranges from 10^{-3} nM to 10^{14} nM, with visible light between 350 nM and 700 nm.

10. **The correct answer is D.** The buoyancy of an object in water or air is determined by its density relative to the surrounding medium: thus, objects less dense than the surrounding medium will float, and those more dense will sink. Salt water is denser than fresh water because of the much greater amount of dissolved substances. Therefore, a person will float more easily in salt water because there is a greater difference between the density of the person's body and that of the water.

11. **The correct answer is B.** Two parameters are directly proportional if their ratio is a mathematical constant $\left(K = \frac{x}{y}\right)$.

12. **The correct answer is A.** Cellular proteins are synthesized by the ribosomes where codon triplets of m-RNA are paired with anticodon triplets of t-RNA to direct amino acid sequences.

13. **The correct answer is C.** Insulin increases the permeability of the cell membrane to glucose, thus increasing the rate of glucose uptake by the cells from the bloodstream. Adrenalin promotes an increase in cardiac activity, respiratory rate, and the breakdown of glycogen (stored in the liver) to glucose, thus raising the glucose level of the blood. With physical activity, glucose is more rapidly utilized by cells, which must remove glucose from the blood, thus reducing the blood level of glucose.

14. **The correct answer is B.** The digestion and absorption of most nutrients occurs in the duodenum, the first portion of the small intestine. Therefore, digestive juices are most active at this site.

15. **The correct answer is C.** The term *cold-blooded* is commonly used in reference to animals such as reptiles that depend on external sources of heat to help regulate their body temperature. Cold-blooded animals, more properly called *ectotherms*, must bask in sunlight or lie on warm ground to raise their body temperature. Conversely, they must lie in the shade or shelter beneath an object such as a rock to cool off their bodies. By contrast, warm-blooded animals, more properly called *endotherms*, are more or less independent of external sources of heat, relying on a combination of heat generated by their metabolism and insulation on the surface of the body to keep their internal temperature constant.

16. **The correct answer is C.** Chromosomes contain genetic material, or carry genes; the separation of the chromosomes of each pair is involved in meiosis, or reduction division, in the production of sexual reproductive cells. The gametes (egg and sperm) will each receive one half the chromosomes carried by the parent, or one chromosome of each pair carried by the parent. Thus, the gametes will be haploid. When fertilization occurs, the zygote becomes diploid, having received one chromosome of each pair from each parent. Therefore, each individual inherits one half of its chromosomes and genes from its father and one half from its mother.

17. **The correct answer is A.** A *hertz* can be defined as the number of wavelengths per second. A wave or wavelength is the distance between successive values, for example, from crest to crest. The diagram shows 4 waves in the one-second period, or 4 hertz.

18. **The correct answer is A.** Light consists of colors of varying wavelengths. Visible light ranges from red, with a wavelength of about 7,000 angstrom units, down to violet, with a wavelength of about 4,000 angstroms. Ultraviolet has shorter wavelengths (150–3,900 Å) and is bactericidal; the highest bactericidal activity occurs between 2,000 Å and 3,000 Å.

19. **The correct answer is B.** The lens is concave; therefore, it is thicker at the edges. Light rays passing through a concave lens are refracted or bent outward, so they spread apart. A light ray passing through the center of the lens is not bent.

20. **The correct answer is B.** The functional group for ethers is R–O–R.

21. **The correct answer is A.** Visible light consists of different colors of light, producing a spectrum of red (with the longest wavelength), orange, yellow, green, blue, indigo, and violet (with the shortest wavelength).

22. **The correct answer is D.** White light consists of the colors or wavelengths of the visible spectrum—red, orange, yellow, green, blue, indigo, and violet. An object appears to be a certain color when it is reflecting light of this wavelength, and absorbing all others. A white object is reflecting all of the colors or wavelengths at the same time.

23. **The correct answer is C.** Liver glycogen, which is a polymer of glucose molecules, is called animal starch.

24. **The correct answer is B.** Persons with sickle cell anemia carry a variant hemoglobin molecule in the red blood cells, instead of the normal hemoglobin A. The production of hemoglobin is under genetic control.

25. **The correct answer is B.** All elements listed are found in cells. Carbon, hydrogen, and phosphorus are three of the six major elements from which most organic molecules are built. Potassium is one of the five essential minor elements.

26. **The correct answer is C.** An ampere (amp) is a unit for measuring the rate of flow of electricity. A watt is the metric unit of power; it is the power produced by 1 amp in a I volt circuit. Thus, the formula *watt = amp × volt*, can be used, or $amp = \dfrac{watt}{volt}$. If the problem is worked using this formula, the answer is choice C, 16 amps.

27. **The correct answer is C.** Photosynthesis is the process by which an organic, energy-containing compound (sugar or glucose) is produced from inorganic materials. This is a process basic to the production of organic compounds that can be used for food. Algae and other green plants exhibit photosynthesis.

28. **The correct answer is B.** A half of the dosage is 5×10^{-5}M.

29. **The correct answer is D.** Cytokinesis is the stage in eukaryotic cell division in which the cytoplasm divides to produce daughter cells.

30. **The correct answer is D.** Efficiency is the ratio of work-out per work-in.

31. **The correct answer is B.** Eukaryotic cells have high efficiency, relative to mechanical device. They are capable of extracting approximately 50 percent of the energy in glucose molecules for biological work.

32. **The correct answer is C.** Vector quantities must have both magnitude and direction for complete description. An object cannot have a velocity without direction.

33. **The correct answer is A.** The equation $E = mc^2$ demonstrates mass and energy are interchangeable and that small amounts of mass can yield large amounts of energy under specific conditions.

34. **The correct answer is B.** The overproduction of the thyroid hormones causes a condition known as exophthalmic goiter, or Graves' disease. The thyroid may or may not be enlarged, but increased metabolic rate, protrusion of eyes (exophthalmus), increased blood pressure, increased heart rate, loss of weight, etc., are symptoms of Graves' disease. This disease may be treated by surgical removal or destruction of part of the thyroid gland.

35. **The correct answer is D.** A person of blood group AB has antigen A and antigen B, but cannot produce antibodies against A or B. Therefore, such a person can receive blood from any of the four blood groups and is often called a "universal recipient."

36. **The correct answer is B.** The Schick test, developed by Bela Schick, is administered by injecting a weak solution of the diphtheria toxin cutaneously. A reddening of the site of injection indicates susceptibility to diphtheria; lack of reddening indicates immunity and the presence of sufficient antitoxin to protect the person against diphtheria.

37. **The correct answer is B.** Evaporation is the physical change of a substance from a liquid to a gas. The rate of movement of gas molecules into the air is more rapid in dry air, or when the humidity is low, and decreases with increased humidity. The movement of air currents (wind) carries away the vapor above the surface of the liquid, thus increasing evaporation rate.

38. **The correct answer is B.** Propane (C_3H_8) satisfies the generic aliphatic hydrocarbon formula (C_nH_{2n+2}).

39. **The correct answer is C.** Of the 17 atoms making up a molecule of $Al_2(SO_4)_3$, there are 2 atoms of aluminum, 3 atoms of sulfur, and 12 atoms of oxygen (4 oxygens in each of the 3 sulfate ions). The weight of the oxygen is 192; the total weight of the molecule is 342. Thus, the percentage of oxygen by weight is $\frac{192}{342}$, or 56 percent.

40. **The correct answer is A.** Backcrossing of a hybrid with one of the parents or a genetically similar individual yields offspring similar to the parent.

41. **The correct answer is C.** A microscope field 2 mm in diameter is $2,000\Phi$. Paramecia (50Φ) could be placed 40Φ side-by-side across the field.

42. **The correct answer is C.** Reptiles do not possess a diaphragm but have the other structures listed.

43. **The correct answer is C.** Sodium chloride is an ionic substance that dissociates in aqueous solutions, to give 2 times the number of particles per mole in molecular substances such as glucose.

44. **The correct answer is B.** Inertia is the tendency of a body at rest or in motion to remain constant unless acted upon by an outside force.

45. **The correct answer is B.** Permeases are cellular proteins that transport substances across plasma membranes.

46. **The correct answer is A.** In a food chain, algae are the primary "producers," occupying the bottom level of the food chain

since they produce organic materials through photosynthetic processes. Insect larvae are some of the animals that can feed on algae; fish, which prey on animals such as insect larvae, are in turn consumed by humans.

47. **The correct answer is A.** Grasses are usually pollinated by wind; the grass flower typically does not attract insects or birds. Since grasses are mostly land plants, water would not play a significant role in their pollination.

48. **The correct answer is A.** The ectoderm is the outer germ layer, which gives rise to the nervous and integumentary systems of the embryo.

49. **The correct answer is B.** Only green plants can produce organic materials (food) from inorganic materials (carbon dioxide and water) through the process of photosynthesis. Oxygen and a by-product are returned to the air by means of this process. Animals may consume green plants (direct dependence) or may consume animals that consume green plants (indirect dependence) for food and energy.

50. **The correct answer is C.** This illustrates the concept of survival-of-the-fittest from a bacterial population.

51. **The correct answer is D.** One mole (gram molecular weight) of nitrogen is 28 grams, since 2 nitrogen atoms form a nitrogen molecule (N_2). One mole of gas occupies a volume of 22.4 liters at standard conditions.

52. **The correct answer is B.** The frequency, or number of vibrations per second, determines pitch, or tone. The greater the frequency, the higher the pitch; the lower the frequency, the lower the pitch.

53. **The correct answer is B.** In DNA and RNA molecules, adenine A must pair with thymine (T) or uracil (U). Guanine (G) always pairs with cytosine (C). This specificity is based on complementarity of molecular geometry, relative to the formation of double or triple bonds.

54. **The correct answer is C.** The NH^+ species has a positive valence, which has affinity for a negative chloride (Cl^-) ion.

55. **The correct answer is A.** Cervical cancer has been determined to be caused by the HPV-16 virus. A vaccine against this virus has been shown to be effective in preventing this disease.

56. **The correct answer is B.** Boyle's Law illustrates the relationship between the pressure and volume of a mass of gas at a fixed temperature. The law can be simply stated: at a given fixed temperature and mass of gas, pressure, and volume are inversely proportional. For example, volume will increase as pressure decreases, or volume will decrease as pressure increases. Therefore, pressure × volume = a constant.

57. **The correct answer is B.** Peas and beans are members of the legume family and have nitrogen-fixing bacteria in nodules on their roots. Nitrogen-fixing bacteria convert atmospheric gaseous nitrogen into nitrates, thus restoring nitrates to the soil. It is only in the form of nitrates that plants generally can obtain nitrogen from the soil.

58. **The correct answer is A.** The male sex chromosome is referred to as the Y chromosome. It is inherited only by male offspring; thus, a male is XY and a female is XX, as far as inheritance of sex is concerned. Therefore, any gene located on the Y chromosome is inherited only by males since females will inherit an X from the male parent.

59. **The correct answer is B.** Oxidation-reduction reactions are those in which one substance is oxidized by the loss of electrons, and another substance is reduced by the gain of electrons. In double replacement reactions, this does not occur. Ions are exchanged between reactants and do not lose or gain electrons.

60. **The correct answer is B.** The cross indicates that the parents were heterozygous blacks (1 black and 1 white allele). The cross would yield 1 homozygous black, 2 heterozygous blacks, and 1 homozygous white offspring.

61. **The correct answer is D.** The mitochondrion is called the powerhouse of the cell; most of the respiratory process involving the release of energy occurs in this organelle.

62. **The correct answer is B.** Reproductive isolation is the major criterion for determination of speciation.

63. **The correct answer is A.** Aerobic metabolism is 19 times more efficient than anaerobic metabolism (which yields 2 mol ATP per 1 mol glucose).

64. **The correct answer is A.** Oxygen is a waste product of photosynthesis. Green plants use carbon dioxide and water as raw materials to produce sugar in the presence of chlorophyll and sunlight as follows:

$$CO_2 + H_2O \xrightarrow[\text{chlorophyll}]{\text{sunlight}} C_6H_{12}O_6 + O_2$$

65. **The correct answer is A.** Chloroplasts contain the chlorophylls, the green pigments, and are characteristic of green plants but not of animals.

66. **The correct answer is A.** In the absence of oxygen, plants and microbes convert pyruvic acid into alcohol and carbon dioxide by a process called fermentation.

67. **The correct answer is A.** The cell wall and plastids are characteristic of plant cells but not of animal cells. A nucleus may not be present in some cells, such as mature human red blood cells. But all cells have cytoplasm surrounded by a plasma or cell membrane.

68. **The correct answer is A.** Digestion in humans occurs primarily in the lumen of the stomach and small intestine where macromolecules are degraded to small molecules capable of being absorbed.

69. **The correct answer is B.** A virus does not exhibit reproduction, synthesis, and other characteristics of life outside a living host cell; thus, it is an obligate intracellular parasite.

70. **The correct answer is A.** At the initiation of the reaction, all substances are reactants (A and B).

71. **The correct answer is A.** The affinity of [C] and [D] is greater than that of [A] and [B], resulting in a greater concentration of products versus reactants at equilibrium.

72. **The correct answer is D.** The reaction is shifted to the right.

73. **The correct answer is C.** The human body is an open system—exchanging nutrients, CO_2 and O_2, nitrogenous waste, water, and heat with the external environment.

74. **The correct answer is D.** The current estimate of genes is about 24,000–40,000 genes.

75. **The correct answer is C.** The smallest chromosome in the human genome is 21.

Reading Comprehension

OVERVIEW

TECHNIQUES

Reading comprehension presents problems for many test takers. To avoid this, make every effort to improve your ability to interpret reading passages.

First, understand that there are two aspects of success in reading interpretation:

1. Reading speed
2. Reading understanding

Too many individuals read with excellent comprehension but read too slowly. Remember, there is a time limit on your test. On the other hand, some people read rapidly, but, for reasons that we shall cite later, do not thoroughly understand what they are reading. Both speed of reading and comprehension of the material read are important during an exam.

Practice Reading Intensively

You were probably taught to read letter-by-letter. Gradually, as you matured, you learned to read word-by-word. As an adult, however, you should be able to read a complete phrase as quickly as you once read just one letter. If you cannot do this, or if you have trouble understanding what you read, you should practice reading intensively.

There is no need to be discouraged if this is the case. Most students can increase the speed of their reading significantly with little effort. The old idea that slow readers make up for their slowness by better comprehension of what they read has been proved untrue. Your ability to comprehend what you read should keep pace with your increase in speed. You can absorb as many ideas per page, and get many more ideas per unit of reading time, by applying specific techniques of reading.

It has been demonstrated that those who read best also read quickly. This is probably due to the fact that heavier concentration is required for rapid reading, and concentration is what enables a reader to grasp important ideas contained in the reading material.

A good paragraph generally has one central thought—that is, a **topic sentence**. Your main task is to locate and absorb that thought while reading the paragraph. The correct interpretation of the paragraph is based upon that thought, and not upon your personal opinions, prejudices, or preferences. If a selection consists of two or more paragraphs, its correct interpretation is based on the central idea of the entire passage. The ability to grasp the central idea of a passage can be acquired by practice—practice that will also increase the speed with which you read.

An important rule to follow in order to improve reading ability is to force yourself to increase your speed. Just as you once stopped reading letter-by-letter, now learn to stop reading word-by-word. Force yourself to read rapidly across the line of type, skimming it. Don't permit your eyes to stop for individual words; try instead to reconstruct the whole idea even if a word has been missed. Proceed quickly through the paragraph in this skimming fashion, without rereading or backtracking to a missed word.

If you find yourself failing to comprehend what you read, read the material over several times rapidly until you do understand. Do *not* slow down on rereading. At first, you may find yourself missing some of the ideas. With persistent practice, however, you will step up both your reading speed and your ability to comprehend.

You may need to overcome certain handicaps or unhelpful reading habits at once. Do not move your lips, pronounce words individually silently or aloud, or think of each word separately as you read. These habits can be overcome almost automatically if you learn to leap from phrase to phrase. You can synchronize your eye movements with your mind, both of which are nimbler than your lips.

Certain physical factors affect reading. You should always read sitting in a comfortable position, erect, with head slightly inclined. The light should be excellent, with both an indirect and a direct source available; direct light should come from behind you and slightly above your shoulder, in such a way that the type is evenly lit. Hold the reading matter at your own best reading distance and at a convenient height, so you don't stoop or squint. If you need reading glasses, you should certainly use them.

How to Increase Reading Speed

Problem: Word-by-word reading

Our earliest reading, since it is done aloud, is, of necessity, word-by-word reading. Unfortunately, this method of reading sometimes becomes so firmly implanted that it persists as a bad reading habit.

Cure: Use the eye-span method.

Look at the first part of a sentence that consists of a thought-unit. Then, look for the next thought-unit, if there is another one in the same sentence—then, look for still another thought-unit. For example, consider this sentence:

Reading maketh a full man, conference a ready man, and writing an exact man. How many ideas are there in the sentence? Three. Now, employ the eye-span method in reading this sentence.

Reading maketh a full man,
EYE-SPAN 1

conference a ready man,
EYE-SPAN 2

and writing an exact man.
EYE-SPAN 3

Problem: Vocalizing

Some readers move their lips or whisper while they read "silently." This practice slows down silent reading time considerably.

Cure

You must consciously refrain from moving your lips or whispering during silent reading. Have someone watch you while you read. Are you vocalizing?

Problem: One-speed reading

You should vary your reading speed according to what you are reading.

Cure

The pace of your reading should change not only from book to book, but even within a reading selection. Be flexible so that you can change speed from paragraph to paragraph, even from sentence to sentence. Adjust your reading rate according to the purpose for which you are reading. Scanning a passage for main ideas may be accomplished with rapid reading. Reading a novel for enjoyment would allow you to read at a medium rate. Reading to obtain detailed information would require you to read at a slower pace.

Increasing Reading Comprehension

The following are ten good techniques to use on *any* reading interpretation question.

1. Read through the selection quickly to get the general sense.
2. Reread the selection, concentrating on the central idea.
3. Attempt to pick out the *topic sentence* in each paragraph.
4. If the selection consists of more than one paragraph, determine the *central idea* of the entire selection.
5. Examine the four choices for each test item carefully yet rapidly. Eliminate immediately those choices that are far-fetched, ridiculous, irrelevant, false, or impossible.

6. Eliminate those choices that may be true but have nothing to do with the sense of the selection.

7. Check those few choices that now remain as possibilities.

8. Refer back to the original selection and determine which one of these remaining possibilities is best in view of

    a. information *stated* in the selection

    b. information *implied* in the selection

9. Be sure to consider only the facts *given* or *definitely implied* in the selection.

10. Be especially careful of trick expressions or catch-words, which sometimes destroy the validity of a seemingly acceptable answer. These include the expressions "under all circumstances," "at all times," "always," "under no conditions," "absolutely," "completely," and "entirely."

Avoid Traps

Trap 1

Sometimes, the questions cannot be answered on the basis of the stated facts. You may be required to make a deduction from the facts given. Making a deduction requires you to draw conclusions from something already known.

Trap 2

Some reading passages are designed to arouse the reader's emotion or describe situations with which the reader can identify. Be certain to base an answer selection on the information presented in the passage. Eliminate your personal opinions.

Trap 3

Many questions, and the appropriate responses to these questions, are based on important details that are nestled in the paragraph. Reread the paragraph as many times as necessary (keeping an eye on your watch) to find significant facts that will provide answers to the questions.

Get Plenty of Practice

Read:

- Editorial pages of various newspapers
- Book, drama, and movie reviews
- Magazine articles

For each selection that you read, do the following:

- Jot down the main idea of the article.
- Look up the meanings of words with which you are unfamiliar or unsure.

A Sample Question

Here is a sample question followed by analysis. Try to understand the process of arriving at the correct answer.

Too often, indeed, have scurrilous and offensive allegations by underworld figures been sufficient to blast the careers of irreproachable and incorruptible executives who, because of their efforts to serve the people honestly and faithfully, incurred the enmity of powerful political forces and lost their positions.

Judging from the contents of the preceding sentence, which conclusion might be most valid?

A. The large majority of executives are irreproachable and incorruptible.

B. Criminals often swear in court that honest officials are corrupt in order to save themselves.

C. Political forces are always clashing with government executives.

D. False statements by criminals sometimes cause honest officials to lose their positions or ruin their careers.

Analysis

Choice A can generally be said to be a true statement, but it cannot be derived from the paragraph. Nothing is said in the paragraph about "the large majority" of executives.

Choice B may also be a true statement and can, to a certain extent, be derived from the paragraph. However, the phrase "in order to save themselves" is not relevant to the sense of the paragraph, but even if it were, this choice does not sum up its central thought.

Choice C cannot be derived from the paragraph. The catch-word *always* makes this choice entirely invalid.

Choice D is the best conclusion that can be drawn from the contents of the paragraph, in light of the four choices given. It is open to no exceptions and adequately sums up the central thought of the paragraph.

Analysis of the Reading Comprehension Test Item

There are standardized tests designed to assess reading comprehension skills and provide an evaluation of the test taker's independent reading level, instructional reading level, frustration reading level, and reading rate. Reading comprehension test items usually elicit a response that would indicate the test taker's ability to identify directly stated details, indirectly stated details, main ideas, inferences, and generalizations. Other target skills may include making judgments, drawing conclusions, and determining the author's purpose.

There are two types of reading comprehension test items. The first type is a long reading passage, usually a few paragraphs in length, followed by a series of questions. The second type is a short passage, usually a single paragraph in length, alongside one question. Several paragraphs in succession may treat the same topic, but the questions will always deal with the adjacent paragraph.

In order to determine your reading rate, the proctor will tell test takers to stop after exactly one minute of exam time. Test takers will then be asked to mark the point at which they were reading when they were told to stop, and this marking will be used for the determination.

Long Reading Passage Sample

This sample long reading passage, followed by a set of six questions, will help you to analyze comprehension test items and to understand why a particular response is the correct or appropriate one.

Studying the questions before reading a passage will cause you to be more alert when reading the passage; that is, you will be aware of what information in the passage will best help you answer the questions. Now read the six questions at the end of the passage, and then read the passage and answer the questions. Note that the questions are followed by explanations that indicate the skill addressed and strategies to use in your approach to a particular type of question.

Passage

"The Land of Frost and Fire" is no misnomer for the elliptic island republic in the North Atlantic known as Iceland. The island is so called because erupting volcanoes and steaming hot springs lie adjacent to its glaciers and ice fields. The official name of the country in Icelandic is Lydveldid Island, or the Republic of Iceland.

The "frost" is frigidly evident in the island's numerous ice fields that traverse the hoary landscape. Approximately one eighth of the island is covered by glaciers. In the southeast, a glacier known as Vatnajokull makes an area of about 8,550 square kilometers (about 3,300 square miles). Iceland, just south of the Arctic Circle, has more than 120 glaciers.

Lydveldid Island's "fire" leaps from the many hot springs and spouting geysers that cloud the panorama of the seventeen-province republic. To add heat to the "fire" are some 100 volcanoes, including at least twenty-five that have erupted and been recorded in the annals of the island's autocratic history. Lava and rocks erupting from volcanoes have contoured much of the land. The central highlands reflect the barren wilderness of lava fields. Hekla, in the southwest, is the best-known Icelandic volcano because of its many eruptions. The years 1766, 1940, 1947, and 1980 mark its explosive appearances.

Thermal springs are also common in Iceland. The springs occur as geysers, sizzling mud lakes, and various other forms. The most famous geyser here is Great Geysir, which is situated in southwest Iceland. The natives of this island of swift-flowing rivers boast of Geysir's spectacular and frequent eruptions occurring at irregular intervals of 5 to 36 hours. The torrid spring reportedly thrusts a column of boiling water upward to about 60 meters, or 200 feet.

Volcanic in origin, Iceland is indeed a land of contrast. Dazzling ice and jet black lava covering most of Iceland's surface attest to the appropriateness of its nickname—"Land of Frost and Fire."

1. Where are Iceland's hot springs and geysers located?
   A. In the central highlands
   B. In the southwest
   C. Next to the glaciers
   D. In the southeast

The correct answer is C. This is a directly stated detail question. When answering this type of question, always consider the *wh* word with which the question begins. *Who* can be answered by the name of a person. *When* is answered by a word or phrase that tells at what time or in what sequence something happens. *Why* is answered by a word or phrase that tells the reason something happens. *What* is usually answered by the name of a thing or event. *Which* is answered by choosing the correct person, place, or thing from two or more persons, places, or things. *Where* is answered by the name of a place or a phrase that describes the location of one person or thing in relation to another (spatial relationships). *How* is answered by the way in which something is done. Question 1 is a *where* question denoting a spatial relationship. Since *adjacent* means "next to" and encompasses the location of both the glaciers and geysers, choice C is the appropriate response. Choices A, B, and D could be ruled out immediately because they do not describe the location of both the hot springs and the geysers.

2. An appropriate title for this passage would be
   A. "Volcanoes and Geysers."
   B. "Iceland: The Island Republic."
   C. "Iceland: A Land of Contrast."
   D. "Thermal Springs."

The correct answer is C. This is a main idea question. This type of question requires the test taker to consider what the passage is mostly about. Read the question first. Then scan the entire passage to find out what it is mostly about. A word of caution: Some answer choices are merely details from the passage. It is not difficult to choose C as the best title.

3. It is apparent that this passage is intended to
   A. inform.
   B. entertain.
   C. persuade.
   D. share an experience.

The correct answer is A. The skill addressed in this question is identifying author's purpose. The test taker must determine what the author is trying to accomplish by writing this selection. What kind of response does he or she want from the reader? If the reader can say that he or she enjoyed this passage or thought it was hilarious, obviously the passage was meant to entertain. If the reader's reaction is, "Well, I think I'll try that," or "I have to agree with that," then the passage was written to persuade. If the passage is a narration or a story-telling written in the first person (*I*, *me*, *my*, *myself*—all references to the writer), the passage is probably aimed at sharing an experience. If the reader's reaction is, "I didn't know that," or "I never heard of this before," there is a good chance that the author intended to inform.

4. The sentiments of people of Iceland toward the presence of geysers in their native land is one of
   A. mixed emotions.
   B. pride.
   C. dread and fear.
   D. indifference.

The correct answer is B. This question requires the test taker to infer a meaning or idea. In other words, "read between the lines." In the fourth paragraph of this passage, it is mentioned that the natives "boast of Geysir's spectacular and frequent eruptions." Usually, people boast about something when they are proud of it. The correct response would therefore be choice B.

5. According to this passage, Iceland's form of government at one time reflected
   A. total rule by the state.
   B. rule by and for the people.
   C. rule by royalty.
   D. rule by dictator.

The correct answer is D. This test question is an example of indirectly stated detail. In paragraph three of this passage the phrase "the annals of the island's autocratic history" appears. The adjective *autocratic*, though irrelevant to the main idea of the passage, and even to the sentence in which it appears, does provide an informational detail. The term *autocratic* suggests government by one person having unlimited power. The correct answer, therefore, would be choice D. In completing this type of question, the test taker should scan the passage to eliminate answer choices that are obviously related to the main idea. In some cases, the reader should also be careful of negative words in the question (*no*, *not*, *not any*).

6. Iceland is a difficult place to
   A. grow crops.
   B. raise a family.
   C. get an education.
   D. start a business.

The correct answer is A. This question requires that you make a judgment or draw a conclusion. Since the passage does not mention family life, education, or industry, it would be safe to eliminate choices B, C, and D. The passage also does not mention agriculture; however, it does describe the land as being "barren wilderness" and "covered by glaciers." These conditions are unsuitable for farming. Therefore, choice A is an appropriate answer.

Short Reading Passage Samples

Here are two sample short reading passages and questions, followed by analyses of the test items. Try to determine the answers on your own before reading the explanations.

A

At birth, you more than likely weighed less than 10 pounds. As an adult, you may weigh anywhere from 90 to 200 pounds or more. Obviously, there is much more of you as an adult. Despite your growth, the cells that make up your adult body are no larger than those that made up your body in infancy. This means that your adult body has billions more cells. You might question the source of these new cells. To satisfy your curiosity, they came from old cells via a process known as cell division.

1. The main idea of Paragraph A:
   A. Most infants weigh less than 10 pounds.
   B. Growth in human beings is accomplished by cell division.
   C. Living cells increase in number by a process called cell division.
   D. The cells that make up an adult body are larger than those of an infant body.

B

At a certain time during its existence, a cell divides into two cells. At the start of cell division, the nucleus becomes more dense and grainier than it was earlier. The grainy material, known as chromatin, eventually divides into short, cordlike structures called chromosomes. The chromosomes travel through the cell, forming a double line near the center of the cell.

2. As a result of the movement of chromosomes through the cell,
   A. a grainy material is formed.
   B. a cell divides into two cells.
   C. the chromatin divides into short, cordlike structures.
   D. a double line of them is formed near the center of the cell.

C

With the growing demand for seafood and the global supply of wild-caught fisheries remaining flat, what does the future of sustainable seafood hold? The solution is not easy and steps need to be taken to strike a balance between wild-capture and farm-raised seafood. Fish and shellfish are renewable resources. If managed, they can be harvested within certain limits, allowing the population to reproduce and replenish naturally, without imminent danger of depletion. U.S. aquaculture is a billion dollar industry that allows for the "farming" of all kinds of fish, shellfish, and plants in all types of aquatic environments, including ponds, lakes, rivers, and oceans. According to NOAA, marine aquaculture is a resource-efficient way of increasing and diversifying U.S. seafood production, helping to stabilize the seafood supply in the face of environmental change and economic uncertainty.

3. *Renewable* may be defined as
   A. paying a donation to help fund a stock pond.
   B. harvesting to extinction.
   C. capable of being replaced by natural ecological cycles.
   D. replenishing through genetic-modification.

Question 1

The correct answer is B. In question 1, you are clearly asked to find the main idea of Paragraph A. This means that you are to consider what the paragraph is mostly about. If you chose choice B, "Growth in human beings is accomplished by cell division," you have cited the correct response. A review or second reading of the paragraph will show that choice A could be supported by the paragraph; however, you should question the word "most." This statement merely provides a detail that leads to the principal concept. Choice C is factual, but it only supplies a major detail to the overall concept. Choice D, according to the paragraph, is incorrect information since the passage states that "despite your growth, the cells that comprise your adult body are no larger than those that made up your body in infancy." Choice B most clearly ties together the two remaining details, choices A and C, and states what the paragraph is mostly about.

Question 2

The correct answer is D. In question 2, the word *result* indicates a cause/effect response (*result* and *effect* are synonymous in this case). The paragraph clearly states that "the chromosomes travel through the cell, forming a double line near the center of the cell" (paraphrase: causing a double line to form). A review of the paragraph would prove that adding any of the activities described in choices A, B, or C to the question stem would not yield the proper sequence of the cell division process.

Question 3

The correct answer is C. If you're thinking Paragraph C is definitely a short passage reading comprehension question, you're right. If you're saying to yourself, "but this looks like a verbal ability question," you're right again. Reading comprehension is closely related to and dependent upon the understanding of words that test makers often include; verbal ability questions are often integrated into reading comprehension test items. This type of question requires you to think in terms of the precise meaning of a word as used in the passage. We call the answer to this question "vocabulary in context."

As for the answer to question 3, you should begin by eliminating choice A. There is clearly no mention of paying money to support stocking a fish pond. Choice B is incorrect because *extinction* is the opposite of *renewable*. Choice D is incorrect because while the meaning of *replenish* is similar to *renewable*, there is no mention of genetic modification. In fact, the passage refers to allowing the fish population to reproduce and replenish "naturally."

Reading in the Content Area

Efficient reading requires that the reader be flexible. As you already read, it is necessary to adjust your reading rate according to the purpose for which you are reading. It is equally important to adapt your reading style to the material being read. Before investigating effective strategies to use in making such reading adjustments, it is necessary to examine and recognize the structure and patterns of writing unique to each subject area. This study of various reading materials will help you get a feel for their differences and determine which reading style to apply to any given reading task.

Reading comprehension test items are frequently designed to reflect the course content of the field of study targeted by the entrance examination. For instance, entrance exams for educational programs leading to health careers may feature reading passages with scientific topics and information.

Unlike the humanities—which deal with emotions, attitudes, and sympathies of human beings via the study of philosophy, religion, music, art, and literature—science is the accumulation of knowledge by means of the study, observation, and classification of data justifiable by general laws or concrete truths. Scientists look for and acquire information regarding forms and processes of nature. They search for an undistorted view of reality and, therefore, cannot allow their values, feelings, attitudes, beliefs, and prejudices—or those of society—to interfere with their work.

Due to the nature of the subject matter, a scientist's writings follow a certain style. Descriptions are very exacting, factual, and detailed. They are void of background mood or setting and are unemotional. As you read scientific material, you must concentrate on the following five reading skills:

ALERT!

Time matters. Don't just keep rereading.

1. Developing vocabulary.

2. Finding the main concepts.

3. Determining and remembering supporting details.

4. Understanding the organization or major pattern of writing in science (examination, classification, generalization, problem solution, comparison or contrast, sequence).

5. Drawing conclusions.

The Verbal Ability section of this book provides strategies for understanding and developing specialized scientific vocabulary. One method encourages vocabulary expansion through the use of a glossary, dictionary, thesaurus, etc., as well as through context clues. Another encourages the recognition of words that stand for concepts instead of facts. Other approaches include the study of word roots and affixes and the recognition of symbols.

The design or style of the text in science reading materials makes finding the main concepts simple. There are usually titles, opening comments in boldface type, headings, a summary, and questions at the end of the chapter or chapter section. In your initial reading, read only the text features just mentioned. This will allow you to explore and get a sense of the main ideas presented in the chapter, article, or selection. It will also prepare you for a second and closer reading.

Once you have identified the main ideas in a scientific passage, the next step in understanding what you are reading is to determine the supporting details. Supporting details answer the *who, what, why, where*, and *when* surrounding the main idea. Ask yourself these questions once you have completed a paragraph. In science, you should also question how much or to what extent.

Understanding the organization or major pattern of writing in science is vital to your reading comprehension. First of all, you should concentrate on examining the material you are about to read *before* you actually read it. Know the topic(s) that will be addressed and sum up the vocabulary in the particular reading selection. Next, identify the writing pattern that stands out in the material. There are four patterns:

1. **Classification** places into groups and subgroups a variety of objects or areas. For instance, in the explanation of plant life, a writer may outline the classification of plants. The breakdown could begin with vascular and nonvascular and seedless nonvascular plants. From here, the author could branch out to descriptions of mosses and liverworts, etc. In this pattern, watching for structural parts in order of importance is a must. Be aware of subheadings and all font treatments.

2. **Process-description** requires you to be aware of what the process is and exactly how it works. Studying illustrations and diagrams is helpful in this pattern.

3. **Factual-statement** involves the presentation of facts to define, compare or contrast, and illustrate. When reading for facts, remember that "fact" in the world of science means a statement that can be supported by scientific observation and experimentation and that has not yet been disproved. A fact defines something or explains its actions.

4. **Problem-solving** usually appears in science passages that give an account of past scientific problems and discoveries achieved through experimentation. There are three helpful

questions that you should ask yourself when analyzing a problem-solving passage: (1) What is the problem or question? (2) How does the author answer or respond to the question? (3) How do I know the question was answered?

Drawing conclusions is basic to the study of the sciences. A sound conclusion is a judgment based on facts. Consider what you need to know in order to make a sound judgment about something you read. Check the given facts. Think about what these facts are based on (experimentation, observation, etc.) to make certain of their reliability. Then consider the facts that are not given. Reread the passage to gather information that may be implied rather than stated. This method should help you in your test-taking venture. Speaking of tests, by now you have probably drawn some conclusions about the entrance exam you are about to take and about the specialized vocabulary that may appear on it. However, do not conclude that scientific reading material is extremely difficult; instead, think of it as a kind of reading material that requires a very different approach.

READING COMPREHENSION ANSWER SHEET

Test 1

1. Ⓐ Ⓑ Ⓒ	4. Ⓐ Ⓑ Ⓒ	7. Ⓐ Ⓑ Ⓒ	10. Ⓐ Ⓑ Ⓒ	13. Ⓐ Ⓑ Ⓒ
2. Ⓐ Ⓑ Ⓒ	5. Ⓐ Ⓑ Ⓒ	8. Ⓐ Ⓑ Ⓒ	11. Ⓐ Ⓑ Ⓒ	14. Ⓐ Ⓑ Ⓒ
3. Ⓐ Ⓑ Ⓒ	6. Ⓐ Ⓑ Ⓒ	9. Ⓐ Ⓑ Ⓒ	12. Ⓐ Ⓑ Ⓒ	15. Ⓐ Ⓑ Ⓒ

Test 2

1. Ⓐ Ⓑ Ⓒ Ⓓ	3. Ⓐ Ⓑ Ⓒ Ⓓ	5. Ⓐ Ⓑ Ⓒ Ⓓ	7. Ⓐ Ⓑ Ⓒ Ⓓ	8. Ⓐ Ⓑ Ⓒ Ⓓ
2. Ⓐ Ⓑ Ⓒ Ⓓ	4. Ⓐ Ⓑ Ⓒ Ⓓ	6. Ⓐ Ⓑ Ⓒ Ⓓ		

Test 3

1. Ⓐ Ⓑ Ⓒ Ⓓ	3. Ⓐ Ⓑ Ⓒ Ⓓ	5. Ⓐ Ⓑ Ⓒ Ⓓ	7. Ⓐ Ⓑ Ⓒ Ⓓ	9. Ⓐ Ⓑ Ⓒ Ⓓ
2. Ⓐ Ⓑ Ⓒ Ⓓ	4. Ⓐ Ⓑ Ⓒ Ⓓ	6. Ⓐ Ⓑ Ⓒ Ⓓ	8. Ⓐ Ⓑ Ⓒ Ⓓ	

Test 4

1. Ⓐ Ⓑ Ⓒ Ⓓ	3. Ⓐ Ⓑ Ⓒ Ⓓ	5. Ⓐ Ⓑ Ⓒ Ⓓ	7. Ⓐ Ⓑ Ⓒ Ⓓ	9. Ⓐ Ⓑ Ⓒ Ⓓ
2. Ⓐ Ⓑ Ⓒ Ⓓ	4. Ⓐ Ⓑ Ⓒ Ⓓ	6. Ⓐ Ⓑ Ⓒ Ⓓ	8. Ⓐ Ⓑ Ⓒ Ⓓ	10. Ⓐ Ⓑ Ⓒ Ⓓ

Test 5

1. Ⓐ Ⓑ Ⓒ Ⓓ	3. Ⓐ Ⓑ Ⓒ Ⓓ	5. Ⓐ Ⓑ Ⓒ Ⓓ	7. Ⓐ Ⓑ Ⓒ Ⓓ	8. Ⓐ Ⓑ Ⓒ Ⓓ
2. Ⓐ Ⓑ Ⓒ Ⓓ	4. Ⓐ Ⓑ Ⓒ Ⓓ	6. Ⓐ Ⓑ Ⓒ Ⓓ		

Test 6

1. Ⓐ Ⓑ Ⓒ Ⓓ	3. Ⓐ Ⓑ Ⓒ Ⓓ	4. Ⓐ Ⓑ Ⓒ Ⓓ	5. Ⓐ Ⓑ Ⓒ Ⓓ	6. Ⓐ Ⓑ Ⓒ Ⓓ
2. Ⓐ Ⓑ Ⓒ Ⓓ				

answer sheet

TEST 1

15 Questions • 35 Minutes

Directions: Carefully read the following paragraphs and then answer the accompanying questions, basing your answer on what is stated or implied in the paragraphs. When you have decided which choice is best, fill in the corresponding space on your answer sheet. There is only one best answer for each question.

Taking It to Heart

A

Prior to 1628, when William Harvey published his book on the circulation of the blood and the operation of the heart, no one really knew or understood the function of the heart or how it worked. There was some speculation about it having something to do with the blood; however, people generally thought of it as the place in the body from which love and courage were generated.

B

Until Harvey's discovery, no one was aware that the heart is one of the toughest muscles in the human body and one of the most awesome pumps in the world. It is the heart that pumps the blood throughout the body night and day. This mighty muscle, though only the size of a clenched fist, does enough work in one 24-hour period to lift a man weighing 150 pounds to an altitude of almost 1,000 feet into the air.

C

Actually, the heart is two pumps, side by side—one on the right and one on the left. The right pump sends blood from the veins to the lungs. Then it pumps blood through the lungs to the pump on the left, which sends it through the body.

1. Based upon paragraph A, which of these statements is true?
   A. One function of the heart is to generate love and courage in a human being.
   B. The purpose and function of the heart was not understood until 1628.
   C. Harvey published a book that dealt with performing operations on the heart.
   D. The fact that the heart is instrumental in the circulation of the blood is merely speculation.

2. According to paragraph B, it is understood that
   A. the heart is a muscle that pumps blood throughout the body.
   B. Harvey discovered the heart.
   C. the heart can lift a man weighing 150 pounds to a height of 1,000 feet.
   D. all muscles in the human body perform as pumps.

3. The main idea of paragraph C is that
   A. the right pump of the heart sends blood from the veins to the lungs.
   B. the pumps that make up the heart are situated side by side.
   C. the left pump sends the blood through the body.
   D. the heart is two pumps that work to send blood throughout the body.

D

Although the right- and left-hand sides of the heart are two different pumps with no direct connection between them, they squeeze and relax in just about the same rhythm. Together they pump approximately 13,000 quarts of blood through the body daily.

E

The most amazing thing about the heart is that it continues beating throughout life, resting only a fraction of a second after each beat. Considering that this entails 100,000 beats per day, the durability of this organ is undoubtedly phenomenal.

4. Paragraph D makes the point that
    A. the human body contains 13,000 quarts of blood.
    B. despite the fact that they squeeze and relax in just about the same rhythm, the two pumps do not have a connection.
    C. the rhythm of the two pumps is synchronized.
    D. the two pumps operate as one.

5. Which statement is supported by paragraph E?
    A. The third part of the heartbeat is a period of rest.
    B. A steady heartbeat is characteristic of a strong and healthy heart.
    C. The heart beats about 70 times per minute.
    D. You can easily detect your own heartbeat.

The Skin You're In

F

The first thing you see when you look at the human body is the skin. The average adult human body is covered with about 18 square feet of skin.

Skin varies in thickness. It is very thin over the eyelids and considerably thicker on the palms of the hands and the soles of the feet.

G

The skin is composed of two layers. The outer layer of skin is called the epidermis. This name comes from ancient Greek meaning "outer layer." This layer is made up of dead, flattened cells that are continually sloughing off as we move around. The bottom of the epidermis is made of live cells that die and replace those that wear off on the surface. Throughout the body's lifetime, the under layer of skin continually creates new cells. This is the reason why cuts and scrapes heal in a short period of time.

H

Beneath the outer layer is another layer called the dermis. This is a much deeper layer made entirely of living cells. There are several small blood vessels and nerve endings in the dermis. There are coiled tubes in this layer that open into the epidermis layer through openings called pores. The pores are openings to the coiled tubes or sweat glands. Hairs, which grow out of the skin, are rooted in the dermis. They grow out of openings called hair follicles. Oil glands in the skin connected with the hair roots constantly oil the outer skin, keeping it supple and strong.

6. From paragraph F, the reader can conclude that
    A. the skin is the one organ readily visible on the human body.
    B. adults have thicker skin than children.
    C. skin on the human body is thicker on parts of the body most likely to come in contact with foreign objects and surfaces.
    D. 18 square feet of skin would be adequate to cover and protect all adult human beings.

7. From paragraph G, it may be inferred that

A. the production of new cells constitutes healing in the human being.

B. the ancient Greeks were probably the first to study skin.

C. the bottom of the epidermis is comprised of flattened cells that gradually wear away.

D. skin is the organ responsible for growth in the human body.

8. Which statement is supported by paragraph H?

A. The skin needs oil to remain pliant and durable.

B. The coiled tubes in the epidermis are actually pores.

C. Dry skin may be an indication of a problem in the hair follicle.

D. The epidermis provides the body with adequate temperature control.

I

The functions of the skin are numerous. The skin is a protective covering for the body that is airtight and waterproof. When it is unbroken it is a barrier to harmful bacteria. The coloring matter of the skin, known as pigment, serves to screen out certain harmful rays of the sun. The skin helps to regulate the temperature of the body and also functions as a sense organ. There are many nerve endings in the skin that caution us to stay away from things that are too hot or too cold and cause us to have a sense of touch. They enable us to detect sensation in our immediate surroundings and transmit impulses to the brain where the sensations are identified.

9. According to paragraph I, it is understood that

A. skin coloring is the result of harmful rays of the sun.

B. sensations are directly perceived by the skin.

C. the function of the skin is merely that of a protective covering.

D. the skin is a deterrent to harmful bacteria only if it is unbroken.

Nursing Interventions

J

The term "nursing interventions" encompasses and describes activities that reflect nursing responsibility in the execution of health treatment. More specifically, it refers to nursing treatments, nursing observations, health teaching, and medical treatment performed by nurses. A nursing intervention is a single course of action intended to fulfill the unmet human needs that are ascertained from the patient's problem. A nursing diagnosis is, therefore, a prerequisite to implementing the appropriate care to meet the needs of the patient. It is apparent that in order to determine and initiate nursing intervention, one must have a scientific background and extensive education in nursing.

10. The main idea of paragraph J is that

A. the role of an individual who has a scientific and nursing education background, and who performs a single course of action to satisfy the unmet human needs of a patient, is known as nursing intervention.

B. a nursing diagnosis is synonymous with nursing intervention.

C. nursing responsibility includes health teaching.

D. nursing assessment is necessary for effective nursing intervention.

Blood Donors Available—No Thanks! I'll Do It Myself!

K

With the advent of AIDS and other communicable diseases, people are reluctant to submit to blood transfusions as a measure of medical treatment, even in emergency situations. Many individuals are opting to store their own blood in case it is ever needed.

L

New blood cells are constantly being produced in the body. This is the reason that lost blood in a healthy person is replaced quickly. This rapid production of blood cells also enables a person to donate to others who might need blood. When blood is taken from one person and given to another, the procedure is called a homologous blood transfer. When a person's own blood is used for transfusion, having been stored in anticipation of surgery, the procedure is known as autologous blood transfer. This blood is collected prior to surgery.

M

Though the concept of being transfused with one's own blood is very comforting, there are many factors that discourage the use of this technology. First is the expense of storing the blood. Another drawback is that a patient may be thousands of miles away from his or her blood supply or blood bank when the need for blood arises.

11. The accelerated interest in autologous transfusion is due to

   A. a lack of blood donors.

   B. an attempt to stimulate rapid production of new blood cells.

   C. the time-saving element in the event of emergency surgery.

   D. a rise in fear of communicable diseases.

N

In an attempt to satisfy patients' requests to be transfused with their own blood, regardless of the medical emergency, doctors have developed two forms of autologous blood transfusion. One form utilizes suction devices to collect blood lost during surgery. After this blood has been cleansed, it may be put back into the body. Blood lost during surgery can also be collected with sponges. The sponges are then squeezed out into a container of saline solution, a kind of salt solution. This blood is processed within 15 minutes and is again introduced into the patient's circulation. Doctors believe that by using both methods they can retrieve up to 90 percent of blood that would otherwise be lost.

O

Despite these efforts to make autologous blood transfer feasible for most patients, there still remain those situations that make it virtually impossible to collect blood. For instance, in the case of an auto accident victim, much blood is often lost before medical treatment is obtainable. To help in an incident such as this, doctors are researching ways to develop artificial hemoglobin that would temporarily transport oxygen and carbon dioxide throughout the body. Another solution being explored is the reproduction of a hormone that causes the body to produce blood cells much more rapidly than it would normally. This would mean that the body could replace most of its own blood and therefore reduce the need for transfusion. Even though researchers are doing extensive work to develop new techniques to protect people from blood tainted by disease, reserving one's own blood for future use seems to be the safest method of transfusion for now.

12. This passage supports the concept that
    A. autologous transfer is a practical and easily accessible alternative to blood transfusion.
    B. any type of blood transfusion places a patient in a high-risk health situation.
    C. hemoglobin carries oxygen and carbon dioxide throughout the body.
    D. lost blood, even in a healthy person, is replaced only after a long period of time.

13. From this passage it may be inferred that
    A. saline is a cleansing or sterilizing agent.
    B. the storing of one's own blood supply is affordable for all.
    C. homologous transfusion requires blood typing and matching.
    D. the option of autologous transfusion is not feasible in instances of elective surgery.

14. A fact expressed in this passage is that
    A. artificial hemoglobin could permanently supply the body with oxygen and carbon dioxide.
    B. suction devices and sponges are two surgical implements used in the collection of blood lost during surgery.
    C. laser surgery is being used more frequently in an effort to minimize blood loss during surgery.
    D. autologous transfusion, in the event of surgery, requires that the blood always be collected prior to surgery.

15. This article suggests that
    A. homologous transfusions are on the decline.
    B. the effort by researchers to protect patients from blood contaminated by disease cannot guarantee safe blood transfusion.
    C. autologous transfusion is impractical.
    D. surgical patients who are transfused autonomously are assured a more rapid recovery.

STOP

IF YOU FINISH BEFORE TIME IS CALLED, YOU MAY CHECK YOUR WORK ON THIS SECTION ONLY. DO NOT TURN TO ANY OTHER SECTION IN THE TEST.

TEST 2

8 Questions • 12 Minutes

> **Directions:** Carefully read the following passage and then answer the accompanying questions, basing your answers on what is stated or implied in the passage. When you have decided which choice is best, fill in the corresponding space on your answer sheet. There is only one best answer for each question.

Live and Learn

A

It has been a difficult year. As our country and the world continue to cope with the aftermath of September 11, 2001, some people have boldly chosen to take their lives back. Many others, though, are finding it extremely difficult to move on.

1. Paragraph A implies that the events of September 11, 2001 were
   A. devastating.
   B. unavoidable.
   C. pragmatic.
   D. intolerable.

2. The event(s) alluded to impacted
   A. nationally.
   B. globally.
   C. positively.
   D. moderately.

B

It is troubling that thousands of lives were taken in a heartbeat, and now we're witnessing a domino effect across the globe as a result of the attacks on America. It's no secret that the U.S. is an ally of Israel and that this position has been the fuel for terrorist attacks on our soil. But war in the Middle East has been brewing for years, so now we explore other issues that contribute to the conflict.

3. According to the writer, the loss of lives was
   A. instantaneous.
   B. by heart malfunction.
   C. ephemeral.
   D. predictable.

C

Are immigration and integration in Palestine to blame? What about U.S. dollars going to Israel? Or Muslim extremists? Whatever the reasons, every nation is adjusting its policies to ready themselves for what might be coming. Recently, the United States and a bloc of Southeast Asian nations signed a treaty aimed at making the region—a second front in the war against terrorism—more responsive to future threats. Sadly, it took a tragedy of this magnitude to get America to realize that it's not invincible and that we really are living in an interdependent world.

4. It is suggested that the attacks of 9/11 may be directly related to
   A. the ongoing Middle East oil dispute.
   B. the absence of a treaty between the United States and Southeast Asian nations.
   C. Palestinians' hatred of the United States.
   D. U.S. aid to and friendship with Israel.

5. America's realization of its vulnerability

    A. has prompted Middle East peace talks.

    B. has resulted in more gun control laws.

    C. is a significant outcome of 9/11.

    D. has resulted in relaxed national security.

6. The author mentions "domino effect" to describe

    A. the falling of the towers.

    B. the mass physical destruction that came out of this event.

    C. the far-reaching consequences that stem from 9/11.

    D. the political turmoil that was caused by 9/11.

D

The nation's economy is in a serious slump. The failures of such high-performing companies as Enron, and the government investigations of others, including AOL Time Warner and MCI WorldCom, Inc., which was charged with fraud after the company admitted to hiding almost $4 billion in costs, has contributed to the stock market nosedive.

E

The ripple effects of the U.S. economic woes are widespread. Stress is on the rise for good reasons. The Dow Jones industrial average recently reached its largest weekly decline (nearly 700 points) since last September. Retirees are having to re-enter the work force, and who doesn't know someone who's recently lost his or her job? People continue to file claims for unemployment insurance, and a study released roughly four months after the attacks predicted that the effects of the more than 1.6 million jobs that will probably be lost in 2002 will reverberate through the U.S. economy for years to come.

F

The jobless are penny-pinching and postponing vacations, which is a dire dilemma for many tourism-dependent nations. Caribbean countries like Jamaica and St. Lucia are expected to lose $3 billion tourism revenue—money that is normally used for health care and other services and accounts for roughly 70 percent of the gross domestic product of many Caribbean countries.

G

Everyone has been affected by September 11 in one way or another. Even though we've struggled through the past year, we, as Americans, are truly blessed. What is most important now is to accept what has taken place, and to learn and grow from it. It takes faith, and it is that faith that has guided our people for centuries. So take pride in this country and help make it a better place for you and your children.

—Reprinted with permission of *Upscale* from "Founder's Desk, Live and Learn," by Bernard Bronner, Founder. *Upscale*, October 2002.

7. The tragedy of 9/11 has

    A. left all of humankind emotionally scarred.

    B. drastically changed our lives and the way we view life.

    C. helped the economy rally.

    D. strengthened relations between the United States and the Middle East.

8. The attitude of the author is one of

    A. defeat.

    B. hopefulness.

    C. indifference.

    D. despair.

STOP

IF YOU FINISH BEFORE TIME IS CALLED, YOU MAY CHECK YOUR WORK ON THIS SECTION ONLY. DO NOT TURN TO ANY OTHER SECTION IN THE TEST.

TEST 3

9 Questions • 12 Minutes

Directions: Carefully read the following passage and then answer the accompanying questions, basing your answers on what is stated or implied in the passage. When you have decided which choice is best, fill in the corresponding space on your answer sheet. There is only one best answer for each question.

Is It Your Fault If You're Fat?

A

Why are more Americans overweight and developing diabetes? Is it fast food? No regular meals and precious little exercise? Our love affair with the TV and computer? The wrong advice about what to eat?

B

Very likely it's all these things—combined with something about the genetic make-up in many of us. Genes may program some to feel hungry when they aren't and others to be less able to tell when they are full.

1. The generalization could be made that obesity is caused by
   - **A.** eating fast foods.
   - **B.** lack of exercise.
   - **C.** lack of education as to which foods to eat.
   - **D.** lifestyle and genetic makeup.

2. People are programmed to feel hungry (when they actually are not) by
   - **A.** therapists.
   - **B.** genes.
   - **C.** nutritional counseling.
   - **D.** dining trends.

C

Some extreme obesity in children is caused by an identifiable, single gene defect. Obesity is no more their "fault" than developing cystic fibrosis is the "fault" of a child who has the CF gene. Admittedly, perhaps only 5 percent of obesity is purely genetic. But research suggests that multiple genes control appetite and metabolism, and defects in one or more may make someone more prone to being overweight. Fat cells, particularly in the abdomen, in turn release substances that can make people more prone to insulin resistance, which leads to Type 2 diabetes.

D

Some people are genetically blessed and never gain much weight. Those with gene defects must expend huge effort to overcome messages their bodies are sending their brains to eat more.

3. People who are more prone to insulin resistance are
   - **A.** candidates for stomach problems.
   - **B.** those with no weight problem.
   - **C.** those who are likely to develop Type 2 diabetes.
   - **D.** in danger of becoming obese.

4. When great effort is put forth, people with gene defects can
   - **A.** overcome urges to eat more.
   - **B.** overcome diabetes.
   - **C.** live a normal life.
   - **D.** be overweight.

5. The author's purpose in this passage is to
   - **A.** inform.
   - **B.** persuade.
   - **C.** entertain.
   - **D.** analyze.

E

For example, research at Rockefeller University and elsewhere suggests that people who lack leptin or lack receptors to make their cells sensitive to leptin have uncontrolled hunger, overeat, and become extremely obese. The melanocortin pathway in the brain has recently been identified by scientists at Beth Israel Deaconess Medical Center and elsewhere as another target influencing both obesity and anorexia.

F

In addition, some researchers have shown that the absence of a peptide called MSH, which suppresses eating, leads to obesity. Research at Joslin Diabetes Center in Boston and elsewhere suggests that another peptide, MCH, which stimulates eating, may also play a role.

6. Researchers have found that
   A. an overabundance of leptin causes obesity.
   B. the absence of a certain substance in the body results in uncontrolled eating.
   C. MHS is a peptide.
   D. overeating is a habit.

7. Obesity may be defined as
   A. fat.
   B. a state of being significantly overweight.
   C. a genetic condition.
   D. a disease related to overeating.

G

Ghrelin, a stomach hormone that signals hunger, is another potential target. Interestingly, extremely obese individuals who undergo stomach bypass surgery (stomach stapling) may be less inclined to eat afterwards because food no longer passes through the section of the stomach that produces ghrelin.

H

Some overeating may be trigged by stress, boredom, or depression. For example, food smells may stimulate production of certain peptides that make one want to eat—even if not hungry. Behavior modification may be needed to combat these stimulants of weight gain.

I

As our genes haven't changed in the last 20–30 years, societal influences are still the major culprit for growing obesity. We are more sedentary. Super-sizing meals makes it harder not to eat for those trying mightily to ignore the errant signals their bodies are sending. Until we can identify who has what gene defects, and the medications are developed to treat them, we must remember that it is much easier to prevent weight gain than to lose weight once gained. Your body adjusts quickly to these extra calories.

J

Life as overweight adults often has its roots in life as a child. For the moment, the best approach to obesity, and the Type 2 diabetes it causes, is prevention—in ourselves and our children. As nationwide studies show, even modest weight loss—15 pounds—and 30 minutes of daily exercise, are the best ways to prevent diabetes in those most likely to develop it.

—Copyright © Joslin Diabetes Center.
Reprinted with permission from *Time*,
"Is It Your Fault If You're Fat?"
by Eleftheria Marasthos-Flier, M.D.,
and Jeffrey S. Flier, M.D.
Time Magazine Special Advertising
Section, November 4, 2002.

8. The main idea of this passage is that
   A. overeating can be controlled with diet and exercise.
   B. diabetes is related to obesity.
   C. current research reveals a number of contributing factors to obesity.
   D. there are cures for obesity.

9. From this passage one can draw the conclusion that
   A. being overweight is unhealthy.
   B. children, too, can have weight problems.
   C. being fat may not necessarily be the fault of the obese individual.
   D. obesity can be attributed solely to genetics.

STOP

IF YOU FINISH BEFORE TIME IS CALLED, YOU MAY CHECK YOUR WORK ON THIS SECTION ONLY. DO NOT TURN TO ANY OTHER SECTION IN THE TEST.

TEST 4

10 Questions • 13 Minutes

> **Directions:** Carefully read the following passage and then answer the accompanying questions, basing your answers on what is stated or implied in the passage. When you have decided which choice is best, fill in the corresponding space on your answer sheet. There is only one best answer for each question.

With the use of DNA (deoxyribonucleic acid) as a means of providing evidence in a number of world-renowned criminal cases, the general public views this carrier of genetic information as a modern-day scientific discovery. However, a glimpse at the history of DNA will prove the notion of a "modern-day miracle" quite to the contrary.

To investigate the discovery of DNA, one would have to research the laboratory and work of the Swiss biochemist, Johan Friedrich Miescher, back in 1868. Miescher had been involved in the study of the cell nucleus, the round control center that contains the chromosomes as well as other elements. He believed that cells were made of protein and attempted to break down this protein with a digestive enzyme. As Miescher continued this investigation, he was perplexed by the fact that the enzyme would break down the cell but not the nucleus. He then launched an investigation of the substance that comprised the cell. As he analyzed it, he saw that it contained large amounts of a strange material that was very unlike protein. Miescher chose to call this substance nuclein. He had no idea of its significance, nor did he recognize that he had discovered what came to be known in later years as nucleic acid. Nucleic acid is the chemical family to which DNA belongs.

In 1944, a team of scientists from the Rockefeller Institute proved for the first time that DNA was the carrier of hereditary information. Oswald T. Avery, Colin M. MacLeod, and Maclyn McCarty accomplished this by extracting some of the DNA in pure form from a bacterium and substituting it for a defective gene in another related bacterium.

Some ten years later, the intricate molecular structure of DNA was described by Harvard biochemist James D. Watson and physicist Francis Crick of Great Britain. However, prior to this, scientist Rosalind Franklin discovered that the DNA molecule was a strand of molecules in a spiral form. Dr. Franklin demonstrated that the spiral was so large that it was most likely formed by two spirals. Ultimately, Franklin determined that the structure of DNA is similar to the handrails and steps of a spiral staircase.

Equipped with the work and findings of Rosalind Franklin and others, Watson and Crick were able to construct a model of a DNA molecule. This model depicted the sides or "handrails" of the DNA molecules as being made up of two twisted strands of sugar and phosphate molecules. The "stairs" that hold the two sugar phosphate strands apart are made up of molecules called nitrogen bases.

All of this data supports the fact that DNA is by no means a "new discovery"; however, what is the significance of it at all? Why is DNA important to you? The answer is that all of the characteristics you possess are affected by the DNA in your cells. It controls the color of your eyes, the color of your hair, and whether or not you have a tolerance for dairy products. These characteristics are known as traits. The way your traits appear depends on the kinds of proteins your cells make. DNA stores the blueprints for making the proteins. Your DNA is uniquely different from that of anyone else on earth, and you are identifiable by these proteins.

1. It could be concluded that
   A. Watson and Crick discovered DNA.
   B. the strands of DNA take the form of a double hexagon.
   C. DNA is as unique to individuals as a fingerprint.
   D. Miescher's analysis of nuclein resulted directly in the discovery of DNA.

2. From this passage, it may be deduced that enzymes are
   A. unstable.
   B. ineffective.
   C. catalysts.
   D. solutions.

3. It may be inferred that an individual's DNA determines
   A. whether or not he or she can digest milk.
   B. whether or not he or she is immune to the common cold.
   C. an individual's choice of residential location.
   D. a person's inclination toward dishonesty.

4. The types of protein produced by a cell are controlled by the DNA contained in its
   A. nitrogen bases.
   B. nucleus.
   C. cell wall.
   D. sugar phosphate bands.

5. It is implied that proteins are the
   A. control center of the cell.
   B. blueprint of the cell.
   C. storage center of the cell.
   D. building blocks of a cell.

6. A reference to the "spiral staircase" constitutes a description of the molecular structure of
   A. proteins.
   B. digestive enzymes.
   C. RNA.
   D. DNA.

7. Digestive enzymes are effective in breaking up
   A. nuclein.
   B. DNA.
   C. all chemical compounds.
   D. protein.

8. The word *nucleus* refers to
   A. the round control center of the cell.
   B. the walls of the cell.
   C. a strand of molecules.
   D. a helix.

9. The scientific disciplines used in determining the structure of the DNA molecule include biology, chemistry, and
   A. genealogy.
   B. serology.
   C. physics.
   D. embryology.

10. As described in this passage, *model* means

   A. an exhibitor of fashion.

   B. a physical form representing a concept.

   C. a miniature version of an existing object.

   D. a person on whom an artist bases his or her rendition.

STOP

> IF YOU FINISH BEFORE TIME IS CALLED, YOU MAY CHECK YOUR WORK ON THIS SECTION ONLY. DO NOT TURN TO ANY OTHER SECTION IN THE TEST.

TEST 5

8 Questions • 8 Minutes

> **Directions:** Carefully read the following passage and then answer the accompanying questions, basing your answers on what is stated or implied in the passage. When you have decided which choice is best, fill in the corresponding space on your answer sheet. There is only one best answer for each question.

Computer Watch Your Step

A

Can a computer spot a criminal or a terrorist infiltrating an airport tarmac? Face-recognition programs are useless if a person's face is obscured, unlit, or just too far away. So a number of researchers are trying to identify a person simply by the way he or she walks.

B

One approach is to collect video images of the surveillance area and analyze everybody passing through. "We've been trying to measure things like stride length and body shapes," says Aaron Bobick, a computer vision researcher at Georgia Tech in Atlanta. Video cameras still require good light and a clear view, however, so Gene Greneker at the Georgia Tech Research Institute is experimenting with radar. "It can see through clothes, at night, at long ranges," he says.

1. The title of this article
   A. cautions computers to watch their step.
   B. cautions readers to watch their step.
   C. implies that computers will be able to observe the way people walk.
   D. implies that computers are a threat.

2. *Surveillance* means
   A. hidden.
   B. obscure.
   C. large surface.
   D. observed.

3. It is implied that
   A. radar may be an alternative to problems encountered with video cameras.
   B. good light and clear vision are attainable with video cameras.
   C. computer vision researchers at Virginia Tech are advancing surveillance technology.
   D. it will be a long time before this technology is available.

4. The video cameras
   A. sweep a designated area.
   B. view the perimeter of the area to be inspected.
   C. collect images that pass through the surveillance area.
   D. have zoom lenses that capture close-ups of people in the surveillance area.

C

Greneker and his team use a device that sends out a signal and measures the echo. If the return waves shift to higher frequencies, that means they reflected off something approaching. "There are different shifts for different body parts, because they are moving at different velocities," Greneker says. A computer program analyzes these shifts and creates a radar fingerprint for each person's walk. So far, researchers have collected gait profiles of about 100 test subjects, which the program can identify up to 80 percent of the time. That is not nearly good enough for airport security, but

Bobick is convinced gait recognition can be made to work. "If I show you moving light displays of people walking, you can distinguish one person from the next. We know the information is there."

—Reprinted with permission from *Discover*, "Computer Watch Your Step" by Fenella Saunders, *Discover* Special Issue: The Year in Science, January 2003.

5. The device used by Greneker and his team

   A. lowers the frequencies.

   B. sends out a signal and measures the echo.

   C. shifts different body parts.

   D. changes the velocities.

6. The identification accuracy is

   A. very high.

   B. moderately low.

   C. average.

   D. moderately high.

7. The researchers have

   A. approved the device for airport security.

   B. not been able to distinguish one person from the next.

   C. completed their study.

   D. gathered gait profiles of subjects.

8. *Gait* most nearly means

   A. style of walking.

   B. fence.

   C. door.

   D. speed of walking.

STOP

IF YOU FINISH BEFORE TIME IS CALLED, YOU MAY CHECK YOUR WORK ON THIS SECTION ONLY. DO NOT TURN TO ANY OTHER SECTION IN THE TEST.

TEST 6

6 Questions • 8 Minutes

> **Directions:** Carefully read the following passage and then answer the accompanying questions, basing your answers on what is stated or implied in the passage. When you have decided which choice is best, fill in the corresponding space on your answer sheet. There is only one best answer for each question.

A

During my stay at an expensive hotel in New York City, I woke up in the middle of the night with an upset stomach. I called room service and ordered some soda crackers. When I looked at the charge slip, I was furious. I called room service and fumed, "I know I'm in a luxury hotel, but $11.50 for six crackers is outrageous!"

B

"The crackers are complimentary," the voice at the other end coolly explained. "I believe you are complaining about your room number."

> —Reprinted with permission from the
> January 2003 *Reader's Digest*,
> "Life in these United States"
> by Robert Menchim.

1. The purpose of this reading selection is to
   A. persuade.
   B. explain.
   C. entertain.
   D. inform.

2. It may be assumed that
   A. the writer does not have sufficient reading comprehension skills.
   B. the format of the bill included several numbers and was difficult to interpret.
   C. room service had made an error.
   D. the hotel guest is frugal.

3. The word *complimentary* means that the crackers were
   A. well suited to the hotel guest.
   B. served with other crackers.
   C. free.
   D. not to be ordered.

4. The author's tone in the call to room service is
   A. humorous.
   B. one of outrage.
   C. sarcastic.
   D. bland.

5. The author implies that
   A. the anticipated services were costly at this particular hotel.
   B. all New York hotels are expensive.
   C. the hotel was substandard.
   D. the hotel was not one of his choice.

6. An appropriate title for this story would be
   A. "Things Are Not Always What They Seem."
   B. "Quality and Price Are Synonymous."
   C. "A Room at the Top."
   D. "Look Before You Leap."

STOP

IF YOU FINISH BEFORE TIME IS CALLED, YOU MAY CHECK YOUR WORK ON THIS SECTION ONLY. DO NOT TURN TO ANY OTHER SECTION IN THE TEST.

ANSWER KEYS AND EXPLANATIONS

Test 1

1. B	4. B	7. A	10. A	13. A
2. A	5. C	8. A	11. D	14. B
3. D	6. C	9. D	12. C	15. B

1. **The correct answer is B.** Sentence 1 states that "Prior to 1628, . . . no one really knew or understood the function of the heart."

2. **The correct answer is A.** Sentence 2 states, "It is the heart that pumps the blood throughout the body night and day."

3. **The correct answer is D.** You are looking for the answer that restates what the paragraph is generally about. Choice D is the best, most all-encompassing statement. The other choices restate just one or two details mentioned in the paragraph.

4. **The correct answer is B.** Choice B restates sentence 1, so it is the correct answer. Choice A is incorrect because the paragraph states that "approximately 13,000 quarts of blood are pumped through the body daily," not that the body contains 13,000 quarts of blood. Choice C is incorrect because the paragraph indicates that the two sides of the heart pump "in about the same rhythm" but this does not mean they are synchronized. Choice D is not mentioned in the paragraph.

5. **The correct answer is C.** A simple mental math calculation verifies that choice C is correct. This question asks you to infer an answer from the information given. You can eliminate Choice A because the paragraph doesn't divide heartbeats into thirds. The paragraph doesn't provide or imply information about steady heartbeats (choice B), or being able to detect your own heartbeat (choice D).

6. **The correct answer is C.** The question has the word *conclude* in it, which is a signal that you will need to figure out the answer from the information given; the answer is not directly stated. The only answer that fulfills this requirement is choice C. Choice A is directly stated, so rule it out. There is nothing stated or implied to conclude that choice B is correct. Choice D is incorrect because while the paragraph states that the average adult human body is covered by 18 square feet of skin, you cannot accurately conclude that this amount of skin would be adequate to cover and protect *all* adult human beings.

7. **The correct answer is A.** The answer can be inferred from the information presented in sentences 6 and 7. Mentioning that the Greeks named the epidermis doesn't necessarily mean they were the first to study skin. Choices C and D are neither implied nor directly stated.

8. **The correct answer is A.** Choice A paraphrases the last sentence in paragraph H. Choice B misstates information in the paragraph, and choices C and D provide information neither stated nor implied.

9. **The correct answer is D.** Choice D paraphrases sentence 3. Choices A, B, and C misstate information in the paragraph.

10. **The correct answer is A.** Only choice A provides an overview of the details in paragraph J. The other answer choices state just a single detail each.

11. **The correct answer is D.** Choice D restates sentence 1 in paragraph K. Choices A, B, and C do not correctly restate information in the paragraphs.

12. **The correct answer is C.** The answer is found in paragraph O, sentence 3. Choices A and D are the opposite of what the passage says. Choice B is not mentioned in either paragraph.

13. **The correct answer is A.** Sentence 5 in paragraph N is the basis for selecting choice A. There is no information in the passage to support choices B, C, or D as valid inferences.

14. **The correct answer is B.** Sentences 1, 2, and 4 in paragraph N provide the basis for selecting choice B. Choice A is the opposite of what the paragraph states, and choice D is the opposite of what the paragraph implies. Choice C has no basis in any paragraph.

15. **The correct answer is B.** If you weren't sure of the answer, you could use the process of elimination. Nothing in the article supports choices A, C, or D.

Test 2

1. A	**3.** A	**5.** C	**7.** B
2. B	**4.** D	**6.** C	**8.** B

1. **The correct answer is A.** *Devastating*, meaning "causing destruction including physical and mental destruction," best fits the sense of paragraph A. *Intolerable* (choice D), may seem like a good choice, but it means "more than can be put up with, irritating" and doesn't fit the sense as well as *devastating*. *Unavoidable* (choice B) makes no sense and neither does *pragmatic* (choice C), meaning "practical."

2. **The correct answer is B.** Sentence 2 states that the world had to cope, so *globally* is the correct answer.

3. **The correct answer is A.** "In a heartbeat," sentence 1, implies *instantaneously* (choice A). Be careful of trick answers like choice B, *by heart malfunction*. On a quick reading of the passage, you might choose this answer.

4. **The correct answer is D.** You can infer choice D based on sentence 2 in the paragraph. Neither choice A nor choice C is either stated directly or implied. Choice B misstates information in the passage.

5. **The correct answer is C.** Only choice C accurately restates information in the paragraph; the answer is in the final sentence.

6. **The correct answer is C.** The answer can be found in paragraph B and in sentences 1 to 5 in paragraph C. No mention is made in the passage of information in choices A or B. Choice C is a better answer than choice D because it contains a wider range of consequences than simply political turmoil.

7. **The correct answer is B.** Choice B can be inferred from the information in paragraphs C, D, E, and F. Nothing in the article supports choices A or D, and choice C is the opposite of what the article says.

8. **The correct answer is B.** Paragraph G supports choice B as the correct answer.

Test 3

1. D	3. C	5. A	7. B	
2. B	4. A	6. B	8. C	9. C

1. **The correct answer is D.** A generalization is defined as "a principle or theory with general application." The only answer that fits this definition is choice D because it includes two large, or general, ideas: lifestyle and genetic makeup. The other answers are too narrow in their descriptions of the problem.

2. **The correct answer is B.** Sentence 2 in paragraph B directly states the answer.

3. **The correct answer is C.** The final sentence in paragraph C states this answer directly.

4. **The correct answer is A.** The final sentence in paragraph D states this answer directly.

5. **The correct answer is A.** The author is stating facts, so *inform* (choice A) is the best answer. Choices B and C are incorrect because there is nothing persuasive or entertaining about the passage. While you may be tempted to choose *analyze* (choice D), this answer is incorrect because the passage is explaining, not analyzing the data.

6. **The correct answer is B.** The answer is directly stated in paragraph E, sentence 1.

7. **The correct answer is B.** If you didn't know this, you could infer it from paragraph C, especially sentence 4, which discusses obesity and being overweight.

8. **The correct answer is C.** To find a main idea statement, you need to look for the statement that encompasses the most information in the passage. Only choice C satisfies this criterion.

9. **The correct answer is C.** To draw a conclusion about the passage in its entirety, you need to consider what the passage is mainly about. Choices A and B are only two points made in the passage. Choice D can be eliminated because it contradicts what the passage says. That leaves only choice C, which is the correct answer.

Test 4

1. C	**3.** A	**5.** D	**7.** D	**9.** C
2. C	**4.** B	**6.** D	**8.** A	**10.** B

1. **The correct answer is C.** The analogy is not stated in the passage, but the last sentence in the article describes DNA as unique and you can infer the analogy from that. The other statements are incorrect and inaccurate.

2. **The correct answer is C.** This answer can be inferred from information in sentences 3 and 4 in paragraph 2.

3. **The correct answer is A.** The answer is stated in the last paragraph, sentence 4.

4. **The correct answer is B.** The answer is found in paragraph 2 in sentences 2 through 4.

5. **The correct answer is D.** This answer can be inferred from the information in the final paragraph.

6. **The correct answer is D.** The answer is the last sentence of paragraph 4.

7. **The correct answer is D.** The answer is in sentence 3 of paragraph 2.

8. **The correct answer is A.** The answer is in sentence 2 of paragraph 2.

9. **The correct answer is C.** The answer is in sentence 1 of paragraph 4. Francis Crick is referred to as a physicist.

10. **The correct answer is B.** The answer can be inferred from the use of the word *construct* in sentence 1 of paragraph 5.

Test 5

1. C	**3.** A	**5.** B	**7.** D
2. D	**4.** C	**6.** D	**8.** A

1. **The correct answer is C.** The answer can be inferred from paragraphs 1 and 2. Paragraph 1 sets up the problem and paragraph 2 explores a solution.

2. **The correct answer is D.** *Surveillance* means "observed, watched over," so choice D is the correct answer. Choice C makes no sense in the sentence, and while *hidden* and *obscure* (choices A and B) may be tempting, *observed* is the more precise word.

3. **The correct answer is A.** The answer is stated in paragraph B, sentences 3 and 4.

4. **The correct answer is C.** The answer is stated in sentence 1 of paragraph B.

5. **The correct answer is B.** The answer is stated in sentence 1 of paragraph C.

6. **The correct answer is D.** An 80 percent accuracy rate, stated in sentence 5 of paragraph C, can be categorized as moderately high.

7. **The correct answer is D.** The answer is stated in sentence 5 of paragraph C.

8. **The correct answer is A.** If you didn't know the answer, you could infer that *gait* means "style of walking" from sentences 2 through 4 in paragraph C. Choice D is close, but not as accurate as choice A.

Test 6

| 1. C | 3. C | 4. B | 5. A | 6. A |
| 2. B | | | | |

1. **The correct answer is C.** The emphasis is on humor in this passage, so choice C is the best answer. There is nothing persuasive, explanatory, or informative about the piece.

2. **The correct answer is B.** Try using the process of elimination if you aren't sure of the answer. You can eliminate choice A immediately because there is nothing to indicate a lack of reading skill by the author, especially since the piece is well written and builds to a climax. Choice C is incorrect because the piece indicates that there was no error. While choice D may be tempting to choose, choice B makes more sense in the context of the passage.

3. **The correct answer is C.** Only choice C makes sense based on the context of the passage.

4. **The correct answer is B.** *Outrage* is a near synonym for *furious,* which is how the writer describes himself in paragraph A, sentence 3.

5. **The correct answer is A.** The answer can be inferred from sentence 4 in paragraph A.

6. **The correct answer is A.** A title should reflect the main idea of a passage, and choice A best describes the scenario recounted in the passage. Choice D may be tempting, but the writer did look before he called, but as the answer to question 2 indicates, the bill was confusingly written.

Vocational Adjustment Index

OVERVIEW

- **Matching Aptitude and Profession**
- **Sample Vocational Adjustment Questions**

MATCHING APTITUDE AND PROFESSION

All three of the Psychological Services Bureau (PSB) examinations include a final section titled "Vocational Adjustment Index," which includes 90 agree/disagree questions, to be answered in 15 minutes. Unlike all other questions on the PSB exams—or any of the other entrance exams, for that matter—these questions do not test your knowledge or ability to think logically. Rather, they assess your attitudes and feelings toward different aspects of a career in nursing or allied health care, as well as your personality and typical behavioral patterns, and whether your responses indicate a good fit for working in health care.

Because these questions are based on your own feelings and personality traits, you cannot study for them in the same way you do other questions. Instead, take some time to evaluate your desire to pursue a career in health care. Reflect on the following questions and write responses to them in a journal:

- Why do I want to be a nurse or other healthcare professional?
- How settled am I on this career path?
- What traits do I have that would make me a good fit for this career?
- What traits do I have that would make me a poor fit for this career?
- How motivated am I to serve others in this field?
- Are there other careers, outside of healthcare, that I should consider?

The better you know yourself and your own perceived aptitude for working in healthcare, the easier it will be to answer the Vocational Adjustment Index questions.

When answering these questions on the test itself, try to go with your immediate, "gut" reaction. Answer the questions quickly and honestly. If you do, your responses and test results will be a more accurate indicator of whether you are a good fit for working in health care. Avoid just giving the response you think the test is asking for. It would be better to find out now that are not likely to be a good fit than after you've already enrolled in school or, worse, graduated and gotten a job in the field.

SAMPLE VOCATIONAL ADJUSTMENT QUESTIONS

Below are some questions much like those found on the Vocational Adjustment Index portion of the PSB exam. The answer choices are either *agree* or *disagree*. For official samples, visit the Test Resources section of PSB's website at **http://psbtests.com/test-resources/**.

> **Directions:** This section is not really a test. It is an inventory of feelings, attitudes, and opinions designed to evaluate whether your personality traits are desirable for a career in health care. There are no right or wrong answers—some feel one way; others feel another way. Agreement or disagreement with the statements that follow simply indicates what you usually think, how you usually feel, or what you usually do about things. Mark accordingly as you agree or disagree with the statement. Choose the answer that is really true for you, and answer immediately.

1. Planning for the future is a worthwhile plan.

2. It's important to have a definite choice of vocations.

3. The possibility of unemployment after graduation is a source of concern.

4. I prefer to work alone.

5. My friends disapprove of my choice of vocations.

6. Working alone rather than with others is preferable.

7. Working with strangers is demanding.

8. Having friends is a key ingredient to happiness.

9. Meeting new people can be a source of severe anxiety.

10. Helping sick and elderly ones can be a source of fulfillment.

11. Working with old people is not too rewarding.

12. Too often, persons in positions of authority abuse those they supervise.

13. Taking orders from an authoritative figure is difficult.

14. To speak up in class discussions is quite easy.

15. Studying takes up too much time in a young person's life.

16. Most teachers will gladly offer students extra help.

17. Teachers are often biased when grading assignments.

18. A job in which continuous learning was expected would be ideal.

19. Stressful situations are upsetting to most people.

20. Highly stressful occupations are the most satisfying.

Results of the Vocational Adjustment Index are not provided to you; the answers you provide will provide admissions personnel an idea of your suitability for a career in health care based on your personality traits.

PART IV

PRACTICE FOR ALLIED HEALTH SCHOOL ENTRANCE EXAMINATIONS

Verbal and Nonverbal Ability

OVERVIEW

Unit 9

VERBAL AND NONVERBAL ABILITY ANSWER SHEET

Test 1: Synonyms

1. Ⓐ Ⓑ Ⓒ Ⓓ	8. Ⓐ Ⓑ Ⓒ Ⓓ	15. Ⓐ Ⓑ Ⓒ Ⓓ	22. Ⓐ Ⓑ Ⓒ Ⓓ	29. Ⓐ Ⓑ Ⓒ Ⓓ
2. Ⓐ Ⓑ Ⓒ Ⓓ	9. Ⓐ Ⓑ Ⓒ Ⓓ	16. Ⓐ Ⓑ Ⓒ Ⓓ	23. Ⓐ Ⓑ Ⓒ Ⓓ	30. Ⓐ Ⓑ Ⓒ Ⓓ
3. Ⓐ Ⓑ Ⓒ Ⓓ	10. Ⓐ Ⓑ Ⓒ Ⓓ	17. Ⓐ Ⓑ Ⓒ Ⓓ	24. Ⓐ Ⓑ Ⓒ Ⓓ	31. Ⓐ Ⓑ Ⓒ Ⓓ
4. Ⓐ Ⓑ Ⓒ Ⓓ	11. Ⓐ Ⓑ Ⓒ Ⓓ	18. Ⓐ Ⓑ Ⓒ Ⓓ	25. Ⓐ Ⓑ Ⓒ Ⓓ	32. Ⓐ Ⓑ Ⓒ Ⓓ
5. Ⓐ Ⓑ Ⓒ Ⓓ	12. Ⓐ Ⓑ Ⓒ Ⓓ	19. Ⓐ Ⓑ Ⓒ Ⓓ	26. Ⓐ Ⓑ Ⓒ Ⓓ	33. Ⓐ Ⓑ Ⓒ Ⓓ
6. Ⓐ Ⓑ Ⓒ Ⓓ	13. Ⓐ Ⓑ Ⓒ Ⓓ	20. Ⓐ Ⓑ Ⓒ Ⓓ	27. Ⓐ Ⓑ Ⓒ Ⓓ	34. Ⓐ Ⓑ Ⓒ Ⓓ
7. Ⓐ Ⓑ Ⓒ Ⓓ	14. Ⓐ Ⓑ Ⓒ Ⓓ	21. Ⓐ Ⓑ Ⓒ Ⓓ	28. Ⓐ Ⓑ Ⓒ Ⓓ	35. Ⓐ Ⓑ Ⓒ Ⓓ

Test 2: Antonyms

1. Ⓐ Ⓑ Ⓒ Ⓓ Ⓔ	7. Ⓐ Ⓑ Ⓒ Ⓓ Ⓔ	13. Ⓐ Ⓑ Ⓒ Ⓓ Ⓔ	19. Ⓐ Ⓑ Ⓒ Ⓓ Ⓔ	25. Ⓐ Ⓑ Ⓒ Ⓓ Ⓔ
2. Ⓐ Ⓑ Ⓒ Ⓓ Ⓔ	8. Ⓐ Ⓑ Ⓒ Ⓓ Ⓔ	14. Ⓐ Ⓑ Ⓒ Ⓓ Ⓔ	20. Ⓐ Ⓑ Ⓒ Ⓓ Ⓔ	26. Ⓐ Ⓑ Ⓒ Ⓓ Ⓔ
3. Ⓐ Ⓑ Ⓒ Ⓓ Ⓔ	9. Ⓐ Ⓑ Ⓒ Ⓓ Ⓔ	15. Ⓐ Ⓑ Ⓒ Ⓓ Ⓔ	21. Ⓐ Ⓑ Ⓒ Ⓓ Ⓔ	27. Ⓐ Ⓑ Ⓒ Ⓓ Ⓔ
4. Ⓐ Ⓑ Ⓒ Ⓓ Ⓔ	10. Ⓐ Ⓑ Ⓒ Ⓓ Ⓔ	16. Ⓐ Ⓑ Ⓒ Ⓓ Ⓔ	22. Ⓐ Ⓑ Ⓒ Ⓓ Ⓔ	28. Ⓐ Ⓑ Ⓒ Ⓓ Ⓔ
5. Ⓐ Ⓑ Ⓒ Ⓓ Ⓔ	11. Ⓐ Ⓑ Ⓒ Ⓓ Ⓔ	17. Ⓐ Ⓑ Ⓒ Ⓓ Ⓔ	23. Ⓐ Ⓑ Ⓒ Ⓓ Ⓔ	29. Ⓐ Ⓑ Ⓒ Ⓓ Ⓔ
6. Ⓐ Ⓑ Ⓒ Ⓓ Ⓔ	12. Ⓐ Ⓑ Ⓒ Ⓓ Ⓔ	18. Ⓐ Ⓑ Ⓒ Ⓓ Ⓔ	24. Ⓐ Ⓑ Ⓒ Ⓓ Ⓔ	30. Ⓐ Ⓑ Ⓒ Ⓓ Ⓔ

Test 3: English Grammar and Usage

1. Ⓐ Ⓑ Ⓒ	4. Ⓐ Ⓑ Ⓒ	7. Ⓐ Ⓑ Ⓒ	10. Ⓐ Ⓑ Ⓒ	13. Ⓐ Ⓑ Ⓒ
2. Ⓐ Ⓑ Ⓒ	5. Ⓐ Ⓑ Ⓒ	8. Ⓐ Ⓑ Ⓒ	11. Ⓐ Ⓑ Ⓒ	14. Ⓐ Ⓑ Ⓒ
3. Ⓐ Ⓑ Ⓒ	6. Ⓐ Ⓑ Ⓒ	9. Ⓐ Ⓑ Ⓒ	12. Ⓐ Ⓑ Ⓒ	15. Ⓐ Ⓑ Ⓒ

Test 4: Spelling

1. Ⓐ Ⓑ Ⓒ	4. Ⓐ Ⓑ Ⓒ	7. Ⓐ Ⓑ Ⓒ	10. Ⓐ Ⓑ Ⓒ	13. Ⓐ Ⓑ Ⓒ
2. Ⓐ Ⓑ Ⓒ	5. Ⓐ Ⓑ Ⓒ	8. Ⓐ Ⓑ Ⓒ	11. Ⓐ Ⓑ Ⓒ	14. Ⓐ Ⓑ Ⓒ
3. Ⓐ Ⓑ Ⓒ	6. Ⓐ Ⓑ Ⓒ	9. Ⓐ Ⓑ Ⓒ	12. Ⓐ Ⓑ Ⓒ	15. Ⓐ Ⓑ Ⓒ

Test 5: Nonverbal Ability

1. Ⓐ Ⓑ Ⓒ Ⓓ Ⓔ	4. Ⓐ Ⓑ Ⓒ Ⓓ Ⓔ	7. Ⓐ Ⓑ Ⓒ Ⓓ Ⓔ	10. Ⓐ Ⓑ Ⓒ Ⓓ Ⓔ	13. Ⓐ Ⓑ Ⓒ Ⓓ Ⓔ
2. Ⓐ Ⓑ Ⓒ Ⓓ Ⓔ	5. Ⓐ Ⓑ Ⓒ Ⓓ Ⓔ	8. Ⓐ Ⓑ Ⓒ Ⓓ Ⓔ	11. Ⓐ Ⓑ Ⓒ Ⓓ Ⓔ	14. Ⓐ Ⓑ Ⓒ Ⓓ Ⓔ
3. Ⓐ Ⓑ Ⓒ Ⓓ Ⓔ	6. Ⓐ Ⓑ Ⓒ Ⓓ Ⓔ	9. Ⓐ Ⓑ Ⓒ Ⓓ Ⓔ	12. Ⓐ Ⓑ Ⓒ Ⓓ Ⓔ	15. Ⓐ Ⓑ Ⓒ Ⓓ Ⓔ

answer sheet

TEST 1: SYNONYMS

35 Questions • 20 Minutes

Review Unit 4, Synonyms, before attempting this test.

> **Directions:** In each of the following sentences, one word is italicized. For each sentence, select the option that best (or most nearly) corresponds in meaning with the italicized word.

1. It has been recommended that this system should be used in place of *traditional* systems that have been in place for decades.
   A. unfamiliar
   B. usual
   C. flexible
   D. general

2. In our society, irresponsible behavior often leads to a monetary *penalty*.
   A. arrangement
   B. gratification
   C. punishment
   D. precaution

3. He spent the *allotted* study time completing his assignments.
   A. authorized
   B. designated
   C. agreed
   D. alerted

4. The Senate passed the farmland *preservation* bill.
   A. maintenance
   B. stratagem
   C. storage
   D. incumbency

5. It was apparent that he had attempted to *concoct* an alibi.
   A. inculcate
   B. conceal
   C. reveal
   D. fabricate

6. The City Council could have avoided this *scenario* by passing the ordinance.
   A. situation
   B. setting
   C. summation
   D. deficiency

7. The Superior Court judge *imposed* the sentence.
   A. indicated
   B. granted
   C. perpetuated
   D. prescribed

8. The study was considered *flawed* because the data was self-reported.
   A. subjective
   B. inaccurate
   C. objective
   D. unscientific

9. Geologists *assure* us that our Earth is a few billion years old.
   A. guarantee
   B. instruct
   C. inform
   D. advise

10. He was determined to *foil* the scheme of his opponent.
    A. heighten
    B. secure
    C. disencumber
    D. thwart

11. The examiner *purported* to be an official representative.
    A. addressed
    B. claimed
    C. propitiated
    D. conciliated

12. The ship carried a *diverse* crowd of vacationers who had come from many countries.
    A. multitude
    B. varied
    C. discrepant
    D. multiplicity

13. The child could not *recollect* the incident.
    A. remember
    B. doubt
    C. interrogate
    D. illumine

14. The governor *rescinded* the state of emergency as soon as the roads were cleared of snow.
    A. negated
    B. maneuvered
    C. revoked
    D. accepted

15. The implementation of the plan was given *scant* consideration.
    A. audacious
    B. fervid
    C. little
    D. clothed

16. The key speaker, in his lengthy presentation, *scoffed at* the notion of marketing as a public service.
    A. exonerated
    B. amplified
    C. confuted
    D. mocked

17. She completed the *sprint* with a sudden surge of energy.
    A. relaxation
    B. adventure
    C. run
    D. convergence

18. The content of the message was *urgent*.
    A. privileged
    B. amendable
    C. pressing
    D. absolved

19. A *simulated* rescue mission was conducted by the forest rangers.
    A. pretended
    B. superficial
    C. stimulated
    D. simultaneous

20. Through the course of the day, she became more *agitated* by the noise of the demolition and less focused on her work.
    A. worried
    B. upset
    C. convulsed
    D. composed

21. Her quickening gait seemed regulated by the *pulse* of the big city.
    A. utility
    B. pace
    C. reverence
    D. solace

22. The language of the publication is *unsophisticated* but informative.
    A. ponderous
    B. elaborate
    C. simple
    D. artificial

23. All the evidence presented pointed to *willful* execution of a crime.
    A. deliberate
    B. eminent
    C. amicable
    D. remorseful

24. There is no *provision* for deadlines in the contract.
    A. improvement
    B. convenience
    C. aggregation
    D. stipulation

25. The furnishings *impart* an air of elegance to the room.
    A. communicate
    B. indemnify
    C. reinforce
    D. disguise

26. She exhibited great *valor* in handling the emergency.
    A. ingeniousness
    B. courage
    C. discretion
    D. optimism

27. Various courses were *fused* in the revision of the curriculum.
    A. required
    B. implicated
    C. combined
    D. involved

28. He was able to *duplicate* his work even though his hard drive failed.
    A. replicate
    B. synthesize
    C. fixate
    D. replenish

29. The task of choosing one from so many qualified applicants *bewildered* the employer.
    A. perplexed
    B. aggravated
    C. subdued
    D. infuriated

30. The revision of the city plan incorporated adjustments in the projected *modes* of transportation.
    A. increments
    B. expenditures
    C. means
    D. modifications

31. The politician sought to *aggrandize* himself at the expense of the people.
    A. exhaust
    B. subjugate
    C. sacrifice
    D. enrich

32. The newcomer made an effort to *mingle* with the crowd.

A. argue

B. mix

C. disrupt

D. flout

33. If an organization's programs were described as *philanthropic*, the programs would be

A. primitive.

B. deleterious.

C. extraneous.

D. benevolent.

34. If the traits of a nation's leader were *covetous*, they would be

A. greedy.

B. exemplary.

C. disparate.

D. adventitious.

35. Rabbits *breed* offspring rapidly.

A. raise

B. gather

C. propagate

D. destroy

STOP

IF YOU FINISH BEFORE TIME IS CALLED, YOU MAY CHECK YOUR WORK ON THIS SECTION ONLY. DO NOT TURN TO ANY OTHER SECTION IN THE TEST.

TEST 2: ANTONYMS

30 Questions • 15 Minutes

Review Unit 4, Antonyms, before attempting this test.

Directions: For each of the following questions, select the word opposite in meaning to the word printed in capital letters.

1. IMMUTABLE
   A. erudite
   B. abject
   C. changeable
   D. fantastic
   E. aura

2. DUCTILE
   A. feted
   B. aloof
   C. stubborn
   D. abnormal
   E. belabored

3. FASTIDIOUS
   A. factitious
   B. absurd
   C. indifferent
   D. sloppy
   E. chary

4. TEMERITY
   A. affinity
   B. cherubim
   C. cautiousness
   D. degenerate
   E. scanty

5. ITINERANT
   A. animosity
   B. metaphor
   C. perpetrator
   D. resident
   E. cerebrum

6. TACITURN
   A. malevolent
   B. loquacious
   C. paltry
   D. opaque
   E. morbid

7. NEFARIOUS
   A. grotesque
   B. virtuous
   C. jovial
   D. pious
   E. ceremonious

8. OBSEQUIOUS
   A. harbinger
   B. bold
   C. heredity
   D. quaff
   E. fashionable

9. OSTENTATION
   A. emulsion
   B. languid
   C. modesty
   D. kilogram
   E. showy

10. CONTENTION
   A. equation
   B. guild
   C. oblivion
   D. friendliness
   E. assertion

11. IMPUTATION
    A. assiduous
    B. radiant
    C. accusation
    D. raiment
    E. vindication

12. BENIGN
    A. defensive
    B. relevant
    C. robot
    D. pernicious
    E. precarious

13. COHERENT
    A. perspicacious
    B. organized
    C. weal
    D. rational
    E. chaotic

14. DEPREDATION
    A. plethoric
    B. gloss
    C. restoration
    D. usher
    E. devastation

15. PROVOCATIVE
    A. sedentary
    B. capricious
    C. vindictive
    D. tawny
    E. unexciting

16. SUBMISSION
    A. authorized
    B. defiance
    C. assignment
    D. defeat
    E. criticism

17. AFFLUENT
    A. immigrant
    B. junction
    C. insufficient
    D. kindred
    E. clandestine

18. CHURLISH
    A. exiguous
    B. laudable
    C. cheerful
    D. maternal
    E. sympathetic

19. SYMMETRY
    A. invocation
    B. synopsis
    C. distortion
    D. satyr
    E. portrayal

20. DULCET
    A. extrinsic
    B. optimistic
    C. unanimous
    D. disagreeable
    E. sweet

Directions: In the following sets of words, choose the word that is most different in meaning from the others.

21. **A.** pungent
    B. piquant
    C. insipid
    D. spicy
    E. zesty

22. **A.** opportune
    B. suitable
    C. advantageous
    D. prudent
    E. inexpedient

23. **A.** irascible
    B. good-humored
    C. petulant
    D. peevish
    E. sullen

24. **A.** savory
    B. delectable
    C. scrumptious
    D. unpalatable
    E. potable

25. **A.** satiated
    B. glutted
    C. gorged
    D. surfeited
    E. rapacious

26. **A.** reserved
    B. reclusive
    C. gregarious
    D. taciturn
    E. misanthropic

27. **A.** courteous
    B. gracious
    C. insolent
    D. polite
    E. urbane

28. **A.** usurp
    B. seize
    C. highjack
    D. appropriate
    E. relinquish

29. **A.** acrimonious
    B. belligerent
    C. truculent
    D. harmonious
    E. peevish

30. **A.** discernible
    B. cryptic
    C. obvious
    D. perceptible
    E. evident

STOP

IF YOU FINISH BEFORE TIME IS CALLED, YOU MAY CHECK YOUR WORK ON THIS SECTION ONLY. DO NOT TURN TO ANY OTHER SECTION IN THE TEST.

TEST 3: ENGLISH GRAMMAR AND USAGE

15 Questions • 10 Minutes

Review Unit 4, English Grammar and Usage, before attempting this test.

> **Directions:** In the following questions, select the answer that completes the sentence in a grammatically correct manner or that represents the most grammatically correct of all options.

1. I _____ taller than you _____, but she _____ taller than we _____.
   - **A.** is; are; is; are
   - **B.** is; is; is; are
   - **C.** am; is; is; are
   - **D.** am; are; is; are

2. Jay usually _____ on the street, whereas you all usually _____ in the garage.
   - **A.** parks; park
   - **B.** park; parks
   - **C.** parks; parks
   - **D.** park; park

3. Somebody _____ my car door; everybody in the neighborhood _____ it happen; nobody _____ me who did it.
   - **A.** dents; see; tell
   - **B.** dent; see; tells
   - **C.** dents; sees; tells
   - **D.** dents; sees; tell

4. I will take _____ dog to the park, and you will take _____.
   - **A.** mine; yours
   - **B.** my; yours
   - **C.** my; your
   - **D.** mine; your

5. My Dad and I are close competitors in ping-pong; yesterday _____ beat _____, but today _____ beat _____.
   - **A.** him; me; me; him
   - **B.** he; I; I; he
   - **C.** he; I; I; him
   - **D.** he; me; I; him

6. _____ are you calling? _____ is that?
   - **A.** Whom; Whom
   - **B.** Whom; Who
   - **C.** Who; Who
   - **D.** Who; Whom

7. Which of the following sentences is the clearest?
   - **A.** While the man was driving down the road, the dog stuck its head out of the open window.
   - **B.** Driving down the road, the dog stuck its head out of the open window.
   - **C.** The dog stuck its head out of the open window driving down the road.
   - **D.** Driving down the road, the man's dog stuck its head out of the open window.

8. He asked his mom for his childhood baseball card collection, but she had already _____ it out.
   - **A.** thrown
   - **B.** threw
   - **C.** throwed
   - **D.** threwn

9. They love their house; they _____ there for over 25 years.
   - **A.** are living
   - **B.** lived
   - **C.** had lived
   - **D.** have lived

10. Identify the part of speech of the italicized word in the following sentence: The Thompsons found a family of snakes living *beneath* their house.
    A. Adjective
    B. Adverb
    C. Preposition
    D. Conjunction

11. Identify the part of speech of the italicized word in the following sentence: Ruth is the *slowest* swimmer on her team.
    A. Adjective
    B. Adverb
    C. Preposition
    D. Conjunction

12. This hiking trail is _____ than that one.
    A. less challenging
    B. not challenging
    C. least challenging
    D. unchallenginger

13. Which of the following sentences is grammatically correct?
    A. The rain falling on the tin roof, nervous cat.
    B. The rain falling on the tin roof alarms the cat.
    C. The rain falls on the tin roof, the cat is alarmed.
    D. Alarmed by the rain falling on the tin roof.

14. Today we'll do some gardening _____ and tomorrow we'll paint the fence.
    A. ;
    B. :
    C. ,
    D. –

15. When Zack is in Vermont, he will stay at the _____ house; you remember Barb and Larry Schneider, don't you?
    A. Schneider's
    B. Schneiders'
    C. Schneider
    D. Schneiders's

TEST 4: SPELLING

15 Questions • 5 Minutes

Review Unit 4, Spelling, before attempting this test.

Directions: In the following sets of words, choose the word that is spelled correctly.

---

1. A. actually
   B. acktually
   C. accually

2. A. bradiecardia
   B. bradycardia
   C. bradycardea

3. A. cromosome
   B. chromosome
   C. khromosome

4. A. dispnea
   B. dysponea
   C. dyspnea

5. A. euphoria
   B. youphoria
   C. euforia

6. A. fashia
   B. phacia
   C. fascia

7. A. jestation
   B. gestation
   C. justation

8. A. hipothalamus
   B. hypothalmus
   C. hypothalamus

9. A. jaundus
   B. jaundice
   C. jandace

10. A. kyphosis
    B. kiphosus
    C. kyfosis

11. A. longevity
    B. longjevity
    C. longgevity

12. A. neglijence
    B. negligence
    C. neglagence

13. A. retena
    B. rettina
    C. retina

14. A. sensitivity
    B. sensativity
    C. sensitivitie

15. A. thrombosus
    B. thrambosis
    C. thrombosis

TEST 5: NONVERBAL ABILITY

15 Questions • 15 Minutes

Review Unit 4, Nonverbal Ability, before attempting this test.

> **Directions:** In the following questions, determine the relationship between the first pair of shapes and then decide which of the answer choices shares a similar relationship with the third shape.

1. ⊂ is to ⊄ as ⊢ is to?
   - A. ⊬
   - B. ⊪⊬
   - C. ⊪⊬
   - D. ⊅
   - E. ⊬

2. ⊼ is to ⊼̄ as ⊤ is to?
   - A. ⊤̄
   - B. ⊤̈
   - C. ⊕
   - D. ⊥
   - E. ⊪⊢

3. ⊛ is to ✵ as ◎ is to?
   - A. �̈
   - B. ◎
   - C. ö
   - D. ⊤̈
   - E. ⛬

4. ○ is to ⬡ as | is to?
   - A. ---
   - B. ▪▪▪
   - C. ⌐
   - D. ┊
   - E. ▪

5. D is to ⬗ as ꓷ is to?
   - A. ꝺ
   - B. ⬥
   - C. ◉
   - D. ◙
   - E. C

6. † is to † as ‡ is to?
   - A. ‡
   - B. ⊦
   - C. ⊢
   - D. ⊥
   - E. ⊹

7. C is to Ɔ as ꞓ is to?
   - A. Ɔ
   - B. C
   - C. Ɔ
   - D. D
   - E. ꝺ

8. 2 is to Ɛ as J is to?
   - A. 2
   - B. Ɛ
   - C. Ɐ
   - D. ʞ
   - E. ꓘ

9. ৎ is to ?? as (is to?

   A. ?

   B.))

   C.)

   D. ((

   E. ||

10. ?¡ is to ‼ as ⊣| is to?

    A. ⊩

    B. ||

    C. ⊣⊢

    D. ⊞

    E. ⊤

11. C is to © as + is to?

    A. +∪

    B. ∪̈

    C. ∪̇

    D. ⊘

    E. ⊙

12. ∪ is to ∪̇ as ← is to?

    A. ↖

    B. ↑

    C. ↗

    D. →

    E. ↔

13. ◆ is to ❖ as ✝ is to?

    A. ⊫

    B. ÷

    C. ╪

    D. ⊣⊢

    E. ⊤

14. ▬ is to ••• as ⌐ is to?

    A. ÷

    B. ¬

    C. ⌐

    D. ⌐

    E. ¬

15. ● is to ◯ as ⦙⦙⦙ is to?

    A. ▦

    B. ▦

    C. ▦

    D. ⁝

    E. ⁝

ANSWER KEYS AND EXPLANATIONS

Test 1: Synonyms

1. B	8. B	15. C	22. C	29. A
2. C	9. A	16. D	23. A	30. C
3. B	10. D	17. C	24. D	31. D
4. A	11. B	18. C	25. A	32. B
5. D	12. B	19. A	26. B	33. D
6. A	13. A	20. B	27. C	34. A
7. D	14. C	21. B	28. A	35. C

1. **The correct answer is B.** *Usual* is a near synonym for *traditional*. A near synonym means almost the same, but not quite. *Unfamiliar* (choice A) doesn't work because the systems to be replaced have been around for years. *Traditional* typically means something is not adaptable, which is one meaning of *flexible*, so the words are antonyms, not synonyms. *General* doesn't relate to *traditional* in any way.

2. **The correct answer is C.** *Penalty* and *punishment* are synonyms. Choice A is not strong enough for something that is "irresponsible behavior." Choice B is the opposite of a penalty. *Precaution* (choice D) doesn't make sense in the sentence and is not a synonym of *penalty*.

3. **The correct answer is B.** *Designated* means "allocated, assigned" and so is the correct answer. Nothing indicates that someone gave the person permission to use his study time to do the assignment, so eliminate choice A. Choice C can be eliminated because there is no indication that the person had *agreed* with someone to use the study time for the assignment. Choice D makes no sense.

4. **The correct answer is A.** *Maintenance* is a synonym for *preservation*. Choice B might be tempting, but a *stratagem* is "a trick, an

underhanded scheme" and that doesn't fit the context nor it is a synonym for *preservation*. Choice C doesn't make sense because how do you store land? Choice D doesn't make sense either because an *incumbency* means "a term of office," which is not the same as maintaining something.

5. **The correct answer is D.** *Concoct* means "to make up" and so does *fabricate*. *Inculcate* (choice A) means "to instill or drill something into someone's mind by forceful repetition" and doesn't make sense. The same goes for *conceal* (choice B) meaning "to hide." *Reveal* (choice C) might be tempting, but the word is not a synonym for *concoct*.

6. **The correct answer is A.** *Situation* is the best choice among the answers. *Setting* (choice A) would fit if the test item were about a play or book, but it isn't, so *setting* doesn't make sense in the sentence. *Summation* (choice C) is another word for *summary* and doesn't make sense either. *Deficiency* (choice D) isn't the right usage of the word, which typically is used to mean "a shortage, a lack of something essential."

7. **The correct answer is D.** *Prescribe* means "to order, assign" and fits the sense of the sentence. Choice A is not strong enough;

the judge didn't show or suggest the sentence, but imposed it. A judge doesn't grant a sentence because *grant* has a positive connotation, giving something pleasant to someone, so eliminate choice B. Choice C doesn't make sense because *perpetuate* is "to make last for a long time."

8. **The correct answer is B.** *Inaccurate* is a synonym for *flawed*. *Subjective* and *objective* (choices A and C) are opposites of each other, but neither is a synonym for *flawed*. Something may be *unscientific* but still accurate, so choice D is also incorrect.

9. **The correct answer is A.** *Instruct*, *inform*, and *advise* (choices B, C, and D) all make sense in the sentence, but only *guarantee* (choice A) is a synonym for *assure*.

10. **The correct answer is D.** *Thwart* is a synonym for *foil*, meaning "to prevent from occurring." *Heighten* (choice A) means "to increase in quality or intensity." *Secure* (choice B) makes no sense because how would someone take possession of a scheme or connect a scheme securely, both meanings of the word? Choice C is incorrect because *disencumber* means "to take away someone's burden, to untangle someone from obligations."

11. **The correct answer is B.** *Claimed* is a synonym for *purported*. *Addressed* (choice A) means "to speak to." *Propitiated* (choice C), means "to appease, to reconcile" and doesn't make sense. For the same reason, *conciliated* (choice D) doesn't make sense; it means "to reconcile" or "to overcome distrust."

12. **The correct answer is B.** *Varied* and *diverse* are synonyms. Choices A and D are incorrect for similar reasons. Both mean "a large number," but neither includes the idea of diversity. Choice C is incorrect because *discrepant* means "not in agreement."

13. **The correct answer is A.** *Remember* is a synonym for *recollect*. None of the other words make sense in the context. *Illumine* (choice D) means "to shed light on," and might tempt you, but it doesn't have the same or a similar meaning to *recollect*.

14. **The correct answer is C.** To *rescind* is "to *revoke*." Choice A is incorrect because typically an official order such as a declaration of a state of emergency is revoked, not *negated*. *Maneuver* (choice B) means "to carry out a military action," "to change tactics," or "to alter the placement of troops," none of which are synonymous with *rescind*. Choice D is incorrect because the governor is ending the state of emergency, not *accepting* it.

15. **The correct answer is C.** *Scant* means "*little*." Choice A is incorrect because *audacious* means "bold, fearless, spirited." Choice B is incorrect because *fervid* means "impassioned, intense emotion." Choice D is incorrect because *clothed* makes no sense, even in a metaphorical sense.

16. **The correct answer is D.** To *scoff at* is "to *mock* or make fun of." Choice A makes no sense because *exonerate* is "to free someone from blame or responsibility." Choice B is incorrect because *amplify* is "to increase," "to exaggerate," or "to make complete." *Confute* (choice C) is "to prove something or someone wrong."

17. **The correct answer is C.** *Run* and *sprint* can be synonyms and are in this case. Choice A makes no sense because you don't need a surge of energy to *relax*. Choice B is incorrect because while *adventure* makes some sense, it is not a synonym for *run*. *Convergence* (choice D), meaning "where two things come together," makes no sense.

18. **The correct answer is C.** *Pressing* means "demanding immediate attention," in

other words, *urgent*. *Privileged* (choice A), meaning "confidential," isn't correct. *Amendable* (choice B), meaning "capable of being changed," is also incorrect. *Absolved* (choice D), meaning "pronounced not guilty," is also incorrect.

19. **The correct answer is A.** *Simulated* is something made to resemble something else; in other words, it is *pretended*. Choice B is incorrect because something superficial is something that may be frivolous, perfunctory, or on the surface, none of which are the same simulated. Choice C is incorrect because *stimulated* means "aroused or excited emotionally." Choice D is incorrect because *simultaneous* means "at the same time."

20. **The correct answer is B.** Both *worried* and *upset* can be synonyms of *agitated*, but in this sentence, *upset* fits the context better. Choice C is incorrect because *convulsed* means "shaking violently"; it can be a synonym of *agitate*, but not in this context. Choice D is incorrect because *composed*, meaning "calm," is the opposite of *agitated*.

21. **The correct answer is B.** A *pulse* is beat or *pace*. Choice A is incorrect because *utility* means either "usefulness" or "a power company." Choice C is incorrect because *reverence* is a feeling of profound awe or respect and makes no sense and is no a synonym of *pulse*. Choice D is incorrect because *solace* is the same as comfort, not a pulse.

22. **The correct answer is C.** One synonym for *unsophisticated* is *simple*. Choice A is incorrect because *ponderous* means "heavy, dull, tedious," none of which is the same as *unsophisticated*. Choice B is incorrect because *elaborate* tends to the opposite of *unsophisticated*. Choice D is incorrect because *artificial* means "contrived,

inauthentic, forced, affected," in other words, the opposite of *unsophisticated*.

23. **The correct answer is A.** *Willful* and *deliberate* are synonyms. Choice B is incorrect because *eminent* means "prominent, great, well-known"; don't confuse it with *imminent*, meaning "about to happen." *Amicable* (choice C) means "friendly" and makes no sense. Choice D is incorrect because *remorseful* means "sorry," and while someone caught for a crime may feel remorseful, it is not a synonym for *willful* and makes no sense.

24. **The correct answer is D.** *Stipulation* is a synonym for *provision*, meaning "arrangement or plan." Choice A is incorrect because *improvement* is not the same as a stipulation and doesn't fit the sense. Choice B is incorrect because *convenience* means "benefit, advantage" or "suitability." Choice C is incorrect because *aggregation* means "a collection of several things taken as a whole."

25. **The correct answer is A.** *Impart* and *communicate* are synonyms. *Reinforce* (choice C) may seem like a good choice, and in terms of context could work, except that *impart* and *reinforce* aren't synonyms. Choice B is incorrect because *indemnify* means "to protect against damage or loss." Choice D is incorrect because *disguise* isn't a synonym for transmitting information, in this case, a feeling or sense of style.

26. **The correct answer is B.** *Valor* and *courage* are the same thing. Choice A is incorrect because *ingeniousness* is "cleverness," "inventiveness," and "creative thinking." Choice C is incorrect because *discretion* is "tactfulness." Choice D is incorrect because *optimism* means "expecting that the best will happen.

27. **The correct answer is C.** To *fuse* is "to mix together," but also "to unite, to join," and among the answer choices, *combine* is the closest in meaning. Choice A is incorrect because *required* is not a synonym for *joining*, though courses can be required. Choice B is incorrect because *implicated*, meaning "to involve or incriminate someone," makes no sense. Choice D is incorrect because while *involved* may make sense in the context, it is not a synonym for *fuse*.

28. **The correct answer is A.** To *duplicate* is "to *replicate*," or "to make an exact copy." Choice B is incorrect because *synthesize* means "to combine pieces to form something new." Choice C is incorrect because *fixate* is "to make something stable" or "to focus attention on something or someone." *Replenish* (choice D) means "to make something full or complete again."

29. **The correct answer is A.** To *bewilder* is "to *perplex*," meaning "to confuse." Choice B is incorrect because *aggravated* means "made angry" or "made something worse." Choice C is incorrect because *subdued* means "conquered, brought under control." Choice D is incorrect because *infuriated* means "angry, enraged."

30. **The correct answer is C.** *Means* can be a synonym of *modes* when they both mean "method, way, or variety," which fits the context of the sentence. Choice A is incorrect because *increments* means "the process of increasing in number, size, or quantity." Choice B is incorrect because *expenditures* refers to the disbursement of money. Choice D is incorrect because *modifications* refers to changes.

31. **The correct answer is D.** One meaning of *aggrandize* is "to enrich one's self." Choice A is incorrect because *exhaust*, "to tire," is not a synonym and doesn't make sense. Choice B is incorrect because *subjugate* means "to conquer, to make subservient." This is not only not a synonym, but the politician isn't about to subjugate himself. Choice C is incorrect because *sacrifice* is not a synonym, and a politician aggrandizing himself is the opposite of one sacrificing himself for his constituents.

32. **The correct answer is B.** To *mingle* is "to mix." Choice A is incorrect because *argue* is not the same as mingle. Choice C is incorrect because *disrupt* is "to interrupt" or "to break up." Choice D is incorrect because *flout* is "to show contempt for" or "to brush off, to ignore."

33. **The correct answer is D.** *Philanthropic* programs are *benevolent*, meaning "generous in helping others, showing kindness." Choice A is incorrect because *primitive* means "basic, simple." Choice B is incorrect because *deleterious* means "harmful," the opposite of *philanthropic*. Choice C is incorrect because *extraneous* means "not essential, unnecessary."

34. **The correct answer is A.** A *covetous* person is a *greedy* person. Choice B is incorrect because *exemplary* means "worthy of being imitated, a model." Choice C is incorrect because *disparate* means "something that is very different, unlike." Choice D is incorrect because *adventitious* means "added to something by chance or accidentally."

35. **The correct answer is C.** To *breed* is "to *propagate*" or "to reproduce." Choice A is incorrect because *raise* is not the same as *reproduce*. *Gather* (choice B) is not only not a synonym but makes no sense. *Destroy* (choice D) is not a synonym for *reproducing*.

Test 2: Antonyms

1. C	**7.** B	**13.** E	**19.** C	**25.** E
2. C	**8.** B	**14.** C	**20.** D	**26.** C
3. D	**9.** C	**15.** E	**21.** C	**27.** C
4. C	**10.** D	**16.** B	**22.** E	**28.** E
5. D	**11.** E	**17.** C	**23.** B	**29.** D
6. B	**12.** D	**18.** C	**24.** D	**30.** B

1. **The correct answer is C.** *Immutable* means "not subject to change," so *changeable* (choice C) is its antonym. *Erudite* (choice A) means "learned, highly educated," so eliminate it. *Abject* (choice B) means "wretched, forlorn" as well as "despicable," none of which are antonyms for *immutable*. *Fantastic* (choice D) has nothing to do with being able to change. *Aura* (choice E) is incorrect because it is a quality that someone possesses or a bright light around someone's head.

2. **The correct answer is C.** *Ductile* means "capable of being persuaded or influenced easily," so *stubborn* (choice C) is an antonym. Choice A is incorrect because *feted* means "honored by a celebration." Choice B is incorrect because *aloof* means "reserved, remote, distant either physically or emotionally." Choice D is incorrect because *abnormal* doesn't relate to being either ductile or stubborn. Choice E is incorrect because *belabored* means "having worked at something for an unusually long period of time" or "having criticized someone harshly."

3. **The correct answer is D.** Being *fastidious* is paying close attention to detail, being fussy, so the opposite is being *sloppy* (choice D). Choice A is incorrect because *factitious* means "lacking in authenticity or genuineness." Choice B is incorrect because *absurd* means "ridiculous" or "unreasonable." Choice C is incorrect because being indifferent, or not caring or feeling for or against something, is not the opposite of being *fastidious*. Choice E is incorrect because *chary* means "wary, cautious."

4. **The correct answer is C.** *Temerity* means "foolhardiness, recklessness, daring," which is the opposite of *cautiousness*. *Affinity* (choice A) means "a natural attraction to" as well as "relationship by marriage" and "an inherent similarity between persons and things"; none of the meanings are opposite in meaning to *temerity*. Choice B is incorrect because *cherubim* is a category of angels. Choice D is incorrect because a *degenerate* means "depraved, perverted, debauched," which isn't the same as *temerity*, but closer to it than opposite of it. Choice E is incorrect because *scanty* means "limited, insufficient, small."

5. **The correct answer is D.** An *itinerant* is someone who moves around from place to place, whereas a *resident* is someone who has a permanent place to stay. Choice A is incorrect because *animosity* is hostility. Choice B is incorrect because a *metaphor* is a figure of speech implying a comparison. Choice C is incorrect because *perpetrator* is someone who commits some act; the connotation is negative. Choice E is incorrect because the *cerebrum* is a part of the brain.

6. **The correct answer is B.** *Taciturn* means "untalkative by habit," whereas *loquacious* means "very talkative." *Malevolent* (choice A) is incorrect because it means "evil." Choice C is incorrect because *paltry* means "insignificant" or "worthless." Choice D is incorrect because something that is *opaque* doesn't transmit light through it. Choice E is incorrect because *morbid* means "having an unusual interest in death" or "gruesome, ghoulish."

7. **The correct answer is B.** *Nefarious* means "evil, wicked," so *virtuous*, meaning "morally excellent," is its opposite. Choice A is incorrect because *grotesque* means "fantastically distorted" or "bizarre." Choice C is incorrect because a *jovial* person is a very happy, jolly person. Choice D is incorrect because *pious* means "reverent toward God; religious; devout," none of which are exactly the same as being virtuous or the opposite of nefarious. Choice E is incorrect because *ceremonious* means "very polite" or "observing formalities."

8. **The correct answer is B.** *Obsequious* means "obedient or attentive in an ingratiating or flattering way; attempting to gain favor by flattery." Its opposite is being *bold*. Choice A is incorrect because *harbinger* means "someone or something that precedes and indicates the approach of someone or something else." Choice C is incorrect because *heredity* is the genetic transmission of characteristics from one generation to the next. Choice D is incorrect because *quaff* is "to drink." Choice E is incorrect because *fashionable*, or stylish, is not an antonym of *obsequious*. Note that *obsequious* is an adjective, and *harbinger* (choice C) is a noun and *quaff* (choice D) is a verb. None of these would be an antonym for an adjective.

9. **The correct answer is C.** *Ostentation* means "pretentious display, flamboyance," so *modesty* is an antonym. Choice A is incorrect because an *emulsion* is a light-sensitive coating on paper or film, or a chemical colloid. Choice B is incorrect because *languid* means "weak, lacking energy or force." Choice D is incorrect because *kilogram* is a unit of measure of mass. Choice E is incorrect because *showy* is a synonym for *ostentatious*, the adjectival form of *ostentation*.

10. **The correct answer is D.** A *contention* may be a competition, a dispute, or a point made in an argument. The only answer choice that is an antonym of any of these meanings is *friendliness*. Choice A is incorrect because an *equation* is a mathematical statement or a state of equality. Choice B is incorrect because a *guild* is an association of workers or merchants. Choice C is incorrect because *oblivion* means "the condition of being forgotten or disregarded." Choice E is incorrect because an *assertion* is a positive statement and a synonym for *contention*.

11. **The correct answer is E.** An *imputation* is a statement attributing blame or dishonesty to someone. The opposite is a *vindication*, exonerating or absolving someone of blame. Choice A is incorrect because *assiduous* means "diligent": note that this is an adjective and the word for which you need to find an antonym is a noun. That eliminates both choices A and B. *Radiant* (choice B) is also incorrect because it is not an antonym of assigning blame to someone. Choice C is incorrect because *accusation* is a synonym for *imputation*. Choice D is incorrect because *raiment* means "any piece of clothing."

12. **The correct answer is D.** *Benign* means "favorable," "showing kindness and mildness," or "harmless, not life-threatening." The only answer choice that is the opposite of any of these definitions is *pernicious*, meaning "deadly" or "destructive." Choice A is incorrect because *defensive* is not an antonym of *benign*, and neither is relevant (choice B). *Robot* (choice C) has no connection with being benign. Choice E is incorrect because *precarious* means "insecure, dangerous, uncertain."

13. **The correct answer is E.** To be *coherent* is "to be organized, clear, rational," so *chaotic* is an antonym. Choices B and D are incorrect because both *organized* and *rational* are synonyms for *coherent*. Choice A is incorrect because *perspicacious* means "having extreme insight and wisdom." Choice C is incorrect because *weal* means "general welfare of the community" or "happiness or prosperity."

14. **The correct answer is C.** *Depredation* means "a raid or attack" or "loss." *Restoration* fits as an antonym for the meaning of loss. Choice A is incorrect because *plethoric*, the adjectival form of *plethora*, means "an overabundance. Choice B is incorrect because *gloss* means either "a shininess on the surface of something" or "to give a shine to something." Choice D is incorrect because an *usher* is someone who shows you to your seat. Choice E is incorrect because *devastation* is a near synonym for *depredation*.

15. **The correct answer is E.** *Provocative* means "serving to stimulate, excite, or anger someone," so its antonym is *unexciting*. Choice A is incorrect because *sedentary* means "accustomed to sitting, getting little exercise." Choice B is incorrect because *capricious* means "impulsive, unpredictable." Choice C is incorrect because *vindictive*

means "revengeful, spiteful." Choice D is incorrect because *tawny* is a light brownish orange color.

16. **The correct answer is B.** Submission is the act of submitting to the power of someone else; it's being compliant. *Defiance*, boldly resisting, is an antonym. Choice A is incorrect because *authorized* means "having been given power or authority." Choice C is incorrect because an *assignment* isn't an antonym for *submission*. Choice D is incorrect because *defeat* isn't an antonym for *submission*. *Criticism* (choice E), meaning "a critical, or unfavorable, judgment" is not the same as bold resistance.

17. **The correct answer is C.** *Affluent* can be a wealthy person or it can mean "having wealth, both money and possessions." The only word that fits as an antonym is *insufficient*, meaning "not having enough." Choice A is incorrect because an *immigrant* is a person who moves permanently to another country. Choice B is incorrect because a *junction*, or place where two or more points meet or join, is not antonym for *affluent*. Choice D is incorrect because *kindred* means either "a group of related people" or "having the same family." Choice E is incorrect because *clandestine* means "done in secret, meant to conceal."

18. **The correct answer is C.** A *churlish* person is one who is surly, difficult, and/or rude. *Cheerful* is the only word that fits as an antonym. Choice A is incorrect because *exiguous* means "meager, stingy." Choice B is incorrect because *laudable* means "commendable, worthy of praise." Choice D is incorrect because *maternal* is an adjective derived from the word for *mother*. Choice E is incorrect because *sympathetic* means "showing sympathy, compassion, or understanding."

19. **The correct answer is C.** *Symmetry* is the similar or balanced arrangement of parts on opposite sides of something. *Distortion*, or misrepresentation or malformation, is the closest to being the opposite of *symmetry*. An invocation (choice A) is an appeal to someone for help, often in the form of a prayer. A synopsis (choice B) is a summary of a report, story, place, etc. A satyr (choice D) is a mythical creature. A portrayal (choice E) is a representation, description, or performance.

20. **The correct answer is D.** Dulcet describes something soothing or pleasant, sweet, especially sounds. *Disagreeable* is the only word among the answers that fits as a antonym. Choice A is incorrect because *extrinsic* means "not essential" or "coming from outside, external." Choice B is incorrect because *optimistic* means "typically expecting the best to occur." Choice C is incorrect because *unanimous* means "being in complete agreement." Choice E is incorrect because *sweet* is a synonym for *dulcet*, not an antonym.

21. **The correct answer is C.** *Pungent*, *piquant*, *spicy*, and *zesty* all mean "flavorful," "interesting," or "provocative." *Insipid* (choice C), meaning "lacking in flavor" or "lacking in anything that excites or stimulates," is the opposite, and thus is the word most different from the others.

22. **The correct answer is E.** *Opportune*, *suitable*, *advantageous*, and *prudent* all mean "advisable" or "beneficial." *Inexpedient* (choice E) means "not suitable, inadvisable," so it is the word most different from the others.

23. **The correct answer is B.** *Irascible*, *petulant*, *peevish*, and *sullen* all mean "irritable, impatient, ill-humored," so *good-humored*

(choice B) is the word most different from the others.

24. **The correct answer is D.** *Savory*, *delectable*, and *scrumptious* all mean "delicious" and *potable* means "drinkable" or "palatable." *Unpalatable* (choice D), meaning "not pleasing to the taste," is the word most different from the others.

25. **The correct answer is E.** *Satiated*, *glutted*, *gorged*, and *surfeited* all mean "filled to satisfaction" or even beyond satisfaction, whereas *rapacious* (choice E) means the opposite, or "famished, hungry."

26. **The correct answer is C.** *Reclusive* (choice B) means "withdrawing from people, living in isolation." *Reserved* and *taciturn* (choices A and D) mean "silent, unsociable." *Misanthropic* (choice E) means "hating humankind, cynical." All of these terms relate to being unsociable. The opposite of these is *gregarious* (choice C), which means "seeking out and enjoying the company of others, sociable."

27. **The correct answer is C.** *Courteous*, *gracious*, *polite*, and *urbane* all relate to being well-mannered. *Insolent*, on the other hand, means "arrogant, rude, disrespectful," and therefore is the word most different from the others.

28. **The correct answer is E.** *Usurp*, *seize*, *highjack*, and *appropriate* all mean "to seize, take over, take control," often illegitimately. *Relinquish*, however, means "to give up," and therefore is the word most different from the others.

29. **The correct answer is D.** *Acrimonious* (choice A) means "bitterness or sharpness in terms of speech, tone, manner, or temper." *Belligerent* and *truculent* (choices B and C) mean "antagonistic." *Peevish* (choice E)

means "testy." All of these terms relate to being difficult to get along with, whereas *harmonious* (choice D) means "being in agreement, cordial, friendly," and thus is the word most different from the others.

30. **The correct answer is B.** *Discernable*, *obvious*, *perceptible*, and *evident* all relate to something that is apparent or easily detected. *Cryptic* (choice B) is the opposite, meaning "having a secret or hidden meaning, mysterious," and thus is the word most different from the others.

Test 3: English Grammar and Usage

1. D	4. B	7. A	10. C	13. B
2. A	5. D	8. A	11. A	14. C
3. C	6. B	9. D	12. A	15. B

1. **The correct answer is D.** The verb *to be* is irregular and is conjugated in the present tense as follows: I am, you are, he/she/it is, we are, you (all) are, they are. Choice A is incorrect because *am* is the correct form to follow *I* in the first blank. Choice B is incorrect because *am* should appear in the first blank (following *I*) and *are* should appear in the second blank (following *you*). Choice C is incorrect because *are* should appear in the second blank (following *you*).

2. **The correct answer is A.** *To park* is a regular verb and is conjugated in the present tense as follows: I park, you park, he/she/it parks, we park, you (all) park, they park. Choice B is incorrect because *parks* should appear in the first blank (following *Jay usually*) and *park* should appear in the second blank (following *you all usually*). Choice C is incorrect because *park* should appear in the second blank (following *you all usually*). Choice D is incorrect because *parks* should appear in the first blank (following *Jay usually*).

3. **The correct answer is C.** The indefinite pronouns *somebody*, *everybody*, and *nobody* are always singular and thus require the verbs *dents*, *sees*, and *tells* in this sentence, respectively.

4. **The correct answer is B.** Possessive pronouns have two forms. One form (i.e., my, your, his, her, and its) is used as an adjective, to modify a noun, as in "my house" or "your house." The other form (i.e., mine, yours, his, hers, and its) is used as a true pronoun, to take the place of a noun, as in the following: "Mine [taking the place of "my house"] is for sale." In this sentence, the first blank calls for the adjective form of the possessive pronoun, *my*, to modify *dog*. The second blank calls for the pronoun form, *yours*, to take the place of "your dog."

5. **The correct answer is D.** The nominative case of a pronoun is used when the pronoun is the subject of a sentence; the objective case of a pronoun is used when the pronoun is the object of a verb or of a preposition. In this sentence, the first and third blanks call for subjects, and thus the nominative case forms of the pronouns should be used (i.e., *he* and *I*). The second and fourth blanks call for direct objects of the verb *beat*, and thus the objective case forms of the pronouns should be used (i.e., *me* and *him*).

6. **The correct answer is B.** The pronoun *who* takes the nominative case (*who*) when it functions as the subject or predicate nominative of a sentence and the objective case (*whom*) when it functions as the object of a verb. In the first sentence, *you* is the subject, *are calling* is the action verb, and the blank requires a direct object of the verb; thus, the objective form, *whom*, should be used. In the second sentence, *that* is the subject, *is* is the linking verb, and the blank requires a predicate nominative; thus, the nominative form, *who*, should be used.

7. **The correct answer is A.** Dangling modifiers occur when a modifying phrase or clause within a sentence does not clearly or sensibly modify any word in the sentence. In choices B, C, and D, the phrase "driving down the road" seems to modify the dog,

which of course is absurd. Thus this phrase is a dangling modifier. Only choice A avoids a dangling modifier by clarifying that it is while the *man* is driving that the dog sticks his head out of the window.

8. **The correct answer is A.** The verb *throw* is irregular, with its past tense form being *threw* and its past participle—which is used to form the present perfect, past perfect, and future perfect tenses—being *thrown*. In this sentence, the throwing out of the baseball card collection occurs before some other past event, which is asking the mom, so the past perfect tense is needed. Thus *thrown* is the proper form of the verb in this case. Choice A is incorrect because *threw* is the simple past tense, not the past perfect tense. Choices C and D are not proper forms of the verb *throw*.

9. **The correct answer is D.** The first independent clause in this sentence indicates that the people love the house in which they are currently living. *There* in the second independent clause refers back to this same house. The phrase *for over 25 years* indicates that the people have lived in this house for a long time in the past. Thus, the most appropriate tense to use in the second independent clause is the present perfect. The present perfect of live is *have lived*. Choice A is incorrect because the present progressive tense, *are living*, does not make sense with the phrase *for over 25 years*. Choice B is incorrect because the past tense, *lived*, would indicate that they no longer live in the house, which is not the case. Choice C is incorrect because the past perfect tense, *had lived*, would indicate that they used to live at this house before some other past event and that they no longer live there, which, again, is not the case.

10. **The correct answer is C.** A preposition is a word that shows the relationship of a noun or pronoun to some other word in the sentence. In this sentence, the preposition *beneath* shows the relationship of the family of snakes to the Thompsons' house. Thus, *beneath* is a preposition (choice C) and not an adjective (which modifies a noun or pronoun), an adverb (which modifies a verb, adjective, or other adverb), or a conjunction (which joins words or groups of words).

11. **The correct answer is A.** An adjective is a word that modifies a noun or pronoun. In this sentence, the word *slowest* modifies the noun *swimmer* and thus is an adjective. More specifically, it is a superlative adjective, indicating that person or thing referred to (Ruth, in this case) has the greatest degree of a certain trait compared with two or more others. *Slowest* is not a preposition (which shows the relationship of a noun or pronoun to some other word in the sentence), an adverb (which modifies a verb, adjective, or other adverb), or conjunction (which joins words or groups of words).

12. **The correct answer is A.** When indicating a lesser degree with an adjective, use *less* plus the adjective for the comparative form (comparing just two items) and *least* plus the adjective for the superlative form (comparing three or more items). In this sentence, the comparison is between two hiking trails; therefore, the comparative form is needed, which is *less challenging*. Choice B is incorrect because *not challenging* is not in the comparative form. Choice C is incorrect because *least challenging* is in the superlative form. Choice D is incorrect because *less* plus the adjective should be used to show a lesser degree with a comparative adjective.

13. **The correct answer is B.** To be grammatically complete, a sentence must have both a subject and a verb, and any independent clauses must be properly joined. Choice A is incorrect because it is missing a verb. Choice C is incorrect because the two independent clauses are improperly joined by a comma. Choice D is incorrect because it is missing a subject.

14. **The correct answer is C.** When two independent clauses are joined by a coordinating conjunction, a comma should immediately precede the conjunction. Choice A is incorrect because a semicolon should be used alone when joining two independent clauses, not in combination with a coordinating conjunction. Choice B is incorrect because a colon is not used together with a coordinating conjunction to join two independent clauses. Choice D is incorrect because a dash is not used together with a coordinating conjunction to join two independent clauses.

15. **The correct answer is B.** To make a plural noun that ends in *s* possessive, simply add an apostrophe. By this sentence's context, we see that the house (mentioned in the statement) belongs to at least two people, Barb and Larry Schneider. The plural form of *Schneider* is *Schneiders*; thus, the possessive plural would be *Schneiders'*.

Test 4: Spelling

1. A	4. C	7. B	10. A	13. C
2. B	5. A	8. C	11. A	14. A
3. B	6. C	9. B	12. B	15. C

1. **The correct answer is A.** The correct spelling is *actually*.

2. **The correct answer is B.** The correct spelling is *bradycardia*.

3. **The correct answer is B.** The correct spelling is *chromosome*.

4. **The correct answer is C.** The correct spelling is *dyspnea*.

5. **The correct answer is A.** The correct spelling is *euphoria*.

6. **The correct answer is C.** The correct spelling is *fascia*.

7. **The correct answer is B.** The correct spelling is *gestation*.

8. **The correct answer is C.** The correct spelling is *hypothalamus*.

9. **The correct answer is B.** The correct spelling is *jaundice*.

10. **The correct answer is A.** The correct spelling is *kyphosis*.

11. **The correct answer is A.** The correct spelling is *longevity*.

12. **The correct answer is B.** The correct spelling is *negligence*.

13. **The correct answer is C.** The correct spelling is *retina*.

14. **The correct answer is A.** The correct spelling is *sensitivity*.

15. **The correct answer is C.** The correct spelling is *thrombosis*.

Test 5: Nonverbal Ability

1. E	4. D	7. A	10. B	13. A
2. A	5. B	8. E	11. C	14. C
3. C	6. A	9. B	12. D	15. B

1. **The correct answer is E.** The relationship between the first two shapes is that the second is the same as the first except that it has a slash through it. So, in the second pair, we begin with a T pointing right and are looking for a T pointing right with a slash through it. Therefore, U pointing right is to U pointing right with a slash through it as T pointing right is to T pointing right with a slash through it.

2. **The correct answer is A.** The relationship between the first two shapes is that the second is the same as the first except that a horizontal line segment has been added above it. So, in the second pair, we begin with a T and are looking for a T with a horizontal line segment above it. Therefore, inverted V with a horizontal line segment above it is to inverted V with two parallel horizontal line segments above it as T is to T with a horizontal line segment above it.

3. **The correct answer is C.** The relationship between the first two shapes is that the same form embedded in a circle in the first shape appears in the second shape without the circle and with two dots above it. So, in the second pair, we begin with a circle embedded in a larger circle and are looking for a circle with two dots above it. Therefore, star embedded in circle is to star with two dots above it as circle embedded in larger circle is to circle with two dots above it.

4. **The correct answer is D.** The relationship between the first two shapes is that the second is a dashed version of the first. So, in the second pair, we begin with a vertical

line and are looking for a dashed vertical line. Therefore, circle is to dashed circle as vertical line is to dashed vertical line.

5. **The correct answer is B.** The relationship between the first two shapes is that the second shape is the first shape joined with its mirror image. So, in the second pair, we begin with D with a smaller D embedded within it and are looking for the same shape joined with its mirror image. Therefore, D is to D joined with its mirror image as D with smaller D embedded within it is to D with smaller D embedded within it joined to its mirror image.

6. **The correct answer is A.** The relationship between the first two shapes is that the second is a duplicate of the first. So, in the second pair, we begin with a double dagger symbol and are looking for the same symbol. Therefore, dagger symbol is to dagger symbol as double dagger symbol is to double dagger symbol.

7. **The correct answer is A.** The relationship between the first two shapes is that the second is a mirror image of the first with a dot embedded within it. So, in the second pair, we begin with a lower case C and are looking for a mirror image of lower case C with a dot embedded in it. Therefore, Capital C is to mirror image of capital C with dot embedded in it as lower case C is to mirror image of lower case C with dot embedded in it.

8. **The correct answer is E.** The relationship between the first two forms is that the second immediately follows the first in a

series two which both belong and is rotated 180 degrees from its normal position. So, in the second pair, we begin with a J and are looking for a K rotated 180 degrees. Therefore, 2 is to 3 rotated 180 degrees as J is to K rotated 180 degrees.

9. **The correct answer is B.** The relationship between the first two shapes is that the second is the mirror image of the first doubled. So, in the second pair, we begin with an opening parenthesis and are looking for the mirror image of an opening parenthesis (which is a closing parenthesis) doubled. Therefore, backward question mark is to two regular question marks as opening parenthesis is to two closing parentheses.

10. **The correct answer is B.** The relationship between the first two forms is that each consists of two elements side by side, but the first has two different elements side by side whereas the second has identical elements side by side, and that element is the second element in the first form. So, in the second pair, we begin with intersecting perpendicular line segments next to a vertical line segment and are looking for two vertical line segments. Therefore, question mark and exclamation point is to exclamation point and exclamation point as intersecting perpendicular line segments and vertical line segment is to vertical line segment and vertical line segment.

11. **The correct answer is C.** The relationship between the first two shapes is that the second is a smaller version of the first that has been embedded in another shape. So, in the second pair, we begin with plus sign and are looking for a smaller plus sign embedded in another shape. Therefore, C is to smaller C embedded in circle as plus sign is to smaller plus sign embedded in U.

12. **The correct answer is D.** The relationship between the first two shapes is that the second indicates a direction of movement

that is the opposite of that indicated by the first. So, in the second pair, we begin with a left arrow and are looking for a right arrow. Therefore, left rotational arrow is to right rotational arrow as left arrow is to right arrow.

13. **The correct answer is A.** The relationship between the first two shapes is that the second is the same as the first except that it is divided into quarters. So, in the second pair, we begin with a cross and are looking for a cross divided into quarters. Therefore, diamond is to diamond divided into quarters as cross is to cross divided into quarters. You might be tempted to choose choice B, as it is similar to a cross divided into quarters. However, it is smaller and of different proportions than the first shape in the second pair; the shape in choice A is much more similar in size and proportion to the first shape in the second pair.

14. **The correct answer is C.** The relationship between the first two shapes is that the second is a dashed version of the first. So, in the second pair, we begin with an upper left corner of a square and are looking for a dashed upper left corner of a square. Therefore, horizontal line segment is to dashed horizontal line segment as upper left corner of square is to dashed upper left corner of square.

15. **The correct answer is B.** The relationship between the first two shapes is that the second is the negative image of the first. This means that the colors in the first shape are switched to their opposites. So, in the second pair, we begin with a group of tiny squares and are looking for the negative image of that same group of tiny squares. Therefore, circle is to negative image of circle as group of tiny squares is to negative image of group of tiny squares.

Mathematics

OVERVIEW

- **Mathematics Answer Sheet**
- **Test 1: Arithmetic**
- **Test 2: Problem Solving**
- **Test 3: Algebra**
- **Answer Keys and Explanations**

Unit 10

MATHEMATICS ANSWER SHEET

Test 1: Artithmetic

1. Ⓐ Ⓑ Ⓒ Ⓓ   4. Ⓐ Ⓑ Ⓒ Ⓓ   7. Ⓐ Ⓑ Ⓒ Ⓓ   10. Ⓐ Ⓑ Ⓒ Ⓓ   13. Ⓐ Ⓑ Ⓒ Ⓓ
2. Ⓐ Ⓑ Ⓒ Ⓓ   5. Ⓐ Ⓑ Ⓒ Ⓓ   8. Ⓐ Ⓑ Ⓒ Ⓓ   11. Ⓐ Ⓑ Ⓒ Ⓓ   14. Ⓐ Ⓑ Ⓒ Ⓓ
3. Ⓐ Ⓑ Ⓒ Ⓓ   6. Ⓐ Ⓑ Ⓒ Ⓓ   9. Ⓐ Ⓑ Ⓒ Ⓓ   12. Ⓐ Ⓑ Ⓒ Ⓓ

Test 2: Problem Solving

1. Ⓐ Ⓑ Ⓒ Ⓓ   4. Ⓐ Ⓑ Ⓒ Ⓓ   7. Ⓐ Ⓑ Ⓒ Ⓓ   10. Ⓐ Ⓑ Ⓒ Ⓓ   13. Ⓐ Ⓑ Ⓒ Ⓓ
2. Ⓐ Ⓑ Ⓒ Ⓓ   5. Ⓐ Ⓑ Ⓒ Ⓓ   8. Ⓐ Ⓑ Ⓒ Ⓓ   11. Ⓐ Ⓑ Ⓒ Ⓓ   14. Ⓐ Ⓑ Ⓒ Ⓓ
3. Ⓐ Ⓑ Ⓒ Ⓓ   6. Ⓐ Ⓑ Ⓒ Ⓓ   9. Ⓐ Ⓑ Ⓒ Ⓓ   12. Ⓐ Ⓑ Ⓒ Ⓓ   15. Ⓐ Ⓑ Ⓒ Ⓓ

Test 3: Algebra

1. Ⓐ Ⓑ Ⓒ Ⓓ   3. Ⓐ Ⓑ Ⓒ Ⓓ   5. Ⓐ Ⓑ Ⓒ Ⓓ   7. Ⓐ Ⓑ Ⓒ Ⓓ   8. Ⓐ Ⓑ Ⓒ Ⓓ
2. Ⓐ Ⓑ Ⓒ Ⓓ   4. Ⓐ Ⓑ Ⓒ Ⓓ   6. Ⓐ Ⓑ Ⓒ Ⓓ

answer sheet

TEST 1: ARITHMETIC

14 Questions • 20 Minutes

> **Directions:** Read each question carefully and consider all possible answers. When you have decided which choice is best, fill in the corresponding space on your answer sheet. There is only one best answer for each question.

1. What fraction of the whole is the shaded area in the figure below?

   SHOW YOUR WORK HERE

   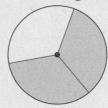

   A. $\dfrac{1}{2}$

   B. $\dfrac{3}{4}$

   C. $\dfrac{2}{3}$

   D. $\dfrac{2}{5}$

2. Which of the following equations demonstrates that the two figures are equivalent?

   A. $\dfrac{3}{9} = \dfrac{1}{3}$

   B. $\dfrac{9}{3} = \dfrac{3}{1}$

   C. $\dfrac{3}{9} = \dfrac{3}{3}$

   D. $\dfrac{9}{3} = \dfrac{1}{3}$

3. Select the answer that represents reduction of the fraction $\frac{630}{140}$ to the lowest term.

SHOW YOUR WORK HERE

  A. $\frac{70}{2}$

  B. $\frac{70}{4}$

  C. $\frac{2}{9}$

  D. $\frac{9}{2}$

4. Which one of the following equations is correct for converting the fraction $\frac{3}{8}$ to an equivalent fraction with a a denominator of 24?

  A. $\frac{3}{8} = \frac{3 \times 3}{3 \times 8} = \frac{9}{24}$

  B. $\frac{3}{8} = 3 \times \frac{24}{8} \times \frac{1}{24} \times \frac{9}{24}$

  C. $8 \times \frac{3}{1} \times \frac{1}{24} = \frac{24}{24}$

  D. $\frac{3}{24} = 3 \times \frac{1}{3} \times \frac{1}{8} = \frac{1}{24}$

5. Which of the following equations expresses the whole number 6 as an equivalent fraction with a denominator of 5?

  A. $\frac{6}{5} = 6 \times \frac{5}{5} \times \frac{1}{5} = \frac{30}{25}$

  B. $\frac{6}{5} = 6 \times \frac{1}{5} \times 1 = \frac{6}{5}$

  C. $\frac{6}{1} = \frac{6 \times 5}{1 \times 5} = \frac{30}{5}$

  D. $\frac{6}{1} = 5 \times \frac{1}{6} \times 1 = \frac{5}{6}$

6. What is the product of $\frac{5}{3} \times \frac{2}{7}$?

SHOW YOUR WORK HERE

    A. $\frac{6}{35}$

    B. $\frac{35}{6}$

    C. $\frac{21}{10}$

    D. $\frac{10}{21}$

7. What is the product of $\frac{25}{36} \times \frac{16}{20}$?

    A. $\frac{10}{8}$

    B. $\frac{8}{10}$

    C. $\frac{9}{5}$

    D. $\frac{5}{9}$

8. What is $\frac{3}{4}$ divided by $\frac{5}{2}$?

    A. $\frac{10}{3}$

    B. $\frac{3}{10}$

    C. $\frac{20}{6}$

    D. $\frac{6}{20}$

9. Select the correct answer for $\frac{72}{50} \div \frac{200}{35}$.

    A. $\frac{63}{250}$

    B. $\frac{250}{63}$

    C. $\frac{288}{35}$

    D. $\frac{35}{288}$

10. A 12-ounce bottle has 7 ounces of liquid in it. What fraction of the bottle is filled?

   A. $\frac{3}{4}$

   B. $\frac{1}{2}$

   C. $\frac{7}{12}$

   D. $\frac{12}{7}$

11. What is the solution to the problem

$\frac{2}{9}+\frac{5}{6}-\frac{3}{8}$?

   A. $\frac{72}{60}$

   B. $\frac{60}{72}$

   C. $\frac{72}{49}$

   D. $\frac{49}{72}$

12. When you multiply $2\frac{1}{3}\times1\frac{1}{2}$, what is the product?

   A. $3\frac{1}{3}$

   B. $3\frac{1}{2}$

   C. $2\frac{1}{5}$

   D. $2\frac{2}{6}$

SHOW YOUR WORK HERE

13. Change $2\frac{1}{2} \div 3\frac{1}{3}$ to a simple fraction.

    SHOW YOUR WORK HERE

    A. $\frac{3}{4}$

    B. $\frac{4}{3}$

    C. $\frac{1}{3}$

    D. $\frac{1}{4}$

14. What is the solution to the problem

    $5\frac{3}{4} + 6\frac{5}{9}$?

    A. $12\frac{5}{12}$

    B. $11\frac{15}{36}$

    C. $12\frac{11}{36}$

    D. $11\frac{8}{13}$

STOP

IF YOU FINISH BEFORE TIME IS CALLED, YOU MAY CHECK YOUR WORK ON THIS SECTION ONLY. DO NOT TURN TO ANY OTHER SECTION IN THE TEST.

TEST 2: PROBLEM SOLVING

15 Questions • 20 Minutes

> **Directions:** Read each question carefully and consider all possible answers. When you have decided which choice is best, fill in the corresponding space on your answer sheet. There is only one best answer for each question.

1. If there are 245 sections in a city containing five boroughs, the average number of sections for each of the five boroughs is

   A. 50 sections.

   B. 49 sections.

   C. 47 sections.

   D. 59 sections.

2. If, in that same city, a section has 45 miles of street to plow after a snowstorm, and nine plows are used, each plow will cover an average of how many miles?

   A. 7 miles

   B. 6 miles

   C. 8 miles

   D. 5 miles

3. If a crosswalk plow engine is run 5 minutes a day for ten days in a given month, how long will it run in the course of this month?

   A. 50 minutes

   B. $1\frac{1}{2}$ hours

   C. 1 hour

   D. 30 minutes

4. If the city uses 1,500 laborers in manual street cleaning and half as many more to load and drive trucks, the total number of laborers used is

   A. 2,200.

   B. 2,520.

   C. 2,050.

   D. 2,250.

SHOW YOUR WORK HERE

5. Of 186 summonses issued, 100 were issued to first offenders. How many summonses were issued to non–first offenders?

   A. 68

   B. 90

   C. 86

   D. 108

6. A sanitation worker is 40 feet behind a sanitation truck. There is a second sanitation truck 90 feet behind the first truck. How much closer is the worker to the first truck than to the second?

   A. 30 feet

   B. 50 feet

   C. 10 feet

   D. 70 feet

7. If a flushing machine has a capacity of 1,260 gallons, how many gallons will it contain when it is two-thirds full?

   A. 809 gallons

   B. 750 gallons

   C. 630 gallons

   D. 840 gallons

8. If a part-time employee earns $160.00 a week and has deductions of $8.00 for the pension fund, $12.00 for medical insurance, and $29.60 withholding tax, his take-home pay is

   A. $110.40.

   B. $108.60.

   C. $102.00.

   D. $98.40.

9. A city department uses 25 twenty-cent, 35 thirty-cent, and 350 forty-cent metered postage units each day. The total cost of stamps used by the department in a five-day period is

   A. $29.50.

   B. $155.00.

   C. $290.50.

   D. $777.50.

SHOW YOUR WORK HERE

SHOW YOUR WORK HERE

10. In 2015, a school bought 500 dozen pencils at $0.40 per dozen. In 2018, only 75 percent as many pencils were bought as had been bought in 2015, but the price per dozen was 20 percent higher than the 2015 price. The total cost of the pencils bought in 2018 was

    A. $180.00.

    B. $187.50.

    C. $240.00.

    D. $250.00.

11. If the average cost of sweeping a square foot of a small town's street is $0.75, the cost of sweeping 100 square feet is

    A. $7.50.

    B. $750.

    C. $75.

    D. $70.

12. If a sanitation department scow is towed at the rate of 3 miles per hour, how many hours will it need to go 28 miles?

    A. 10 hours, 30 minutes

    B. 12 hours

    C. 9 hours, 20 minutes

    D. 9 hours, 15 minutes

13. A man is 60 feet away from a sanitation truck. How many feet nearer is he to the sanitation truck than a second truck is, if the second truck is 100 feet away from the sanitation truck?

    A. 60 feet

    B. 40 feet

    C. 50 feet

    D. 20 feet

14. Six gross of special drawing pencils were purchased for use in a city department. If the pencils were used at the rate of 24 a week, the maximum number of weeks that the six gross of pencils would last is

    A. 6 weeks.

    B. 12 weeks.

    C. 24 weeks.

    D. 36 weeks.

15. A cogwheel having eight cogs plays into another cogwheel having 24 cogs. When the small wheel has made 42 revolutions, how many has the larger wheel made?

    A. 14

    B. 20

    C. 16

    D. 10

SHOW YOUR WORK HERE

STOP

IF YOU FINISH BEFORE TIME IS CALLED, YOU MAY CHECK YOUR WORK ON THIS SECTION ONLY. DO NOT TURN TO ANY OTHER SECTION IN THE TEST.

TEST 3: ALGEBRA

8 Questions • 20 Minutes

Directions: Read each question carefully and consider all possible answers. When you have decided which choice is best, fill in the corresponding space on your answer sheet. There is only one best answer for each question.

---

1. In the equation $4a + 5 = 13$, a equals

   A. 4.

   B. 2.

   C. 7.

   D. 6.

   SHOW YOUR WORK HERE

2. In the equation $\dfrac{10}{m} - 8 = \dfrac{5}{3}$, m equals

   A. $\dfrac{10}{3}$.

   B. $\dfrac{3}{10}$.

   C. $\dfrac{30}{29}$.

   D. $\dfrac{29}{30}$.

3. In the equation $3c^2 = 75d^4$, c equals

   A. $\pm 5d^2$.

   B. $\pm 5d^4$.

   C. $\pm 25d^2$.

   D. $\pm 25d^4$.

4. If 2 moles of compound A react with 5 moles of compound B to form compound C, then how many moles of A are required to react completely with 7 moles of B to form compound C?

   A. 5.7

   B. 2.8

   C. 7.5

   D. 8.2

5. A car traveling at x mph takes 5 hours to go from city A to city B. Traveling at $x - 15$ mph, the car makes the return trip in $6\frac{2}{3}$ hours. What was the speed of the car on the return trip?
   A. 60 mph
   B. 55 mph
   C. 50 mph
   D. 45 mph

6. In 2016, item A cost $2,500. In 2017, the price of A went up 20 percent because of inflation, while in early 2018 there was a 10 percent increase in the price of A over its 2017 price. In June 2018, A was put on sale with a 30 percent decrease in price. What was the sale price of A?
   A. $2,500
   B. $2,400
   C. $2,310
   D. $2,110

7. In the expression $\log_4 \frac{1}{16} = x$, what is the value of x?
   A. −2
   B. −4
   C. +2
   D. +4

8. What is the volume of a sphere of a radius 3 centimeters?
   A. 119.05 c^3
   B. 113.04 c^3
   C. 106.00 c^3
   D. 101.08 c^3

STOP

IF YOU FINISH BEFORE TIME IS CALLED, YOU MAY CHECK YOUR WORK ON THIS SECTION ONLY. DO NOT TURN TO ANY OTHER SECTION IN THE TEST.

ANSWER KEYS AND EXPLANATIONS

Test 1: Arithmetic

1. C	4. A	7. D	10. C	13. A
2. A	5. C	8. B	11. D	14. C
3. D	6. D	9. A	12. B	

1. **The correct answer is C.** Since the whole is divided into 3 units, the denominator is 3. There are 2 units shaded, so the numerator is 2. The shaded part is $\frac{2}{3}$ of the whole.

2. **The correct answer is A.** The left-hand figure is divided into 9 parts, and is a square. The shaded part can be represented by the fraction $\frac{3}{9}$. The right-hand figure is divided in 3 parts, and is also a square. The fraction $\frac{1}{3}$ represents the shaded part; $\frac{3}{9}$ and $\frac{1}{3}$ represent the same part of the whole and are therefore equivalent, $\frac{3}{9} = \frac{1}{3}$.

3. **The correct answer is D.**

$$\frac{630}{140} = \frac{63}{14} = \frac{63 \div 7}{14 \div 7} = \frac{9}{2}$$

4. **The correct answer is A.** Multiply both parts by the same number. 8 multiplied by what number will give 24? Answer: divide 24 by 8 to get 3. The denominator and the numerator are multiplied by 3 to get $\frac{9}{24}$.

$$\frac{3}{8} = \frac{3 \times 3}{3 \times 8} = \frac{9}{24}$$

5. **The correct answer is C.** Write 6 as $\frac{6}{1}$, and use the same process as in answer number 4.

$$\frac{6}{1} = \frac{6}{1} \times \frac{5}{5} = \frac{30}{5}$$

6. **The correct answer is D.** Multiply numerators and denominators.

$$\frac{5}{3} \times \frac{2}{7} = \frac{5 \times 2}{3 \times 7} = \frac{10}{21}$$

7. **The correct answer is D.** Reduce and perform the multiplication.

$$\frac{25}{36} \times \frac{\cancel{16}}{\cancel{20}} = \frac{25}{36} \times \frac{4}{5} \quad \text{(divide by 4)}$$

$$\frac{\cancel{25}}{36} \times \frac{4}{\cancel{5}} = \frac{5}{36} \times \frac{4}{1} \quad \text{(divide by 5)}$$

$$= \frac{5}{36} \times \frac{4}{1} \quad \text{(divide by 4)}$$

$$= \frac{5}{9} \times \frac{1}{1}$$

$$= \frac{5}{9}$$

8. **The correct answer is B.** Invert the divisor and change the operation to multiplication, reduce, and perform the multiplication.

$$\frac{3}{4} \div \frac{5}{2} = \frac{3}{4} \times \frac{2}{5}$$

$$\frac{3}{4} \times \frac{2}{5} \quad \text{(divide by 2)}$$

$$\frac{3}{2} \times \frac{1}{5} = \frac{3}{10}$$

9. **The correct answer is A.** Use the same procedure as in answer number 8.

$$\frac{72}{50} \div \frac{200}{35} = \frac{72}{50} \times \frac{35}{200}$$

$$\frac{72}{50} \times \frac{35}{200} \quad \text{(divide by 8)}$$

$$\frac{9}{50} \times \frac{35}{25} \quad \text{(divide by 5)}$$

$$\frac{9}{10} \times \frac{7}{25} = \frac{63}{250}$$

10. **The correct answer is C.** The bottle (whole) is divided into 12 ounces (the denominator) of which 7 ounces (the numerator) is filled. Thus, $\frac{7}{12}$ of the bottle is filled.

11. **The correct answer is D.** Find the lowest common denominator (LCD), which is 72, build up each fraction to have 72 as denominator, and perform addition and subtraction as indicated.

    The least common multiple (LCM) of 9 and 6 is 18.

    The LCM of 18 and 8 is 72.

    Therefore, LCD = 72.

    $$\frac{2}{9} = \frac{2}{9} \times \frac{8}{8} = \frac{16}{72}$$

    $$\frac{5}{6} = \frac{5 \times 12}{6 \times 12} = \frac{60}{72}$$

    $$\frac{3}{8} = \frac{3 \times 9}{8 \times 9} = \frac{27}{72}$$

    $$\frac{2}{9} + \frac{5}{6} - \frac{3}{8} = \frac{16}{72} + \frac{60}{72} - \frac{27}{72} = \frac{76}{72} - \frac{27}{72} = \frac{49}{72}$$

12. **The correct answer is B.** Change both mixed numbers into improper fractions and multiply.

    $$2\frac{1}{3} \times 1\frac{1}{2} = \frac{7}{3} \times \frac{3}{2}$$

    $$\frac{7}{3} \times \frac{3}{2} = \frac{7}{2} = 3\frac{1}{2}$$

13. **The correct answer is A.** Use the same procedure as in answer number 12, then change ÷ to × and invert the second fraction.

    $$2\frac{1}{2} \div 3\frac{1}{3} = \frac{5}{2} \div \frac{10}{3}$$

    $$\frac{\overset{1}{\cancel{5}}}{2} \times \frac{3}{\underset{2}{\cancel{10}}} = \frac{1}{2} \times \frac{3}{2} = \frac{3}{4}$$

14. **The correct answer is C.** Add the whole numbers and fractional parts separately. Change the improper fraction to a mixed number. Find common denominators for fractional parts, then add.

    $$5\frac{3}{4} + 6\frac{5}{9} = 5 + \frac{3}{4} + 6 + \frac{5}{9}$$

    $$= 11 + \frac{3}{4} + \frac{5}{9}$$

    $$= 11 + \frac{27}{36} + \frac{20}{36}$$

    $$= 11 + \frac{47}{36}$$

    $$= 11 + 1 + \frac{11}{36}$$

    $$= 12 + \frac{11}{36}$$

    $$= 12\frac{11}{36}$$

Test 2: Problem Solving

1. B	**4.** D	**7.** D	**10.** A	**13.** B
2. D	**5.** C	**8.** A	**11.** C	**14.** D
3. A	**6.** C	**9.** D	**12.** C	**15.** A

1. **The correct answer is B.** To find the *average* number of sections per borough, take:

   245 sections divided by 5 boroughs = 49

   49 sections/borough

2. **The correct answer is D.**

   Total miles = 45

   Number of plows = 9

   To find the *average* number of miles, divide:

   45 miles by 9 plows = 5 miles/plow

   Average = 5 miles

3. **The correct answer is A.**

   Total time per day = 5 minutes
   Total days per month = 10 days
   Total time per month =

   $$\frac{5 \text{ minutes}}{\text{day}} \times \frac{10 \text{ days}}{\text{month}} = \frac{50 \text{ minutes}}{\text{month}}$$

4. **The correct answer is D.**

   Total number for street cleaning = 1,500
   half that number load and drive = +750
   2,250

   2,250 laborers used

5. **The correct answer is C.**

Total issued =	186
subtract:	
first offenders =	−100
non-first offenders	86

6. **The correct answer is C.** The second truck is 90 feet − 40 feet = 50 feet from the man. The first truck is 40 feet from the man. The first truck is 50 feet − 40 feet = 10 feet closer than the second truck.

7. **The correct answer is D.**

   Total capacity = 1,260 gallons

   $$\frac{2}{3} \text{ of } 1,260 = \frac{2}{3} \times 1,260$$
   $$= \frac{2,520}{3}$$
   $$= 840 \text{ gallons}$$

8. **The correct answer is A.**

Total earnings	=	$160.00
Deductions	=	$8.00 pension
		$12.00 medical insurance
+		$29.60 withholding tax
		$49.60 total deductions

   The take-home pay can be found by subtracting the total deductions from the salary.

   $160.00 − $49.60 = $110.40

   Take-home pay = $110.40

9. **The correct answer is D.**

Stamps per day	Cost per day
25 / day × $0.20 =	5.00
35 / day × $0.30 =	10.50
350 × $0.40 =	140.00
Total cost/day	$155.50

   For five days, 5 × $155.50 = $777.50

   Total cost = $777.50

10. **The correct answer is A.** Total number of pencils bought in 2015 was 500 dozen at $0.40 a dozen; in 2018, 75 percent of the 500 dozen were bought at a 20 percent increase in price.

First, find how many pencils were bought in 2018. Do this by multiplying:

$500 \times 0.75 = 375$ dozen were bought in 2018

Now find the price per dozen. You know that it was 20 percent more than $0.40:

0.40×0.20 increase = $0.08, or 8¢, increase in price

So the price per dozen is:

40¢ + 8¢ = 48¢, or $0.48

To find the cost, multiply the number of dozens of pencils by the cost per dozen.

375 dozen × $0.48/dozen = $180

Total cost for 2018 = $180

11. **The correct answer is C.** If it costs $0.75 to sweep 1 square foot, to find the cost for 100 square feet, multiply:

100 square feet × 0.75 per square foot = $75.00

Total cost = $75

12. **The correct answer is C.** It takes 1 hour to tow a scow 3 miles. Find the time to tow the scow 28 miles by dividing:

28 miles ÷ 3 miles/hour = $9\frac{1}{3}$ hours

Note: 1 hour = 60 minutes. To change hours to minutes, multiply the fraction of an hour by

$$\frac{60 \text{ minutes}}{\text{hour}}$$

$\frac{1}{3}$ hour × 60 minutes/hour = 20 minutes

It takes 9 hours, 20 minutes to tow the scow 28 miles.

13. **The correct answer is B.**

Truck to the other truck	100 feet
Truck to the man	− 60 feet
	40 feet

The difference is 40 feet.

14. **The correct answer is D.**

One gross = 144 pencils

6 gross = 144 pencils/gross × 6 gross = 864 pencils (on hand)

If 24 pencils are used each week, divide to find the number of weeks they will last:

864 divided by 24/week = 36 weeks

Supplies would last 36 weeks.

15. **The correct answer is A.** If the cogs on two wheels are sized and spaced the same, the smaller of the two wheels will turn faster than the larger one—the fewer cogs a wheel has, the more revolutions it makes. The number of cogs is, therefore, inversely proportional to the number of revolutions.

The smaller wheel will make 3 revolutions for every 1 revolution the larger wheel makes. So when the smaller wheel makes 42 revolutions, the larger wheel will make 42 divided by 3 = 14 revolutions.

Test 3: Algebra

1. B	3. A	5. D	7. A	8. B
2. C	4. B	6. C		

1. **The correct answer is B.**

$$4a + 5 - 5 = 13 - 5$$
$$4a = 8$$
$$\frac{4a}{4} = \frac{8}{4}$$
$$a = 2$$

2. **The correct answer is C.**

$$\frac{10}{m} - 8 = \frac{5}{3} \quad \text{(multiply by } 3m\text{)}$$
$$3m \times \frac{10}{m} - (3m)(8) = \frac{(3m)(5)}{3}$$
$$\frac{30m}{m} - 24m = \frac{15m}{3}$$
$$30 - 24m = 5m$$
$$30 = 29m$$
$$m = \frac{30}{29}$$

3. **The correct answer is A.**

$$\frac{3c^2}{3} = \frac{75d^4}{3}$$
$$c^2 = 25d^4$$
$$\sqrt{c^2} = \sqrt{25d^4}$$
$$c = \pm 5d^2$$

4. **The correct answer is B.** In a chemical reaction, the quantities of reactants/products are directly proportional.

$$\frac{y_1}{x_1} = \frac{y_2}{x_2}$$

Let $x_1 = 2$ moles of A and $y_1 = 5$ moles of B.

Then $x_2 =$ number of moles of A and $y_2 = 7$ moles of B such that:

$$\frac{5}{2} = \frac{7}{x_2}; x_2 = 2.8 \text{ moles of A.}$$

5. **The correct answer is D.** Since displacement = (speed)(time), $d = vt$, speed and time are inversely proportional for a constant displacement. Let $v_1 = x$ mph and $t_1 = 5$ hours; $v_2 = x - 15$ mph and $t_2 = 6\frac{2}{3}$ hours $= \frac{20}{3}$ hours. Since both displacements (the distance between the two towns) are the same, we have $v_1 t_1 = v_2 t_2$. Substitute and solve.

$$5x = 6\frac{2}{3}(x - 15)$$
$$5x = \frac{20}{3}(x - 15)$$
$$3(5x) = 3\left(\frac{20}{3}\right)(x - 15)$$
$$15x = 20(x - 15)$$
$$15x = 20x - 300$$
$$300 = 5x$$

$x = 60$ mph, speed from A to B

$x - 15 = 45$ mph is the speed on the return trip

6. **The correct answer is C.**

2016: Cost of A = \$2,500

2017: Cost of A $= \$2,500 + \frac{20}{100} \times \$2,500 = \$3,000$

2018: Cost of A $= \$3,000 + \frac{10}{100} \times \$3,000 = \$3,300$

Sale Price (2018) $= \$3,300 - \frac{30}{100} \times \$3,300 = \$2,310$

7. **The correct answer is A.**

$$\log_4 \frac{1}{16} = x$$
$$4^x = \frac{1}{16}$$
$$x = -2$$

8. **The correct answer is B.** $v = \frac{4}{3}\pi r^3$

    (Note: because $r = 3$ and $\pi = 3.14$)

    $$v = \frac{4}{3}\pi r^3$$
    $$= \frac{4}{3}(3.14)(3^3)$$
    $$= \frac{4}{3}(3.14)(27)$$
    $$= \frac{4(3.14)(27)}{3}$$
    $$= 4(3.14)(9)$$
    $$= 113.04\ c^3$$

Science

HUMANS AND THEIR ENVIRONMENT

Organisms must adapt to the environment in which they live in order to survive. Organisms may possess or develop certain traits that enable them to live or thrive in a specific environment. These adaptations, or changes, may originate in an individual and spread throughout a population, making the survival rate of that population greater. The changes that are most conducive to survival are preserved in the next generation and may eventually lead to a new species or subspecies.

Energy in Ecosystems

Humans—like other species—have a complex relationship with their environment. Organisms in any given environment can be divided into three categories: producers, consumers, and decomposers.

1. **Producers:** Producers are organisms that are able to use energy from the sun to make complex organic molecules from simple inorganic substances, such as nitrogen and phosphorous, in their environment. Plants are producers that carry out the process of photosynthesis. All other organisms rely upon producers as a food source, either directly or indirectly.

2. **Consumers:** Consumers are organisms that either eat producers or other consumers to obtain energy. Humans are classified as consumers. In particular, humans are omnivores because they eat both producers (plants) and consumers (animals).

3. **Decomposers:** Decomposers are organisms that rely upon nonliving organic matter as a source of energy and material for growth. When an organism dies, sheds, or excretes waste, it provides a source of food for decomposers.

587

Unit 11

Biomes

The kinds and amounts of life found in each environment are dependent upon abiotic (nonliving) factors such as temperature, moisture (rainfall), sunlight, soil conditions, and climate. Environments with different conditions form **biomes**. Each biome is characterized by its temperature and amount of precipitation. Some of the biomes in which humans and animals live in include deserts, grasslands, savannas, Mediterranean shrublands, tropical dry forests, tropical rainforests, temperate deciduous forests, northern coniferous forests (taiga), and tundra.

The more specific or localized type of environment where a species naturally lives and finds everything it needs for survival is its **habitat**. Biomes are much larger scale. All of the variety of life, including all species, genetic resources, habitats, and ecosystems, is the **biodiversity** of Earth.

Food Webs

Because only organisms that contain chlorophyll—such as plants—can make their own food, food webs exist in all environments so that all organisms can obtain energy. Energy from the sun is passed on to the producers in the environment. In turn, producers pass on the energy to primary consumers that eat the plants. A simple food chain continues to pass on energy as shown below.

producer → primary consumer → secondary consumer → tertiary consumer → decomposer

Each step in the flow of energy through an ecosystem is known as a **trophic level**. Because most consumers rely upon two or more types of organisms at different trophic levels for their energy, multiple food chains can overlap and intersect, forming a complex **food web**. Complex food webs are more stable than a simple food chain because the organisms are all dependent on more than one source of energy. The survival of humankind and other species is influenced by other species in the same environment. If one species struggles for survival or dies off, then due to the nature of a food web, many other species may also struggle for an energy source.

In addition to its position in the food web, every species has a **niche**. The niche is all of the biotic and abiotic features a species needs to survive in its environment. A simplified way to view a niche is as the particular role or job of a species in its ecosystem. For example, one tree might have several different types of birds in it. Some eat the fruit, some feed on insects near the trunk, others eat flying insects at the top branches, etc. Each bird has a niche in its environment—the tree where it lives.

When two organisms or individuals use each other's resources (e.g., both trying to occupy the same niche) and each has a negative effect on the other, they are said to be in **competition**. Many organisms have evolved defense mechanisms to give themselves an advantage against predators or competitors, such as thorns, warning colors, or toxins. Poison ivy, for example, is a widespread plant in North America that secretes an irritating clear compound from its leaves to avoid being eaten by herbivores.

Symbiosis

Symbiosis is a close, long-lasting physical relationship between two species. In a given environment, living organisms form an interrelated community in which many species live in close association with one another. There are three different categories of symbiotic relationships:

1. **Mutualism:** Mutualism is a relationship between organisms that is beneficial to both species. Most symbiotic relationships are mutualistic.

2. **Commensalism:** Commensalism is a relationship between organisms in which one organism benefits from the relationship and the other is not affected.

3. **Parasitism:** Parasitism is a relationship in which one organism (known as a parasite) lives in or on another organism called the host. The parasite derives energy and nourishment from the host, but the host is harmed by the relationship.

Conservation of Resources

The supply of natural resources in the environment is limited. Soil, wind, water, and fossil fuels are all examples of natural resources. A **renewable resource** can be formed or generated by natural processes and will not be used up, unless the resource is used more quickly than it can be renewed. A **nonrenewable resource** is not replaced by natural processes. In relation to the human time scale, fossil fuels and mountain ranges are examples of resources that are not renewable. Humans often practice conservation in order to limit use of natural resources, so that these resources are preserved for future generations.

Population growth can reduce the amount of resources available to individuals in an environment. A renewable resource can be formed, generated, or replenished by natural biological, chemical, mechanical, or physical processes. Population control may be another way to ensure adequate amounts of food, energy, and other resources upon which humans depend.

A population of an organism will, barring other factors, continue to grow until it reaches the maximum population an area can sustain, known as **carrying capacity**, or **K**. When a population undergoes **exponential growth**, the rate of growth continues to increase as the population grows. Consider bacteria; each one splits into two, than each of those splits into 2, leaving 4, which split into 8, and then into 16, etc. Before long the population is extremely large, and if it exceeds K, it will crash. Contrast that with **logistic growth**, where the growth rate levels off as the population size approaches K.

Human Interaction with the Environment

Organisms within an environment may cause changes to the environment because of exploitation or overpopulation. The changes made to the environment may be to the extent that the environment then becomes suitable for a different group or species. In this way, succession occurs as the environment continues to change under the influence of different species, in turn causing other species to adapt or invade the environment. **Succession** is a series of recognizable and predictable changes over time that act to restabilize a community. When an ecosystem or environment is disturbed in some manner, either through natural disaster or overuse of land, succession can occur, and a new species may become better adapted to an environment than the existing species.

As humans move around more easily through improved transportation networks, they often transport species of plants and animals from one continent to another. For example, gingko trees are native to China, but now exist widely across North America and other areas. These species would not be able to reach this new area without human interference. When these species start to reproduce rapidly in their new range and become an economic nuisance or a threat to local eco-systems, they are considered to be an **invasive species** (in water, they are **aquatic invasive species**). The species indigenous to an area are called **native species**. Invasive species can be plants or animals. Some examples of invasive species are zebra mussels in North American lakes and lionfish in the Caribbean.

In addition to protecting the environment, humans must also protect themselves from biological, chemical, physical, and radiological hazards. Vaccines are one way in which humans can protect themselves from certain biological hazards. Acquiring a natural immunity to viruses is another form of protection. Other biological hazards can be controlled through the use of antibiotics (to fight bacterial infections), antitoxins, and disinfectants. Sterilization, pasteurization, and refrigeration are all ways in which humans can keep their food supply safe from biological hazards.

Staying healthy and following safety precautions are ways in which humans can avoid biological, chemical, and physical hazards. Radiological hazards can be avoided by practicing safe laboratory and industrial methods.

Evolution

Since the beginning of life on Earth around 3.5 billion years ago, organisms have changed over time in a process called **evolution**. Some species permanently die out (**extinction**) while new species emerge (**speciation**).

The mechanism for evolution is **natural selection**. The theory of evolution by natural selection, proposed independently by Charles Darwin and Alfred Russell Wallace, operates on the following premises:

- not every individual will survive,
- there is variation in the number of offspring,
- some individuals will have traits (characteristics) that help them survive and reproduce better than others, and
- those changes are heritable.

Eventually, individuals with beneficial traits will become a completely new species. An individual that is more successful at passing its genes on to the next generation, usually by producing more surviving offspring, has higher **fitness**.

Evolution can occur quite rapidly, especially in a small population that is subjected to rapid environmental changes (e.g., a population of butterflies gets blown off course to an isolated island). Anything that reproduces quickly is also capable of rapid evolution. When bacteria are exposed to antibiotics, most die, but a few sometimes survive. Those survivors can quickly grow into a population of **antibiotic-resistant** bacteria, and may share the genes for resistance with other bacteria. A similar process occurs when insects or plants evolve resistance to pesticides or herbicides.

There have been several milestones in evolution and speciation throughout the history of life on Earth. Mass extinction events, where rapid changes lead to the widespread die-off of organisms, are often followed by a rapid increase in new species. The extinction of dinosaurs at the end of the Cretaceous Period, for example, was followed by an increase in the number of mammal and bird species. Geologic time can be divided into blocks based on which organisms dominated at the time.

The entire range is known as the **Geologic Time Scale**. The types of fossils discovered in a rock layer will help establish the age of those rocks. Deeper layers are often older, but not always.

As life evolved, the earth itself was changing as well. All the continents sit on top of massive plates that float on the earth's semisolid lower mantle (asthenosphere). Convection currents in the mantle cause small movements in these plates, forcing the continents to move. Around 175 million years ago, all the continents were together in one giant land mass called Pangaea until they began slowly moving apart. Certain creatures, like the now extinct Lystrosaurus, lived on Pangaea before the continents split, so today their fossils are found on different continents.

It is theorized that life on Earth almost certainly evolved in water, and life first diversified in the oceans. Small unicellular organisms evolved and diversified first, then multicellular organisms, followed by marine invertebrates and eventually fish. Plants first colonized the land, and the earliest insects, which often helped to pollinate plants, appeared on land shortly after. Insects are the most diverse group of animals on Earth; the largest order, the Coleoptera (beetles and weevils), currently consists of hundreds of thousands of species. Spiders (arachnids), distinguished by eight legs in four pairs, are important small predators and evolved shortly after insects.

Amphibians, which can breathe in both land and water but lay eggs in water, were the first terrestrial vertebrates. **Reptiles**, capable of laying eggs on land and breathing through lungs, came next (although only certain groups of reptiles have a diaghragm). Dinosaurs and primitive mammal-like reptiles, part of the **synapsid** group that eventually became **mammals**, followed the reptiles. Birds are direct descendants of theropod dinosaurs. Note that there was significant overlap between some of these groups; they didn't occur in a rigid sequence.

Evolution can be traced based on characteristics. These characteristics can help illustrate relationships between different organisms by tracing a characteristic back to a common ancestor, or the most basic animal from which two species are related. Humans belong to a lineage of mammals called primates, which includes monkeys and apes. Apes and humans share a common ancestor, so humans are more closely related to the great apes than to any other primate group. Different hominids, the group leading to humans, evolved after humans and apes split off from one another. Today, only our species, *Homo sapiens*, is still in existence; all other hominid species have gone extinct.

ASTRONOMY

Billions of years ago, a huge mass of gas and dust particles called a **nebula** began to collapse in upon itself. All the material coalesced at the center to form a star. The mass of the star forced the remaining material in the nebula to swirl around it. In a process called **accretion**, tiny particles grouped together to form slightly larger particles, which kept collecting into ever-larger pieces, eventually forming large bodies such as planets. There are many nebulas, some so huge that many stars are forming at once.

The **solar system** is comprised of a star and all the objects gravitationally connected to it, such as all the planets, their moons, and any other smaller bodies. The sun is the largest body in our solar system, and the radiation it produces reaches Earth in the form of light and heat. Light travels extremely fast (186,000 miles per second), but the sun is still 92.96 million miles from Earth. At that distance, light takes a little more than eight minutes to reach Earth from the sun. In other words, you see the sun as it appeared about eight minutes ago, not as it is right this second.

An orbit occurs any time a smaller body moves around a larger body. Earth, for example, orbits the sun, taking 365 days to do so; this movement defines one year. The orbit of Earth and the other planets is **elliptical**, not circular, meaning it is shaped much like a running track. **Aphelion** is the point of orbit where a planet is farthest from the star it orbits (the sun, in our solar system); the closest point is **perihelion**.

Any smaller object orbiting a larger one is called a **satellite**. The moon is a satellite of Earth, moving around the planet in an elliptical orbit. The moon is closest to Earth at **perigee**, and farthest away at **apogee**. Since any object with mass has gravity, and the moon is a large, nearby mass, the moon's gravity affects Earth and vice versa. Tides, for example, are partially a result from influence of the moon's gravity. As part of this gravitational interplay between the two bodies, the time it takes the moon to rotate on its axis is exactly the same as the time it takes to complete one rotation around Earth. Since these two motions are in sync, only one side of the moon faces Earth at any point in time, a condition known as **tidal locking**. The far side of the moon is sometimes called the dark side, but it is metaphorical. Sunlight hits all sides of the moon.

When the moon's position is just right, the moon is directly between Earth and the sun, casting a shadow over part of Earth in a partial or total **solar eclipse**. A more common event is a **lunar eclipse**, where the sun, moon, and Earth are aligned and the moon passes into Earth's shadow. During a lunar eclipse, the moon appears darkened or red.

Like the moon, Earth also spins around on its axis; one spin takes 24 hours, or one day. Different sides of Earth face the sun at different times, resulting in different time of day depending where on Earth an observer is located. While a side of Earth is facing away from the sun, it is night on that side.

Earth's axis tilts at a constant angle of 23.5 degrees, so the Northern Hemisphere points toward the sun at Earth's aphelion and away from the sun at Earth's perihelion. It is warmer where sunlight hits Earth's surface more directly. It's counterintuitive, but Earth is closer to the sun during the winter. Because of the earth's tilt, when the sun shines directly on Earth in one hemisphere, it shines indirectly on the other hemisphere. So winter in the Northern Hemisphere is summer in the Southern Hemisphere, and vice versa. In the tropics, the area between 23.5°N and 23.5°S, the angle of the sun is fairly constant, and seasons are less pronounced.

Planets

According to the International Astronomical Union, a **planet** is any object that orbits a star, has enough mass to be spherical, does not itself orbit another body (i.e., it isn't a moon) and clears its immediate orbit of debris or other materials. Starting closest from the sun and moving outward, the planets are Mercury, Venus, Earth, Mars, Jupiter, Saturn, Uranus, and Neptune. Mercury, Venus, Earth, and Mars are known as the **inner planets**, and Jupiter, Saturn, Uranus, and Neptune are called the **outer planets**. The farther a planet is from the sun, the longer it takes to complete one orbit. Mercury, the closest planet, takes 88 days to complete one orbit of the sun (one Mercury year). Distant Neptune takes 165 Earth years to circle the sun once.

Size is important to the nature of a planet. In decreasing order of size, the largest planet is Jupiter, followed by Saturn, Uranus, Neptune, Earth, Venus, Mars, and finally tiny Mercury. The outer planets are larger, are composed primarily of gas, and are often referred to as the **gas giants**. Larger objects have higher gravity, so these huge outer planets have higher gravity than the inner planets and attract more debris and other materials into their orbits. As a result, all of the gas giants have numerous moons. The smaller inner planets are rockier, since the high temperatures in the inner solar system at the time these planets formed vaporized any gas, leaving behind only rock and metals. Of the inner planets, only Earth and Mars have moons.

Some of the outer planets, especially Mars and Saturn, have some very large moons that may have primitive **atmospheres** (a layer of gas surrounding a planet or other body) of their own. Some moons, such as Enceladus (a moon of Saturn) or Europa (a moon of Jupiter) have huge oceans of liquid water underneath their surface. There are a few other gas giant moons, as well as the planet Mars, that might have liquid water; liquid water is considered the most likely place for life outside of Earth to evolve.

Other Objects in the Solar System

Between Mars and Jupiter is the asteroid belt, a band of numerous leftover pieces (asteroids) from the formation of the solar system. These irregular objects range in size from tiny to nearly planet-sized. Occasionally one of these objects hits the earth's atmosphere, becoming a **meteor**. This meteor becomes a **meteorite** if enough of the object survives to reach the surface of the earth. Most meteorites come from the asteroid belt. The oldest objects are **comets**, frozen chunks of ice and rock that have very elongated orbits and only pass close to the sun at long intervals. The distinctive tail of a comet occurs only as the comet approaches the sun, temporarily vaporizing some of the ice into an atmosphere called a **coma**. Solar radiation pushes the coma backwards to form the tail.

Beyond Neptune

Beyond Neptune lies the Kuiper Belt, a very distant and cold region extremely far beyond the sun. The Kuiper Belt is mostly composed of comets, asteroids, and other small icy bodies. Occasionally larger bodies are discovered, called **Trans-Neptunian Objects** or TNOs. Pluto is a TNO, classified as a **dwarf planet**. Dwarf planets are smaller than "true planets," are usually spherical or close to spherical, and they do not meet all three of the IAU definitions of a planet. In addition to Pluto, the Kuiper Belt dwarf planets are Makemake, Haumea, Eris, and several other objects awaiting official confirmation. Ceres is a dwarf planet in the asteroid belt.

Beyond the Solar System

Beyond the solar system, there are large, practically empty regions of space until the next star. The nearest star (other than the sun) to Earth is Alpha Centauri, 4.367 light years from Earth. A **light year** is the distance light can travel in a year, so it takes more than four years for light to reach Earth from the nearest other star. It might take light thousands or even millions of years to reach Earth from extremely distant stars. Since the light left these stars so long ago, observing these stars is like observing the distant past.

Many, if not most, of these stars are orbited by planets (called **exoplanets** since they are beyond the solar system). Initially, exoplanets were detected by searching for the slight wobble in a star when the gravity of a large planet pulled on the star; the Hubble Space Telescope was sometimes used for this purpose. The recently decommissioned Kepler telescope discovered thousands of exoplanets by detecting the slight decrease in the light from a distant star when a planet passed between it and the telescope, casting a shadow. This method allowed detection of much smaller planets, and many of these orbit stars at a distance that might support life.

Stars are classified based on their size and brightness. Stars burn hydrogen as fuel, and **main sequence** stars are still comfortably burning their hydrogen. The sun is a main sequence star. The most common star type is the **red dwarf**. Red dwarfs are smaller, low-mass main sequence stars. Most stars tend to expand as they age, like **red giant** stars. After a red giant uses up all its hydrogen fuel, it collapses into a **white dwarf** star. Some stars explode in a huge ejection of mass and particles called a **supernova**. A **black hole** is a region of space with such high gravity that no radiation, even light, can escape. Since light can't escape, black holes are invisible.

Two stars that circle around each other are called **binary stars**. Stars can also accumulate into groups connected by each other's gravity called **clusters**; huge accumulations of stars and star clusters are called **galaxies**. Galaxies can even bind together in galactic clusters. Our solar system is part of the Milky Way Galaxy.

Many of these distant objects can be studied with a variety of telescopes. Traditional **optical telescopes** simply magnify the visible light reflecting from distant objects, resulting in a direct image. **Radio telescopes** receive emissions from stars and distant objects in the radio end of the electromagnetic (EM) spectrum; many astronomical instruments work by detecting emissions outside the visible range. To avoid interference from the atmosphere, most telescopes are built in high altitude or very clear areas. The Kepler and the Hubble Space Telescopes are located in space, bypassing the atmosphere altogether. Within the solar system, unmanned probes have flown near or even landed on all the planets in the solar system, as well as Pluto, Ceres, asteroids, comets, and several moons. Some missions, like NASA's Mars Exploration Rovers, landed vehicles on other planets to collect more detailed images and geological data.

ENVIRONMENTAL SCIENCE

Like Earth, the environment is not static. The essential nutrients and materials necessary for life such as carbon, nitrogen, water, and other inorganic minerals are constantly shifting through different parts of the ecosystem and becoming available to different organisms at different stages. These movements of abiotic materials through the ecosystem are called **biogeochemical cycles**, and human activities have begun to have a major impact on the movement of materials. Take a moment to consider the human impact on the air we breathe.

The composition of air is approximately 78% nitrogen, 21% oxygen, 1% argon, 0.04% carbon dioxide (CO_2), and traces of other gases. In the **carbon cycle**, CO_2 is taken from the atmosphere by plants during photosynthesis. That carbon then becomes part of an animal's body when an animal eats a plant. Decomposition returns some carbon to the atmosphere as methane and other gases while a large portion of carbon is buried deep in the earth as **fossil fuels** or stored in the trunks of trees. Humans are disrupting the carbon cycle by burning fossil fuels and cutting trees, thereby returning carbon to the atmosphere faster.

In the case of the **nitrogen cycle**, atmospheric nitrogen is in a form that living organisms cannot use. Through a process called nitrogen fixation, which is carried out by certain plants, fungi, and lightning strikes, atmospheric nitrogen is transferred to soil, where it can be taken up in small amounts by plants. The mass production of fertilizer for farms speeds up the transfer of nitrogen from air to soil. Humans have altered all of the major geochemical cycles.

Human disruption to carbon cycling also has an effect on the climate of the planet. Beginning in the industrial revolution of the 1700s, when people began widespread burning of coal as fuel, excess carbon has returned to the atmosphere at an accelerated rate. The main gas is CO_2, but methane also contributes to an overall warming of the planet, called **Global Climate Change**. Heat from the sun is absorbed at the earth's surface, but a large proportion is also reflected back into space. CO_2, methane, and a few other gases trap some of the reflected solar heat in the atmosphere, rather than let it go harmlessly into space. This is called the **greenhouse effect**, and as these heat-trapping gases, called **greenhouse gases**, build up in the atmosphere, they trap more and more heat. The major sources of CO_2 emissions are transportation and power generation; agriculture and natural gas production are the major sources of methane.

Even though the global atmosphere is warming, the actual effect on the weather in any given place is variable. Some places may experience cooling or increases in snowfall, while others are measurably hotter. Deforestation speeds the process as the carbon stored in trees is released. Some excess CO_2 is absorbed in the ocean, slowly lowering the pH of the ocean in a process called **ocean acidification**. The ocean absorbs heat as well and, as the ocean warms, its chemistry and ecology can suffer.

Beyond fossil fuels, air pollution in general is responsible for a number of environmental and health problems. According the World Health Organization, in 2017, as many as 7 million people worldwide may have died as a direct or indirect result of air pollution.

There are two major types of air pollutants: **primary pollutants**, which are released directly into the air, and **secondary pollutants**, which result from reactions between primary pollutants and the atmosphere.

There are many different types of primary pollutants. Two major concerns are sulfur dioxides and nitrogen oxides (also products of fossil fuel combustion), both of which can react with moisture in the atmosphere to produce **acidic precipitation**, commonly known as **acid rain**. Acid rain can kill forests and aquatic life as well as damage buildings and historic structures. **Particulate matter**, such as ash from forest fires, are small particles that irritate the lungs. Ground-level ozone is a secondary pollutant that forms from a reaction between nitrogen oxides and sunlight. It can be irritating to breathe and dangerous for those with health conditions. Visible air pollution is smog, a combination of smoke and fog. Smog is made of a number of air pollutants in high enough concentrations to obscure the air. Smog is a greater risk when air cannot circulate freely, such as in cities surrounded by mountains. Atmospheric conditions called **inversions** can keep pollution at low altitudes, where it is dangerous to human health.

Fortunately, there are ways to reduce and even prevent air pollution. Coal, one of the most polluting fuel sources, is now used much less than somewhat cleaner natural gas. Technologies such as solar, wind, or hydropower can produce electricity with no emissions at all. However, even with zero emissions, steps need to be taken to avoid harm to wildlife such as obstruction of migratory pathways. **Catalytic converters**, devices using platinum and other metals to remove pollutants from vehicle tailpipes are now standard. Scrubbers and other technologies can limit harmful smokestack emissions. Sulfur emissions have been greatly reduced, and acid rain is much less of a problem now than a few decades ago.

Sometimes, world leaders are able to cooperate to reduce air pollution. In 1987, every country signed the Montreal Protocol. That agreement, later amended a few times, banned the production of chemicals like CFCs that depleted the **ozone layer**, a layer of ozone surrounding the earth that protects it from harmful cosmic radiation. Before 1987, ozone-depleting chemicals caused a large hole in the ozone layer, which is now closing. More recently, the Kyoto Protocols and Paris Accords are international agreements to reduce greenhouse gases, but their effectiveness has been limited as emissions continue to increase. Legislation such as the Clean Air Act has also been instrumental in reducing air pollution.

Water pollution is an issue as well. Water pollution can come from an identified source (e.g., a pipe) called a **point source** or it may have no particular point of origin (a **nonpoint source**). Examples of nonpoint source pollution are the runoff of oil and gasoline from a parking lot and rainfall or snowmelt moving over and through the ground. Some water pollution, such as PCPs, sink into the sediment at the bottom of water bodies, accumulating until the sediments are physically removed.

In general, water pollution is monitored around drinking water sources, but pollution occurs to plant and animal life as well. Pesticides and herbicides can flow from where they are sprayed into nearby water bodies, harming aquatic life. As an example, DDT was a pesticide initially used in World War II to control malaria, typhus, body lice, and bubonic plague. It was also used worldwide on a variety of food crops and in buildings for pest control. It was often sprayed near or in water where mosquitoes bred. Small fish and other organisms would eat mosquitos that had DDT in their systems. These small fish and organisms would in turn be eaten by larger fish, and the amount of DDT in an organism's system increased on up the food chain. This process is called **bioaccumulation**, and it can occur with any pollutant taken in by small animals. Eventually, predatory birds such as bald eagles had so much DDT in their system that their eggs' shells became too thin, killing their chicks. The population of eagles and other birds plummeted until DDT was banned by the U.S. Environmental Protection Agency in 1972.

Another water pollution problem that affects plant and aquatic life is **eutrophication**. Excess nitrogen and phosphorus used in fertilizers is not absorbed by plants and can run into the water, causing algae and small plants to bloom. These plants clog the water and use up the oxygen in the water as they decompose, killing aquatic life from lack of oxygen. Eutrophication can be prevented by using less fertilizer. Permeable surfaces like grass that can absorb fertilizer runoff before it hits the water can also reduce eutrophication. Plantings near the edges of ponds and streams called **buffers** can absorb fertilizer runoff before it enters the water. Too much concrete or other impermeable surfaces that do not allow water to drain encourage pollutants to run directly into the water.

The last type of pollution is **solid waste**, such as municipal waste, food waste, or construction debris. This waste is stored in designated dumping spaces called landfills, although a lot of it winds up in the ocean. Once buried in a landfill, even waste such as paper, which easily decomposes under normal circumstances, can take decades to break down. Decomposition in landfills can produce the greenhouse gas methane, although some areas are capturing this gas to use as fuel in a process called waste to energy (WtE). Plastics are a huge problem because the material is produced using fossil fuels and does not fully decompose. Plastic only breaks into tiny pieces called **microplastics**. Single-use plastics such as bottles or packaging fill up landfills and often wind up in the ocean where they can harm aquatic life.

The best way to decrease solid waste is to **reduce** the amount of waste produced by limiting consumption, making smaller packages, etc. **Reuse**, or using objects like glass bottles repeatedly, instead of relying on disposable items is also a good way to reduce solid waste. A third way to reduce waste is to **recycle**, which involves converting waste materials into new materials. Recycling is not as efficient as reducing or reusing as it takes more energy and some material is still lost. Together, reducing, reusing, and recycling are sometimes called the **three Rs**. In addition, a good way to prevent organic waste from entering landfills is to **compost**, which is collecting and storing organic material so it can decay into soil.

Finally, a very important issue is land use. Improper use of land can result in erosion, or the gradual destruction of land. Overgrazing, or grazing too many livestock in one place, can destroy all the vegetation that holds the soil in place, rendering the land unusable. **Deforestation** or over-development, especially on steep slopes, also destabilizes the soil and can result in erosion or even destructive landslides. Preserving forests on slopes and shorelines can help reduce erosion. Farming practices can also contribute to destruction of farmland. Too much plowing exposes soil to wind and rain, causing topsoil loss. No-till agriculture, which minimizes plowing time, reduces the exposure and loss of soil. Cover crops and crop rotation, or planting different crops in different seasons and years, can help prevent the loss of soil and soil nutrients while reducing the need for fertilizer. Poor agricultural practices, especially coupled with climate change, fire, or drought, can cause **desertification**, or the conversion of fertile land into desert.

SCIENCE ANSWER SHEET

Test 1: General Science

1. Ⓐ Ⓑ Ⓒ Ⓓ   11. Ⓐ Ⓑ Ⓒ Ⓓ   21. Ⓐ Ⓑ Ⓒ Ⓓ   31. Ⓐ Ⓑ Ⓒ Ⓓ   41. Ⓐ Ⓑ Ⓒ Ⓓ
2. Ⓐ Ⓑ Ⓒ Ⓓ   12. Ⓐ Ⓑ Ⓒ Ⓓ   22. Ⓐ Ⓑ Ⓒ Ⓓ   32. Ⓐ Ⓑ Ⓒ Ⓓ   42. Ⓐ Ⓑ Ⓒ Ⓓ
3. Ⓐ Ⓑ Ⓒ Ⓓ   13. Ⓐ Ⓑ Ⓒ Ⓓ   23. Ⓐ Ⓑ Ⓒ Ⓓ   33. Ⓐ Ⓑ Ⓒ Ⓓ   43. Ⓐ Ⓑ Ⓒ Ⓓ
4. Ⓐ Ⓑ Ⓒ Ⓓ   14. Ⓐ Ⓑ Ⓒ Ⓓ   24. Ⓐ Ⓑ Ⓒ Ⓓ   34. Ⓐ Ⓑ Ⓒ Ⓓ   44. Ⓐ Ⓑ Ⓒ Ⓓ
5. Ⓐ Ⓑ Ⓒ Ⓓ   15. Ⓐ Ⓑ Ⓒ Ⓓ   25. Ⓐ Ⓑ Ⓒ Ⓓ   35. Ⓐ Ⓑ Ⓒ Ⓓ   45. Ⓐ Ⓑ Ⓒ Ⓓ
6. Ⓐ Ⓑ Ⓒ Ⓓ   16. Ⓐ Ⓑ Ⓒ Ⓓ   26. Ⓐ Ⓑ Ⓒ Ⓓ   36. Ⓐ Ⓑ Ⓒ Ⓓ   46. Ⓐ Ⓑ Ⓒ Ⓓ
7. Ⓐ Ⓑ Ⓒ Ⓓ   17. Ⓐ Ⓑ Ⓒ Ⓓ   27. Ⓐ Ⓑ Ⓒ Ⓓ   37. Ⓐ Ⓑ Ⓒ Ⓓ   47. Ⓐ Ⓑ Ⓒ Ⓓ
8. Ⓐ Ⓑ Ⓒ Ⓓ   18. Ⓐ Ⓑ Ⓒ Ⓓ   28. Ⓐ Ⓑ Ⓒ Ⓓ   38. Ⓐ Ⓑ Ⓒ Ⓓ   48. Ⓐ Ⓑ Ⓒ Ⓓ
9. Ⓐ Ⓑ Ⓒ Ⓓ   19. Ⓐ Ⓑ Ⓒ Ⓓ   29. Ⓐ Ⓑ Ⓒ Ⓓ   39. Ⓐ Ⓑ Ⓒ Ⓓ   49. Ⓐ Ⓑ Ⓒ Ⓓ
10. Ⓐ Ⓑ Ⓒ Ⓓ   20. Ⓐ Ⓑ Ⓒ Ⓓ   30. Ⓐ Ⓑ Ⓒ Ⓓ   40. Ⓐ Ⓑ Ⓒ Ⓓ   50. Ⓐ Ⓑ Ⓒ Ⓓ

answer sheet

TEST 1: GENERAL SCIENCE

50 Questions • 45 Minutes

> **Directions:** For each of the following items, select the choice that best answers the question or completes the statement. Fill in the corresponding space on your answer sheet.

1. A tree native to China and NOT to the United States is the
   A. silvery maple.
   B. chestnut.
   C. gingko.
   D. tulip tree.

2. Mammals are believed to have evolved directly from
   A. fish.
   B. amphibians.
   C. reptiles.
   D. birds.

3. In a series of rock layers arranged one on top of another, fossils found in the lowest layers are
   A. completely different from fossils found in the upper layers.
   B. older than the fossils found in the upper layers.
   C. of organisms simpler than the organisms fossilized in the upper layers.
   D. of organisms more complex than the organisms fossilized in the upper layers.

4. Which of the following groups, in primate phylogeny, includes the primate most closely related to humans?
   A. Old World monkeys
   B. Great apes
   C. New World monkeys
   D. Lemurs

5. Stanley Miller obtained evidence supporting the possibility of spontaneous generation by achieving laboratory synthesis of
   A. amino acids.
   B. DNA.
   C. RNA.
   D. glucose.

6. The part of a compound light microscope that focuses light before it passes through the specimen is the
   A. objective.
   B. micrometer.
   C. ocular.
   D. condenser.

7. The Hubble telescope is able to produce images of very distant celestial objects more clearly than other telescopes because
   A. its reflector is able to concentrate more light on the lens.
   B. its images are enhanced by computer.
   C. its view is not obstructed by atmosphere.
   D. it has a larger lens.

8. We can see only one side of the moon because the
   A. earth rotates on its own axis.
   B. moon makes one rotation as it makes one revolution around the earth.
   C. moon has no refractive atmosphere.
   D. sun does not shine on the moon's unseen side.

9. Which of the following is NOT an essential biotic element of all ecosystems?
   A. Producers
   B. Water
   C. Consumers
   D. Decomposers

10. The deadly property of carbon monoxide, if inhaled, is due to its
    A. high affinity for O_2.
    B. low affinity for hemoglobin.
    C. high affinity for hemoglobin.
    D. conversion to cyanide gas.

11. Of the following, vitamin B_{12} is most useful in combating
    A. pernicious anemia.
    B. night blindness.
    C. rickets.
    D. goiter.

12. Continental drift is caused by
    A. fluctuations in the earth's magnetic field.
    B. tectonic movement of floating plates.
    C. fragmentation of larger land masses into smaller ones.
    D. the Coriolis force generated by the rotation of the earth.

13. An emission device in modern cars that uses platinum beads to oxidize carbon monoxide and hydrocarbons to carbon dioxide and water is the
    A. carburetor.
    B. catalytic converter.
    C. PCV valve.
    D. air filter.

14. Organisms that live on dead organic matter are called
    A. parasites.
    B. carnivorous.
    C. autotrophs.
    D. saprophytes.

15. The relation between termites and their intestinal protozoa is an example of
    A. trophism.
    B. parasitism.
    C. mutualism.
    D. commensalism.

16. Air-polluting sulfur dioxide (SO_2) results primarily from
    A. natural gas furnaces.
    B. leaded gasoline.
    C. paper waste.
    D. coal-burning power plants.

17. The "dark" side of the moon refers to the
    A. craters, into which no sunlight has ever reached.
    B. south pole of the moon's axis.
    C. hemisphere that has never reflected the sun's rays on the earth.
    D. moon itself in the early phases of the month.

18. Of the following, the one NOT characteristic of poison ivy is
    A. milky juice.
    B. shiny leaves.
    C. three-leaflet clusters.
    D. white berries.

Questions 19 and 20 refer to the following diagram.

Exponential growth (I):

$\Delta N/\Delta t = r_N$–change in number per change in time

Logistic growth (II):

$\Delta N/\Delta t = r_N(k- N/K)$

r = intrinsic rate of increase

K = carrying capacity of the environment

19. Choose the correct statement expressed by curve II, as N approaches K.

    A. r approaches maximum.
    B. K expands upward.
    C. $\Delta N/\Delta t$ approaches zero.
    D. Resources remain unlimited.

20. Choose the correct statement about curve I.

    A. It assumes unlimited resources.
    B. It expresses limited growth.
    C. It expresses a K value.
    D. It assumes limited resources.

21. Of the following, the one present in greatest amounts in dry air is

    A. carbon dioxide.
    B. oxygen.
    C. water vapor.
    D. nitrogen.

Questions 22 and 23 refer to the following ecological pyramid of biomass and energy.

22. Select the correct population changes resulting from hunters reducing the hawk population.
    A. Grasshoppers increase → Field mice decrease → Sunflowers increase
    B. Field mice increase → Grasshoppers increase → Sunflowers increase
    C. Field mice increase → Grasshoppers decrease → Sunflowers increase
    D. Sunflowers decrease → Grasshoppers decrease → Field mice decrease

23. The second law of thermodynamics would suggest that the most energy-efficient feeding pattern would be if
    A. field mice ate grasshoppers.
    B. hawks ate sunflowers.
    C. hawks ate field mice.
    D. grasshoppers ate field mice.

24. The most important of the greenhouse gases contributing to global warming and altering the marine carbon cycle is
    A. SO_2.
    B. CO.
    C. NH_3.
    D. CO_2.

25. Rank the planets in order of lowest to highest gravity.
    A. Mars, Earth, Neptune, Saturn
    B. Saturn, Neptune, Earth, Mars
    C. Earth, Mars, Saturn, Neptune
    D. Saturn, Neptune, Mars, Earth

26. The normal height of a mercury barometer at sea level is
    A. 15 inches.
    B. 30 inches.
    C. 32 feet.
    D. 34 feet.

27. One of the necessary parameters for supporting the theory of evolution by natural selection is the age of the earth, which is, by geographical indices, approximately (in years)
    A. 1 billion.
    B. 400 million.
    C. 4.5 billion.
    D. 100 million.

28. Of the following, the statement that best describes a "high" on a weather map is that the air
    A. extends farther up than normal.
    B. pressure is greater than normal.
    C. temperature is higher than normal.
    D. moves faster than normal.

29. An owl nesting in a small hole in a tree is an example of which ecological relationship?
    A. Mutualism
    B. Commensalism
    C. Competition
    D. Predation

30. Which international agreement resulted in a ban on CFCs and other ozone-depleting chemicals?
    A. The Kyoto Protocol
    B. The Montreal Protocol
    C. The Paris Accords
    D. The Clean Air Act

31. The development of insecticide-resistant insects is based on
    A. inheritance of acquired characteristics.
    B. gradualism.
    C. natural selection.
    D. sexual selection.

32. Which of the following insects belongs to the order of insects containing the largest number of species?
    A. Housefly
    B. Flour beetle
    C. Grasshopper
    D. Cockroach

33. Which of the following is a harmful impact of plastic pollution?
    A. Plastics break into small pieces but don't decompose.
    B. Plastics can harm marine life.
    C. Plastics require fossil fuels to produce.
    D. All of the above.

34. Black holes are notoriously difficult to detect. However, there are indirect ways to view them. For one, the gravity of a black hole influences stars and other objects nearby. Destruction of matter in a black hole also produces a lot of X-rays. Which instrument would be best suited for detecting a black hole?
    A. Optical Telescope
    B. Kepler Telescope
    C. Radio telescope
    D. Hubble Telescope

35. One-celled eukaryotes belong to the group of living things known as
    A. protistans.
    B. poriferans.
    C. annelids.
    D. arthropods.

36. Spiders can be distinguished from insects because spiders have
    A. hard outer coverings.
    B. large abdomens.
    C. four pairs of legs.
    D. biting mouth parts.

37. The greenhouse effect is believed to be primarily due to
    A. pesticide accumulation in soil.
    B. carbon dioxide increase in the atmosphere.
    C. oxygen increase in the atmosphere.
    D. pesticide increase in the water.

38. Which astronomical phenomenon is also called a "stellar nursery?"
    A. Accretion Disk
    B. Quasar
    C. Binary Star
    D. Nebula

39. What is the ultimate source for all energy in the ecosystem?
    A. The sun
    B. Producers
    C. Decomposers
    D. Consumers

40. Eutrophication is ultimately a result of which problem?
    A. Point source pollution
    B. Nonpoint source pollution
    C. Nitrogen oxide
    D. Too much permeable surface

41. In some species of birds, if resources are scarce, when a baby bird grows up, before moving away, the adult offspring lives with its parents and helps raise its baby siblings for a season. This behavior likely increases the offspring's _____ since it shares 50% of its _____ with its siblings.
    - A. evolution, speciation
    - B. DNA, fitness
    - C. fitness, DNA
    - D. fitness, resistance

42. If the toxicity of a pesticide or an herbicide is in the range that a few drops could be fatal, the label should read
    - A. Warning.
    - B. Caution.
    - C. Avoid.
    - D. Danger.

43. The time it takes for light from the sun to reach the earth is approximately
    - A. four years.
    - B. four months.
    - C. eight minutes.
    - D. sixteen years.

44. The time it takes for the earth to rotate 45 degrees is
    - A. one hour.
    - B. three hours.
    - C. four hours.
    - D. ten hours.

45. The major cause for seasonal changes in temperature and light on the earth is
    - A. distance of the earth from the sun.
    - B. a 23.5° inclination of the earth on its axis.
    - C. alignment between the earth, sun, and moon.
    - D. rotation of the earth on its axis.

46. Of the following planets, the one that has the largest number of satellites is
    - A. Jupiter.
    - B. Mercury.
    - C. Neptune.
    - D. Earth.

47. The deserts of the earth generally occur on the _____ side of the continents.
    - A. west
    - B. north
    - C. east
    - D. south

48. Atmospheric moisture (H_2O) combines with oxides of carbon, nitrogen, and sulfur (CO_2, NO_3, and SO_2) to produce
    - A. alkaline precipitation.
    - B. acid rain.
    - C. alcohol.
    - D. None of the above

49. The chlorinated hydrocarbon pesticide DDT was banned from use in the United States during the 1970s because it
    - A. has high affinity for milk and adipose tissues.
    - B. is deleterious to eggs of several species of birds.
    - C. is a biological concentration in ecosystem food chains.
    - D. All of the above

50. Passive immunity to diphtheria may be achieved by taking an injection of a(n)

- **A.** vaccine.
- **B.** toxin.
- **C.** toxoid.
- **D.** antitoxin.

STOP

IF YOU FINISH BEFORE TIME IS CALLED, YOU MAY CHECK YOUR WORK ON THIS SECTION ONLY. DO NOT TURN TO ANY OTHER SECTION IN THE TEST.

ANSWER KEY AND EXPLANATIONS

Test 1: General Science

1. C	11. A	21. D	31. C	41. C
2. C	12. B	22. C	32. B	42. D
3. B	13. B	23. B	33. D	43. C
4. B	14. D	24. D	34. D	44. B
5. A	15. C	25. A	35. A	45. B
6. D	16. D	26. B	36. C	46. A
7. C	17. C	27. C	37. B	47. A
8. B	18. A	28. B	38. D	48. B
9. B	19. C	29. B	39. A	49. D
10. C	20. A	30. B	40. B	50. D

1. **The correct answer is C.** The gingko is native to the Orient but has been imported into the United States and now is in widespread use as an ornamental tree.

2. **The correct answer is C.** Evidence indicates that a primitive reptile known as a therapsid is the ancestor of mammals. These early reptiles of the Triassic period had acquired some mammalian characteristics, such as warm-bloodedness, hair, and mammary glands. They are sometimes referred to as "premammals."

3. **The correct answer is B.** Fossils found in the lowest rock layers are the oldest because these layers were deposited before the ones above. Fossils in upper layers are not always different from the lower layers. Some species have very long histories and leave fossils in more than one layer. Conversely, fossils in upper layers are never completely the same as fossils in lower layers. At least some species of organisms whose fossils lie in lower layers would have become extinct and been replaced by fossils of different organisms by the time upper layers were deposited. Older organisms were not always simpler than modern organisms and were certainly not more complex.

4. **The correct answer is B.** Fossil evidence indicates that there was an isolation of apelike forms, including hominids (humanlike creatures), during the Pliocene period. These seemingly originated from the same "branch" of the evolutionary "tree." Lemurs, New World monkeys, and Old World monkeys apparently evolved earlier.

5. **The correct answer is A.** It was found that if a mixture of methane, ammonia, and hydrogen is continuously bombarded with spark discharges as an energy source, amino acids are formed. If inorganic phosphate is added to the mixture, ATP, the energy compound of cells, is formed also. The earth, at its very early age, had the inorganic substances, and the sun could have provided the energy source.

6. **The correct answer is D.** The condenser is an adjustable lens that focuses light before it reaches the specimen. This enhances the sharpness of the image produced by the magnifying lenses of the microscope. The objective and the ocular are the lenses used to create a magnified image of the light after it has passed through the specimen. A micrometer is a device used to measure objects viewed through the microscope.

7. **The correct answer is C.** The Hubble telescope is able to produce sharper images of objects than other telescopes because it is in orbit around Earth and does not have its view obstructed by atmosphere. Images seen through telescopes on Earth's surface are always obscured to some degree by the scattering of light as it passes through the atmosphere and by the passage of air currents created by heating of the atmosphere.

8. **The correct answer is B.** As the moon revolves around the earth, it rotates on its axis so that only one side of the moon faces the earth. Because the moon makes one rotation with one revolution around the earth, one side of the moon never faces the earth.

9. **The correct answer is B.** In all ecosystems, producers (green plants or algae) convert CO_2 and H_2O into sugars, which serve as food for consumers (animals) whose bodies are ultimately degraded by decomposers (bacteria and fungi). Water, although vital, is an inorganic substance.

10. **The correct answer is C.** Carbon monoxide has a greater affinity than oxygen for hemoglobin. This binding blocks hemoglobin from binding oxygen for transport to body cells for metabolic needs.

11. **The correct answer is A.** A deficiency of vitamin B_{12} leads to pernicious anemia, a condition in which red blood cells fail to mature. Vitamin B_{12} is essential for the formation of red blood cells.

12. **The correct answer is B.** The continents are parts of massive plates that float on top of the lower mantle. Convection in the currents causes these plates to move slightly every year, over time drifting large distances. Fluctuations in Earth's magnetic field and the Coriolis force are real events, but neither has any effect on continental drift. Fragmentation of large landmasses to make smaller ones has sometimes been a part of continental drift, but it qualifies as a result rather than a cause.

13. **The correct answer is B.** The catalytic converter uses platinum to convert carbon monoxide and hydrocarbons to carbon dioxide and water, resulting in reduced air pollution.

14. **The correct answer is D.** Some bacteria and fungi feed on dead organic matter to get their energy (*saphros* means rotten, putrid).

15. **The correct answer is C.** Any relationship between two individual species is symbiosis. The word *symbiosis* means "life together." There are several kinds of symbiotic relationships, including commensalism, parasitism, and mutualism. A mutualistic relationship is one in which strong bonds exist between the two species, and each member benefits from the relationship. This kind of symbiotic relationship exists between termites and the protozoans (flagellates) of their intestinal tract. There is evidence that some bacteria in the termite's intestinal tract also play a role in the relationship. The flagellates and bacteria digest the cellulose that the termites consume.

16. **The correct answer is D.** Coal is the major source of SO_2 because gasoline, natural gas, and paper waste contain only small amounts of sulfur.

17. **The correct answer is C.** The moon shines by the reflected light of the sun. Because the moon rotates on its axis as it revolves around the earth, one side of the moon never faces the earth. This side, the dark side of the moon, can never reflect the sun's light onto the earth.

18. **The correct answer is A.** Poison ivy has a clear juice rather than a milky sap. Three-leaflet clusters, white berries, and shiny leaves are all characteristic of poison ivy.

19. **The correct answer is C.** With limited resources, as the numbers of individuals produced approach the environmental capacity, reproduction declines and eventually stops.

20. **The correct answer is A.** The assumption of unlimited resources suggests the absence of a K value.

21. **The correct answer is D.** Air is a mixture of gases; dry air consists of about 78% nitrogen and 21% oxygen. The remaining 1% consists of other gases, including carbon dioxide.

22. **The correct answer is C.** Reduction in the hawk population reduced the pressure on the mouse population, which increased and thus suppressed the grasshopper numbers, which allowed the sunflower population to increase.

23. **The correct answer is B.** The highest concentration of energy in an ecological pyramid is at the base (producers). Energy is lost as heat at the successive trophic levels.

24. **The correct answer is D.** Carbon dioxide (CO_2) comprises only approximately 0.04% of the earth's atmospheric gases. When this percentage increases, it prevents sun rays that strike the earth from radiating back into space. This produces warming of the atmosphere and the earth's surface, causing the greenhouse effect.

25. **The correct answer is A.** The larger the planet, the larger its mass and the stronger gravity it has. Of the planets listed, Mars is the smallest, followed by Earth, then Neptune, and finally Saturn, the second most massive planet in the solar system.

26. **The correct answer is B.** Air pressure at sea level is 14.7 pounds/square inch. This pressure, at 0°C, supports a barometer mercury column of 76 centimeters, or 30 inches. This is equivalent to 1 atmosphere of pressure.

27. **The correct answer is C.** Radioactive elements suggest that the earth is 4.5 billion years old.

28. **The correct answer is B.** A high indicates an area of high air pressure, while a low indicates an area of low air pressure. Weather can be predicted by measuring differences between pressures. A high usually indicates fair weather, whereas low pressure areas indicate storms and bad weather.

29. **The correct answer is B.** The owl is living in and deriving an advantage (a home) from the tree, but is not harming the tree in any way; nor is owl being harmed by the tree. These kinds of neutral interactions are called commensalism. Neither the owl nor the tree are harming each other, so choices C and D are incorrect. Only the owl is benefiting, so it cannot be a mutually beneficial arrangement (choice A).

30. **The correct answer is B.** The Montreal Protocol, first signed in 1987, enacted a rapid phase-out of ozone depleting chemicals, especially CFCs. The Kyoto Protocol and the Paris Accords are both agreements intended to limit climate change from greenhouse gas emissions. The Clean Air Act made a huge difference in limiting air pollution in general but did not specifically address CFCs.

31. **The correct answer is C.** Insecticide resistance is acquired and developed through natural selection. Some insects are not affected by the chemical; they are "resistant."

32. **The correct answer is B.** The flour beetle belongs to the Order Coleoptera, which, with approximately 350,000 described species, is the largest order of insects. The

housefly belongs to the Order Diptera, containing approximately 120,000 described species. The grasshopper belongs to the Order Orthoptera, containing approximately 20,000 species. The cockroach belongs to the Order Blattaria, containing only 4,000 species.

33. **The correct answer is D.** Plastics do not ever fully decompose, and they are light enough that they often wind up in the ocean where they can harm marine life. Plastics are also made out of fossil fuels, so they contribute to greenhouse gas emissions both during production and when they break apart.

34. **The correct answer is D.** The Hubble telescope can do a variety of things, but if it can detect the gravitational anomaly caused by a planet interacting with a star, it can detect the far larger disturbances caused by a black hole. An optical telescope is useless, since black holes emit no light. Radio telescopes detect radio waves, on the opposite end of the EM spectrum from X-rays. An X-ray telescope would be more suitable to detect X-ray emissions. The Kepler telescope is specifically designed to look for distant planets, not black holes.

35. **The correct answer is A.** Unicellular eukaryotes, including colonial forms, belong to the Kingdom Protista. The other organisms belong to phyla in the Kingdom Animalia, of which all members are multicellular. Phylum Annelida includes segmented worms, such as the earthworm. Phylum Porifera includes sponges. Phylum Arthropoda includes animals such as insects, spiders, crabs, crayfish, and millipedes that have a chitinous exoskeleton and jointed appendages.

36. **The correct answer is C.** Spiders are characterized by a two-part body and four pairs of legs, while insects have a three-part body and three pairs of legs.

37. **The correct answer is B.** The CO_2 from the burning of fossil fuels prevents heat from escaping the earth's surface, thus raising temperatures.

38. **The correct answer is D.** Stars are formed in nebulae, which are masses of gas and dust. *Stellar* is the word for star, and a nursery is a place where young things are nurtured. Quasars and binary stars are types of stars, while an accretion disk is a phase early in the development of a star or planet.

39. **The correct answer is A.** Except for certain unusual deep sea ecosystems based on chemicals, all energy available to life on earth starts with the sun. The producers (choice B) convert that energy into a useable form, but they don't create it in the first place. Decomposers (choice C) break down dead organic material into component nutrients, again making energy available but not creating it. Consumers (choice D) only intake energy, they take no part in making it available until they themselves are consumed.

40. **The correct answer is B.** Eutrophication is a result of runoff containing nitrogen and phosphorus, which may come from farms, lawns, parks, or any other area where fertilizers are used. There is no defined point of origin like a pipe, which would make it the result of point source pollution. Eutrophication is the result of pure nitrogen; nitrogen oxide, an air pollutant, is a cause of acid rain and can kill plants rather than stimulate excess growth. Permeable sources tend to reduce eutrophication as they allow the capture of runoff in the ground before it enters the water.

41. **The correct answer is C.** Anything that helps an individual carry its genetic

material into the next generation increases that individual's fitness. DNA is genetic material, and siblings share 50% of their DNA. Helping 50% of its DNA reach maturity will still benefit an individual's fitness, especially if direct reproduction might be difficult due to scarce resources. When conditions improve, these birds will make their own nest and lay their own eggs. Evolution does not apply to individuals (choice A). Choice B does not work since DNA does not increase and fitness is an individual quality. In choice D, resistance is the ability to withstand a potential threat, which does not apply in this instance.

42. **The correct answer is D.** The federal government requires that all pesticides have a label with a signal word. The pesticide will read DANGER (highly toxic) if only a few drops could be fatal.

43. **The correct answer is C.** Light travels at a speed of about 186,000 miles per second; the sun is approximately 93,000,000 miles from Earth. Thus, calculations (93,000,000 miles divided by 186,000 miles per second) show that it takes about 500 seconds, or a bit more than eight minutes, for light from the sun to reach Earth.

44. **The correct answer is B.** The earth makes one complete rotation on its axis (360 degrees) in 24 hours; 45 degrees is one-eighth of 360 degrees. Therefore, it would take one-eighth of 24 hours, or three hours, for the earth to rotate 45 degrees.

45. **The correct answer is B.** The 23.5° inclination of the earth on its axis causes it to tilt toward and away from the sun as it revolves around the sun.

46. **The correct answer is A.** As of 2018, Jupiter has 53 named moons and 16 more that have been discovered but not given official status or names, which is the most in the solar system.

47. **The correct answer is A.** Deserts of the earth generally occur on the west side of continents, as influenced by prevailing westerly winds and nearby mountains. As the earth rotates from west to east, winds that approach continents from the west side lose moisture in ascending mountains and evaporate moisture from the opposite side—resulting in dry regions known as deserts.

48. **The correct answer is B.** Atmospheric moisture combines with oxides of carbon, nitrogen, and sulfur to produce acid rain, as illustrated by the following reactions:

$$H_2O + CO_2 \rightarrow H_2CO_3$$
$$H_2O + 2NO_2 \rightarrow 2HNO_3$$
$$H_2O + SO_2 \rightarrow H_2SO_3$$

49. **The correct answer is D.** The pesticide DDT was banned from the United States during the 1970s because research studies had shown it to be present in milk, fatty tissues, and the eggs of eagles and other birds. It was also proven to be a biological concentration—building up to higher concentration in succeeding levels of food chains.

50. **The correct answer is D.** Passive immunity involves administering an antibody (an antitoxin, in the case of diphtheria) to the patient. This immunity is temporary, since the patient's body is not stimulated to form antibodies, as it would be if an antigen were administered. The temporary immunity is considered passive because the body is not active in forming antibodies. If an antigen stimulates the body to form its own antibodies against it, the immunity produced is active. Passive immunity provides temporary protection to one who has been exposed to a disease, or a method of treatment until the patient's body has started producing its own antibodies if the disease has been contracted. Active immunity imparts more lasting protection.

Reading Comprehension

OVERVIEW

Unit 12

READING COMPREHENSION ANSWER SHEET

Test 1

1. Ⓐ Ⓑ Ⓒ Ⓓ   2. Ⓐ Ⓑ Ⓒ Ⓓ   3. Ⓐ Ⓑ Ⓒ Ⓓ   4. Ⓐ Ⓑ Ⓒ Ⓓ

Test 2

1. Ⓐ Ⓑ Ⓒ Ⓓ   2. Ⓐ Ⓑ Ⓒ Ⓓ   3. Ⓐ Ⓑ Ⓒ Ⓓ   4. Ⓐ Ⓑ Ⓒ Ⓓ

Test 3

1. Ⓐ Ⓑ Ⓒ Ⓓ   3. Ⓐ Ⓑ Ⓒ Ⓓ   5. Ⓐ Ⓑ Ⓒ Ⓓ   7. Ⓐ Ⓑ Ⓒ Ⓓ   8. Ⓐ Ⓑ Ⓒ Ⓓ

2. Ⓐ Ⓑ Ⓒ Ⓓ   4. Ⓐ Ⓑ Ⓒ Ⓓ   6. Ⓐ Ⓑ Ⓒ Ⓓ

Test 4

1. Ⓐ Ⓑ Ⓒ Ⓓ   3. Ⓐ Ⓑ Ⓒ Ⓓ   5. Ⓐ Ⓑ Ⓒ Ⓓ   7. Ⓐ Ⓑ Ⓒ Ⓓ   8. Ⓐ Ⓑ Ⓒ Ⓓ

2. Ⓐ Ⓑ Ⓒ Ⓓ   4. Ⓐ Ⓑ Ⓒ Ⓓ   6. Ⓐ Ⓑ Ⓒ Ⓓ

answer sheet

TEST 1

4 Questions • 9 Minutes

> **Directions:** Carefully read the following passage and then answer the accompanying questions, basing your answers on what is stated or implied in the passage. When you have decided which choice is best, fill in the corresponding space on your answer sheet. There is only one best answer for each question.

Communicable means "capable of being transmitted or passed through a medium." A communicable disease is an infection that may be transmitted directly or indirectly from one individual to another. The primary objective of programs for the prevention and control of communicable diseases is to prevent the transmission or spread of the disease by eliminating conditions supportive to infection. Since communicable diseases are caused by microorganisms, the process of infection can be avoided or reversed by eliminating microbial sources, destroying the infectious organisms, creating conditions unfavorable to the growth of infectious microorganisms, and building up the body's defenses against microbial attack.

Any measure designed to control or protect anyone from the hazards of the infectious microbes in the environment is called a barrier. The use of barriers is based upon three factors: time, distance, and shielding. "Time" refers to avoiding prolonged exposure; "distance" refers to keeping away from the infectious source; and "shielding" refers to avoiding bodily contact when exposure cannot be avoided (e.g., wearing a mask). The specific plan for selecting barriers in cases where infection exists and for preventing the occurrence of infection is dependent upon the characteristics of the causative microorganism(s). All of these microbes have a certain structure, a specific way of digesting foods, a system for utilizing oxygen or the oxidation-reduction processes, and a technique for reproducing. These microbes are classified by similarities in life characteristics. Therefore, the approach to prevention and control of communicable disease is to eliminate environmental sources or to identify the kind of organisms (by characteristics) and alter their life processes in order to protect human beings from attack.

1. Infectious diseases are "communicable" because they
   - **A.** attack human beings.
   - **B.** spread from one source to another.
   - **C.** cannot be controlled by barriers.
   - **D.** can cause disease.

2. The goal of programs to control and prevent the spread of communicable diseases is to
   - **A.** eliminate conditions that support the spread of the disease.
   - **B.** shield people from the disease.
   - **C.** avoid contact with people who have the disease.
   - **D.** find the right barrier to the spread of the disease.

3. A barrier that represents "shielding" would be
   - **A.** isolating a child with a cold.
   - **B.** using a stick to pick up infected material.
   - **C.** short visits with a friend who has pneumonia.
   - **D.** looking at a baby through a nursery window.

4. Having knowledge of the characteristics of an infectious microorganism helps in the prevention and control of communicable disease in that it

A. determines how long the infection will last.

B. identifies which methods should be used to counteract the infection.

C. establishes whether or not the organism is a hazard.

D. relates to the severity of the infection.

STOP

IF YOU FINISH BEFORE TIME IS CALLED, YOU MAY CHECK YOUR WORK ON THIS SECTION ONLY. DO NOT TURN TO ANY OTHER SECTION IN THE TEST.

TEST 2

4 Questions • 9 Minutes

> **Directions:** Carefully read the following passage and then answer the accompanying questions, basing your answers on what is stated or implied in the passage. When you have decided which choice is best, fill in the corresponding space on your answer sheet. There is only one best answer for each question.

The "liberated woman" is a phrase that most of us associate with the sixties and seventies. The ERA's and NOW's consciousness-raising and bra-burning blitzed the media with a fury. In reality, the American woman had begun to cast off the restraints of feminine suppression long before the seventies, by snipping the strings of her proverbial apron, if not the straps of her bra. We are referring to both the 1920s and the postwar era.

The flood of labor-saving and time-saving devices pouring from the factories freed women from much of the never-ending drudgery that had been the plight of housewives since the beginning of time.

Women also found new freedom outside the home. The vote was finally rendered to women via the Nineteenth Amendment to the Constitution, and the long-awaited dream of political equality between the sexes was fulfilled. Members of what was once known as the "gentle sex" cast down their brooms, cast forth their ballots, and fled their kitchens to take part in a social freedom that catapulted their grandmothers right out of their rocking chairs. Chaperones no longer made the scene at young people's parties. Fashion editors reported "the American woman has lifted her skirt far beyond any modest limitation." The hemline was being hoisted nine inches from the ground and was heading for the knee.

The boyish look was in, and women everywhere invaded the strictly male territory known as the barbershop to have their beautiful and once-treasured tresses "bobbed." Breast implants, no way! Damsels of every social station were binding their chests to acquire that fashionable look of masculinity. In contrast to this trend of fashion, beautiful debutantes took heed to the cliche "powder and paint will make you what you ain't" and plastered their faces doll-style with rouge and lipstick.

Young ladies no longer puffed secretly into the fireplaces of their homes to conceal the damnable sin of which they were partaking. Women were smoking in public for the first time.

Extensive vicissitudes in lifestyle and values placed women in the workplace. The "Roaring Twenties" were characterized by women finding new opportunities for employment in the booming cities. Though they were limited to a few low-paying jobs hastily labeled "women's work," such as retail clerking and office typing, they were making an impact on the post-war era. A feisty feminist, Margaret Sanger, led a birth-control movement and openly defended the use of contraceptives. To add insult to injury, the women of the twenties deflated many a male ego with the organization of the National Women's Party in 1923.

"You've Come a Long Way Baby" was putting it mildly in the twenties. In all probability, the women of the 1990s recoined the phrase "...and you ain't seen nothin' yet!"

1. This passage would suggest that women of the 1920s were
   A. docile in their attitudes regarding social change.
   B. assertive in their views on women's social and political status.
   C. willing to compromise on political issues concerning women.
   D. eager to return to life in the kitchen.

2. A fitting title for this passage would be
   A. "You've Come a Long Way Baby—Twenties Style."
   B. "Women in the Workplace."
   C. "Women's Political Advancements in the Twenties."
   D. "Male Bashing in the Twenties."

3. The tone of this passage would suggest that the author is
   A. a male chauvinist.
   B. a product of the seventies.
   C. a trendy individual.
   D. a historian of women's changing roles in U.S. society.

4. The message of this passage is that the era known as the "Roaring Twenties" was characterized by
   A. an increase in women's unemployment.
   B. marked social change.
   C. an industrial slump.
   D. an indifference to fashion and style.

STOP

IF YOU FINISH BEFORE TIME IS CALLED, YOU MAY CHECK YOUR WORK ON THIS SECTION ONLY. DO NOT TURN TO ANY OTHER SECTION IN THE TEST.

TEST 3

8 Questions • 10 Minutes

Directions: Carefully read the following passage and then answer the accompanying questions, basing your answers on what is stated or implied in the passage. When you have decided which choice is best, fill in the corresponding space on your answer sheet. There is only one best answer for each question.

Every cell in the body is bathed in water. The substances dissolved in the water provide the immediate environment for the cells' existence, that is, for their respiration, digestion, excretion, and reproduction. This water—70% of our body weight and originally from our food and drink—is carried in the blood and is distributed in three places in the body. In terms of body weight:

- 5% remains in blood
- 15% goes to tissue spaces
- 50% goes inside the cell

Of course, more water is needed in the cell than elsewhere in the body because there are more solutes to be dissolved and because ionization must take place for anabolism and catabolism—two divisions of metabolism—to function.

All of the substances inside the cell and outside the cell in the tissue spaces were at one time a part of the blood. The blood is the transportation system of the body and, therefore, is the recipient of all substances, which include vitamins, nutrients, hormones, oxygen, and carbon dioxide. Substances are "unloaded" by pushing out those that can filter through the tiny openings of the semipermeable membranes of the capillaries into the tissue spaces. These substances, along with water, are then sucked into the semipermeable membranes of the cells. At the same time, the cell has produced waste substances; it now pushes those out into the tissue fluid so that they can be pushed into the capillaries and thereby excreted by the kidneys, skin, respiratory system, etc.

The pushing and sucking forces are regulated by concentrations. The more concentrated a substance is, the more force it has. What determines whether that force will push or suck is whether the substance is primarily water (solvent) or particles dissolved in water (solute). If water is the primary component of a substance, it will be sucked; that is, it will pass from a lesser to a greater concentration. This is called osmosis. The substance that is sucking in the water has the greater force or pull, called osmotic pressure, because it has the greater concentration. If solutes are the primary component, they can be pushed only by diffusion from a greater to a lesser concentration. The sucking and pushing processes go on simultaneously, and that is why we identify this mechanism as being dynamic. The "equilibrium" of body fluids is explained in terms of a balance of forces. This dynamic factor is controlled by three things:

1. How much of the substance is present (solute/solvent)
2. What kind of substance is present (electrolytes/non-electrolytes)
3. The placement and distribution of the substance (cell/tissue space/blood)

The concentration of a solution is determined by the relationship between the solutes and water. "Solutes" may be electrolytes or non-electrolytes. Non-electrolytes do not ionize and, therefore, they affect the concentration of a solution and its diffusion processes, but they do not affect the osmolarity of a solution. Osmotic pressure is determined by "tonic" relationships. "Tonic" refers to the comparison of the number of specific ions per unit volume in two given solutions—*iso* being "the same as," *hypo* being "less than," and *hyper* being "more than."

Given two solutions of the same solute, the more concentrated solution contains more solute particles, has a higher potential osmotic pressure, and is hypertonic as compared with the less concentrated solution. Given two solutions of different solutes, the solution containing more particles has the greater concentration, but there are no "tonic" relationships.

1. Why is an adequate intake of water essential to life?
   A. Solutes will dissolve only in water.
   B. Water is the medium for exchange of solutes.
   C. Osmosis will take place only in water.
   D. Water is necessary for metabolism.

2. The blood is described as "the transportation system of the body" because
   A. blood has the capacity for osmosis and diffusion.
   B. all nutrients and wastes are received by the blood.
   C. blood has a higher concentration than any other body fluid.
   D. all metabolic processes are controlled by the blood.

3. The concentration of a solution is directly determined by
   A. placement of solutes.
   B. distribution of water.
   C. percentage of solute to solvent.
   D. percentage of electrolytes to non-electrolytes.

4. The largest percentage of H_2O in the body is found
   A. intracellularly.
   B. extracelluarly.
   C. intravascularly.
   D. interstitially.

5. In the process of osmosis (sucking), the primary factor is
   A. water.
   B. solute.
   C. ionization.
   D. force.

6. If blood cells were placed in a hypertonic solution of salt, which one of the following blood cell reactions would take place?
   A. Swelling
   B. Shrinkage
   C. Destruction
   D. No change

7. The primary factor in diffusion (pushing) is
   A. water.
   B. solute.
   C. ionization.
   D. force.

8. If there are two solutions of sodium chloride, which of the following factors will determine which solution has the highest potential for osmosis?
   A. Isotonicity
   B. Hypotonicity
   C. Hypertonicity
   D. All of the above

STOP

IF YOU FINISH BEFORE TIME IS CALLED, YOU MAY CHECK YOUR WORK ON THIS SECTION ONLY. DO NOT TURN TO ANY OTHER SECTION IN THE TEST.

TEST 4

8 Questions • 15 Minutes

Directions: Carefully read the following passage and then answer the accompanying questions, basing your answers on what is stated or implied in the passage. When you have decided which choice is best, fill in the corresponding space on your answer sheet. There is only one best answer for each question.

As the world's population grows, the part played by humans in influencing plant life becomes increasingly great. In old and densely populated countries, as in western Europe, humans determine almost wholly what shall grow and what shall not grow. In such regions, the influence of humans on plant life is in large measure a beneficial one. Laws, often centuries old, protect plants of economic value and preserve soil fertility. In newly settled countries, the situation is, unfortunately, quite the reverse. The pioneer's life is too strenuous for him to think of posterity.

Some years ago, Mt. Mitchell, the highest summit east of the Mississippi, was covered with a magnificent forest. A lumber company was given full rights to fell the trees. Those not cut down were crushed. The mountain was left a waste area where fire would rage and erosion complete the destruction. There was no stopping the devastating foresting of the company for the contract had been given. Under a more enlightened civilization, this could not have happened. The denuding of Mt. Mitchell is a minor chapter in the destruction of lands in the United States, and this country is by no means the only sufferer. China, India, Egypt, and East Africa all have their thousands of square miles of wasteland, the result of human indifference to the future.

Deforestation, grazing, and poor farming techniques are the chief causes of the destruction of land fertility. Wasteful cutting of timber is the first step. Grazing follows lumbering, often bringing about ruin. The Caribbean slopes of northern Venezuela are barren wastes, owing first to ruthless cutting of forests and then to destructive grazing. Hordes of goats roamed these slopes until only a few thorny acacias and cacti remained. Erosion completed the devastation. What is illustrated there on a small scale is the story of vast areas in China and India, countries where famines occur regularly.

Humans are not wholly to blame, for nature is often merciless. In parts of India and China, plant life, even when left undisturbed, cannot cope with either the disastrous floods of wet seasons or the destructive winds of the dry season. Humans have learned much; prudent land management has been the policy of the Chinese people since 2700 B.C.E., but even they have not learned enough.

When the American forestry service was in its infancy, it met with much opposition from legislators, who loudly claimed that the protected land would in one season yield a crop of cabbages of more value than all the timber on it. Herein lay the fallacy: that one season's crop is all that need be thought of. Nature, through the years, adjusts crops to the soil and to the climate. Forests usually occur where precipitation exceeds evaporation. If the reverse is true, grasslands are found; where evaporation is still greater, desert or scrub vegetation alone survives. The phytogeographic map of a country is very similar to the climatic map based on rainfall, evaporation, and temperature. Humans ignore this natural adjustment of crops and strive for one "bumper" crop in a single season; it may be produced, but "year in and year out, the yield of the grassland is certain; that of the planted fields, never."

Humans are learning; we spray trees with insecticides and fungicides; import ladybugs to destroy aphids; irrigate, fertilize, and rotate crops; but we are still indifferent to many of the consequences of short-sighted policies.

In spite of the evidence from the experience of this country, the people of other countries still in the pioneer stage farm as wastefully as did our own pioneers. In the interiors of Central and South America, natives fell superb forest trees and leave them to rot in order to obtain virgin soil for cultivation. Where the land is hilly, it readily washes, and after one or two seasons, it is unfit for crops. So the frontier farmer pushes back into the primeval forest, moving his hut as he goes, and fells more monarchs to lay bare another patch of ground for his plantings to support his family. Valuable timber that will require a century to replace is destroyed and the land laid waste to produce what could be supplied for a pittance.

How badly humans can err in the handling of land is shown by the draining of extensive swamp areas, which to the uninformed would seem to be a very good thing to do. One of the first effects of the drainage is the lowering of the water table, which may bring about the death of the dominant species and leave to another species the possession of the soil, even when the difference in water level is little more than an inch. Bog country will frequently yield marketable crops of cranberries and blueberries, but, if drained, will grow neither these nor any other economically useful plant on the fallow soil. Swamps and marshes may have their drawbacks, but humans should beware of disturbing the ecosphere. When drained, wetlands may leave waste land, the surface of which can erode rapidly and be blown away in dust blizzards disastrous to both humans and wild beasts.

1. The best title for this passage might be
   A. "How to Increase Soil Productivity."
   B. "Conservation of Natural Resources."
   C. "Humans' Effect on Soil."
   D. "Soil Conditions and Plant Growth."

2. A policy of good management is sometimes upset by
   A. the indifference of humans.
   B. centuries-old laws.
   C. floods and winds.
   D. grazing animals.

3. Areas in which the total amounts of rain and snow falling on the ground are greater than the moisture evaporated will support
   A. forests.
   B. grasslands.
   C. scrub vegetation.
   D. no plants.

4. Pioneers usually do not have a long-range view on soil problems since they
   A. are not protected by laws.
   B. live under adverse conditions.
   C. use poor methods of farming.
   D. must protect themselves from famine.

5. A *bumper crop* is a crop that
   A. is harvested from grasslands.
   B. is protected from pests.
   C. has to be irrigated.
   D. is unusually large.

6. The first act of prudent land management might be to
   A. prohibit drainage of swamps.
   B. use irrigation and crop rotation in planted areas.
   C. increase use of fertilizers.
   D. prohibit excessive forest lumbering.

7. The results of effective land management may usually be found in
   A. heavily populated areas.
   B. areas not given over to grazing.
   C. underdeveloped areas.
   D. ancient civilizations.

8. The word *monarchs* (paragraph 7) refers to
   A. kings and queens.
   B. forests.
   C. huge, stately trees.
   D. a type of butterfly.

STOP

IF YOU FINISH BEFORE TIME IS CALLED, YOU MAY CHECK YOUR WORK ON THIS SECTION ONLY. DO NOT TURN TO ANY OTHER SECTION IN THE TEST.

ANSWER KEYS AND EXPLANATIONS

Test 1

1. B	2. A	3. D	4. B

1. **The correct answer is B.** The answer is stated in sentence 2 of paragraph 1.

2. **The correct answer is A.** The answer is stated in sentence 3 of paragraph 1. The other answers are specific ways to eliminate conditions that spread communicable diseases, but they are not the goal of the program, only tools or tactics.

3. **The correct answer is D.** Answering this question requires applying information from sentence 3 in paragraph 2 that defines "shielding."

4. **The correct answer is B.** The answer is stated in sentence 4 in paragraph 2.

Test 2

1. B	2. A	3. D	4. B

1. **The correct answer is B.** This answer can be inferred from information in paragraphs 3, 4, 5, and 6.

2. **The correct answer is A.** A title should reflect the main idea of a piece, and choice A best suggests the contents of the passage. Choices B and C suggest only specific information discussed in the passage, not the overall theme. Choice D isn't discussed in the passage.

3. **The correct answer is D.** To answer this question, you need to infer the tone based on the information in the piece. The tone is celebratory of the changes in women's lives in the 1920s. Choice D is the only answer that fits that description. Choice A is incorrect because a male chauvinist would not applaud the changes. Choice B is incorrect because the passage is about the 1920s, not the 1970s, and no connection is made between the 1920s and 1970s. Applauding changes to women's lives doesn't mark someone as trendy, so choice C doesn't make sense.

4. **The correct answer is B.** The passage is mainly about social change, so based on that, you can conclude that the "Roaring Twenties" were characterized by social change. Choice A is the opposite of what the passage says. Choice C is incorrect because the passage doesn't discuss industrial output or employment, either negatively or positively. Choice D is the opposite of what paragraphs 3 and 4 say.

Test 3

1. D	3. C	5. A	7. B
2. B	4. A	6. B	8. C

1. **The correct answer is D.** The answer is found in the final sentence in paragraph 1.

2. **The correct answer is B.** The answer is stated in sentence 2, paragraph 2.

3. **The correct answer is C.** The answer is stated in the first sentence after the enumerated list in paragraph 3. Don't be fooled because the sentence says "relationship" instead of "percentage."

4. **The correct answer is A.** The answer is stated in the list of percentages in paragraph 1. The prefix *intra-* means "within," so the correct answer is "50% goes inside the cell."

5. **The correct answer is A.** The answer is stated in sentence 4 of paragraph 3.

6. **The correct answer is B.** This answer requires drawing a conclusion. If the cell were placed in a hypertonic solution, the water from the cell would move to the solution of greater concentration via osmosis and the cell would therefore shrink.

7. **The correct answer is B.** The answer is stated in sentence 7 in paragraph 3.

8. **The correct answer is C.** This answer requires drawing a conclusion. Based on information in the last sentence in paragraph 3, hypertonicity would determine which solution has the highest potential for osmosis.

Test 4

1. C	3. A	5. D	7. A
2. C	4. B	6. D	8. C

1. **The correct answer is C.** The title of a passage should reflect the main idea of the piece. Choices A, B, and D reflect only parts of the passage, not what the whole piece is about.

2. **The correct answer is C.** The answer is stated in sentence 2 of paragraph 4.

3. **The correct answer is A.** The answer is found in sentence 4 of paragraph 5, which discusses precipitation.

4. **The correct answer is B.** The answer is stated in the final sentence in paragraph 1.

5. **The correct answer is D.** A bumper crop is one that is unusually large or abundant.

This can be inferred from information in paragraph 5, sentences 1, 2, and 7.

6. **The correct answer is D.** This answer can be found in sentence 2 of paragraph 3. If the first step in destroying land fertility is the "wasteful cutting of timber," then the first step in prudent land management would be to prohibit excessive forest lumbering.

7. **The correct answer is A.** The answer is found in paragraph 1, sentence 2.

8. **The correct answer is C.** In paragraph 7, sentence 4, the writer is likening huge and stately trees reaching high in the air to human rulers.

PART V
PRACTICE FOR PRACTICAL/ VOCATIONAL NURSING SCHOOL ENTRANCE EXAMINATIONS

Verbal and Nonverbal Ability

OVERVIEW

Unit 13

VERBAL AND NONVERBAL ABILITY ANSWER SHEET

Test 1: Antonyms

1. Ⓐ Ⓑ Ⓒ Ⓓ	11. Ⓐ Ⓑ Ⓒ Ⓓ	21. Ⓐ Ⓑ Ⓒ Ⓓ	31. Ⓐ Ⓑ Ⓒ Ⓓ	41. Ⓐ Ⓑ Ⓒ Ⓓ
2. Ⓐ Ⓑ Ⓒ Ⓓ	12. Ⓐ Ⓑ Ⓒ Ⓓ	22. Ⓐ Ⓑ Ⓒ Ⓓ	32. Ⓐ Ⓑ Ⓒ Ⓓ	42. Ⓐ Ⓑ Ⓒ Ⓓ
3. Ⓐ Ⓑ Ⓒ Ⓓ	13. Ⓐ Ⓑ Ⓒ Ⓓ	23. Ⓐ Ⓑ Ⓒ Ⓓ	33. Ⓐ Ⓑ Ⓒ Ⓓ	43. Ⓐ Ⓑ Ⓒ Ⓓ
4. Ⓐ Ⓑ Ⓒ Ⓓ	14. Ⓐ Ⓑ Ⓒ Ⓓ	24. Ⓐ Ⓑ Ⓒ Ⓓ	34. Ⓐ Ⓑ Ⓒ Ⓓ	44. Ⓐ Ⓑ Ⓒ Ⓓ
5. Ⓐ Ⓑ Ⓒ Ⓓ	15. Ⓐ Ⓑ Ⓒ Ⓓ	25. Ⓐ Ⓑ Ⓒ Ⓓ	35. Ⓐ Ⓑ Ⓒ Ⓓ	45. Ⓐ Ⓑ Ⓒ Ⓓ
6. Ⓐ Ⓑ Ⓒ Ⓓ	16. Ⓐ Ⓑ Ⓒ Ⓓ	26. Ⓐ Ⓑ Ⓒ Ⓓ	36. Ⓐ Ⓑ Ⓒ Ⓓ	46. Ⓐ Ⓑ Ⓒ Ⓓ
7. Ⓐ Ⓑ Ⓒ Ⓓ	17. Ⓐ Ⓑ Ⓒ Ⓓ	27. Ⓐ Ⓑ Ⓒ Ⓓ	37. Ⓐ Ⓑ Ⓒ Ⓓ	47. Ⓐ Ⓑ Ⓒ Ⓓ
8. Ⓐ Ⓑ Ⓒ Ⓓ	18. Ⓐ Ⓑ Ⓒ Ⓓ	28. Ⓐ Ⓑ Ⓒ Ⓓ	38. Ⓐ Ⓑ Ⓒ Ⓓ	48. Ⓐ Ⓑ Ⓒ Ⓓ
9. Ⓐ Ⓑ Ⓒ Ⓓ	19. Ⓐ Ⓑ Ⓒ Ⓓ	29. Ⓐ Ⓑ Ⓒ Ⓓ	39. Ⓐ Ⓑ Ⓒ Ⓓ	49. Ⓐ Ⓑ Ⓒ Ⓓ
10. Ⓐ Ⓑ Ⓒ Ⓓ	20. Ⓐ Ⓑ Ⓒ Ⓓ	30. Ⓐ Ⓑ Ⓒ Ⓓ	40. Ⓐ Ⓑ Ⓒ Ⓓ	50. Ⓐ Ⓑ Ⓒ Ⓓ

Test 2: Antonyms

1. Ⓐ Ⓑ Ⓒ Ⓓ	5. Ⓐ Ⓑ Ⓒ Ⓓ	9. Ⓐ Ⓑ Ⓒ Ⓓ	13. Ⓐ Ⓑ Ⓒ Ⓓ Ⓔ	17. Ⓐ Ⓑ Ⓒ Ⓓ Ⓔ
2. Ⓐ Ⓑ Ⓒ Ⓓ	6. Ⓐ Ⓑ Ⓒ Ⓓ	10. Ⓐ Ⓑ Ⓒ Ⓓ	14. Ⓐ Ⓑ Ⓒ Ⓓ Ⓔ	18. Ⓐ Ⓑ Ⓒ Ⓓ Ⓔ
3. Ⓐ Ⓑ Ⓒ Ⓓ	7. Ⓐ Ⓑ Ⓒ Ⓓ	11. Ⓐ Ⓑ Ⓒ Ⓓ Ⓔ	15. Ⓐ Ⓑ Ⓒ Ⓓ Ⓔ	19. Ⓐ Ⓑ Ⓒ Ⓓ Ⓔ
4. Ⓐ Ⓑ Ⓒ Ⓓ	8. Ⓐ Ⓑ Ⓒ Ⓓ	12. Ⓐ Ⓑ Ⓒ Ⓓ Ⓔ	16. Ⓐ Ⓑ Ⓒ Ⓓ Ⓔ	20. Ⓐ Ⓑ Ⓒ Ⓓ Ⓔ

Test 3: Synonyms

1. Ⓐ Ⓑ Ⓒ Ⓓ	11. Ⓐ Ⓑ Ⓒ Ⓓ	21. Ⓐ Ⓑ Ⓒ Ⓓ	31. Ⓐ Ⓑ Ⓒ Ⓓ	41. Ⓐ Ⓑ Ⓒ Ⓓ
2. Ⓐ Ⓑ Ⓒ Ⓓ	12. Ⓐ Ⓑ Ⓒ Ⓓ	22. Ⓐ Ⓑ Ⓒ Ⓓ	32. Ⓐ Ⓑ Ⓒ Ⓓ	42. Ⓐ Ⓑ Ⓒ Ⓓ
3. Ⓐ Ⓑ Ⓒ Ⓓ	13. Ⓐ Ⓑ Ⓒ Ⓓ	23. Ⓐ Ⓑ Ⓒ Ⓓ	33. Ⓐ Ⓑ Ⓒ Ⓓ	43. Ⓐ Ⓑ Ⓒ Ⓓ
4. Ⓐ Ⓑ Ⓒ Ⓓ	14. Ⓐ Ⓑ Ⓒ Ⓓ	24. Ⓐ Ⓑ Ⓒ Ⓓ	34. Ⓐ Ⓑ Ⓒ Ⓓ	44. Ⓐ Ⓑ Ⓒ Ⓓ
5. Ⓐ Ⓑ Ⓒ Ⓓ	15. Ⓐ Ⓑ Ⓒ Ⓓ	25. Ⓐ Ⓑ Ⓒ Ⓓ	35. Ⓐ Ⓑ Ⓒ Ⓓ	45. Ⓐ Ⓑ Ⓒ Ⓓ
6. Ⓐ Ⓑ Ⓒ Ⓓ	16. Ⓐ Ⓑ Ⓒ Ⓓ	26. Ⓐ Ⓑ Ⓒ Ⓓ	36. Ⓐ Ⓑ Ⓒ Ⓓ	46. Ⓐ Ⓑ Ⓒ Ⓓ
7. Ⓐ Ⓑ Ⓒ Ⓓ	17. Ⓐ Ⓑ Ⓒ Ⓓ	27. Ⓐ Ⓑ Ⓒ Ⓓ	37. Ⓐ Ⓑ Ⓒ Ⓓ	47. Ⓐ Ⓑ Ⓒ Ⓓ
8. Ⓐ Ⓑ Ⓒ Ⓓ	18. Ⓐ Ⓑ Ⓒ Ⓓ	28. Ⓐ Ⓑ Ⓒ Ⓓ	38. Ⓐ Ⓑ Ⓒ Ⓓ	48. Ⓐ Ⓑ Ⓒ Ⓓ
9. Ⓐ Ⓑ Ⓒ Ⓓ	19. Ⓐ Ⓑ Ⓒ Ⓓ	29. Ⓐ Ⓑ Ⓒ Ⓓ	39. Ⓐ Ⓑ Ⓒ Ⓓ	49. Ⓐ Ⓑ Ⓒ Ⓓ
10. Ⓐ Ⓑ Ⓒ Ⓓ	20. Ⓐ Ⓑ Ⓒ Ⓓ	30. Ⓐ Ⓑ Ⓒ Ⓓ	40. Ⓐ Ⓑ Ⓒ Ⓓ	50. Ⓐ Ⓑ Ⓒ Ⓓ

answer sheet

Test 4: Synonyms

1. Ⓐ Ⓑ Ⓒ Ⓓ	5. Ⓐ Ⓑ Ⓒ Ⓓ	9. Ⓐ Ⓑ Ⓒ Ⓓ	13. Ⓐ Ⓑ Ⓒ Ⓓ	17. Ⓐ Ⓑ Ⓒ Ⓓ
2. Ⓐ Ⓑ Ⓒ Ⓓ	6. Ⓐ Ⓑ Ⓒ Ⓓ	10. Ⓐ Ⓑ Ⓒ Ⓓ	14. Ⓐ Ⓑ Ⓒ Ⓓ	18. Ⓐ Ⓑ Ⓒ Ⓓ
3. Ⓐ Ⓑ Ⓒ Ⓓ	7. Ⓐ Ⓑ Ⓒ Ⓓ	11. Ⓐ Ⓑ Ⓒ Ⓓ	15. Ⓐ Ⓑ Ⓒ Ⓓ	19. Ⓐ Ⓑ Ⓒ Ⓓ
4. Ⓐ Ⓑ Ⓒ Ⓓ	8. Ⓐ Ⓑ Ⓒ Ⓓ	12. Ⓐ Ⓑ Ⓒ Ⓓ	16. Ⓐ Ⓑ Ⓒ Ⓓ	20. Ⓐ Ⓑ Ⓒ Ⓓ

Test 5: English Grammar and Usage

1. Ⓐ Ⓑ Ⓒ	4. Ⓐ Ⓑ Ⓒ	7. Ⓐ Ⓑ Ⓒ	10. Ⓐ Ⓑ Ⓒ	13. Ⓐ Ⓑ Ⓒ
2. Ⓐ Ⓑ Ⓒ	5. Ⓐ Ⓑ Ⓒ	8. Ⓐ Ⓑ Ⓒ	11. Ⓐ Ⓑ Ⓒ	14. Ⓐ Ⓑ Ⓒ
3. Ⓐ Ⓑ Ⓒ	6. Ⓐ Ⓑ Ⓒ	9. Ⓐ Ⓑ Ⓒ	12. Ⓐ Ⓑ Ⓒ	15. Ⓐ Ⓑ Ⓒ

Test 6: Spelling

1. Ⓐ Ⓑ Ⓒ	4. Ⓐ Ⓑ Ⓒ	7. Ⓐ Ⓑ Ⓒ	10. Ⓐ Ⓑ Ⓒ	13. Ⓐ Ⓑ Ⓒ
2. Ⓐ Ⓑ Ⓒ	5. Ⓐ Ⓑ Ⓒ	8. Ⓐ Ⓑ Ⓒ	11. Ⓐ Ⓑ Ⓒ	14. Ⓐ Ⓑ Ⓒ
3. Ⓐ Ⓑ Ⓒ	6. Ⓐ Ⓑ Ⓒ	9. Ⓐ Ⓑ Ⓒ	12. Ⓐ Ⓑ Ⓒ	15. Ⓐ Ⓑ Ⓒ

Test 7: Nonverbal Ability

1. Ⓐ Ⓑ Ⓒ Ⓓ Ⓔ	4. Ⓐ Ⓑ Ⓒ Ⓓ Ⓔ	7. Ⓐ Ⓑ Ⓒ Ⓓ Ⓔ	10. Ⓐ Ⓑ Ⓒ Ⓓ Ⓔ	13. Ⓐ Ⓑ Ⓒ Ⓓ Ⓔ
2. Ⓐ Ⓑ Ⓒ Ⓓ Ⓔ	5. Ⓐ Ⓑ Ⓒ Ⓓ Ⓔ	8. Ⓐ Ⓑ Ⓒ Ⓓ Ⓔ	11. Ⓐ Ⓑ Ⓒ Ⓓ Ⓔ	14. Ⓐ Ⓑ Ⓒ Ⓓ Ⓔ
3. Ⓐ Ⓑ Ⓒ Ⓓ Ⓔ	6. Ⓐ Ⓑ Ⓒ Ⓓ Ⓔ	9. Ⓐ Ⓑ Ⓒ Ⓓ Ⓔ	12. Ⓐ Ⓑ Ⓒ Ⓓ Ⓔ	15. Ⓐ Ⓑ Ⓒ Ⓓ Ⓔ

TEST 1: ANTONYMS

50 Questions • 30 Minutes

Review Unit 4, Antonyms, before attempting this test.

Directions: For each question, select the word that is opposite in meaning to the capitalized word. Fill in the corresponding space on your answer sheet.

1. GARRULOUS
   A. talkative
   B. reserved
   C. unruly
   D. fraternal

2. TRANSLUCENT
   A. patent
   B. transitory
   C. transparent
   D. opaque

3. BENEVOLENT
   A. generous
   B. charitable
   C. malevolent
   D. good

4. LETHARGIC
   A. energetic
   B. sluggish
   C. apathetic
   D. fatal

5. AMICABLE
   A. lonely
   B. reactionary
   C. hostile
   D. laconic

6. TRANQUILITY
   A. complacency
   B. tumult
   C. plagiarism
   D. prophecy

7. PROCRASTINATE
   A. elegiac
   B. mediate
   C. expedite
   D. investiture

8. QUIESCENT
   A. restless
   B. slow
   C. mendicant
   D. malignant

9. DELETERIOUS
   A. fractious
   B. pathetic
   C. salubrious
   D. gullible

10. COGNIZANCE
    A. ignorance
    B. abeyance
    C. anecdote
    D. idiom

11. CLEMENCY
    A. mercy
    B. indulgence
    C. kindness
    D. vindictiveness

12. IGNOBLE
    A. honorable
    B. shameful
    C. disgraceful
    D. humble

13. CURSORY
    A. hasty
    B. superficial
    C. awful
    D. thorough

14. ADMONISH
    A. warn
    B. praise
    C. advise
    D. reprove

15. PHLEGMATIC
    A. energetic
    B. dull
    C. extraordinary
    D. morbid

16. LAMENTABLE
    A. laughable
    B. generous
    C. emotional
    D. doleful

17. PERILOUS
    A. vivacious
    B. unresponsive
    C. safe
    D. hazardous

18. INIQUITOUS
    A. unequaled
    B. unfriendly
    C. righteous
    D. injurious

19. ASSIDUOUS
    A. cooperative
    B. indifferent
    C. active
    D. satisfactory

20. CORROBORATE
    A. fascinate
    B. corrupt
    C. confirm
    D. dispute

21. CONFLUENCE
    A. convention
    B. sympathy
    C. divergence
    D. concurrence

22. DASTARDLY
    A. cowardly
    B. bravely
    C. friendly
    D. sinfully

23. ABSTRUSE
    A. understandable
    B. hidden
    C. absurd
    D. religious

24. ILLUSION
    A. delusion
    B. conception
    C. reality
    D. dramatization

25. AVARICIOUS

   A. greedy

   B. persuasive

   C. generous

   D. gracious

26. COERCE

   A. enforce

   B. cohere

   C. forestall

   D. encourage

27. TEMERITY

   A. recklessness

   B. prudence

   C. support

   D. sanity

28. LACONIC

   A. verbose

   B. concise

   C. serene

   D. interesting

29. CREDULOUS

   A. exuberant

   B. skeptical

   C. dangerous

   D. legible

30. INCARCERATE

   A. immunize

   B. anesthetize

   C. transport

   D. release

31. OBTUSE

   A. oblique

   B. obese

   C. perpendicular

   D. acute

32. MUNIFICENT

   A. political

   B. miserly

   C. liberal

   D. educational

33. DERANGED

   A. unsettled

   B. paralyzed

   C. sane

   D. awkward

34. LEVITY

   A. flippancy

   B. peace

   C. gravity

   D. trickery

35. EQUANIMITY

   A. peace

   B. inflation

   C. agitation

   D. tranquility

36. MARAUD

   A. purchase

   B. plunder

   C. masticate

   D. elevate

37. ENCOMIUM

   A. immorality

   B. praise

   C. egotism

   D. defamation

38. ABOMINABLE

   A. delightful

   B. horrible

   C. meaningful

   D. insane

39. ABSTEMIOUS
   A. frugal
   B. happy
   C. greedy
   D. radiant

40. ADVERTENT
   A. retentive
   B. inconsiderate
   C. empathetic
   D. abnormal

41. ENIGMATIC
   A. perplexing
   B. explicit
   C. persistent
   D. officious

42. EXECRABLE
   A. unusual
   B. detestable
   C. fallible
   D. pleasant

43. IGNOMINIOUS
   A. reputable
   B. shameful
   C. intangible
   D. irascible

44. SAGACITY
   A. sorrowfulness
   B. support
   C. satisfaction
   D. stupidity

45. PROVERBIAL
   A. innovative
   B. current
   C. wise
   D. cautious

46. ANNIHILATE
   A. advertise
   B. destroy
   C. preserve
   D. announce

47. AFFABLE
   A. discourteous
   B. beloved
   C. sociable
   D. debonair

48. CAPRICIOUS
   A. erratic
   B. agreeable
   C. awkward
   D. constant

49. CONTINGENT
   A. conditional
   B. independent
   C. confined
   D. familiar

50. PRETENTIOUS
   A. meddling
   B. modest
   C. emaciated
   D. pompous

STOP

IF YOU FINISH BEFORE TIME IS CALLED, YOU MAY
CHECK YOUR WORK ON THIS SECTION ONLY. DO NOT
TURN TO ANY OTHER SECTION IN THE TEST.

TEST 2: ANTONYMS

20 Questions • 10 Minutes

Review Unit 4, Antonyms, before attempting this test.

Directions: For each question, select the word that is opposite in meaning to the capitalized word. Fill in the corresponding space on your answer sheet.

---

1. DECEIT
   - A. fraud
   - B. truthfulness
   - C. treachery
   - D. imposition

2. DOCILE
   - A. teachable
   - B. compliant
   - C. tame
   - D. inflexible

3. HARMLESS
   - A. safe
   - B. hurtful
   - C. innocent
   - D. innocuous

4. MELANCHOLY
   - A. jolly
   - B. low-spirited
   - C. dreamy
   - D. sad

5. IMPETUOUS
   - A. violent
   - B. furious
   - C. calm
   - D. vehement

6. JOY
   - A. gladness
   - B. grief
   - C. mirth
   - D. delight

7. LUNACY
   - A. sanity
   - B. madness
   - C. derangement
   - D. mania

8. MOIST
   - A. dank
   - B. dry
   - C. damp
   - D. humid

9. PUERILE
   - A. youthful
   - B. weak
   - C. silly
   - D. mature

10. WEIGHT
    - A. gravity
    - B. heaviness
    - C. lightness
    - D. triviality

Directions: In the following sets of words, choose the word that is most different in meaning from the others.

11. A. superfluous
    B. necessary
    C. excessive
    D. gratuitous
    E. dispensable

12. A. reform
    B. amend
    C. correct
    D. better
    E. corrupt

13. A. scanty
    B. bare
    C. ample
    D. insufficient
    E. meager

14. A. misery
    B. happiness
    C. woe
    D. tribulation
    E. affliction

15. A. proper
    B. legitimate
    C. appropriate
    D. wrong
    E. pertinent

16. A. incongruous
    B. compatible
    C. alien
    D. contrary
    E. disparate

17. A. fatigue
    B. lassitude
    C. weariness
    D. malaise
    E. vigor

18. A. hasten
    B. delay
    C. accelerate
    D. dispatch
    E. expedite

19. A. absorb
    B. emit
    C. engulf
    D. engross
    E. consume

20. A. abuse
    B. defilement
    C. shelter
    D. violation
    E. offense

STOP

IF YOU FINISH BEFORE TIME IS CALLED, YOU MAY CHECK YOUR WORK ON THIS SECTION ONLY. DO NOT TURN TO ANY OTHER SECTION IN THE TEST.

TEST 3: SYNONYMS

50 Questions • 30 Minutes

Review Unit 4, Synonyms, before attempting this test.

Directions: In each of the following, choose the word that best corresponds in meaning to the italicized word. Fill in the corresponding space on your answer sheet.

1. Her efforts to revive the child were *futile*.
   - A. strong
   - B. clumsy
   - C. useless
   - D. sincere

2. The supply of pamphlets has been *depleted*.
   - A. exhausted
   - B. delivered
   - C. included
   - D. rejected

3. The *gist* of his speech was that we should strike.
   - A. end
   - B. essence
   - C. strength
   - D. spirit

4. The soldier received a medal in recognition of his *valor* in battle.
   - A. injury
   - B. ability
   - C. cooperation
   - D. courage

5. When Mary arrived in California, her future seemed *auspicious*.
   - A. bleak
   - B. uncertain
   - C. promising
   - D. somber

6. To our *consternation*, the child's bicycle rolled into the busy street.
   - A. dismay
   - B. amazement
   - C. incompetence
   - D. annoyance

7. *Indolence* is a habit that cannot be excused.
   - A. inability
   - B. snoring
   - C. carelessness
   - D. idleness

8. The political candidate made *cogent* remarks.
   - A. pleasing
   - B. convincing
   - C. flattering
   - D. slandering

9. A *prolific* writer is one who is
   - A. productive.
   - B. popular.
   - C. frank.
   - D. effective.

10. He was *meticulous* when performing his work.
    - A. careless
    - B. patient
    - C. scrupulous
    - D. nervous

11. There were *sporadic* outbreaks of food poisoning at the camp.
    A. epidemic
    B. widespread
    C. serious
    D. scattered

12. The motion passed even though there were three *dissenting* votes.
    A. annoying
    B. disagreeing
    C. abstaining
    D. approving

13. It is *traditional* for the bride to wear a white gown.
    A. normal
    B. customary
    C. ordinary
    D. gracious

14. The company has *rescinded* the order.
    A. canceled
    B. revised
    C. confirmed
    D. misinterpreted

15. Although the prisoner was released early, he was *vindictive* toward society.
    A. prejudiced
    B. impatient
    C. revengeful
    D. unreasonable

16. The *sedulous* student worked many hours in the laboratory.
    A. eager
    B. persistent
    C. intelligent
    D. inexperienced

17. The neighbors were *interrogated* by the police.
    A. arrested
    B. detained
    C. investigated
    D. questioned

18. The lifeguard *disparaged* his brave rescue of the child.
    A. explained
    B. belittled
    C. demonstrated
    D. elucidated

19. The water could not *permeate* the rubber apron.
    A. penetrate
    B. wet
    C. harm
    D. discolor

20. The *docile* dog waited at the gate.
    A. mongrel
    B. hungry
    C. intractable
    D. obedient

21. The two hospitals in our town will *amalgamate* next year.
    A. close
    B. expand
    C. relocate
    D. merge

22. She wasted her money on *frivolous* things.
    A. sweet
    B. expensive
    C. unimportant
    D. cheap

23. The teacher *divulged* the test grades.
    A. whispered
    B. disregarded
    C. revealed
    D. averaged

24. The *salary* offered for the job did not match her experience.

    A. reimbursement

    B. remuneration

    C. indemnity

    D. reparation

25. The art dealer *scrutinized* the painting to verify its authenticity.

    A. touched

    B. bought

    C. inspected

    D. measured

26. The bridge was closed because it was *decrepit*.

    A. slippery

    B. weak

    C. swaying

    D. flooded

27. The driver *conceded* that he was at fault.

    A. denied

    B. explained

    C. complained

    D. admitted

28. The machinery in the vocational classroom was *obsolete*.

    A. out-of-date

    B. new

    C. reliable

    D. complicated

29. The speaker made *candid* remarks about the candidate's record.

    A. biased

    B. confidential

    C. frank

    D. insulting

30. When the hostage was released, he was speaking *incoherently*.

    A. disconnectedly

    B. cohesively

    C. prodigiously

    D. sluggishly

31. The mother tried to *pacify* the child.

    A. detain

    B. restrain

    C. accompany

    D. calm

32. The head nurse on 2 West was young and *vivacious*.

    A. kind

    B. lively

    C. short

    D. talkative

33. The town was *devastated* after the earthquake.

    A. rebuilt

    B. deserted

    C. destroyed

    D. saved

34. The teacher *digressed* from her custom and didn't give any homework.

    A. deviated

    B. reposed

    C. alighted

    D. moored

35. The Colonel was a *gallant* man.

    A. rude

    B. fastidious

    C. cowardly

    D. chivalrous

36. The evening *reflected* the host's interest in good food, good wine, and good company.
    A. contemplated
    B. demonstrated
    C. imitated
    D. possessed

37. When I visited her in the nursing home, she was *querulous* and unhappy.
    A. satisfied
    B. cheerful
    C. complaining
    D. painful

38. The FBI agent kept a *vigilant* guard on the suspect.
    A. careful
    B. continuous
    C. observant
    D. reciprocal

39. The play treated current social issues *satirically*.
    A. contemptuously
    B. interminably
    C. musically
    D. ironically

40. She felt an *antipathy* for lizards.
    A. aversion
    B. fondness
    C. interest
    D. fear

41. The hiker had a *premonition* of danger.
    A. vision
    B. forewarning
    C. recurrence
    D. apprehend

42. The policeofficer *confiscated* the illegal drugs.
    A. stored
    B. distributed
    C. destroyed
    D. appropriated

43. John was asked to resign because of his *impropriety*.
    A. age
    B. tardiness
    C. dishonesty
    D. absenteeism

44. There is no *tangible* evidence of damage.
    A. concrete
    B. theoretical
    C. verified
    D. scientific

45. Her *blithe* spirit made her popular.
    A. free
    B. cheerful
    C. kind
    D. insolent

46. The jury *deliberated* for 8 hours.
    A. met
    B. convened
    C. considered
    D. summarized

47. He had a *sinister* motive for entering the building.
    A. practical
    B. treacherous
    C. important
    D. honest

48. The requirements for admission to the school were *stringent*.

   A. unusual

   B. numerous

   C. rigid

   D. lax

49. The students refused to give up their *prerogatives*.

   A. demands

   B. rights

   C. ideals

   D. duties

50. The widow and her children were *destitute*.

   A. impoverished

   B. detained

   C. loathed

   D. ill

STOP

> IF YOU FINISH BEFORE TIME IS CALLED, YOU MAY CHECK YOUR WORK ON THIS SECTION ONLY. DO NOT TURN TO ANY OTHER SECTION IN THE TEST.

TEST 4: SYNONYMS

20 Questions • 10 Minutes

Review Unit 4, Synonyms, before attempting this test.

Directions: For each question, select the word that corresponds in meaning to the capitalized word. Fill in the corresponding space on your answer sheet.

1. COMPETENT
   A. agreeable
   B. inept
   C. vigorous
   D. capable

2. OMNIBUS
   A. threatening
   B. all-embracing
   C. rotund
   D. slow-moving

3. INGENUITY
   A. deceitfulness
   B. appeal
   C. cleverness
   D. innocence

4. CONCAVE
   A. curving inward
   B. curving outward
   C. oval-shaped
   D. rounded

5. CANON
   A. barrier
   B. noisy place
   C. guiding principle
   D. rigorous

6. PROPITIOUS
   A. questionable
   B. well-known
   C. free
   D. favorable

7. VACILLATING
   A. changeable
   B. decisive
   C. equalizing
   D. progressing

8. FORFEIT
   A. exchange
   B. relinquish
   C. protect
   D. withdraw

9. QUERY
   A. question
   B. look over carefully
   C. follow through
   D. act peculiarly

10. STEADFAST
    A. gradual
    B. strong
    C. friendly
    D. unwavering

11. ACCESS
    A. too much
    B. extra
    C. admittance
    D. arrival

12. PERMUTATION
    A. alteration
    B. permission
    C. combination
    D. seepage

13. SPRITZ
    A. spray
    B. bubble
    C. protrude
    D. sail

14. PERSONABLE
    A. intimate
    B. cheerful
    C. attractive
    D. superficial

15. EXPEDITE
    A. dismiss
    B. advise
    C. accelerate
    D. demolish

16. COMPULSORY
    A. imperative
    B. impossible
    C. imminent
    D. logical

17. PRACTICABLE
    A. lenient
    B. feasible
    C. simple
    D. visible

18. AGREE
    A. inquire
    B. acquiesce
    C. discharge
    D. endeavor

19. FLORID
    A. overflowing
    B. ruddy
    C. seedy
    D. flowery

20. NEARNESS
    A. adherence
    B. declivity
    C. worldliness
    D. proximity

STOP

IF YOU FINISH BEFORE TIME IS CALLED, YOU MAY
CHECK YOUR WORK ON THIS SECTION ONLY. DO NOT
TURN TO ANY OTHER SECTION IN THE TEST.

TEST 5: ENGLISH GRAMMAR AND USAGE

15 Questions • 10 Minutes

Review Unit 4, English Grammar and Usage, before attempting this test.

Directions: In the following questions, select the answer that completes the sentence in a grammatically correct manner or that represents the most grammatically correct of all options.

1. _____ rain nor snow _____ Hank from his morning bicycle ride.
   A. Either; keeps
   B. Either; keep
   C. Neither; keeps
   D. Neither; keep

2. Everyone _____ a critic, but no one _____ receiving criticism.
   A. are; likes
   B. is; likes
   C. are; like
   D. is; like

3. Identify the verb type of the italicized word in the following sentence: It *looks* sunny and beautiful outside today.
   A. Transitive verb
   B. Helping verb
   C. Action verb
   D. Linking verb

4. Identify the case of the italicized word in the following sentence: Who are *we*?
   A. Nominative
   B. Objective
   C. Possessive
   D. Subjunctive

5. Identify the indirect object in the following sentence: Megan handed Dillon the keys, and he put them in his pocket.
   A. keys
   B. them
   C. Dillon
   D. pocket

6. Which sentence is in the subjunctive mood?
   A. If Thomas were my partner in Spades, we'd win every time.
   B. Come over to my house and play Spades with us tonight.
   C. Thomas and I were partners in Spades every summer at camp.
   D. Do you know whether Thomas plays Spades?

7. Which of the following is the present participle of the verb *walk*?
   A. walk
   B. walking
   C. walked
   D. walks

8. We are currently driving on Route 66 toward Flagstaff; we _____ this same route every summer for the past 25 years.
   A. drove
   B. have drove
   C. have driven
   D. had driven

9. By the time she turns 30 next May, Alice _____ in over 100 triathlons.
   A. will compete
   B. will have competed
   C. has competed
   D. had competed

10. Identify the part of speech of the italicized word in the following sentence: Before the storm arrived, state officials acted *quickly* to prepare residents for the worst.

- **A.** Adverb
- **B.** Adjective
- **C.** Preposition
- **D.** Verb

11. Gymnasts are _____ than badminton players but _____ than weightlifters.

- **A.** stronger; less strong
- **B.** more stronger; not strong
- **C.** strongest; least strong
- **D.** more strongly; less strongly

12. Although the car did not run _____ it looked nice sitting in Todd's driveway, he thought.

- **A.** :
- **B.** .
- **C.** ;
- **D.** ,

13. Which of the following sentences is grammatically correct?

- **A.** People really value homemade jewelry, therefore, Kelly figured her business would be a success.
- **B.** People really value homemade jewelry, therefore; Kelly figured her business would be a success.
- **C.** People really value homemade jewelry; therefore, Kelly figured her business would be a success.
- **D.** People really value homemade jewelry, therefore Kelly figured her business would be a success.

14. Which sentence is grammatically correct in terms of capitalization?

- **A.** Next Friday, maggie and i are driving south to Mexico, where we'll stay in la Paz, the city that is the setting of Steinbeck's novel, *the Pearl*.
- **B.** Next Friday, Maggie and I are driving south to Mexico, where we'll stay in La Paz, the city that is the setting of Steinbeck's novel, *The Pearl*.
- **C.** Next Friday, Maggie and I are driving South to Mexico, where we'll stay in la paz, the city that is the setting of Steinbeck's novel, *the pearl*.
- **D.** next friday, Maggie and I are driving south to Mexico, where we'll stay in La Paz, the city that is the setting of steinbeck's novel, *The pearl*.

15. Which sentence is grammatically correct?

- **A.** Our waiter: if I'm not mistaken: is the brother of my former college roommate, Evie.
- **B.** Our waiter, if I'm not mistaken—is the brother of my former college roommate, Evie.
- **C.** Our waiter—if I'm not mistaken—is the brother of my former college roommate, Evie.
- **D.** Our waiter; if I'm not mistaken; is the brother of my former college roommate, Evie.

STOP

IF YOU FINISH BEFORE TIME IS CALLED, YOU MAY CHECK YOUR WORK ON THIS SECTION ONLY. DO NOT TURN TO ANY OTHER SECTION IN THE TEST.

TEST 6: SPELLING

15 Questions • 5 Minutes

Review Unit 4, Spelling, before attempting this test.

Directions: In the following sets of words, choose the word that is spelled correctly.

---

1. A. accessible
   B. acsessible
   C. accesible

2. A. benine
   B. benign
   C. binign

3. A. conchusness
   B. consciousness
   C. contiousness

4. A. dialisis
   B. dyalisis
   C. dialysis

5. A. efficacy
   B. eficacy
   C. efficasy

6. A. floroscopy
   B. florosscopy
   C. fluoroscopy

7. A. guage
   B. gauge
   C. gaige

8. A. hereditery
   B. heredetary
   C. hereditary

9. A. lukocyte
   B. leukocyte
   C. leukocite

10. A. misspelled
    B. mispelled
    C. misspeled

11. A. myocardial
    B. maiocardial
    C. myocartial

12. A. nuron
    B. neuron
    C. nouron

13. A. optholmologist
    B. opthalmologist
    C. ophthalmologist

14. A. susceptible
    B. suseptible
    C. susseptable

15. A. unnesessary
    B. unnescessary
    C. unnecessary

STOP

IF YOU FINISH BEFORE TIME IS CALLED, YOU MAY
CHECK YOUR WORK ON THIS SECTION ONLY. DO NOT
TURN TO ANY OTHER SECTION IN THE TEST.

TEST 7: NONVERBAL ABILITY

15 Questions • 15 Minutes

Review Unit 4, Nonverbal Ability, before attempting this test.

> **Directions:** In the following questions, determine the relationship between the first pair of shapes and then decide which of the answer choices shares a similar relationship with the third shape.

1. ⊬ is to ⊢ as ¢ is to?
   - A. ¢
   - B. ⊂
   - C. ⊃
   - D. ⊅
   - E. ⊔

2. ⊤̄ is to ⊤ as ⊼ is to?
   - A. ∨
   - B. ⊼̄
   - C. ∧
   - D. >
   - E. <

3. Ö is to ◎ as ✶ is to?
   - A. ⊛
   - B. ö
   - C. ★
   - D. ☨
   - E. ✳

4. ⦙ is to │ as ◌ is to?
   - A. ⑪
   - B. ◉
   - C. ⌣
   - D. ⌢
   - E. ○

5. ⊕⊕ is to Ð as ◑ is to?
   - A. Ð
   - B. ◉
   - C. ⊃
   - D. D
   - E. C

6. ‡ is to ‡ as † is to?
   - A. ‖
   - B. ⊓
   - C. ✝
   - D. †
   - E. ⊤

7. Ɔ is to C as ◠ is to?
   - A. Ⓒ
   - B. C
   - C. ⊃
   - D. D
   - E. C

8. J is to K as 2 is to?

A. ट

B. Ɛ

C. ε

D. K

E. A

9.)) is to (as ?? is to?

A. ꜱ

B. ?

C.)

D. ((

E. ?!

10. ‖ is to ⊣ as ‼ is to?

A. ?!

B. !?

C. ?

D. !

E. ¡

11. ⊎ is to ✚ as Ⓒ is to?

A. Ⓡ

B. ◯

C. Ɔ

D. C

E. Ɔ

12. → is to ← as ↻ is to?

A. ↰

B. ↱

C. ↺

D. ↗

E. ↔

13. ╪ is to ✚ as ❖ is to?

A. ⊞

B. ✚

C. ◈

D. ■

E. ◆

14. ⌐ is to ⌈ as --- is to?

A. ─

B. ╎

C. │

D. □

E. =

15. ▦ is to ⸬ as ◖ is to?

A. ▨

B. ●

C. ◙

D. □

E. ■

STOP

IF YOU FINISH BEFORE TIME IS CALLED, YOU MAY
CHECK YOUR WORK ON THIS SECTION ONLY. DO NOT
TURN TO ANY OTHER SECTION IN THE TEST.

ANSWER KEYS AND EXPLANATIONS

Test 1: Antonyms

1. B	11. D	21. C	31. D	41. B
2. D	12. A	22. B	32. B	42. D
3. C	13. D	23. A	33. C	43. A
4. A	14. B	24. C	34. C	44. D
5. C	15. A	25. C	35. C	45. A
6. B	16. A	26. D	36. A	46. C
7. C	17. C	27. B	37. D	47. A
8. A	18. C	28. A	38. A	48. D
9. C	19. B	29. B	39. C	49. B
10. A	20. D	30. D	40. B	50. B

1. **The correct answer is B.** *Garrulous* means "talkative," so its antonym is *reserved* (choice B), meaning "marked by self restraint, silent, formal." Choice A is incorrect because *talkative* is a synonym for *garrulous*. Choice C is incorrect because *unruly*, means "difficult to control." Fraternal (choice D) means both "brotherly" and "relating to a fraternity," making it incorrect.

2. **The correct answer is D.** *Translucent* means "allowing some light to pass through, semitransparent," so *opaque*, meaning "something that does not allow light to pass through," is its antonym. It is also an antonym of *transparent* (choice C), which is closer to the meaning of *translucent* than to an opposite meaning. Choice A is incorrect because *patent* may mean "the grant of sole rights to an inventor of his or her invention" or "obvious, clear." *Transitory* (choice B) is incorrect because it means "fleeting, short-lived."

3. **The correct answer is C.** *Benevolent* means "generous in helping others, showing kindness," whereas *malevolent* (choice C) means "evil, wicked." Choice A is incorrect because *generous* is similar in meaning to *benevolent*. Choice B is incorrect because *charitable* is also similar in meaning to *benevolent*. The same goes for *good* (choice D).

4. **The correct answer is A.** To be lethargic is to be sluggish, so choice B is incorrect. However, being full of energy is to be energetic, which is the opposite of *lethargic*, so choice A is the correct answer. *Apathetic* (choice C) is incorrect because it means "showing or feeling a lack of interest or little or no emotion; being indifferent," which is not the right antonym for *lethargic*, which is lacking in energy. Choice D is incorrect because *fatal* means "causing death" or "causing destruction."

5. **The correct answer is C.** To be *amicable* is "to be friendly," so *hostile* is the correct answer. Choice A is incorrect because *lonely* is not an antonym for *amicable*, and neither is *reactionary* (choice B), meaning "someone opposed to progress or change" or the adjective meaning "characterized by opposition to progress or change." *Laconic* (choice D) is incorrect because it means "using few words, terse, to the point."

6. **The correct answer is B.** *Tranquility* means "a state or condition of peace and calm," so *tumult*, meaning "a great amount of noise and confusion, a violent disturbance," is the opposite and the correct answer. Choice A is incorrect because *complacency* means "a feeling of satisfaction, contentment," or "smugness" and is neither the same as nor the opposite of *tranquility*. Choice C is incorrect because *plagiarism* is stealing someone else's writing and calling it your own. *Prophecy* (choice D) is a prediction or knowledge of the future which makes this answer incorrect.

7. **The correct answer is C.** To *procrastinate* is "to put off doing something," whereas to *expedite* is "to speed something up, to do something quickly and efficiently." Choice A is incorrect because *elegiac* means "characteristic of an elegy," which is a sad or melancholy poem or song often composed for someone who has died. Choice B is incorrect because *mediate* is "to intervene, to work to bring about an agreement between disputing parties." Choice D is incorrect because an *investiture* is a formal ceremony bestowing certain authority and symbols of that authority on a person.

8. **The correct answer is A.** *Quiescent* means "being quiet, inactive, or still," so *restless* is an antonym. Choice B is incorrect because *slow* is closer in meaning to *quiescent* than to its opposite. Choice C is incorrect because a *mendicant* is a beggar. Choice D is incorrect because *malignant* means "dangerous to health" or "tending to cause harm."

9. **The correct answer is C.** *Deleterious* means "having a harmful effect," whereas *salubrious* means "favorable to health." Choice A is incorrect because *fractious* means "unruly, inclined to troublemaking." Choice B is incorrect because *pathetic* means "deserving of pity" or "inspiring a mix of contempt and pity." *Gullible* (choice D) is incorrect because it means "easily taken advantage of, easily tricked."

10. **The correct answer is A.** *Cognizance* is having knowledge of something, being aware, whereas *ignorance* is the lack of knowledge. Choice B is incorrect because to be in *abeyance* is "to temporarily set aside or suspend." Choice C is incorrect because an *anecdote* is a short account of something that happened and may be humorous. Choice D is incorrect because an *idiom* is an expression whose meaning can't be predicted from the meanings of the individual words.

11. **The correct answer is D.** *Clemency* is mercy or leniency, often in a legal sense, whereas *vindictiveness*, seeking revenge, is the opposite. Choice A is incorrect because *mercy* is the same as *clemency*. Choice B is incorrect because *indulgence* means "extravagance," "yielding to someone else's wishes," or "the act of indulging or gratifying a desire." Choice C is incorrect because *kindness* is not the opposite of *clemency*.

12. **The correct answer is A.** *Ignoble* means "the opposite of noble," that is, "dishonorable, despicable," so *honorable* is an antonym. Choice B is incorrect because *shameful* is closer to the meaning of *ignoble* than to an antonym, which is also true for *disgraceful* (choice C). Choice D is incorrect because *humble* means "meek, modest" or "showing deference and respect."

13. **The correct answer is D.** A *cursory* glance is a quick, superficial or hasty glance, so *thorough* is an appropriate antonym. Choice A is incorrect because *hasty* means the same as *cursory*. Choice B is incorrect because *superficial* is also a meaning of *cursory*. Choice C is incorrect because *awful* doesn't relate to *cursory*.

14. **The correct answer is B.** *Admonish* means "to reprove firmly, but not harshly," that is, "to express disapproval of." The word can also mean "to counsel or warn against." *Praise* is the opposite of "speaking against." Choices A and D are incorrect because both *warn* and *reprove* are meanings of *admonish*. Choice C is incorrect because *advise* means "to offer advice or counsel," which is similar to one meaning of admonish.

15. **The correct answer is A.** *Phlegmatic* means "not easily excited," "not showing a great amount of emotion, or "a calm, sluggish temperament," so *energetic* is an antonym. Choice B is incorrect because *dull* is similar to *phlegmatic*. Choice C is incorrect because *extraordinary* does not relate to *phlegmatic*. Choice D is incorrect because *morbid* means "having an unusual interest in death" or "gruesome, ghoulish."

16. **The correct answer is A.** *Lamentable* means "regrettable, unfortunate, sad," whereas *laughable* is the opposite. Choice B is incorrect because *generous* has no relation to *lamentable*. Choice C is incorrect because *emotional* is not an antonym for *lamentable*. *Doleful* (choice D) is incorrect because it means "causing grief" of "filled with sadness."

17. **The correct answer is C.** *Perilous* means "dangerous, hazardous," so its antonym is *safe*. Choice A is incorrect because *vivacious* means "lively, full of life and spirit." Choice B is incorrect because *unresponsive* means "not responding or reacting." Choice D is incorrect because *hazardous* is a synonym for *perilous*.

18. **The correct answer is C.** *Iniquitous* means "wicked, evil," so *righteous*, meaning "virtuous, without guilt" is its antonym. Choice A is incorrect because *unequaled* has no relation to *iniquitous*, and neither does *unfriendly* (choice B). Choice D is

incorrect because *injurious* means "harmful, causing injury."

19. **The correct answer is B.** *Assiduous* means "diligent, hardworking, persevering," whereas *indifferent* means "apathetic, have no great interest in or for or against something or someone," so it is an antonym of *assiduous*. Choice A is incorrect because *cooperative* has no relation to *assiduous*. *Active* (choice C) is incorrect because it's similar in meaning to *assiduous*. Choice D is incorrect because *satisfactory* has no relation to *assiduous*.

20. **The correct answer is D.** *Corroborate* means "to confirm or support," whereas *dispute* is the opposite—to disagree. Choice A is incorrect because *fascinate* has no relation to *corroborate*; neither does *corrupt* (choice B). Choice C is incorrect because *confirm* is a synonym rather than an antonym for *corroborate*.

21. **The correct answer is C.** *Confluence* means "a point where things merge, often two rivers," whereas a *divergence* is the act or result of diverging, that is, moving apart. Choice A is incorrect because a *convention* is a gathering together, so it's close in meaning to *confluence*, rather than being opposite in meaning. Choice B is incorrect because *sympathy* means "sharing another's feelings or emotions." Choice D is incorrect because *concurrence* means "agreement," "cooperation," or "coincidence."

22. **The correct answer is B.** *Dastardly* means "cowardly, mean, malicious," whereas *bravely* is the opposite. Choice A is incorrect because *cowardly* is one of the definitions of *dastardly*. Choice C is incorrect because *friendly* has no relation to *dastardly*. Choice D is incorrect because *sinfully* is not the same as *dastardly* but is close in meaning.

23. **The correct answer is A.** *Abstruse* means "difficult to understand, incomprehensible to ordinary people," so *understandable* is the opposite. Choice B is incorrect because *hidden* is similar in meaning to *abstruse*. Choice C is incorrect because *absurd*, meaning "ridiculously or completely false," has no relation to *abstruse*. Choice D is incorrect because *religious* has no relation to *abstruse*.

24. **The correct answer is C.** An *illusion* is a false idea or belief, or a false or misleading perception, so *reality* is the opposite. Choice A is incorrect because a delusion is a false belief that a person holds despite evidence to the contrary, so it is similar to an *illusion*, rather than being an antonym. Choice B is incorrect because a conception is the creation of something, such as an idea, plan, or design. Choice D is incorrect because a dramatization is acting out a scene or play or the conversion of a piece of writing into a dramatic presentation.

25. **The correct answer is C.** To be *avaricious* is to be greedy, so its antonym is *generous*. Choice A is incorrect because *greedy* is a definition of *avaricious*. Choice B is incorrect because *persuasive* has no relation to *avaricious*, and neither does *gracious* (choice D).

26. **The correct answer is D.** *Coerce* means "to force someone to do or think in a certain way by means of threats or violence," whereas *encourage* means "to inspire with courage, spirit, or hope." Choice A is incorrect because *enforce*, "to compel obedience," is similar to *coerce* rather than being an antonym. *Cohere* (choice B) meaning "to stick or hold together" is incorrect. Choice C is incorrect because *forestall* means "to delay or stop something from happening" or "to anticipate."

27. **The correct answer is B.** *Temerity* means "foolhardiness, recklessness, daring," which is the opposite of *prudence*, meaning "caution" and "care taken in managing one's resources." Choice A is incorrect because *recklessness* is a definition of *temerity*. Choice C is incorrect because *support* has no relation to *temerity*, nor does *sanity* (choice D).

28. **The correct answer is A.** *Laconic* means "terse, using few words," whereas *verbose*, meaning "wordy," is the opposite. Choice B is incorrect because *concise*, meaning "brief, using few words," is a synonym. Choice C is incorrect because *serene*, meaning "calm," has no relation to *laconic*. Choice D is incorrect because *interesting* has no relation to *laconic*.

29. **The correct answer is B.** A *credulous* person is someone who believes too easily what people say without evidence, whereas a *skeptical* person is one who tends to doubt what people say. Choice A is incorrect because *exuberant* means "full of joy," "full of life or vitality," or "lavish;" none of these definitions bears a relation to *credulous*, nor does *dangerous* (choice C). *Legible* (choice D), meaning "apparent" or "able to read," has no relation to *credulous*.

30. **The correct answer is D.** To incarcerate someone is "to imprison" the person, so to *release* a person is the opposite. Choice A is incorrect because *immunize* is either "to grant a person protection from prosecution" or "to vaccinate against disease." Choice B is incorrect because *anesthetize* is "to administer anesthesia." *Transport* (choice C) meaning "to move or carry" is incorrect.

31. **The correct answer is D.** *Obtuse* means "insensitive emotionally" or "not sharp or pointed," whereas *acute*, meaning "perceptive" or "having a sharp point or end," is the antonym. Choice A is incorrect

because *oblique* means "slanting, sloping." Choice B is incorrect because *obese* means "excessively overweight." Choice C is incorrect because *perpendicular* means "being at right angles to a horizontal plane."

32. **The correct answer is B.** *Munificent* means "very generous," whereas *miserly* means "very stingy." Choice A is incorrect because *political* has no relation to *munificent*. Choice C is incorrect because *liberal* may mean "generous, munificent," so it is a synonym. Choice D is incorrect because *educational* has no relation to *munificent*.

33. **The correct answer is C.** *Deranged* means "driven insane, insane," whereas *sane* is the opposite. Choice A is incorrect because *unsettled*, meaning "disturbed, unpredictable," is closer to the meaning of *deranged* than to its opposite. Choice B is incorrect because *paralyzed* has no relation to *deranged*, and neither does *awkward* (choice D).

34. **The correct answer is C.** *Levity* means "lack of appropriate seriousness, lighthearted behavior," whereas *gravity*, meaning "seriousness," is the opposite. Choice A is incorrect because *flippancy* means "disrespectful and inappropriate levity," so it is a synonym. Choice B is incorrect because *peace* has no relation to *levity*, and neither does *trickery* (choice D).

35. **The correct answer is C.** *Equanimity* means "calmness of temperament and/or mind," whereas *agitation*, being in a state of excitement or worry, is the opposite. Choice A is incorrect because *peace* is similar to *equanimity*. Choice B is incorrect because *inflation* means "being pompous" or "a general increase in prices." Choice D is incorrect because *tranquility* means "free from stress or emotion" and so is close in

meaning to *equanimity* rather than being an antonym.

36. **The correct answer is A.** To *maraud* is "to raid and rob, to attack and rob," whereas to *purchase* is the opposite. Choice B is incorrect because *plunder*, meaning "to rob, especially in time of war" is a synonym. Choice C is incorrect because *masticate* is "to chew." Choice D is incorrect because *elevate* is "to raise up."

37. **The correct answer is D.** An encomium is warm praise of someone, a tribute, whereas *defamation* is falsely accusing someone or falsely attacking a person's character. Choice A is incorrect because *immorality* is the lack of moral qualities or behaving without morals. While choice A may be tempting, *defamation* is a better choice for the answer. Choice B is incorrect because *praise* is a synonym for *encomium*. *Egotism* (choice C), meaning "an inflated sense of self-worth," has no relation to *ecomium*.

38. **The correct answer is A.** *Abominable* means "hateful, detestable" or "very bad or displeasing," so the antonym is *delightful*. Choice B is incorrect because *horrible* is closer to being a synonym for *abominable* as it means "dreadful" or "very unpleasant, disagreeable." Choices C and D are incorrect because *meaningful* and *insane* have no relation to *abominable*.

39. **The correct answer is C.** *Abstemious* means "moderate or sparing, especially in regard to eating and drinking." *Greedy*, on the other hand, means "excessively desirous of acquiring wealth, avaricious, acquisitive." Choice A is incorrect because *frugal* means "thrifty" or "not costly," so it's a synonym of *abstemious*. Choice B is incorrect because *happy* has no relation to *abstemious*. Choice D is incorrect because *radiant* has no relation to *abstemious*.

40. **The correct answer is B.** *Advertent* means "paying or giving attention or care to," whereas *inconsiderate* means "lacking in care or thought or others, thoughtless." Choice A is incorrect because *retentive*, meaning "having the power or capacity to retain information, good at remembering," is a synonym for *advertent*. Choice C is incorrect because *empathetic* means "understanding and identifying with others' feelings." *Abnormal* (choice D) is incorrect because it has no relation to *advertent*.

41. **The correct answer is B.** Something that is *enigmatic* is mysterious or puzzling, whereas something that is *explicit* is clearly expressed, not implied. Choice A is incorrect because *perplexing* is similar to *enigmatic*. Choice C is incorrect because *persistent* means "refusing to give up" and has no relation to *enigmatic*. Choice D is incorrect because *officious* means "unnecessarily or excessively eager" or "intruding in an offensive way."

42. **The correct answer is D.** *Execrable* means "hateful," "disgusting, unpleasant," or "of very poor quality," whereas *pleasant* is its opposite. Choice A is incorrect because *unusual* has no relation to *execrable*. The same goes for choice C because *fallible* means "capable of error or mistakes." Choice B is incorrect because *detestable* is a synonym for *execrable*, not an antonym.

43. **The correct answer is A.** *Ignominious* means "shameful or disgraceful" or "deserving of shame or disgrace," whereas *reputable* means "honorable, having a good reputation." Choice B is incorrect because *shameful* is a definition of *ignominious*. Choice C is incorrect because *intangible* means "not able to be perceived by touch" or "unclear," and neither definition relates to *ignominious*. Choice D is incorrect because *irascible* means "easily angered."

44. **The correct answer is D.** *Sagacity* is wisdom, whereas *stupidity* is its opposite. Choice A is incorrect because *sorrowfulness* has no relation to sagacity. Choices B and C are incorrect because *support* and *satisfaction* have no relation to *sagacity*.

45. **The correct answer is A.** *Proverbial* means "widely known" and also "conventional, traditional," so *innovative* is its opposite. Choice B is incorrect because *current* means "in the here and now." Choice C is incorrect because *wise* has no relation to *proverbial*. Choice D is incorrect because *cautious* has no relation to *proverbial*.

46. **The correct answer is C.** *Annihilate* means "to destroy completely, to wipe out, to abolish," whereas *preserve* is the opposite. Choice A is incorrect because *advertise* has no relation to *annihilate*. Choice B is incorrect because *destroy* is a synonym for *annihilate*. Choice D is incorrect because *announce* has no relation to *annihilate*.

47. **The correct answer is A.** An *affable* person is kind, easy to talk to, and approachable. The opposite is a *discourteous* person, one lacking in courtesy. Choice B is incorrect because *beloved* has no relation to *affable*. Choice C is incorrect because *sociable* is a near synonym for *affable*. Choice D is incorrect because *debonair* means "refined, urbane" and also "affable," so it also is a synonym.

48. **The correct answer is D.** *Capricious* means "liable to sudden and unpredictable changes in behavior or attitude," whereas *constant* is the opposite. Choice A is incorrect because *erratic* is a synonym for *capricious*. Choices B and C are incorrect because *agreeable* and *awkward* have no relation to *capricious*.

49. **The correct answer is B.** *Contingent* means "dependent on events or circumstances," whereas *independent* is the opposite. Choice A is incorrect because *conditional* means "depending on other factors," so it's a synonym. Choice C is incorrect because *confined* means "restricted within certain bounds" or "kept in." Choice D is incorrect because *familiar* has no relation to *contingent*.

50. **The correct answer is B.** *Pretentious* means "trying to be something that one isn't, claiming a distinction or importance that is not deserved," whereas *modest*, or humble, is the opposite. Choice A is incorrect because *meddling* means "intruding on others' lives, interfering." *Emaciated* (choice C) means "excessively thin, especially from disease or hunger" making it incorrect. Choice D is incorrect because *pompous*, meaning "arrogant" or "egotistic," is a synonym.

Test 2: Antonyms

1. B	5. C	9. D	13. C	17. E
2. D	6. B	10. D	14. B	18. B
3. B	7. A	11. B	15. D	19. B
4. A	8. B	12. E	16. B	20. C

1. **The correct answer is B.** *Deceit* means "a trick, fraud" or "misleading someone deliberately, a misrepresentation," whereas *truthfulness* is the opposite. Choice A is incorrect because *fraud* is a definition of *deceit*. Choice C is incorrect because *treachery* is also a synonym for *deceit*. Choice D is incorrect because *imposition* means "something forced on a person," which has no relation to *deceit*.

2. **The correct answer is D.** *Docile* means "teachable" or "willing to be managed or supervised," so *inflexible*, meaning "unwilling, obstinate" as well as "rigid, stiff," is the opposite. Choice A is incorrect because *teachable* is a definition of *docile*. *Compliant* (choice B) means "willing to be managed, to agree to do something as requested or required by someone else," so it's a synonym for *docile*. Choice C is incorrect because *tame* means "docile."

3. **The correct answer is B.** *Hurtful* is the opposite of *harmless*. Choice A is incorrect because *safe* is not an antonym for *harmless*. Choice C is incorrect because *innocent* is not an antonym, and neither is *innocuous* (choice D), meaning "harmless," making it a synonym instead.

4. **The correct answer is A.** *Melancholy* means "tendency to depression, gloominess," whereas the opposite is *jolly*. Choice B is incorrect because *low-spirited* is similar to *melancholy*. Choice C is incorrect because *dreamy* means "impractical, vague," "lacking liveliness," or "gentle, relaxing," none of which fits as an opposite of *melancholy*. Choice D is incorrect because *sad* is closer in meaning to *melancholy* than to an antonym.

5. **The correct answer is C.** *Impetuous* means "impulsive, acting quickly without a great amount of thought," whereas *calm* is its opposite. Choice A is incorrect because *violent* is not an antonym. *Furious* (choice B) and *vehement* (choice D) are incorrect because both have an element of intensity, and neither is an antonym of *impetuous*.

6. **The correct answer is B.** The opposite of *joy* is *grief*. Choice A is incorrect because *gladness* is similar to joy, not the opposite. Choice C is incorrect because *mirth*, meaning "gladness and laughter," may express a feeling of joy. Choice D is incorrect because *delight* is closer in meaning to *joy* than to an opposite idea.

7. **The correct answer is A.** *Lunacy* means "insanity," so *sanity* is its opposite. Choices B, C, and D are all synonyms for *lunacy*, rather than being antonyms.

8. **The correct answer is B.** *Moist* and *dry* are antonyms. Choice A is incorrect because *dank* means "*damp* or *humid*" (choices C and D).

9. **The correct answer is D.** *Puerile* means "juvenile" or "immature, childish," so the opposite is *mature*. Choice A is incorrect because *youthful* is a synonym for the first meaning. Choice B is incorrect because *weak* has no relation to *puerile*. Choice C is incorrect because *silly* is closer in meaning to *puerile* than its opposite.

10. **The correct answer is D.** *Weight* may mean "emphasis, importance" so *triviality*, meaning "something unimportant, frivolous" can be its antonym. Choice A is incorrect because *gravity* means "seriousness, importance," so it's a synonym. Choices B and C are incorrect because *heaviness* and *lightness* are qualities of weight.

11. **The correct answer is B.** *Superfluous*, *excessive*, *gratuitous*, and *dispensable* all mean "beyond what is needed," whereas *necessary* (choice B) is the opposite and, therefore, the most different from the others.

12. **The correct answer is E.** *Reform*, *amend*, *correct*, and *better* all mean "to improve." *Corrupt* (choice E), meaning "to pervert, to cause someone to become dishonest, to destroy someone's integrity," is the word most different from the others.

13. **The correct answer is C.** *Scanty*, *bare*, *insufficient*, and *meager* all mean "limited, not enough, small," whereas *ample* means "large, more than sufficient, abundant" and thus is the word most different from the others.

14. **The correct answer is B.** *Misery*, *woe*, *tribulation*, and *affliction* all relate to a state of trouble or suffering. *Happiness* (choice B) is the opposite of all of these and so is the word most different from the others.

15. **The correct answer is D.** *Proper*, *legitimate*, *appropriate*, and *pertinent* all mean "correct, fitting," and are the opposite of *wrong*. Choice D is the word most different from the others.

16. **The correct answer is B.** *Incongruous*, *alien*, *contrary*, and *disparate* all mean "incompatible, different from," so *compatible* (choice B) is the antonym and the word most different from the others.

17. **The correct answer is E.** *Fatigue*, *lassitude*, *weariness*, and *malaise* all mean "tiredness, weariness." *Vigor*, meaning "mental or physical strength, energy" or "enthusiasm, intensity," is the opposite of these and the word most different from the others.

18. **The correct answer is B.** *Hasten*, *accelerate*, *dispatch*, and *expedite* all relate to doing something in a hurry, whereas *delay* (choice B) is "to postpone," "to hinder, to cause to be late," or "to linger" and so is the word most different from the others.

19. **The correct answer is B.** *Absorb*, *engulf*, *engross*, and *consume* all relate to taking in, enveloping, or occupying, whereas *emit* (choice B) means "to give out or off, to release, to discharge," and so is the word most different from the others.

20. **The correct answer is C.** *Abuse*, *defilement*, *violation*, and *offense* all mean "misuse" as well as "maltreatment," whereas *shelter* (choice C) relates to protection and, therefore, is the word most different from the others.

Test 3: Synonyms

1. C	11. D	21. D	31. D	41. B
2. A	12. B	22. C	32. B	42. D
3. B	13. B	23. C	33. C	43. C
4. D	14. A	24. B	34. A	44. A
5. C	15. C	25. C	35. D	45. B
6. A	16. B	26. B	36. B	46. C
7. D	17. D	27. D	37. C	47. B
8. B	18. B	28. A	38. C	48. C
9. A	19. A	29. C	39. D	49. B
10. C	20. D	30. A	40. A	50. A

1. **The correct answer is C.** *Futile* and *useless* are synonyms. Choices A, B, and D are incorrect because *strong*, *clumsy*, and *sincere* have no relation to *futile*.

2. **The correct answer is A.** *Exhausted* may mean "used up," which makes it a synonym for *depleted* in this sentence. *Delivered* and *rejected* (choices B and D) make sense in the sentence, but are not synonyms, so they are incorrect. Choice C is incorrect because *included* is not a synonym.

3. **The correct answer is B.** *Essence* means "essential part, central meaning" and is a synonym for *gist*. Choices A, C, and D could fit the sense of the sentence, but *end*, *strength*, and *spirit* are not synonyms for *gist*.

4. **The correct answer is D.** *Valor* and *courage* are synonyms. Although choices A and B may fit the sense of the sentence, *injury* and *ability* are not synonyms for *valor*. *Cooperation* (choice C) isn't a synonym and doesn't make sense.

5. **The correct answer is C.** *Auspicious* and *promising* are synonyms. Choice A is incorrect because *bleak*, meaning "gloomy, somber, with little hope" or "cold and damp," is an antonym. The same goes for *somber* (choice D). Choice B is incorrect because *uncertain* is also an antonym.

6. **The correct answer is A.** *Consternation* and *dismay* are synonyms. *Amazement* (choice B); *incompetence* (choice C), meaning "lack of physical or intellectual ability;" and *annoyance* (choice D) all work in the context but are incorrect because none of these words are synonyms for *consternation*.

7. **The correct answer is D.** *Indolence* and *idleness*, or being inactive, are synonyms. Choice A is incorrect because *inability* is not a habit. Choice B is incorrect because *snoring* makes no sense. Choice C is incorrect because, although *carelessness* may be a habit, it's not a synonym for *indolence*.

8. **The correct answer is B.** *Cogent*, meaning "convincing, persuasive," and *convincing* are synonyms. The other choices fit the sense of the sentence, but *pleasing, flattering,* and *slandering* aren't synonyms for *cogent*.

9. **The correct answer is A.** *Prolific* means "producing a great amount of work," so *productive* is a synonym. Choices B, C, and D could all fit the sense of the sentence, but *popular, frank,* and *effective* aren't synonyms.

10. **The correct answer is C.** *Meticulous* means "very careful" or "excessively concerned with details," so *scrupulous*, meaning "painstaking, conscientious," is a synonym. Choice A is incorrect because *careless* is an antonym. Choice B is incorrect because *patient*, while tempting, is not a synonym. Choice D is incorrect because *nervous* is not a synonym.

11. **The correct answer is D.** *Sporadic* means "intermittent, occurring at irregular intervals" so *scattered*, meaning "to occur at widely spaced time periods," is a synonym. Choice A is incorrect because *epidemic* may mean "spreading an infection rapidly and over a wide area to infect many people" and thus is an antonym. Choice B is incorrect because *widespread* has no relation to *sporadic*. Choice C is incorrect because *serious* fits the sense but is not a synonym.

12. **The correct answer is B.** Even if you didn't know the meaning of *dissent*, the context tells you that you're looking for a negative word. That rules out *approving* (choice D). You can eliminate choice A because "annoying votes" doesn't make sense. If you're not sure about the meaning of *abstaining* ("choosing not to vote, refraining from voting"), go on to the next word, *disagreeing*, which does make sense and is the best answer.

13. **The correct answer is B.** *Traditional* and *customary* are synonyms. *Normal* (choice A) is tempting but is incorrect because it means "regular, typical" and doesn't quite have the same connotation as *traditional*, meaning "conventional, standard, what is commonly accepted." Although also a tempting choice, *ordinary* (choice C) is incorrect for the same reason. Choice D is incorrect because *gracious* has no relation to *traditional*.

14. **The correct answer is A.** *Rescinded* and *canceled* are synonyms. Choice B is incorrect because *revised* is "to rework" or "to rewrite," which is not the same as *rescinding* something. Choice C is incorrect because *confirmed* is an antonym. Choice D is incorrect because *misinterpreted* has no relation to *rescinded*.

15. **The correct answer is C.** *Vindictive* and *revengeful* are synonyms. Choice A is incorrect because *prejudiced* means "being biased, having an opinion or belief based on emotions." *Vindictive* is a more intense word. Choice B is incorrect because *impatient* has no relation to *vindictive*, but the sentence might lead you incorrectly to choose this answer because of the phrase "released early," which is why it's important to read questions quickly but carefully. Choice D is incorrect because *unreasonable* has no relation to *vindictive*.

16. **The correct answer is B.** *Sedulous* means "persevering, persistent," so *persistent* is a synonym. Choices A, C, and D are incorrect because *eager*, *intelligent*, and *inexperienced* are not synonyms.

17. **The correct answer is D.** To *interrogate* is "to *question*." *Arrested*, *detained*, and *investigated* all make sense in the context but aren't synonyms for *interrogate*.

18. **The correct answer is B.** To *disparage* is "to speak in disapproving terms, to belittle," so *belittled* is a synonym. *Explained*, *demonstrated*, and *elucidated* could fit the sentence but these words are not synonyms for *disparage*. *Elucidate* (choice D) means "to explain in order to clarify, to make clear."

19. **The correct answer is A.** To *permeate* is "to pass through, to penetrate," or ""to spread throughout," so *penetrate* and *permeate* in this sentence are synonyms. *Wet*, *harm*, and

discolor may seem to make sense but they're not synonyms.

20. **The correct answer is D.** *Docile* means "easy to manage, submissive," so *obedient* is a synonym. Choice A is incorrect because *mongrel* refers to a type of dog. Choice B is incorrect because *hungry* has no relation to *docile*. Choice C is incorrect because *intractable* means "difficult to manage" and so is an antonym.

21. **The correct answer is D.** To *amalgamate* is "to combine, unite, merge," so *merge* is a synonym. The other choices, *close, expand,* and *relocate,* make sense in the sentence, but aren't synonyms for *amalgamate*.

22. **The correct answer is C.** *Frivolous,* meaning "trivial, not serious, silly" and *unimportant* are synonyms. Choice A is incorrect because *sweet* has no relation to *frivolous*. Both choices B and D may be tempting because frivolous things can be cheap or expensive. However, in this case, *unimportant* is the best answer choice.

23. **The correct answer is C.** To *divulge* is "to reveal." Choice A is incorrect because, while the teacher might for some reason *whisper* the grades, it is not a synonym. Choice B is incorrect because *disregarded* has no relation to *divulged*. Choice D is incorrect because *averaged* has no relation to *divulged*, though it does make sense in the context.

24. **The correct answer is B.** A *salary* is the same as *remuneration*. Choice A is incorrect because a *reimbursement* is a repayment of money spent, not a wage for a job done. Choice C is incorrect because *indemnity* means "money compensation for damage, loss, or injury." Choice D is incorrect because a *reparation* is money paid to compensate for an injury or insult.

25. **The correct answer is C.** *Scrutinized* means "to examine closely," so *inspected* is a synonym. *Touched* and *measured* (choices A and D) make sense in the context but neither is a synonym for *scrutinized*. Choice B is incorrect because *bought* has no relation to *scrutinized*.

26. **The correct answer is B.** *Decrepit* means "weakened, worn out, or broken down," so *weak* is a synonym. The other choices, *slippery, swaying,* and *flooded,* make sense in context, but are not synonyms and, therefore, are incorrect.

27. **The correct answer is D.** *Conceded* is the same as *admitted*. Choice A is incorrect because *denied* is an antonym. Choice B is incorrect because *explained* means merely "to make something understandable"; it doesn't include the idea of admitting something. Choice C is incorrect because *complained* has no relation to *conceded*.

28. **The correct answer is A.** *Obsolete* means "out-of-date." Choice B is incorrect because *new* is an antonym. *Reliable* and *complicated* (choices C and D) make sense in context but are not synonyms.

29. **The correct answer is C.** *Candid* means "frank, outspoken, open, unreserved," so *frank* is a synonym. *Biased, confidential,* and *insulting* make sense in context but are not synonyms for *candid*. *Confidential* may tempt you, but it means "something spoken, written, or given in confidence" as well as "secret."

30. **The correct answer is A.** *Incoherently* means the same as *disconnectedly*. Choice B is incorrect because *cohesively* means "sticking together" or "consistent, logically connected," so it's an antonym rather than a synonym. Choice C is incorrect because *prodigiously* means "extraordinary" or "huge in size, extent, or force." Choice D is

incorrect because *sluggishly* means "slowly" or "lacking in energy."

31. **The correct answer is D.** To *pacify* is "to calm." Choice A is incorrect because *detain*, meaning "to stop," is not a synonym. Choice B is incorrect because *restrain* is "to hold back, to control." Choice C is incorrect because *accompany* has no relation to *pacify*.

32. **The correct answer is B.** *Vivacious* and *lively* are synonyms. *Kind*, *short*, and *talkative* work in the sentence but are not synonyms for *vivacious*.

33. **The correct answer is C.** *Devastated* means "destroyed." Choice A is incorrect because *rebuilt* is an antonym. Choice B is incorrect because a devastated town may be *deserted*, but that is not a synonym. Choice D is incorrect because *saved* is not a synonym.

34. **The correct answer is A.** One meaning of *digress* is "to deviate or depart from a direct course," so *deviated* is a synonym. Choice B is incorrect because *repose* means "to put something somewhere" or "to lie down for rest." Choice C is incorrect because *alight* means "to come to rest, to settle." Choice D is incorrect because *moored* is what one does with a boat, that is, make it fast or tie it up at a dock.

35. **The correct answer is D.** *Gallant* and *chivalrous*, meaning "gallant, courteous, gentlemanly," are synonyms. Choice A is incorrect because *rude* is the opposite. Choice B is incorrect because *fastidious* means "showing careful attention to detail," "difficult to please," or "fussy." Choice C is incorrect because *cowardly* has no relation to *gallant*.

36. **The correct answer is B.** *Reflect* can mean the same as *demonstrate*. Choice A is incorrect because *contemplate* means "to

think about intently." Choice C is incorrect because *imitate* means "to use something as a model, to reproduce," and the context doesn't suggest this meaning. Choice D is incorrect because *possessed* has no relation to *reflect*.

37. **The correct answer is C.** *Querulous* means "*complaining*, grumbling." A *satisfied* or *cheerful* person wouldn't be complaining, so choices A and B are incorrect. Choice D is incorrect because pain might make a person complain, but *painful* is not a synonym.

38. **The correct answer is C.** To be *vigilant* is "to be watchful, *observant*." Choice A is incorrect because *careful* may tempt you, but it is not as close a synonym as *observant* is. Choice B is incorrect because *continuous* is not a synonym. Choice D is incorrect because *reciprocal* means "something concerning two or more people or things."

39. **The correct answer is D.** *Satirically* and *ironically* are synonyms when they mean "witty, humorous language used to convey insults or ridicule." Choice A is incorrect because *contemptuously* means "without respect, scornfully," and while close in meaning to *satirically*, *ironically* is the closer match. Choice B is incorrect because *interminably* means "seemingly endless" or "tedious." Choice C is incorrect because *musically* is not a synonym.

40. **The correct answer is A.** An *antipathy* is an *aversion*, or strong dislike, disgust, loathing. Choice B is incorrect because *fondness* is the opposite. Choice C is incorrect because an *interest* implies a positive feeling, which makes it closer to an antonym than a synonym. Choice D is incorrect because *fear* may tempt you, but that is not a synonym.

41. **The correct answer is B.** A premonition is a *forewarning*, a sense or feeling of evil about the future. Choice A is incorrect because a premonition is a feeling, not a *vision*. Choice C is incorrect because *recurrence* means "something that happens again" or "a returning thought or memory." Choice D is incorrect because *apprehend* means "to understand" as well as "to arrest."

42. **The correct answer is D.** To *appropriate* means "to seize, to confiscate." Choice A is incorrect because *stored* has no relation to *confiscated*. Choice B is incorrect because *distributed* is an antonym for *confiscated*. Choice C is incorrect because *destroyed* makes sense in the context but is not a synonym for *confiscated*.

43. **The correct answer is C.** *Impropriety* means "an improper act or behavior," so *dishonesty* is its synonym. Choice A is incorrect because *age* has no relation to *impropriety*. Choices B and D are incorrect because tardiness and absenteeism may be improper, but being late or absent is not a synonym for *impropriety*.

44. **The correct answer is A.** *Tangible*, meaning "possible to touch" or "real and concrete," and *concrete*, meaning "able to be perceived, real," are synonyms. Choice B is incorrect because *theoretical* is an antonym. Choice C is incorrect because *verified* means "having determined the truth of something." Choice D is incorrect because *scientific* might work in the context but is not a synonym.

45. **The correct answer is B.** *Blithe* means "happy, *cheerful*," as well as "carefree." Choice A is incorrect because *free* is not the same as *carefree*, meaning "without any worries or responsibilities." Choice C is incorrect because *kind* has no direct relation to *blithe*. Choice D is incorrect because *insolent* means "arrogant, disrespectful."

46. **The correct answer is C.** To *deliberate* is "to think carefully, often with a group," that is, "to *consider*." All the other choices, *met, convened,* and *summarized,* make sense in context, but they are not synonyms for *deliberated*.

47. **The correct answer is B.** *Sinister* means "ominous," "threatening," or "*treacherous*." *Practical, important,* and *honest* make sense in the context but are not synonyms.

48. **The correct answer is C.** *Stringent* means "severe," "tight," or "*rigid*." *Unusual, numerous,* and *lax* work in the sentence, but they are not synonyms.

49. **The correct answer is B.** *Prerogative* means "exclusive *right* or privilege." *Demands* and *ideals* (choices A and C) make sense in the context, but they are not synonyms. Choice D can be eliminated because it is not a synonym.

50. **The correct answer is A.** *Destitute* means "poverty-stricken," in other words, *impoverished*. Choice B is incorrect because *detained* means "stopped, not allowed to leave" or "confined in custody." Choice C is incorrect because *loathed* means "hated." Choice D is incorrect because *ill* is not a synonym for *destitute*.

Test 4: Synonyms

1. D	**5.** C	**9.** A	**13.** A	**17.** B
2. B	**6.** D	**10.** D	**14.** C	**18.** B
3. C	**7.** A	**11.** C	**15.** C	**19.** B
4. A	**8.** B	**12.** A	**16.** A	**20.** D

1. **The correct answer is D.** A *competent* person is a *capable* person. Choice A is incorrect because being *agreeable* has no relation to being competent. Choice B is incorrect because *inept* is an antonym. Choice C is incorrect because *vigorous* has nothing to do with competence.

2. **The correct answer is B.** *Omnibus* means "providing for many things at once, comprehensive," so *all-embracing* is a synonym. Choice A is incorrect because *threatening* has no relation to *omnibus*. Neither does *rotund* (choice C), meaning "round," and *slow-moving* (choice D).

3. **The correct answer is C.** *Ingenuity* means "*cleverness*, inventiveness." *Deceitfulness*, *appeal*, and *innocence* are not synonyms.

4. **The correct answer is A.** *Concave* means "*curving inward*." Choice B is incorrect because it's the reverse of *concave*. Choices C and D are incorrect because they do not describe the shape correctly.

5. **The correct answer is C.** *Canon* means "a *guiding principle*, a collection of such rules or laws." *Barrier*, *noisy place*, and *rigorous* are not synonyms.

6. **The correct answer is D.** *Propitious* means "*favorable*, auspicious." *Questionable*, *well-known*, and *free* do not have any relation to *propitious*.

7. **The correct answer is A.** *Vacillating* means "indecisive, uncertain, moving back and forth from one opinion or course of action to another," so *changeable* is a synonym. Choice B is incorrect because *decisive* is an antonym. Choice C is incorrect because *equalizing*, "making things equal," is not a synonym. Choice D is incorrect because *progressing* may be movement, but it's not a synonym.

8. **The correct answer is B.** To *forfeit* is "to give up something as a penalty, to surrender something," in other words, to *relinquish* something. Choice A is incorrect because *exchange* is not a synonym. Neither *protect* nor *withdraw* (choices C and D) is a synonym.

9. **The correct answer is A.** To *query* is "to *question*." Choice B is incorrect because you might come up with a query after *looking over something carefully*, but choice B is not a synonym. Choice C is incorrect because *following through* is not a synonym, and neither is *acting peculiarly* (choice D).

10. **The correct answer is D.** *Steadfast* means "dependable, especially in terms of loyalty" or "determined, resolute," so *unwavering*, meaning "resolute, determined," is a synonym. *Strong* (choice B) may be tempting, but it is not as close in meaning as *unwavering*. Choices A and C are incorrect because *gradual* and *friendly* have no relation to *steadfast*.

11. **The correct answer is C.** *Access* is *admittance*. Choice A is incorrect because *too much* is not a synonym, but on a quick read you might think that *access* was *excess*. Read quickly but with concentration, so you don't fall into a trap like this. Choices

B and D are incorrect because *extra* and *arrival* are not synonyms.

12. **The correct answer is A.** *Permutation* means "a complete change," or "one thing is substituted for another," so the word that is the closest in meaning is *alteration*, meaning "a change, a modification." Choice B is incorrect because *permission* is not the same. Choice C is incorrect because *combination* is not a synonym either. Choice D is incorrect because *seepage* means "process of leaking or oozing."

13. **The correct answer is A.** To *spritz* is "to spray." *Bubble*, *protrude*, and *sail* do not have any relation to *spritz*. *Protrude* (choice C) means "to stick out."

14. **The correct answer is C.** *Personable* means "*attractive*, pleasing." Choice A is incorrect because *intimate* means "deeply personal," or "characteristic of a close or warm personal relationship." Choice B is incorrect because *cheerful* is not a synonym. Choice D is incorrect because *superficial* means "on the surface, insignificant" and is closer to being an antonym than a synonym.

15. **The correct answer is C.** *Expedite* means "to hurry up something, to speed up," so *accelerate* is its synonym. Choices A and B are incorrect because *dismiss* and *advise* are not synonyms. Choice D is incorrect because *demolish* means "to tear down, to destroy."

16. **The correct answer is A.** *Compulsory* means "required, obligatory" and *imperative* means "obligatory" as well as "urgent." Choice B is incorrect because *impossible* has no relation to *compulsory*. Choice C is incorrect because *imminent* means "about to occur." Choice D is incorrect because *logical* has no relation to *compulsory*.

17. **The correct answer is B.** *Practicable* means "*feasible*, able to happen." Choice A is incorrect because *lenient* means "generous, not harsh." Choice C is incorrect because *simple* has no relation to *practicable*, and neither does *visible* (choice D).

18. **The correct answer is B.** *Agree* and *acquiesce* are synonyms. *Inquire, discharge,* and *endeavor* have no relation to *agree* and are, therefore, incorrect answers. *Endeavor* (choice D) means "to attempt to do something by great effort" or "an activity undertaken with great purpose and industry, that is, hard work."

19. **The correct answer is B.** *Florid* is similar to *ruddy*, meaning "flushed, rosy colored." *Overflowing, seedy,* and *flowery*, are not synonyms.

20. **The correct answer is D.** *Nearness* and *proximity* are synonyms. Choice A is incorrect because *adherence* means "attachment to something, loyal support." Choice B is incorrect because *declivity* means "downward slope." Choice C is incorrect because *worldliness* has no relation to *nearness*.

Test 5: English Grammar and Usage

1. C	4. A	7. B	10. A	13. C
2. B	5. C	8. C	11. A	14. B
3. D	6. A	9. B	12. D	15. C

1. **The correct answer is C.** *Neither* functions in this sentence as a correlative conjunction joining the words *rain* and *snow*, which serve as the compound subject. As a correlative conjunction, *neither* is always paired with *nor*. This allows us to rule out choices A and B. Singular subjects joined by *or* or *nor* take a singular verb, which allows us to rule out choice D.

2. **The correct answer is B.** The indefinite pronouns *everyone* and *no one* are in third-person singular and thus require third-person singular verb forms (*is* and *likes*). Therefore, choices A, C, and D cannot be correct.

3. **The correct answer is D.** In this sentence, *looks* functions as a linking verb, linking the subject *it* to the predicate adjectives *sunny* and *beautiful*. Choice A is incorrect because transitive verbs have an object, which *looks* does not. Choice B is incorrect because a helping verb is used together with another verb to express an action or make a statement, but *looks* is used alone in this sentence. Choice C is incorrect because action verbs express an action, whereas *looks* does not.

4. **The correct answer is A.** *We* is the subject of this sentence and thus is in the nominative case. Choice B is incorrect because *we* is not the object of a verb or preposition and thus is not in the objective case. Choice C is incorrect because *we* is not showing possession and thus is not in the possessive case. Choice D is incorrect because *we* is not expressing a wish or something contrary to reality and thus is not in the subjunctive (which is a mood, not a case).

5. **The correct answer is C.** An indirect object is a person or thing for which or to which an action is taken and is used in conjunction with a direct object. In this sentence, Megan is handing the keys *to* Dillon; thus, choice A is incorrect because *keys* is the direct object, and choice C is correct because *Dillon* is the indirect object. Choice B is incorrect because *them*, which refers back to *keys*, is the direct object of the verb *put*. Choice D is incorrect because *pocket* is the object of the preposition *in*.

6. **The correct answer is A.** The subjunctive mood is used to express a wish or something contrary to reality. In choice A, Thomas is not the speaker's partner in Spades, so the subjunctive (which is formed in the past tense by adding if before the subject and using were as the verb) is used to express this hypothetical situation that is actually contrary to fact. Choice B is incorrect because it represents the imperative mood, which is used to give a command or make a request. Choices C and D are incorrect because they are in the indicative mood, which is used to make a statement or ask a question.

7. **The correct answer is B.** The present participle of *walk* is *walking*, which is used to form the progressive aspect of a verb (e.g., I am going, I was going, I will be going), which shows an action that is continuous. *Walk* is the infinitive and the simple present tense form for all but third-person singular nouns, which allows us to rule out choice

A. Choice C is incorrect because *walked* is the past participle, which is used to form the present perfect and past perfect tenses. Choice D is incorrect because *walks* is the third-person singular form for the present tense.

8. **The correct answer is C.** The context of this sentence indicates that the subjects not only drove this route many times in the past but continue to do so every summer. Thus, the present perfect tense is the most appropriate tense to use here. It is formed by using *have* plus the past participle of the verb. The past participle of *drive* is *driven*; thus *have driven* is the correct answer. Choice A is incorrect because *drove* is the simple past tense of the verb *drive*, and only indicates that the subjects performed the action at some point in the past, not that they continue to perform it in the present. Choice B is incorrect because the past participle of *drive* is *driven*, not *drove*. Choice D is incorrect because the past perfect (i.e., *had driven*) is used to indicate a past action that occurred before some other past action, not to indicate a past action that continues to be performed in the present.

9. **The correct answer is B.** The context of this sentence indicates that an action will occur in the future before some other future event; specifically, before she turns 30 years old next May, Alice *will have competed* in over 100 triathlons. This represents the future perfect tense (formed by using *will* plus the past participle of the verb). Choice A is incorrect because the simple future tense only refers to an event that is expected to occur at some point in the future, not before some other future event. Choice C is incorrect because *has competed* is the present perfect tense, referring to something that occurred in the past and continues to occur in the present. Choice D is incorrect because *had competed* is in

the past perfect tense, referring to something that occurred in the past before some other past event.

10. **The correct answer is A.** *Quickly* is an adverb because it modifies the verb *acted*. Choices B, C, and D are incorrect because *quickly* is not modifying a noun or pronoun (the role of an adjective), describing the relationship of a noun to some other word in the sentence (the role of a preposition), or expressing an action or making a statement (the role of a verb).

11. **The correct answer is A.** Two comparisons are made in this sentence, one positive and one negative. One-syllable adjectives typically form the positive comparative by adding *–er* to the end of the adjective and the negative comparative by adding *less* before the adjective. Choice B is incorrect because *more stronger* is a double comparative (which is incorrect) and because *not strong* is not a comparative form. Choice C is incorrect because *strongest* and *least strong* are superlatives, not comparatives. Choice D is incorrect because *more strongly* and *less strongly* are adverb comparisons, whereas what are needed are adjective comparisons.

12. **The correct answer is D.** A comma is used after an introductory adverb clause, such as "Although the car did not run," to set it off from the rest of the sentence. Choice A is incorrect because a colon indicates "note what follows" and is not used to set off introductory clauses. Choice B is incorrect because a period is used to end a complete sentence, not to set off a dependent clause from the rest of the sentence. Choice C is incorrect because a semicolon is used to join two independent clauses, not to set off an introductory dependent clause from an independent clause.

13. **The correct answer is C.** Here we have two independent clauses, the second of which

is introduced by a conjunctive adverb, *therefore*. Independent clauses may be joined by either a coordinating conjunction preceded by a comma or a semicolon, but not simply by a comma alone. This allows us to rule out choices A and D. Choice B is incorrect because the semicolon should come before *therefore*, not after, as *therefore* is introducing the second independent clause and should be followed by a comma.

14. **The correct answer is B.** The first word in a sentence, all proper nouns (names of particular people, places, things, or ideas), the pronoun *I*, and the first word and all important words in the titles of books should be capitalized, as shown in choice B. Choice A is incorrect because the proper noun *Maggie* and the pronoun *I* should be capitalized, as well as *La* in the city name *La Paz* and *The* in the title of the novel, *The Pearl*. Choice C is incorrect because

south is not a proper noun and thus should not be capitalized, whereas *La Paz* and *The Pearl* should be capitalized. Choice D is incorrect because the first word of the sentence, *Next*, the proper nouns *Friday* and *Steinbeck's*, and *Pearl* in the title of the novel, *The Pearl*, should all be capitalized.

15. **The correct answer is C.** A dash or pair of dashes is used to set off an abrupt change in thought from the rest of the sentence, as shown in choice C. Choice A is incorrect because a colon is used to indicate "note what follows" and is only used alone, not in pairs. Choice B is incorrect because either two commas or two dashes should be used to set off the interrupting clause, not a combination of the two. Choice D is incorrect because a semicolon is used to join two independent clauses, not to set off an interrupting subordinate clause.

Test 6: Spelling

1. A	4. C	7. B	10. A	13. C
2. B	5. A	8. C	11. A	14. A
3. B	6. C	9. B	12. B	15. C

1. **The correct answer is A.** The correct spelling is *accessible*.

2. **The correct answer is B.** The correct spelling is *benign*.

3. **The correct answer is B.** The correct spelling is *consciousness*.

4. **The correct answer is C.** The correct spelling is *dialysis*.

5. **The correct answer is A.** The correct spelling is *efficacy*.

6. **The correct answer is C.** The correct spelling is *fluoroscopy*.

7. **The correct answer is B.** The correct spelling is *gauge*.

8. **The correct answer is C.** The correct spelling is *hereditary*.

9. **The correct answer is B.** The correct spelling is *leukocyte*.

10. **The correct answer is A.** The correct spelling is *misspelled*.

11. **The correct answer is A.** The correct spelling is *myocardial*.

12. **The correct answer is B.** The correct spelling is *neuron*.

13. **The correct answer is C.** The correct spelling is *ophthalmologist*.

14. **The correct answer is A.** The correct spelling is *susceptible*.

15. **The correct answer is C.** The correct spelling is *unnecessary*.

Test 7: Nonverbal Ability

1. B	**4.** E	**7.** E	**10.** A	**13.** E
2. C	**5.** D	**8.** C	**11.** D	**14.** A
3. A	**6.** D	**9.** A	**12.** C	**15.** B

1. **The correct answer is B.** The relationship between the first two shapes is that the second is the same as the first except that the diagonal slash through it has been removed. So, in the second pair, we begin with a U pointing right with a slash through it and are looking for a U pointing right without a slash through it. Therefore, T pointing right with a slash through it is to T pointing right as U pointing right with a slash through it is to U pointing right.

2. **The correct answer is C.** The relationship between the first two shapes is that the second is the same as the first except that the horizontal line segment has been removed. So, in the second pair, we begin with an inverted V with a horizontal line segment above it and are looking for an inverted V without a horizontal line segment above it. Therefore, T with a horizontal line segment above it is to T as inverted V with a horizontal line segment above it is to inverted V.

3. **The correct answer is A.** The relationship between the first two shapes is that the two dots above the inner shape are replaced by a circle in the second shape. So, in the second pair, we begin with a star with two dots above it and are looking for a star in the center of a circle. Therefore, circle with two dots above it is to circle embedded in larger circle as star with two dots above it is to star embedded in circle.

4. **The correct answer is E.** The relationship between the first two shapes is that the first is a dashed version of the second. So,

in the second pair, we begin with a dashed circle and are looking for a regular circle. Therefore, dashed vertical line is to vertical line as dashed circle is to circle.

5. **The correct answer is D.** The relationship between the first two shapes is that the first shape is the second shape joined with its mirror image. So, in the second pair, we begin with D joined with its mirror image and are looking for just D. Therefore, D with smaller D embedded within it joined to its mirror image is to D with smaller D embedded within it as D joined with its mirror image is to D.

6. **The correct answer is D.** The relationship between the first two shapes is that the second is an exact duplicate of the first. So, in the second pair, we begin with a dagger symbol and are looking for its exact duplicate. Therefore, double dagger symbol is to double dagger symbol as dagger symbol is to dagger symbol.

7. **The correct answer is E.** The relationship between the first two shapes is that the first is a mirror image of the second with a dot embedded within it. So, in the second pair, we begin with a mirror image of a capital C with a dot embedded in it and are looking for a capital C. Therefore, mirror image of lower case C with dot embedded in it is to lower case C as mirror image of capital C with dot embedded in it is to capital C.

8. **The correct answer is C.** The relationship between the first two forms is that the second immediately follows the first in a series to which both belong and is rotated

180 degrees from its normal position. So, in the second pair, we begin with a 2 and are looking for a 3 rotated 180 degrees. Therefore, J is to K rotated 180 degrees as 2 is to 3 rotated 180 degrees.

9. **The correct answer is A.** The relationship between the first two shapes is that the second is a single, mirror-image version of the first. So, in the second pair, we begin with two regular question marks and are looking for a single, mirror-image question mark (which is a backward question mark). Therefore, two closing parentheses are to opening parenthesis as two regular question marks are to backward question mark.

10. **The correct answer is A.** This one is a little tricky! Vertical line segment and vertical line segment are to intersecting perpendicular line segments and vertical line segment as exclamation point and exclamation point are to question mark and exclamation point. The relationship between the first two forms is that each consists of two elements side by side, but the first has identical elements whereas the second has two different elements, with the first element being new and the second element being the same as the two identical elements in the first form. So, in the second pair, we begin with two exclamation points and are looking for a new element (such as the question mark) followed by an exclamation point.

11. **The correct answer is D.** The relationship between the first two shapes is that the second is a larger version of the element that is embedded in another element in the first. So, in the second pair, we begin with a C embedded in a circle and are looking for a larger C. Therefore, plus sign embedded in U is to larger plus sign as C embedded in circle is to larger C.

12. **The correct answer is C.** The relationship between the first two shapes is that the second indicates a direction of movement that is the opposite of that indicated by the first. So, in the second pair, we begin with a right rotational arrow and are looking for a left rotational arrow. Therefore, right arrow is to left arrow as right rotational arrow is to left rotational arrow.

13. **The correct answer is E.** The relationship between the first two shapes is that the first is the same as the second except that it is divided into quarters. So, in the second pair, we begin with a diamond divided into quarters and are looking for a solid diamond. Therefore, cross divided into quarters is to solid cross as diamond divided into quarters is to solid diamond.

14. **The correct answer is A.** The relationship between the first two shapes is that the first is a dashed version of the second. So, in the second pair, we begin with a dashed horizontal line segment and are looking for a solid horizontal line segment. Therefore, dashed upper left corner of square is to solid upper left corner of square as dashed horizontal line segment is to solid horizontal line segment.

15. **The correct answer is B.** The relationship between the first two shapes is that the first is the negative image of the second. This means that the colors in the second shape are switched to their opposites. So, in the second pair, we begin with a negative image of a circle and are looking for a circle. Therefore, negative image of group of tiny squares is to group of tiny squares as negative image of circle is to circle.

Mathematics

OVERVIEW

- Fractions
- Decimals
- Ratios and Proportions
- Percentages and Roman Numerals
- Solutions to Practice Exercises
- Mathematics Answer Sheet
- Test 1: Arithmetic
- Test 2: Mathematics
- Answer Keys and Explanations
- Mathematics Answer Sheet
- Final Mathematics Examination
- Answer Key and Explanations

Arithmetic is an important part of the study of pharmacology and the related sciences. In this section, practice exercises on fractions, decimals, ratios, proportions, and percentages are included with a review of the appropriate processes. Solutions to the practice exercises are presented before the practice tests. If you have made numerous errors in a specific area, review the appropriate section again before moving on to take the practice tests. After you have completed all the exercises and practice tests, take the Final Mathematics Test.

FRACTIONS

Reduction of Fractions

To reduce fractions to lowest terms, divide both the numerator and the denominator by the same number (a common factor).

Example:

$$\frac{4}{8} = \frac{4 \div 4}{8 \div 4} = \frac{1}{2}$$

Practice Exercise A

Reduce the following fractions to their lowest terms.

1. $\frac{8}{16} =$ _____

2. $\frac{3}{12} =$ _____

3. $\frac{5}{10} =$ _____

7. $\frac{27}{54} =$ _____

4. $\frac{25}{100} =$ _____

8. $\frac{4}{64} =$ _____

5. $\frac{18}{72} =$ _____

9. $\frac{12}{144} =$ _____

6. $\frac{50}{60} =$ _____

10. $\frac{25}{150} =$ _____

Improper Fractions

To change an **improper fraction** to a **mixed number**, divide the denominator into the numerator to get the whole part. The remainder will be the numerator, and the divisor will be the denominator of the fractional part. Reduce to the lowest terms.

Examples:

$$\frac{21}{7} = 21 \div 7 = 3$$

21 divided by 7 gives a quotient of 3 and no remainder.

$$\frac{15}{9} = 1\frac{6}{9} = 1\frac{2}{3}$$

15 divided by 9 gives a quotient of 1 and a remainder of six. The fraction $\frac{9}{6}$ reduces to $\frac{2}{3}$.

To change a mixed number to an improper fraction, divide the denominator into the numerator to get the whole number. The remainder will be the numerator of the fraction, and the divisor will be the denominator.

Example:

$$4\frac{3}{8} = \frac{(4 \times 8) + 3}{8} = \frac{32 + 3}{8} = \frac{35}{8}$$

Practice Exercise B

Change the following improper fractions to mixed numbers and vice versa.

1. $\frac{15}{4} =$ _____

6. $2\frac{1}{9} =$ _____

2. $\frac{13}{6} =$ _____

7. $6\frac{4}{5} =$ _____

3. $\frac{27}{5} =$ _____

8. $8\frac{3}{4} =$ _____

4. $\frac{17}{3} =$ _____

9. $3\frac{7}{8} =$ _____

5. $\frac{99}{10} =$ _____

10. $2\frac{1}{6} =$ _____

Addition of Fractions

To add two or more fractions, the denominators must be the same. Rewrite each fraction as an equivalent fraction with the **Least (smallest) Common Multiple (LCM)** as the common denominator. Then add the numerators and reduce the answer to lowest terms.

Example:

Add $\dfrac{2}{3} + \dfrac{3}{4}$.

Multiples of 3 = 3, 6, 9, 12, 15, 18, 21, 24, . . .

Multiples of 4 = 4, 8, 12, 16, 20, 24, . . .

Common multiples are 12 and 24

LCM = 12 (the common denominator)

To make an equivalent fraction, divide the common denominator by the original denominator and multiply the original numerator and denominator by the result.

$12 \div 3 = 4; 2 \times 4 = 8$

$12 \div 4 = 3; 3 \times 3 = 9$

Add and reduce to lowest terms. $\qquad \dfrac{2}{3} + \dfrac{3}{4} = \dfrac{8}{12} + \dfrac{9}{12} = \dfrac{17}{12} = 1\dfrac{5}{12}$

Practice Exercise C

Add the following fractions.

1.
$$\dfrac{1}{2}$$
$$\dfrac{1}{3}$$
$$+\dfrac{1}{6}$$

4.
$$1\dfrac{1}{4}$$
$$5\dfrac{3}{16}$$
$$+2\dfrac{5}{12}$$

2.
$$\dfrac{3}{4}$$
$$\dfrac{1}{12}$$
$$+\dfrac{2}{3}$$

5.
$$26\dfrac{3}{5}$$
$$14\dfrac{1}{5}$$
$$+5\dfrac{7}{8}$$

3.
$$7\dfrac{2}{3}$$
$$3\dfrac{5}{24}$$
$$+\dfrac{5}{12}$$

6.
$$7\dfrac{5}{8}$$
$$\dfrac{1}{32}$$
$$+3\dfrac{1}{10}$$

7. $4\frac{1}{2}$

    $3\frac{1}{4}$

    $+9\frac{3}{8}$

9. $1\frac{3}{24}$

    $8\frac{1}{3}$

    $+3\frac{5}{6}$

8. $7\frac{11}{12}$

    $16\frac{3}{4}$

    $+2\frac{4}{18}$

10. $5\frac{5}{6}$

    $7\frac{3}{8}$

    $+2\frac{3}{10}$

Subtraction of Fractions

Rewrite each fraction as an equivalent fraction with the LCM as the common denominator. If the fraction of the mixed number to be subtracted is larger than the one from which it is to be subtracted, you must borrow 1 from the whole number of the larger mixed number. Add the numerator and denominator of the larger mixed number to make a new numerator. Subtract and reduce to lowest terms.

Example:

$9\frac{1}{2} = 9\frac{3}{6} = 8\frac{9}{6}$ Find the common denominator and make equivalent fractions. Borrow from the whole number of the larger mixed number ($9 - 1 = 8$)

$-1\frac{2}{3} = 1\frac{4}{6} = 1\frac{4}{6}$ Add the numerator and denominator to make a new numerator ($3 + 6 = 9$).

$\overline{\phantom{-1\frac{2}{3} = 1\frac{4}{6} = }\;7\frac{5}{6}}$ Subtract and reduce to lowest terms.

Practice Exercise D

Subtract the following fractions.

1. $\frac{5}{8}$

    $-\frac{3}{16}$

3. $\frac{1}{2}$

    $-\frac{1}{8}$

2. $7\frac{5}{12}$

    $-3\frac{1}{4}$

4. $3\frac{1}{8}$

    $-1\frac{3}{4}$

5. $\dfrac{7}{9}$

$-\dfrac{1}{6}$

6. $\dfrac{17}{20}$

$-\dfrac{3}{4}$

7. $5\dfrac{3}{8}$

$-1\dfrac{7}{16}$

8. $\dfrac{2}{5}$

$-\dfrac{2}{9}$

9. $4\dfrac{3}{4}$

$-2\dfrac{2}{3}$

10. $11\dfrac{7}{8}$

$-1\dfrac{3}{4}$

Multiplication of Fractions

To multiply fractions, multiply the numerators, then multiply the denominators. You may be able to simplify the fractions before multiplying, which allows you to work with smaller numbers. To simplify, divide the numerator of one fraction and the denominator of another fraction by the same number. Multiply and reduce to lowest terms.

Example:

$$\frac{12}{25} \times \frac{5}{9} = \frac{\overset{4}{\cancel{12}}}{\underset{5}{\cancel{25}}} \times \frac{\overset{1}{\cancel{5}}}{\underset{3}{\cancel{9}}} = \frac{4}{15}$$

To multiply a fraction by a whole number, change the whole number to a fraction by placing the whole number over 1. Multiply, simplify, if possible, and reduce to lowest terms.

Example:

$$4 \times \frac{1}{12} = \frac{4}{1} \times \frac{1}{12} = \frac{\overset{1}{\cancel{4}}}{1} \times \frac{1}{\underset{3}{\cancel{12}}} = \frac{1}{3}$$

To multiply mixed numbers, change the mixed number to an improper fraction. Simplify, if possible, and then multiply. Reduce answer to lowest terms.

Example:

$$3\frac{1}{2} \times \frac{6}{21} = \frac{7}{2} \times \frac{6}{21} = \frac{\overset{1}{\cancel{7}}}{\underset{1}{\cancel{2}}} \times \frac{\overset{3}{\cancel{6}}}{\underset{3}{\cancel{21}}} = \frac{3}{3} = 1$$

Practice Exercise E

Multiply the following fractions.

1. $\frac{2}{3} \times \frac{1}{8} =$ _____

2. $\frac{2}{5} \times \frac{5}{12} =$ _____

3. $\frac{4}{21} \times \frac{7}{8} =$ _____

4. $\frac{15}{16} \times \frac{9}{10} =$ _____

5. $\frac{4}{6} \times \frac{2}{4} =$ _____

6. $3\frac{3}{8} \times \frac{27}{8} =$ _____

7. $\frac{1}{2} \times 8 =$ _____

8. $6\frac{1}{2} \times 5\frac{4}{8} =$ _____

9. $3\frac{2}{3} \times \frac{3}{4} =$ _____

10. $9 \times 3\frac{1}{3} =$ _____

Division of Fractions

To divide fractions, invert the divisor (the second fraction) and change the sign from division ($\div$) to multiplication ($\times$). Then follow the rules for multiplication. Whole numbers are written as fractions with denominator of 1. Mixed numbers are written as improper fractions.

Examples:

$$\frac{2}{3} \div \frac{3}{4} = \frac{2}{3} \times \frac{4}{3} = \frac{8}{9}$$

$$5 \div 6\frac{2}{3} = \frac{5}{1} \div \frac{20}{3} = \frac{\overset{1}{\cancel{5}}}{1} \times \frac{3}{\underset{4}{\cancel{20}}} = \frac{3}{4}$$

Practice Exercise F

Divide the following fractions.

1. $2\frac{1}{5} \div 11 =$ _____

2. $\frac{1}{50} \div \frac{1}{200} =$ _____

3. $6\frac{3}{5} \div 8\frac{3}{10} =$ _____

4. $\frac{3}{4} \div \frac{1}{8} =$ _____

5. $\frac{5}{12} \div \frac{5}{60} =$ _____

6. $10\frac{1}{2} \div \frac{1}{3} =$ _____

7. $\frac{1}{60} \div \frac{1}{2} =$ _____

8. $8 \div \frac{2}{3} =$ _____

9. $\frac{1}{6} \div \frac{1}{3} =$ _____

10. $\frac{7}{8} \div \frac{3}{4} =$ _____

DECIMALS

The decimal system is based on the number 10. All numbers to the right of the decimal point are decimal fractions whose denominator is 10 or a multiple of 10. *Tenths* are directly after the decimal point, *hundredths* two places after, *thousandths* three places after, *ten-thousandths* four places after, etc. Whole numbers are written to the left of the decimal point, and the decimal point is read as "and."

Changing Fractions to Decimals

To change a fraction to a decimal, divide the numerator by the denominator. Write a decimal after the numerator and add as many zeros as needed. The division ends when the remainder is zero.

Example:

$$\frac{3}{4} = 4\overline{)3.00}$$

$$
\begin{array}{r}
.75 \\
4\,\overline{)3.00} \\
\underline{28} \\
20 \\
\underline{20} \\
0
\end{array}
$$

Sometimes, the division is not exact and a remainder may repeat itself. Draw a bar over the number in the answer that repeats.

$$
\frac{1}{12} = 12\,\overline{)1.0000} = .08\overline{3}
$$

$$
\begin{array}{r}
.0833 \\
12\,\overline{)1.0000} \\
\underline{96} \\
40 \\
\underline{36} \\
40 \\
\underline{36} \\
4
\end{array}
$$

Practice Exercise G

Change the following fractions to decimals.

1. $\frac{1}{4} =$ _____

2. $\frac{7}{8} =$ _____

3. $\frac{5}{6} =$ _____

4. $\frac{5}{125} =$ _____

5. $\frac{5}{16} =$ _____

6. $\frac{3}{25} =$ _____

7. $\frac{9}{20} =$ _____

8. $\frac{1}{75} =$ _____

9. $\frac{3}{8} =$ _____

10. $\frac{3}{10} =$ _____

Changing Decimals to Fractions

Decimals may be changed to fractions by dropping the decimal point and using the proper denominator. The number of decimal places to the right of the decimal point represents the number of zeros to be used in the denominator preceded by the number 1. Remove the decimal point from the number that you are converting and this becomes the numerator.

Example:

Change 0.025 to a fraction. There are 3 places to the right of the decimal point. Therefore, the denominator is 1 followed by 3 zeros (1,000). Next, remove the decimal point from 0.025; this number (25) becomes the numerator.

$$0.025 = \frac{25}{1,000}$$

Practice Exercise H

Change the following decimals to fractions and reduce to lowest terms.

1. 0.16 = _____
2. 0.04 = _____
3. 0.125 = _____
4. 0.06 = _____
5. 0.257 = _____

6. 0.75 = _____
7. 0.250 = _____
8. 0.525 = _____
9. 0.2 = _____
10. 4.75 = _____

Adding Decimals

To add decimals, place the numbers in columns so that the decimal points are directly under one another. Then add in the same manner that you would add columns of whole numbers. Place a decimal point in your answer directly under the others.

Example:

Add 22.05 + 1.375 + 10.2

22.05
 1.375
10.2
———
33.625

Practice Exercise I

Add the following decimals.

1. 7.2 + 3.57 + 10.8 = _____
2. 48.3 + 18.25 + 4.002 = _____
3. 6.3 + 0.005 + 2.67 = _____

4. 25.4 + 37.06 + 41 = _____
5. 8.50 + 19.625 + 0.17 = _____
6. 29.042 + 2.6 + 3.120 = _____

7. $5.4 + 8.62 + 0.95 =$ _____   **9.** $16.1 + 1.12 + 3.525 =$ _____

8. $2.246 + 16.8 + 4.26 =$ _____   **10.** $30.7 + 4.05 + 20.5 =$ _____

Subtracting Decimals

To subtract decimals, use the same rule as for adding decimals: place decimal points directly under one another. Then subtract in the same manner you would subtract whole numbers, placing the decimal point in your answer directly under the others.

Example:

$$50.789$$
$$-24.19$$
$$\overline{26.599}$$

Practice Exercise J

Subtract the following decimals.

1. $5.67 - 3.9 =$ _____   **6.** $15 - 7.82 =$ _____

2. $37.2 - 25.37 =$ _____   **7.** $205.6 - 105.23 =$ _____

3. $17.4 - 13.262 =$ _____   **8.** $246.52 - 107.988 =$ _____

4. $58.94 - 27.363 =$ _____   **9.** $35.25 - 17.0 =$ _____

5. $2.425 - 0.675 =$ _____   **10.** $1,725.5 - 50.6325 =$ _____

Multiplying Decimals

To multiply decimals, multiply the numbers as if they were whole numbers. Then place the decimal point in the answer by counting from the right the combined number of decimal places in the multiplier and the multiplicand.

Example:

$$2.56 \quad \text{(2 decimal places)}$$
$$\times \quad 0.6 \quad \text{(1 decimal place)}$$
$$\overline{1.536} \quad \text{(2 + 1 = 3 decimal places)}$$

Practice Exercise K

Multiply the following decimals.

1. $5.64 \times 1.2 =$ _____   **6.** $28.6 \times 8.16 =$ _____

2. $4.25 \times 12 =$ _____   **7.** $50.06 \times 2.15 =$ _____

3. $35.6 \times 2.5 =$ _____   **8.** $32.2 \times 3.15 =$ _____

4. $4.92 \times 9.5 =$ _____   **9.** $21.0 \times 41.6 =$ _____

5. $51 \times 0.92 =$ _____   **10.** $8.06 \times 3.654 =$ _____

Dividing Decimals

To divide decimals, the divisor must always be a whole number. If the divisor is a decimal, move the decimal to the right as many places as necessary to make the decimal a whole number. Then move the decimal point in the dividend the same number of places to the right to avoid changing the value of the quotient. The decimal point in the quotient is placed directly above the decimal point in the dividend.

Example:

$$.25)\overline{28} = .25.)\overline{28.00.}$$

$$
\begin{array}{r}
112 \\
\underline{25} \\
30 \\
\underline{25} \\
50 \\
\underline{50} \\
0
\end{array}
$$

Practice Exercise L

Divide the following decimals.

1. $100 \div 2.5 =$ _____

2. $0.9 \div 0.3 =$ _____

3. $38.59 \div 1.7 =$ _____

4. $115 \div 1.5 =$ _____

5. $5.5 \div 2.5 =$ _____

6. $3.22 \div 0.46 =$ _____

7. $4.65 \div 1.5 =$ _____

8. $15 \div 7.5 =$ _____

9. $0.042 \div 0.3 =$ _____

10. $0.006 \div 0.05 =$ _____

RATIOS AND PROPORTIONS

Ratio

A ratio is the comparison of two numbers by division. A ratio can be written using the symbol (:) or can be written as a fraction. The ratio 1 : 8 shows the relationship between 1 and 8. The ratio 1 : 8 can be written as the fraction $\frac{1}{8}$.

Example:

$$2 : 50 = 1 : 25$$

$$2 : 50 = \frac{2}{50} = \frac{1}{25}$$

$$\therefore 2 : 50 = 1 : 25$$

Practice Exercise M

Write the following fractions as ratios and reduce to lowest terms.

1. $\frac{4}{5} =$ _____   6. $\frac{2}{3} =$ _____

2. $\frac{1}{3} =$ _____   7. $\frac{1}{2} =$ _____

3. $\frac{3}{4} =$ _____   8. $\frac{25}{50} =$ _____

4. $\frac{3}{8} =$ _____   9. $\frac{3}{9} =$ _____

5. $\frac{1}{10} =$ _____   10. $\frac{2}{5} =$ _____

Proportion

A proportion states that two ratios are equal. Proportions may be expressed in two ways:

$$\frac{1}{2} = \frac{50}{100} \text{ or } 1 : 2 :: 50 : 100$$

Both are read: *One is to two as fifty is to one hundred.* The product of the means equals the product of the extremes.

If one number is not known, substitute an alphabet letter and solve for the unknown number by multiplying the means and the extremes, or multiplying the diagonals.

Example:

$$5 : y = 25 : 125$$

$$\frac{5}{y} = \frac{25}{125}$$

$$25 \times y = 5 \times 125$$
$$25y = 625$$
$$y = 25$$

Practice Exercise N

Solve for x in the following proportions.

1. $8 : 10 = x : 30$ _____

2. $\dfrac{9}{15} = \dfrac{x}{5}$ _____

3. $x : 80 = 3 : 12$ _____

4. $\dfrac{3}{x} = \dfrac{8}{24}$ _____

5. $2 : 3 = x : 63$ _____

6. $5 : 15 = x : 60$ _____

7. $\dfrac{7}{x} = \dfrac{4}{28}$ _____

8. $0.2 : 8 = 25 : x$ _____

9. $\dfrac{5}{7} = \dfrac{x}{28}$ _____

10. $\dfrac{1}{10} x : 2,000 = 1 : 100$ _____

PERCENTAGES AND ROMAN NUMERALS

Percentages

To change a decimal to a percentage, multiply the decimal by 100 (move the decimal point two places to the right), and then add the percent sign.

Example:

$$0.25 = .25\!\!\nearrow$$
$$= 25\%$$

To find the percentage of a number, change the percentage to its decimal equivalent, or to a fraction, and multiply.

Example:

Find 7% of 40. (Note: "of" means multiply.)

$$\begin{array}{r} 40 \\ \times .07 \\ \hline 2.80 \end{array} \quad \text{or} \quad \dfrac{7}{\cancel{100}_{10}} \times \dfrac{\cancel{40}^{4}}{1} = \dfrac{28}{10} = 2.8$$

To find the percent one number is of another, use the is/of method. The "is" number is the numerator, and the "of" number is the denominator.

Example:

18 is what percent of 24?

$$\dfrac{18}{24} = \dfrac{3}{4} \qquad 4\overline{)3.00} = 75\%$$
$$\underline{28}$$
$$20$$
$$\underline{20}$$
$$0$$

Example:

What percent of 500 is 125?

$$\frac{125}{500} = \frac{1}{4} \qquad 4\overline{)1.00}^{.25} = 25\%$$

$$\frac{8}{20}$$

$$\underline{20}$$

$$0$$

To find the percent of change, subtract to find the amount of change. Then find what the percent is of the original amount using the is/of method.

Example:

A sweater is on sale for $42. The original price was $56. What is the percent of change?

$$\begin{array}{r} \$56 \\ -\,42 \\ \hline \$14 \end{array} \qquad \frac{14}{56} = \frac{1}{4} = 4\overline{)1.00}^{.25} = 25\%$$

$$\frac{8}{20}$$

$$\underline{20}$$

$$0$$

Practice Exercise O

Solve the following percentage problems.

1. 0.225 = _____%

2. 3.45 = _____%

3. 0.7 = _____%

4. 0.14 = _____%

5. 4.5 = _____%

6. 24 percent of 72 =   _____

7. 5 percent of 12 =   _____

8. 225 is what percent of 300?   _____

9. What percent of 60 is 24?   _____

10. What percent of 45 is 135?   _____

Roman Numerals

Roman numerals are written using letters of the alphabet. The letters used to designate Arabic numbers are:

Roman	Arabic Equivalent
I	1
V	5
X	10
L	50
C	100
D	500
M	1,000

Rules Governing the Use of Roman Numerals

The following are some rules governing the use of Roman numerals:

- Addition
  - Placing one or more Roman numerals after the basic numeral adds to its value.

    Example: VII = 7
  - The same numeral cannot be repeated more than three times in succession. If this seems necessary, the rule for subtraction is used.

    Example: XXX = 30; however, XXXX is not allowed, so use XL = 40.
- Subtraction
  - Placing one or more Roman numerals in front of (before) the basic numeral removes value from it.

    Example: IV = 4
  - The numerals V, D, and L are never used in subtraction.

Practice Exercise P

Convert the following to Roman numerals.

1. 8 _____	**8.** 36 _____	**15.** 18 _____
2. 15 _____	**9.** 56 _____	**16.** 526 _____
3. 50 _____	**10.** 19 _____	**17.** 94 _____
4. 4 _____	**11.** 25 _____	**18.** 39 _____
5. 23 _____	**12.** 100 _____	**19.** 62 _____
6. 44 _____	**13.** 37 _____	**20.** 1,980 _____
7. 93 _____	**14.** 7 _____	

Practice Exercise Q

Convert the following to Arabic numbers.

1. XXIV _____	**8.** XIX _____	**15.** LXIX _____
2. XVII _____	**9.** XXX _____	**16.** XVII _____
3. L _____	**10.** XXIX _____	**17.** XXII _____
4. XL _____	**11.** VI _____	**18.** XI _____
5. V _____	**12.** LXX _____	**19.** CCIV _____
6. III _____	**13.** C _____	**20.** MCXV _____
7. M _____	**14.** XCII _____	

SOLUTIONS TO PRACTICE EXERCISES

Practice Exercise A

1. $\dfrac{8}{16} = \dfrac{1}{2}$

2. $\dfrac{3}{12} = \dfrac{1}{4}$

3. $\dfrac{5}{10} = \dfrac{1}{2}$

4. $\dfrac{25}{100} = \dfrac{1}{4}$

5. $\dfrac{18}{72} = \dfrac{1}{4}$

6. $\dfrac{50}{60} = \dfrac{5}{6}$

7. $\dfrac{27}{54} = \dfrac{1}{2}$

8. $\dfrac{4}{64} = \dfrac{1}{16}$

9. $\dfrac{12}{144} = \dfrac{1}{12}$

10. $\dfrac{25}{150} = \dfrac{1}{6}$

Practice Exercise B

1. $\dfrac{15}{4} = 3\dfrac{3}{4}$

2. $\dfrac{13}{6} = 2\dfrac{1}{6}$

3. $\dfrac{27}{5} = 5\dfrac{2}{5}$

4. $\dfrac{17}{3} = 5\dfrac{2}{3}$

5. $\dfrac{99}{10} = 9\dfrac{9}{10}$

6. $2\dfrac{1}{9} = \dfrac{19}{9}$

7. $6\dfrac{4}{5} = \dfrac{34}{5}$

8. $8\dfrac{3}{4} = \dfrac{35}{4}$

9. $3\dfrac{7}{8} = \dfrac{31}{8}$

10. $2\dfrac{1}{6} = \dfrac{13}{6}$

Practice Exercise C

1.
$$\begin{aligned}
\dfrac{1}{2} &= \dfrac{3}{6} \\
\dfrac{1}{3} &= \dfrac{2}{6} \\
\dfrac{1}{6} &= \dfrac{1}{6} \\
\hline
\dfrac{6}{6} &= 1
\end{aligned}$$

2.
$$\begin{aligned}
\dfrac{3}{4} &= \dfrac{9}{12} \\
\dfrac{1}{12} &= \dfrac{1}{12} \\
\dfrac{2}{3} &= \dfrac{8}{12} \\
\hline
\dfrac{18}{12} &= 1\dfrac{6}{12} = 1\dfrac{1}{2}
\end{aligned}$$

3.
$$\begin{aligned}
7\dfrac{2}{3} &= 7\dfrac{16}{24} \\
3\dfrac{5}{24} &= 3\dfrac{5}{24} \\
\dfrac{5}{12} &= \dfrac{10}{24} \\
\hline
10\dfrac{31}{24} &= 11\dfrac{7}{24}
\end{aligned}$$

4.
$$\begin{aligned}
1\dfrac{1}{4} &= 1\dfrac{12}{48} \\
5\dfrac{3}{16} &= 5\dfrac{9}{48} \\
2\dfrac{5}{12} &= 2\dfrac{20}{48} \\
\hline
8\dfrac{41}{48}
\end{aligned}$$

5. $26\frac{3}{5} = 26\frac{24}{40}$

   $14\frac{1}{5} = 14\frac{8}{40}$

   $\underline{5\frac{7}{8} = 5\frac{35}{40}}$

   $45\frac{67}{40} = 46\frac{27}{40}$

8. $7\frac{11}{12} = 7\frac{33}{36}$

   $16\frac{3}{4} = 16\frac{27}{36}$

   $\underline{2\frac{4}{18} = 2\frac{8}{36}}$

   $25\frac{68}{36} = 26\frac{32}{36} = 26\frac{8}{9}$

6. $7\frac{5}{8} = 7\frac{100}{160}$

   $\frac{1}{32} = \frac{5}{160}$

   $\underline{3\frac{1}{10} = 3\frac{16}{160}}$

   $10\frac{121}{160}$

9. $1\frac{3}{24} = 1\frac{3}{24}$

   $8\frac{1}{3} = 8\frac{8}{24}$

   $\underline{3\frac{5}{6} = 3\frac{20}{24}}$

   $12\frac{31}{24} = 13\frac{7}{24}$

7. $4\frac{1}{2} = 4\frac{4}{8}$

   $3\frac{1}{4} = 3\frac{2}{8}$

   $\underline{9\frac{3}{8} = 9\frac{3}{8}}$

   $16\frac{9}{8} = 17\frac{1}{8}$

10. $5\frac{5}{6} = 5\frac{100}{120}$

    $7\frac{3}{8} = 7\frac{45}{120}$

    $\underline{2\frac{3}{10} = 2\frac{36}{120}}$

    $14\frac{181}{120} = 15\frac{61}{120}$

Practice Exercise D

1. $\frac{5}{8} = \frac{10}{16}$

   $\underline{-\frac{3}{16} = \frac{3}{16}}$

   $\frac{7}{16}$

4. $3\frac{1}{8} = 3\frac{1}{8} = 2\frac{9}{8}$

   $\underline{-1\frac{3}{4} = 1\frac{6}{8} = 1\frac{6}{8}}$

   $1\frac{3}{8}$

2. $7\frac{5}{12} = 7\frac{5}{12}$

   $\underline{-3\frac{1}{4} = 3\frac{3}{12}}$

   $4\frac{2}{12} = 4\frac{1}{6}$

5. $\frac{7}{9} = \frac{14}{18}$

   $\underline{-\frac{1}{6} = \frac{3}{18}}$

   $\frac{11}{18}$

3. $\frac{1}{2} = \frac{4}{8}$

   $\underline{-\frac{1}{8} = \frac{1}{8}}$

   $\frac{3}{8}$

6. $\frac{17}{20} = \frac{17}{20}$

   $\underline{-\frac{3}{4} = \frac{15}{20}}$

   $\frac{2}{20} = \frac{1}{10}$

7.

$$5\frac{3}{8} = 5\frac{6}{16} = 4\frac{22}{16}$$

$$-1\frac{7}{16} = 1\frac{7}{16} = 1\frac{7}{16}$$

$$3\frac{15}{16}$$

9.

$$4\frac{3}{4} = 4\frac{9}{12}$$

$$-2\frac{2}{3} = 2\frac{8}{12}$$

$$2\frac{1}{12}$$

8.

$$\frac{2}{5} = \frac{18}{45}$$

$$-\frac{2}{9} = \frac{10}{45}$$

$$\frac{8}{45}$$

10.

$$11\frac{7}{8} = 11\frac{7}{8}$$

$$-1\frac{3}{4} = 1\frac{6}{8}$$

$$10\frac{1}{8}$$

Practice Exercise E

1. $\dfrac{\overset{1}{\cancel{2}}}{3} \times \dfrac{1}{\underset{4}{\cancel{8}}} = \dfrac{1}{12}$

2. $\dfrac{\overset{1}{\cancel{2}}}{\underset{1}{\cancel{3}}} \times \dfrac{\overset{1}{\cancel{3}}}{\underset{6}{\cancel{12}}} = \dfrac{1}{6}$

3. $\dfrac{\overset{1}{\cancel{4}}}{\underset{3}{21}} \times \dfrac{7}{\underset{2}{\cancel{8}}} = \dfrac{1}{6}$

4. $\dfrac{\overset{3}{\cancel{15}}}{16} \times \dfrac{9}{\underset{2}{\cancel{10}}} = \dfrac{27}{32}$

5. $\dfrac{\overset{1}{\cancel{4}}}{\underset{3}{\cancel{6}}} \times \dfrac{\overset{1}{\cancel{2}}}{\underset{1}{\cancel{4}}} = \dfrac{1}{3}$

6. $3\frac{3}{8} \times \frac{27}{8} = \frac{27}{8} \times \frac{27}{8} = \frac{729}{64} = 11\frac{25}{64}$

7. $\frac{1}{2} \times 8 = \frac{1}{\underset{1}{\cancel{2}}} \times \frac{\overset{4}{\cancel{8}}}{1} = 4$

8. $6\frac{1}{2} \times 5\frac{4}{8} = \frac{13}{2} \times \frac{\overset{11}{\cancel{44}}}{\underset{2}{\cancel{8}}} = \frac{143}{4} = 35\frac{3}{4}$

9. $3\frac{2}{3} \times \frac{3}{4} = \frac{11}{\underset{1}{\cancel{3}}} \times \frac{\overset{1}{\cancel{3}}}{4} = \frac{11}{4} = 2\frac{3}{4}$

10. $9 \times 3\frac{1}{3} = \frac{\overset{3}{\cancel{9}}}{1} \times \frac{10}{\underset{1}{\cancel{3}}} = 30$

Practice Exercise F

1. $2\frac{1}{5} \div 11 = \frac{11}{5} \div \frac{11}{1} = \frac{\cancel{11}^1}{5} \times \frac{1}{\cancel{11}_1} = \frac{1}{5}$

2. $\frac{1}{50} \div \frac{1}{200} = \frac{1}{\cancel{50}_1} \times \frac{\cancel{200}^4}{1} = \frac{4}{1} = 4$

3. $6\frac{3}{5} \div 8\frac{3}{10} = \frac{33}{5} \div \frac{83}{10} = \frac{33}{\cancel{5}_1} \times \frac{\cancel{10}^2}{83} = \frac{66}{83}$

4. $\frac{3}{4} \div \frac{1}{8} = \frac{3}{\cancel{4}_1} \times \frac{\cancel{8}^2}{1} = \frac{6}{1} = 6$

5. $\frac{5}{12} \div \frac{5}{60} = \frac{\cancel{5}^1}{\cancel{12}_1} \times \frac{\cancel{60}^5}{\cancel{5}_1} = \frac{5}{1} = 5$

6. $10\frac{1}{2} \div \frac{1}{3} = \frac{21}{2} \times \frac{3}{1} = \frac{63}{2} = 31\frac{1}{2}$

7. $\frac{1}{60} \div \frac{1}{2} = \frac{1}{\cancel{60}_{30}} \times \frac{\cancel{2}^1}{1} = \frac{1}{30}$

8. $8 \div \frac{2}{3} = \frac{\cancel{8}^4}{1} \times \frac{3}{\cancel{2}_1} = \frac{12}{1} = 12$

9. $\frac{1}{6} \div \frac{1}{3} = \frac{1}{\cancel{6}_2} \times \frac{\cancel{3}^1}{1} = \frac{1}{2}$

10. $\frac{7}{8} \div \frac{3}{4} = \frac{7}{\cancel{8}_2} \times \frac{\cancel{4}^1}{3} = \frac{7}{6} = 1\frac{1}{6}$

Practice Exercise G

1. **The correct answer is 0.25.**

$$\frac{1}{4} = 4)\overline{1.00}^{\,.25}$$

2. **The correct answer is 0.875.**

$$\frac{7}{8} = 8)\overline{7.000}^{\,.875}$$
$$\underline{64}$$
$$60$$
$$\underline{56}$$
$$40$$
$$\underline{40}$$
$$0$$

3. **The correct answer is $0.8\overline{3}$.**

$$\frac{5}{6} = 6)\overline{5.00}^{\,.08\overline{3}}$$
$$\underline{48}$$
$$20$$
$$\underline{18}$$
$$2$$

4. **The correct answer is 0.04.**

$$\frac{5}{125} = 125)\overline{5.00}^{\,.04}$$
$$\underline{500}$$
$$0$$

5. **The correct answer is 0.3125.**

$$\frac{5}{16} = 16)\overline{5.000}^{\,.3125}$$
$$\underline{48}$$
$$20$$
$$\underline{16}$$
$$40$$
$$\underline{32}$$
$$80$$
$$\underline{80}$$
$$0$$

6. **The correct answer is 0.12.**

$$\frac{3}{25} = 25)\overline{3.00}^{\,.12}$$
$$\underline{25}$$
$$50$$
$$\underline{50}$$
$$0$$

7. The correct answer is 0.45.

$$\frac{9}{20} = 20\overline{)9.00} \quad \begin{array}{r} .45 \\ \hline \end{array}$$

$$\begin{array}{r} 80 \\ \hline 100 \\ \underline{100} \\ 0 \end{array}$$

8. The correct answer is $0.01\overline{3}$.

$$\frac{1}{75} = 75\overline{)1.000} \quad \begin{array}{r} .01\overline{3} \\ \hline \end{array}$$

$$\begin{array}{r} 75 \\ \hline 250 \\ \underline{225} \\ 25 \end{array}$$

9. The correct answer is 0.375.

$$\frac{3}{8} = 8\overline{)3.000} \quad \begin{array}{r} .375 \\ \hline \end{array}$$

$$\begin{array}{r} 24 \\ \hline 60 \\ \underline{56} \\ 40 \\ \underline{40} \\ 0 \end{array}$$

10. The correct answer is 0.3.

$$\frac{3}{10} = 10\overline{)3.00} \quad \begin{array}{r} .30 \\ \hline \end{array}$$

$$\begin{array}{r} 30 \\ \hline 00 \end{array}$$

Practice Exercise H

1. $0.16 = \frac{16}{100} = \frac{4}{25}$

2. $0.04 = \frac{4}{100} = \frac{1}{25}$

3. $0.125 = \frac{125}{1,000} = \frac{1}{8}$

4. $0.06 = \frac{6}{100} = \frac{3}{50}$

5. $0.257 = \frac{257}{1,000}$

6. $0.75 = \frac{75}{100} = \frac{3}{4}$

7. $0.250 = \frac{250}{1,000} = \frac{1}{4}$

8. $0.525 = \frac{525}{1,000} = \frac{21}{40}$

9. $0.2 = \frac{2}{10} = \frac{1}{5}$

10. $4.75 = 4\frac{75}{100} = 4\frac{3}{4}$

Practice Exercise I

1.
$$\begin{array}{r} 7.2 \\ 3.57 \\ + 10.8 \\ \hline 21.57 \end{array}$$

2.
$$\begin{array}{r} 48.3 \\ 18.25 \\ + 4.002 \\ \hline 70.552 \end{array}$$

3.
$$\begin{array}{r} 6.3 \\ 0.005 \\ + 2.67 \\ \hline 8.975 \end{array}$$

4.
$$\begin{array}{r} 25.4 \\ 37.06 \\ + 41.0 \\ \hline 103.46 \end{array}$$

5.
$$\begin{array}{r} 8.50 \\ 19.625 \\ + 0.17 \\ \hline 28.295 \end{array}$$

6.
$$\begin{array}{r} 29.042 \\ 2.6 \\ + 3.12 \\ \hline 34.762 \end{array}$$

7.	5.4	9.	16.1
	8.62		1.12
	+ 0.95		+ 3.525
	14.97		20.745

8.	2.246	10.	30.7
	16.8		4.05
	+ 4.26		+ 20.5
	23.306		55.25

Practice Exercise J

1.	5.67	6.	15.00
	− 3.90		− 7.82
	1.77		7.18

2.	37.20	7.	205.60
	− 25.37		− 105.23
	11.83		100.37

3.	17.400	8.	246.520
	− 13.262		− 107.988
	4.138		138.532

4.	58.940	9.	35.25
	− 27.363		− 17.00
	31.577		18.25

5.	2.425	10.	1,725.5000
	− 0.675		− 50.6325
	1.750		1,674.8675

Practice Exercise K

1.	5.64	3.	35.6
	× 1.2		× 2.5
	1128		1780
	564		712
	6.768		89.00

2.	4.25	4.	4.92
	× 12		× 9.5
	850		2460
	425		4428
	51.00		46.740

5.

```
      51
 × 0.92
     102
    459
   46.92
```

6.

```
     28.6
  ×  8.16
     1716
      286
    2288
  233.376
```

7.

```
    50.06
  ×  2.15
    25030
     5006
    10012
  107.6290
```

8.

```
     32.2
  ×  3.15
     1610
      322
      966
  101.430
```

9.

```
     21.0
  ×  41.6
     1260
      210
      840
   873.60
```

10.

```
     8.06
  ×  3.654
     3224
     4030
     4836
     2418
  29.45124
```

Practice Exercise L

1. The correct answer is 40.

```
        40.
2.5.)100.0.
```

2. The correct answer is 3.

```
      3.
.3.).9.
```

3. The correct answer is 22.7.

```
       22.7
1.7.)38.5.9
       34
       45
       34
      119
      119
        0
```

4. The correct answer is 76.6̄.

```
        76.66
1.5.)115.0.00
       105
       100
        90
       100
        90
        10
```

5. The correct answer is 2.2.

```
       2.2
2.5.)5.5.0
       50
       50
       50
```

6. The correct answer is 7.

$$
\begin{array}{r}
7. \\
.46.)\overline{3.22.} \\
\underline{322} \\
0
\end{array}
$$

7. The correct answer is 3.1.

$$
\begin{array}{r}
3.1 \\
1.5.)\overline{4.6.5} \\
\underline{45} \\
15 \\
\underline{15}
\end{array}
$$

8. The correct answer is 2.

$$
\begin{array}{r}
2. \\
7.5.)\overline{15.0.} \\
\underline{150} \\
0
\end{array}
$$

9. The correct answer is 0.14.

$$
\begin{array}{r}
.14 \\
.3.)\overline{0.42} \\
\underline{3} \\
12 \\
\underline{12}
\end{array}
$$

10. The correct answer is 0.12.

$$
\begin{array}{r}
.12 \\
.05.)\overline{00.60} \\
\underline{5} \\
10
\end{array}
$$

Practice Exercise M

1. $\frac{4}{5} = 4 : 5$

2. $\frac{1}{3} = 1 : 3$

3. $\frac{3}{4} = 3 : 4$

4. $\frac{3}{8} = 3 : 8$

5. $\frac{1}{10} = 1 : 10$

6. $\frac{2}{3} = 2 : 3$

7. $\frac{1}{2} = 1 : 2$

8. $\frac{25}{50} = 25 : 50 = 1 : 2$

9. $\frac{3}{9} = 3 : 9 = 1 : 3$

10. $\frac{2}{5} = 2 : 5$

Practice Exercise N

1. $8 : 10 = x : 30$
   $10x = 240$
   $x = 24$

2. $9 : 15 = x : 5$
   $15x = 45$
   $x = 3$

3. $x : 80 = 3 : 12$
   $12x = 240$
   $x = 20$

4. $3 : x = 8 : 24$
   $8x = 72$
   $x = 9$

5. $2 : 3 = x : 63$
   $3x = 126$
   $x = 42$

6. $5 : 15 = x : 60$
   $15x = 300$
   $x = 20$

7. $7 : x = 4 : 28$

$4x = 196$

$x = 49$

8. $0.2 : 8 = 25 : x$

$0.2x = 200$

$x = 1,000$

9. $5 : 7 = x : 28$

$7x = 140$

$x = 20$

10. $\frac{1}{10} x : 2,000 = 1 : 100$

$10x = 2,000$

$x = 200$

Practice Exercise O

1. $0.225 = 22.5\%$

2. $3.45 = 345\%$

3. $0.7 = 70\%$

4. $0.14 = 14\%$

5. $4.5 = 450\%$

6.
$$\begin{array}{r} 72 \\ \times\ .24 \\ \hline 17.28 \end{array}$$

7.
$$\begin{array}{r} 12 \\ \times\ .05 \\ \hline .60 \end{array}$$

8. $\dfrac{\overset{3}{\cancel{225}}}{\underset{4}{\cancel{300}}} = \dfrac{3}{4} = 4\overline{)3.00}^{.75} = 75\%$

$$\begin{array}{r} \underline{28} \\ 20 \\ \underline{20} \\ 0 \end{array}$$

9. $\dfrac{24}{60} = \dfrac{2}{5} = 5\overline{)2.0}^{.4} = 40\%$

$$\begin{array}{r} \underline{20} \\ 0 \end{array}$$

10. $\dfrac{135}{45} = 3. = 300\%$

Practice Exercise P

1. The correct answer is VIII.

2. The correct answer is XV.

3. The correct answer is L.

4. The correct answer is IV.

5. The correct answer is XXIII.

6. The correct answer is XLIV.

7. The correct answer is XCIII.

8. The correct answer is XXXVI.

9. The correct answer is LVI.

10. The correct answer is XIX.

11. The correct answer is XXV.

12. The correct answer is C.

13. The correct answer is XXXVII.

14. The correct answer is VII.

15. The correct answer is XVIII.

16. The correct answer is DXXVI.

17. The correct answer is XCIV.

18. The correct answer is XXXIX.

19. The correct answer is LXII.

20. The correct answer is MCMLXXX.

Practice Exercise Q

1. The correct answer is 24.

2. The correct answer is 17.

3. The correct answer is 50.

4. The correct answer is 40.

5. The correct answer is 5.

6. The correct answer is 3.

7. The correct answer is 1,000.

8. The correct answer is 19.

9. The correct answer is 30.

10. The correct answer is 29.

11. The correct answer is 6.

12. The correct answer is 70.

13. The correct answer is 100.

14. The correct answer is 92.

15. The correct answer is 69.

16. The correct answer is 17.

17. The correct answer is 22.

18. The correct answer is 11.

19. The correct answer is 204.

20. The correct answer is 1,115.

MATHEMATICS ANSWER SHEET

Test 1: Arithmetic

Fill in your answers in the spaces provided on the test.

Test 2: Mathematics

1. Ⓐ Ⓑ Ⓒ Ⓓ   5. Ⓐ Ⓑ Ⓒ Ⓓ   9. Ⓐ Ⓑ Ⓒ Ⓓ   13. Ⓐ Ⓑ Ⓒ Ⓓ   17. Ⓐ Ⓑ Ⓒ Ⓓ

2. Ⓐ Ⓑ Ⓒ Ⓓ   6. Ⓐ Ⓑ Ⓒ Ⓓ   10. Ⓐ Ⓑ Ⓒ Ⓓ   14. Ⓐ Ⓑ Ⓒ Ⓓ   18. Ⓐ Ⓑ Ⓒ Ⓓ

3. Ⓐ Ⓑ Ⓒ Ⓓ   7. Ⓐ Ⓑ Ⓒ Ⓓ   11. Ⓐ Ⓑ Ⓒ Ⓓ   15. Ⓐ Ⓑ Ⓒ Ⓓ   19. Ⓐ Ⓑ Ⓒ Ⓓ

4. Ⓐ Ⓑ Ⓒ Ⓓ   8. Ⓐ Ⓑ Ⓒ Ⓓ   12. Ⓐ Ⓑ Ⓒ Ⓓ   16. Ⓐ Ⓑ Ⓒ Ⓓ   20. Ⓐ Ⓑ Ⓒ Ⓓ

answer sheet

TEST 1: ARITHMETIC

30 Questions • 30 Minutes

Directions: Perform the specified computation and fill in your answer sheet in the space provided.

Reduce to lowest terms:

SHOW YOUR WORK HERE

1. $\dfrac{3}{6} =$ _____

2. $\dfrac{10}{12} =$ _____

3. $\dfrac{40}{1,000} =$ _____

4. $\dfrac{15}{50} =$ _____

5. $\dfrac{75}{90} =$ _____

Change to improper fractions:

6. $2\dfrac{3}{5} =$ _____

7. $10\dfrac{3}{5} =$ _____

8. $6\dfrac{5}{6} =$ _____

9. $17\dfrac{1}{2} =$ _____

10. $9\dfrac{1}{3} =$ _____

Add:

11. $\begin{aligned}&\dfrac{2}{3}\\&\dfrac{1}{4}\\+&\dfrac{5}{6}\\\hline\end{aligned}$

12.
$$\frac{5}{9}$$
$$\frac{3}{8}$$
$$+ \frac{1}{4}$$

13.
$$\frac{4}{5}$$
$$\frac{3}{8}$$
$$+ \frac{1}{20}$$

14.
$$17\frac{2}{3}$$
$$\frac{8}{9}$$
$$+ 2\frac{1}{12}$$

15.
$$1\frac{9}{10}$$
$$8\frac{4}{5}$$
$$+ 9\frac{2}{3}$$

Subtract

16. $\dfrac{7}{8}$

    $-\dfrac{1}{3}$

17. $\dfrac{11}{18}$

    $-\dfrac{2}{9}$

18. $7\dfrac{1}{3}$

    $-2\dfrac{3}{4}$

19. $2\dfrac{5}{6}$

    $-\dfrac{8}{9}$

20. $17\dfrac{1}{3}$

    $-8\dfrac{5}{15}$

Multiply:

21. $\frac{1}{5} \times \frac{25}{50} =$ _____

22. $\frac{1}{3} \times \frac{3}{4} =$ _____

23. $\frac{7}{10} \times \frac{5}{6} =$ _____

24. $15 \times 2\frac{1}{3} =$ _____

25. $\frac{2}{3} \times \frac{9}{16} =$ _____

Divide:

26. $\frac{1}{2} \div \frac{1}{50} =$ _____

27. $\frac{1}{2} \div 6 =$ _____

28. $2\frac{1}{4} \div 3\frac{1}{2} =$ _____

29. $2\frac{4}{5} \div 7 =$ _____

30. $\frac{1}{2} \div \frac{3}{50} =$ _____

STOP

IF YOU FINISH BEFORE TIME IS CALLED, YOU MAY
CHECK YOUR WORK ON THIS SECTION ONLY. DO NOT
TURN TO ANY OTHER SECTION IN THE TEST.

TEST 2: MATHEMATICS

20 Questions • 20 Minutes

> **Directions:** Solve the following problems and choose the correct answer from the four choices provided. Fill in the corresponding space on your answer sheet.

1. 23 + 4.67 + 19.2 + 0.365 =
   A. 1047.0
   B. 47.235
   C. 1172.4
   D. 46.235

2. 2.37 × 0.6 =
   A. 14.22
   B. 1.282
   C. 1.422
   D. 12.82

3. The freshman nursing class consists of 40 students. Of the class, $\frac{7}{8}$ are women. How many women are in the class?
   A. 35
   B. 38
   C. 21
   D. 24

4. What percent of 20 is 12?
   A. 12 percent
   B. 60 percent
   C. 14 percent
   D. 8 percent

5. What is the value of x in the proportion
   $1 : 5 = x : 1,500$?
   A. 5
   B. $\frac{1}{3}$
   C. 750,000
   D. 300

SHOW YOUR WORK HERE

SHOW YOUR WORK HERE

6. Of the 900 students who attend a school, 3 percent of them went on a trip. How many students remained in school?

    A. 27

    B. 30

    C. 873

    D. 773

7. What is the fraction $\frac{7}{16}$ expressed as a decimal?

    A. .1120

    B. .2286

    C. .4850

    D. .4375

8. If 30 is divided by .06, what is the result?

    A. 5

    B. 50

    C. 500

    D. 5,000

9. What is most nearly the sum of 637.894, 8352.16, 4.8673, and 301.5?

    A. 8,989.5

    B. 9,021.35

    C. 9,294.9

    D. 9,296.4

10. What is the sum of $82.79, $103.06, and $697.85?

    A. $883.70

    B. $1,628

    C. $791

    D. $873

11. What is 1 percent of $23,000?

    A. $23

    B. $2.30

    C. $230

    D. $2,300

12. If $1\frac{1}{2}$ pounds of candy are required to fill an Easter basket, how many baskets can be filled with $10\frac{1}{2}$ pounds of candy?

   A. 7.5
   B. 2.5
   C. $5\frac{1}{2}$
   D. 7

SHOW YOUR WORK HERE

13. If 1 T-shirt costs $5.60, how many T-shirts can be bought for $61.60?

   A. $8\frac{1}{2}$
   B. 10
   C. 9
   D. 11

14. The decimal 410.07 less 38.49 is equal to:

   A. 372.58
   B. 371.58
   C. 381.58
   D. 382.68

15. Express the fraction $\frac{3}{10}$ as a decimal.

   A. 0.3
   B. 0.03
   C. 0.003
   D. 0.0003

16. Express 12.5 as a fraction.

   A. $\frac{1}{25}$
   B. $12\frac{1}{2}$
   C. $1\frac{1}{2}$
   D. $\frac{125}{100}$

17. What is the product of 8.3 x 80?　　　　　**SHOW YOUR WORK HERE**

    A. 6.64

    B. 66.4

    C. 664

    D. 6,640

18. Which of the following fractions is equal
    to 0.0625?

    A. $\frac{1}{16}$

    B. $\frac{1}{15}$

    C. $\frac{1}{14}$

    D. $\frac{1}{13}$

19. The number 0.03125 is equal to which of
    the following fractions?

    A. $\frac{3}{64}$

    B. $\frac{1}{16}$

    C. $\frac{1}{64}$

    D. $\frac{1}{32}$

20. The quantity 21.70 divided by 1.75
    is equal to:

    A. 124

    B. 12.4

    C. 1.24

    D. .124

STOP

IF YOU FINISH BEFORE TIME IS CALLED, YOU MAY
CHECK YOUR WORK ON THIS SECTION ONLY. DO NOT
TURN TO ANY OTHER SECTION IN THE TEST.

ANSWER KEYS AND EXPLANATIONS

Test 1: Arithmetic

1. $\frac{1}{2}$	7. $\frac{53}{5}$	13. $1\frac{9}{40}$	19. $1\frac{17}{18}$	25. $\frac{3}{8}$
2. $\frac{5}{6}$	8. $\frac{41}{6}$	14. $20\frac{23}{36}$	20. 9	26. 25
3. $\frac{1}{25}$	9. $\frac{35}{2}$	15. $20\frac{11}{30}$	21. $\frac{1}{10}$	27. $\frac{1}{12}$
4. $\frac{3}{10}$	10. $\frac{28}{3}$	16. $\frac{13}{24}$	22. $\frac{1}{4}$	28. $\frac{9}{14}$
5. $\frac{5}{6}$	11. $1\frac{3}{4}$	17. $\frac{7}{18}$	23. $\frac{7}{12}$	29. $\frac{2}{5}$
6. $\frac{13}{5}$	12. $1\frac{13}{72}$	18. $4\frac{7}{12}$	24. 35	30. $8\frac{1}{3}$

1. $\frac{3}{6} = \frac{1}{2}$

2. $\frac{10}{12} = \frac{5}{6}$

3. $\frac{40}{1,000} = \frac{1}{25}$

4. $\frac{15}{50} = \frac{3}{10}$

5. $\frac{75}{90} = \frac{5}{6}$

6. $2\frac{3}{5} = \frac{13}{5}$

7. $10\frac{3}{5} = \frac{53}{5}$

8. $6\frac{5}{6} = \frac{41}{6}$

9. $17\frac{1}{2} = \frac{35}{2}$

10. $9\frac{1}{3} = \frac{28}{3}$

11. $\quad \dfrac{2}{3} = \dfrac{8}{12}$

$\quad\ \dfrac{1}{4} = \dfrac{3}{12}$

$\quad +\dfrac{5}{6} = \dfrac{10}{12}$

$\qquad \dfrac{21}{12} = 1\dfrac{9}{12} = 1\dfrac{3}{4}$

12. $\quad \dfrac{5}{9} = \dfrac{40}{72}$

$\quad\ \dfrac{3}{8} = \dfrac{27}{72}$

$\quad +\dfrac{1}{4} = \dfrac{18}{72}$

$\qquad \dfrac{85}{72} = 1\dfrac{13}{72}$

13. $\quad \dfrac{4}{5} = \dfrac{32}{40}$

$\quad\ \dfrac{3}{8} = \dfrac{15}{40}$

$\quad +\dfrac{1}{20} = \dfrac{2}{40}$

$\qquad \dfrac{49}{40} = 1\dfrac{9}{40}$

14. $17\frac{2}{3} = 17\frac{24}{36}$

$\qquad \frac{8}{9} = \frac{32}{36}$

$\qquad +2\frac{1}{12} = 2\frac{3}{36}$

$\qquad\qquad 19\frac{59}{36} = 20\frac{23}{36}$

15. $1\frac{9}{10} = 1\frac{27}{30}$

$\qquad 8\frac{4}{5} = 8\frac{24}{30}$

$\qquad +9\frac{2}{3} = 9\frac{20}{30}$

$\qquad\qquad 18\frac{71}{30} = 20\frac{11}{30}$

16. $\qquad \frac{7}{8} = \frac{21}{24}$

$\qquad -\frac{1}{3} = \frac{8}{24}$

$\qquad\qquad \frac{13}{24}$

17. $\qquad \frac{11}{18} = \frac{11}{18}$

$\qquad -\frac{2}{9} = \frac{4}{18}$

$\qquad\qquad \frac{7}{18}$

18. $\qquad 7\frac{1}{3} = 7\frac{4}{12} = 6\frac{16}{12}$

$\qquad -2\frac{3}{4} = 2\frac{9}{12} = 2\frac{9}{12}$

$\qquad\qquad\qquad\qquad 4\frac{7}{12}$

19. $2\frac{5}{6} = 2\frac{15}{18} = 1\frac{33}{18}$

$\qquad -\frac{8}{9} = \frac{16}{18} = \frac{16}{18}$

$\qquad\qquad\qquad 1\frac{17}{18}$

20. $17\frac{1}{3} = 17\frac{5}{15}$

$\qquad -8\frac{5}{15} = 8\frac{5}{15}$

$\qquad\qquad\qquad 9$

21. $\frac{1}{5} \times \frac{\overset{1}{\cancel{25}}}{\underset{2}{\cancel{50}}} = \frac{1}{10}$

22. $\frac{1}{\underset{1}{\cancel{3}}} \times \frac{\overset{1}{\cancel{3}}}{4} = \frac{1}{4}$

23. $\frac{7}{\underset{2}{\cancel{10}}} \times \frac{\overset{1}{\cancel{5}}}{6} = \frac{7}{12}$

24. $15 \times 2\frac{1}{3} = \overset{5}{\cancel{15}} \times \frac{7}{\underset{1}{\cancel{3}}} = \frac{35}{1} = 35$

25. $\frac{\overset{1}{\cancel{2}}}{\underset{1}{\cancel{3}}} \times \frac{\overset{3}{\cancel{9}}}{\underset{8}{\cancel{16}}} = \frac{3}{8}$

26. $\frac{1}{2} \div \frac{1}{50} = \frac{1}{\underset{1}{\cancel{2}}} \times \frac{\overset{25}{\cancel{50}}}{1} = \frac{25}{1} = 25$

27. $\frac{1}{2} \div 6 = \frac{1}{2} \times \frac{1}{6} = \frac{1}{12}$

28. $2\frac{1}{4} \div 3\frac{1}{2} = \frac{9}{4} \div \frac{7}{2} = \frac{9}{\underset{2}{\cancel{4}}} \times \frac{\overset{1}{\cancel{2}}}{7} = \frac{9}{14}$

29. $2\frac{4}{5} \div 7 = \frac{14}{5} \div \frac{7}{1} = \frac{\overset{2}{\cancel{14}}}{5} \times \frac{1}{\underset{1}{\cancel{7}}} = \frac{2}{5}$

30. $\frac{1}{2} \div \frac{3}{50} = \frac{1}{\underset{1}{\cancel{2}}} \times \frac{\overset{25}{\cancel{50}}}{3} = \frac{25}{3} = 8\frac{1}{3}$

Test 2: Mathematics

1. B	**5.** D	**9.** D	**13.** D	**17.** C
2. C	**6.** C	**10.** A	**14.** B	**18.** A
3. A	**7.** D	**11.** C	**15.** A	**19.** D
4. B	**8.** C	**12.** D	**16.** B	**20.** B

1. The correct answer is B.

23.0
4.67
19.2
+ 0.365
47.235

2. The correct answer is C.

2.37
× 0.6
1.422

3. The correct answer is A.

$$\frac{7}{\cancel{8}_{1}} \times \frac{\cancel{40}^{5}}{1} = 35$$

4. The correct answer is B.

$$\frac{12}{20} = \frac{3}{5} = .6 = 60\%$$

5. The correct answer is D.

$$1 : 5 = x : 1,500$$
$$5x = 1,500$$
$$x = 300$$

6. The correct answer is C.

900   900
× .03   − 27
27.00   873

7. The correct answer is D.

$$\frac{7}{16} = 16\overline{)7.0000}^{.4375}$$

64
60
48
120
112
80
80

8. The correct answer is C.

$$.06\overline{)30.00.}^{500.}$$

30
00

9. The correct answer is D.

637.8940
8,352.1600
4.8673
+ 301.5000
9,296.4213

10. The correct answer is A.

$ 82.79
103.06
+ 697.85
$883.70

11. The correct answer is C.

$ 230.000
× 0.01
$230.00

12. **The correct answer is D.**

$$\frac{1.5}{1} = \frac{10.5}{x}$$
$$1.5x = 10.5$$
$$x = 7$$

13. **The correct answer is D.**

$$5.60.\overline{)61.60.}$$
$$\underline{560}$$
$$560$$

with quotient 11.

14. **The correct answer is B.**

$$\begin{array}{r} 410.07 \\ -\ 38.49 \\ \hline 371.58 \end{array}$$

15. **The correct answer is A.**

$$\frac{3}{10} = 0.3$$

16. **The correct answer is B.**

$$12.5 = 12\frac{5}{10} = 12\frac{1}{2}$$

17. **The correct answer is C.**

$$\begin{array}{r} 8.3 \\ \times\ 80 \\ \hline 00 \\ \underline{664} \\ 664.0 \end{array}$$

18. **The correct answer is A.**

$$.0625 = \frac{625}{10,000} = \frac{1}{16}$$

19. **The correct answer is D.**

$$0.03125 = \frac{3,125}{100,000} = \frac{1}{32}$$

20. **The correct answer is B.**

$$1.75.\overline{)21.70.0}$$
$$\underline{175}$$
$$420$$
$$\underline{350}$$
$$700$$
$$\underline{700}$$

with quotient 12.4

FINAL MATHEMATICS EXAMINATION
ANSWER SHEET

1. Ⓐ Ⓑ Ⓒ Ⓓ   5. Ⓐ Ⓑ Ⓒ Ⓓ   9. Ⓐ Ⓑ Ⓒ Ⓓ   13. Ⓐ Ⓑ Ⓒ Ⓓ   17. Ⓐ Ⓑ Ⓒ Ⓓ

2. Ⓐ Ⓑ Ⓒ Ⓓ   6. Ⓐ Ⓑ Ⓒ Ⓓ   10. Ⓐ Ⓑ Ⓒ Ⓓ   14. Ⓐ Ⓑ Ⓒ Ⓓ   18. Ⓐ Ⓑ Ⓒ Ⓓ

3. Ⓐ Ⓑ Ⓒ Ⓓ   7. Ⓐ Ⓑ Ⓒ Ⓓ   11. Ⓐ Ⓑ Ⓒ Ⓓ   15. Ⓐ Ⓑ Ⓒ Ⓓ   19. Ⓐ Ⓑ Ⓒ Ⓓ

4. Ⓐ Ⓑ Ⓒ Ⓓ   8. Ⓐ Ⓑ Ⓒ Ⓓ   12. Ⓐ Ⓑ Ⓒ Ⓓ   16. Ⓐ Ⓑ Ⓒ Ⓓ   20. Ⓐ Ⓑ Ⓒ Ⓓ

answer sheet

FINAL MATHEMATICS EXAMINATION

20 Questions • 30 Minutes

> **Directions:** Solve the following problems and choose the correct answer from the four choices provided. Fill in the corresponding space on your answer sheet.

1. Add $\frac{1}{4}$, $\frac{3}{8}$, and $\frac{7}{16}$.

   SHOW YOUR WORK HERE

   A. $\frac{11}{16}$

   B. $1\frac{1}{16}$

   C. $\frac{11}{28}$

   D. $\frac{18}{16}$

2. Multiply 25.5 by 0.326.

   A. 83.13

   B. 25.826

   C. 0.2805

   D. 8.313

3. Subtract 25.246 from 307.401.

   A. 282.155

   B. 54.941

   C. 549.41

   D. 28.2155

4. Add 14.75, 15.1256, and 0.07.

   A. 299.46

   B. 36.8756

   C. 29.946

   D. 268.756

5. Divide 36.36 by 0.0606.

   A. .06

   B. 0.6

   C. 60

   D. 600

6. Write the fraction $\frac{1}{8}$ as a ratio.

   SHOW YOUR WORK HERE

   A. 8 : 1
   B. 0.18
   C. 1 : 8
   D. 0.125

7. Solve for x in 2 : 8 = 11 : x.

   A. 44
   B. $2\frac{3}{4}$
   C. $\frac{11}{16}$
   D. 4.4

8. Change 85 percent to a fraction and reduce to lowest terms.

   A. $\frac{85}{100}$
   B. $\frac{17}{20}$
   C. $\frac{100}{85}$
   D. $\frac{20}{17}$

9. Change 0.12 to a percent.

   A. 0.12%
   B. 0.0012%
   C. .12%
   D. 12%

10. Subtract $\frac{1}{8}$ from $\frac{1}{6}$.

    A. $\frac{2}{8}$
    B. $\frac{3}{24}$
    C. $\frac{1}{24}$
    D. $\frac{1}{12}$

11. How many grains of codeine are there in $1\frac{1}{2}$ tablets of $\frac{1}{8}$ grain each?

   A. $\frac{2}{8}$

   B. $\frac{3}{16}$

   C. $\frac{3}{8}$

   D. $\frac{5}{8}$

SHOW YOUR WORK HERE

12. Mary drank 8 ounces of milk from a quart containing 32 ounces of milk. What part of the quart had she consumed?

   A. $\frac{1}{4}$

   B. $\frac{1}{8}$

   C. $\frac{1}{3}$

   D. $\frac{1}{2}$

13. There are 75 nursing students in the freshman class, and 15 are men. What is the ratio of women to men?

   A. $\frac{1}{4}$

   B. $\frac{1}{5}$

   C. $\frac{4}{1}$

   D. $\frac{5}{1}$

14. If a recipe calls for 5 ounces of sugar for every 15 ounces of flour, what part of the mixture will be sugar?

   A. $\frac{1}{2}$

   B. $\frac{1}{5}$

   C. $\frac{1}{3}$

   D. $\frac{1}{4}$

15. If a suit is on sale for $120, and the
original cost was $150, what percent would
you save by buying it on sale?

    A. 40%

    B. 30%

    C. 10%

    D. 20%

SHOW YOUR WORK HERE

16. A seamstress bought $2\frac{2}{3}$ yards of wool
material and $1\frac{3}{4}$ yards of crepe material.
How many yards of material did she buy?

    A. $4\frac{5}{12}$

    B. $4\frac{2}{3}$

    C. $5\frac{1}{4}$

    D. $4\frac{1}{3}$

17. A sack contained 10 pounds of potatoes.
The chef used $1\frac{3}{4}$ pounds for French fries
yesterday and $2\frac{1}{3}$ pounds for a casserole
today. How many pounds of potatoes does
she have left?

    A. $5\frac{1}{2}$

    B. $5\frac{11}{12}$

    C. $6\frac{2}{3}$

    D. $6\frac{11}{12}$

18. How many ounces is $\frac{3}{8}$ of a pound if a
pound equals 16 ounces?

    A. 6 ounces

    B. 12 ounces

    C. 8 ounces

    D. 10 ounces

19. If John receives $\frac{2}{5}$ of $10, how much does

   he receive?

   SHOW YOUR WORK HERE

   A. $2
   B. $4
   C. $5
   D. $3

20. If there are 3,000 registered voters in

   Center City and $\frac{3}{5}$ of them are

   Democrats, how many Democrats are

   there in Center City?

   A. 500
   B. 600
   C. 1,800
   D. 1,500

STOP

IF YOU FINISH BEFORE TIME IS CALLED, YOU MAY CHECK YOUR WORK ON THIS SECTION ONLY. DO NOT TURN TO ANY OTHER SECTION IN THE TEST.

ANSWER KEY AND EXPLANATIONS

Final Mathematics Examination

1. B	**5.** D	**9.** D	**13.** C	**17.** B
2. D	**6.** C	**10.** C	**14.** D	**18.** A
3. A	**7.** A	**11.** B	**15.** D	**19.** B
4. C	**8.** B	**12.** A	**16.** A	**20.** C

1. **The correct answer is B.**

$$\frac{1}{4} = \frac{4}{16}$$
$$\frac{3}{8} = \frac{6}{16}$$
$$\frac{7}{16} = \frac{7}{16}$$
$$\frac{17}{16} = 1\frac{1}{16}$$

2. **The correct answer is D.**

$$
\begin{array}{r}
25.5 \\
\times\ .326 \\
\hline
1530 \\
510 \\
765 \\
\hline
8.3130
\end{array}
$$

3. **The correct answer is A.**

$$
\begin{array}{r}
307.401 \\
-\ 25.246 \\
\hline
282.155
\end{array}
$$

4. **The correct answer is C.**

$$
\begin{array}{r}
14.75 \\
15.1256 \\
+\ \ 0.07 \\
\hline
29.9456 = 29.946
\end{array}
$$

5. **The correct answer is D.**

$$
\begin{array}{r}
600. \\
0.0606.\overline{)36.3600.} \\
\underline{36.36} \\
00
\end{array}
$$

6. **The correct answer is C.**

$$\frac{1}{8} = 1:8$$

7. **The correct answer is A.**

$$2:8 = 11:x$$
$$2x = 88$$
$$x = 44$$

8. **The correct answer is B.**

$$85\% = 0.85 = \frac{85}{100} = \frac{17}{20}$$

9. **The correct answer is D.**

$$0.12 = 12\%$$

10. **The correct answer is C.**

$$
\begin{array}{r}
\frac{1}{6} = \frac{4}{24} \\
-\ \frac{1}{8} = \frac{3}{24} \\
\hline
\frac{1}{24}
\end{array}
$$

11. **The correct answer is B.**

$$1\frac{1}{2} \times \frac{1}{8} = \frac{3}{2} \times \frac{1}{8} = \frac{3}{16}$$

12. **The correct answer is A.**

$$\frac{8}{32} = \frac{1}{4}$$

13. **The correct answer is C.**

$$\frac{60 \text{ women}}{15 \text{ men}} = \frac{4}{1}$$

14. **The correct answer is D.**

$$\frac{5 \text{ oz. sugar}}{20 \text{ oz. total mixture}} = \frac{1}{4}$$

15. **The correct answer is D.**

$$\frac{30}{150} = 150\overline{)30.00} = 20\%$$
$$\underline{300}$$
$$00$$

16. **The correct answer is A.**

$$2\frac{2}{3} = 2\frac{8}{12}$$
$$+1\frac{3}{4} = 1\frac{9}{12}$$
$$\overline{3\frac{17}{12} = 4\frac{5}{12}}$$

17. **The correct answer is B.**

$$1\frac{3}{4} = 1\frac{9}{12}$$
$$+2\frac{1}{3} = 2\frac{4}{12}$$
$$\overline{3\frac{13}{12} = 4\frac{1}{12}}$$

$$10 \text{ lbs}$$
$$\underline{-4\frac{1}{12} \text{ lbs}}$$
$$5\frac{11}{12} \text{ lbs}$$

18. **The correct answer is A.**

$$\frac{3}{\cancel{8}_{1}} \times \frac{\cancel{16}^{2}}{1} = 6 \text{ ounces}$$

19. **The correct answer is B.**

$$\frac{2}{\cancel{8}_{1}} \times \frac{\cancel{16}^{2}}{1} = \$4.00$$

20. **The correct answer is C.**

$$\frac{3}{\cancel{8}_{1}} \times \frac{\cancel{3000}^{600}}{1} = 1,800 \text{ Democrats}$$

Science

OVERVIEW

The practical nurse needs comprehensive knowledge of basic concepts in order to understand body structure and functions and to recognize deviations from the norm. This unit provides facts and principles related to body structure, how the body functions, nutrition, and factors affecting health.

UNDERSTANDING BODY STRUCTURE AND FUNCTION

Understanding the concepts of anatomy and physiology is an important foundation for nursing. This section gives an overview of the structure and function of cells and each biological system in the human body. Cells, tissue, and organs make up the structure of multicellular organisms such as humans. Structure refers to the arrangement of parts of the organism and function refers to the activity of each part of the organism.

The Cell

Like all living organisms, humans are made up of cells. A cell is the smallest functional and structural unit of a living organism. Some organisms are made up of just one cell, but the human body is composed of trillions of cells. Although there are many types of cells in the human body and each has a specific function and structure, there are basic structures that are common to almost all of the cells in the body.

Cell Membrane

The cell membrane is a protective layer that covers the cell's outer surface. The membrane acts as a protective barrier between the inside of the cell and the cell's environment. There are small channels in the cell membrane that allow for substances such as water, oxygen, sodium, potassium, proteins, and other macromolecules to pass into and out of the cell.

The Cytoplasm

The region inside the cell membrane that includes the cellular fluids and all the organelles except the nucleus is called the **cytoplasm**. The cytoplasm is a watery substance that helps to maintain the shape of the cell and the concentration of various substances, such as sodium and potassium, in the cell.

The Nucleus

The nucleus is the control center of the cell. It is a membrane-bound organelle that contains the genetic information of the cell. Genetic information is packaged into molecules of DNA (deoxyribonucleic acid) that provide instruction for all the cell's processes. The DNA is responsible for the cell's ability to reproduce itself. Inside the nucleus is another structure called the **nucleolus**, and this is where RNA (ribonucleic acid) is made.

The Organelles

An organelle is a small structure in the cell's cytoplasm that performs a specific function for the cell. The following are typical organelles found in human cells.

- **Ribosomes:** Ribosomes are structures that are assembled in the nucleolus from proteins and RNA and are then transported to the cytoplasm. Ribosomes are the sites of protein synthesis.

- **Endoplasmic reticulum (ER):** The ER is the site of protein production and transportation. Some ER organelles are coated with ribosomes. These are called **rough ER** and are the structures in which proteins are made. Another type of ER has a smooth outer surface and is called **smooth ER**. It functions to break down toxic chemicals in the body and make lipids (fats), steroids, and hormones.

- **Golgi apparatus:** The Golgi apparatus, or Golgi body, plays a role in protein synthesis by making modifications to proteins, processing and sorting them, and then packaging the final protein product in a small sac called a **vesicle**. The vesicle leaves the Golgi body and transports the protein to the cell membrane where it can leave the cell to carry out its function in the body.

- **Mitochondria:** The mitochondria are known as the powerhouse of the cell. Their function is to convert energy from organic molecules into adenosine triphosphate (ATP), which is a form of energy that can be used by the cell.

- **Lysosomes:** Lysosomes are the "clean-up" crew of cells. They are tiny sacs that contain enzymes that can digest other molecules and substances. In the lysosome, old worn-out organelles, cell debris, and large molecules are broken down and digested.

- **Cytoskeleton:** The cytoskeleton helps to maintain the shape of the cell. It is made up of a network of fibers called **microtubules** and **microfilaments**.

- **Vacuoles:** Vacuoles are storage sacs filled with fluid. They store water, food, salts, waste, and pigments.

- **Centrioles:** Centrioles are the center of microtubule production in animal and human cells.

The Respiratory System

The respiratory system exchanges oxygen from the air with carbon dioxide in the body. The exchange of gases takes place in the lungs. When a person inhales air through the mouth or nose, it is drawn into the lungs. In the lungs, the oxygen is transferred into the blood. The oxygen-rich blood in the lungs exits through capillaries and enters cells in the body. The oxygen is used in each cell for cellular respiration. During cellular respiration, energy that is stored in food molecules is released to form ATP, which is the energy source all cells use to maintain function and growth. Therefore, without oxygen, cells would not be able to produce energy to survive.

When a person exhales air out of the lungs, carbon dioxide is released from the body. Carbon dioxide is a waste product of cellular respiration, and the body needs to rid itself of it. Blood containing carbon dioxide moves from the cells in the body into capillaries that carry the blood back to the lungs. As the lungs relax, they expel the carbon dioxide.

The quantity of available oxygen determines the effectiveness of respiration. In addition, oxygen consumption by the body is directly proportional to the rate of energy use and the level of physical activity of the body. Changes in oxygen consumption caused by an increase or decrease in physical activity have a temporary effect on the concentration of oxygen in the blood. Blood oxygen levels are restored to normal by a change in the respiratory rate. Metabolic processes are also affected by the level of oxygen in the blood.

The human respiratory system consists of the following parts:

- **Nasal / Oral Cavity:** The nasal cavity (nose) and the oral cavity (mouth) are the openings through which air is drawn into the body. Both cavities moisten and warm the air that enters the body. Nose hairs help to filter inspired air by trapping some particulate matter.

- **Pharynx (throat):** The pharynx is the passageway that connects the oral and nasal cavities to the esophagus and larynx. It serves both respiratory and digestive functions. When food is not being ingested, the air passage to the pharynx remains open so air can travel to the larynx. The pharynx also branches into the esophagus, which leads to the stomach.

- **Larynx (voice box):** The larynx contains vocal cords, and when air passes across the vocal cords, they vibrate, making vocal sounds.

- **Trachea (windpipe):** The trachea, or windpipe, is encircled by rings of cartilage so that it always remains open. Mucus in the trachea prevents dust and pollutants from entering the lungs.

- **Bronchi:** The trachea branches into two bronchi leading to the right and left lungs. The bronchi branch into narrower and narrower tubes called bronchioles.

- **Lungs:** Lungs are large sacs of air space and connective tissue. The lungs expand when air is taken in and contract when air is expelled.

- **Alveoli:** The alveoli are small clusters of sacs within the lungs that allow oxygen and carbon dioxide to move between the lungs and bloodstream. Alveoli are surrounded by blood vessels (capillaries), and oxygen moves across the thin walls of the alveoli into the blood vessels. As you breathe, air is sucked in and out of the alveoli.

- **Diaphragm:** The diaphragm, a dome-shaped muscle below the lungs, is responsible for the mechanical process of breathing. The diaphragm contracts to expand the chest when air is taken in and relaxes to decrease the volume of the lungs as air is expelled.

Blood that contains a lot of carbon dioxide is carried back to the lungs through blood vessels, and carbon dioxide travels back across the membrane of the capillaries and the alveoli where it can be expelled out through the respiratory structures (trachea, larynx, pharynx, mouth, or nose).

The Circulatory System

The circulatory system includes the cardiovascular system (heart and blood) and the lymphatic system (lymph nodes and lymphatic organs). Both systems work in connection with each other to move fluids around the body and protect the body from disease. Both systems are made up of a network of vessels, and both systems are part of the body's defense against bacteria, viruses, and other pathogens. The circulatory system in humans delivers oxygen and nutrients to cells throughout the body and carries carbon dioxide to the lungs and metabolic waste to the excretory system.

The Cardiovascular System

The heart, blood, and blood vessels make up the cardiovascular system.

The Heart

The heart is a four-chambered organ that pumps blood throughout the body by contracting and creating a pressure that moves the blood through vessels. The upper chambers of the heart are called the right and left atria (singular: atrium), and the lower chambers are called the right and left ventricles. Flap-like structures called valves are located between the atria and the ventricles. These valves ensure that blood flows in only one direction. The left atrium of the heart receives oxygen-rich blood from the lungs. The left ventricle of the heart pumps oxygen-rich blood through the body. The right atrium receives oxygen-poor blood from the body, and the right ventricle pumps oxygen-poor blood to the lungs.

Blood

Blood consists of four components: plasma, red blood cells (erythrocytes), white blood cells (leukocytes), and platelets.

- **Plasma** is a fluid component in the blood that is a mixture of proteins, enzymes, nutrients, wastes, hormones, and gases, which it carries and delivers throughout the body. It makes up the largest component of blood, at about 55 percent. The other three blood components float in the plasma.

The remaining blood components are made in the marrow of the bone. Blood formation begins in pluripotent stem cells that mature to become red blood cells, white blood cells, or platelets.

- **Red blood cells** are small, disc-shaped cells. Their size and shape help them to squeeze through capillaries to deliver oxygen to and pick up carbon dioxide from body tissue. Red blood cells contain an iron-rich protein called **hemoglobin**, which binds to oxygen and carries it through the bloodstream and throughout the body.

- **White blood cells** serve to fight infection in the body. They keep the body healthy by fighting infection from pathogens such as bacteria and viruses. Some white blood cells, called **phagocytes**, destroy pathogens by consuming toxins or infectious material; others, called **lymphocytes**, participate in cell defense and immunity by forming antibodies against the pathogens. **B-cells** are a type of lymphocyte that produces antibodies against foreign antigens. **Helper T-cells** help the B-cells and other T-cells. **Killer T-cells** destroy cells that have been infected with a virus.

- **Platelets** are tiny fragments of bone marrow cells in the blood that are important in minimizing blood loss through three mechanisms: vascular constriction, which slows the bleeding of an injured blood vessel; platelet plug formation, during which platelets adhere to an injury site and to other platelets to form a plug that can stop or reduce minor bleeding; and blood clotting.

Blood can be further characterized by blood type. There are four blood types found in humans: A, B, AB, and O. These are based on the antigen found in the red blood cells. Knowing a person's blood type is important for two reasons: 1) if he or she needs to receive blood, or 2) if the person wishes to donate blood.

- A person with type A blood will have the A antigen and will have white blood cells that produce antibodies against the B antigen (anti-B). People with this blood type can donate blood to others with type A blood or to someone with type AB blood. They can receive blood from type A or type O individuals.

- Blood type B contains B antigens and anti-A antibodies. A person with blood type B can donate to type B or AB individuals and can receive blood from type B and O donors.

- Type AB blood contains A and B antigens and no antibodies. These individuals can donate blood only to AB individuals and can receive blood from all blood types.

- Type O blood contains no antigens and has both anti-A and anti-B antibodies. Type O blood can be donated to others of any blood type and is called the **universal donor**. Individuals with type O blood can receive only type O blood.

Blood Vessels

There are three types of blood vessels that carry blood through the body: arteries, capillaries, and veins.

An **artery** is a blood vessel that has thick walls containing a layer of smooth muscle and carries blood away from the heart. Blood is pumped into the arteries at high pressure when the heart contracts. This is known as **blood pressure**. The pressure pushes blood through the arteries. Artery walls are strong and able to stretch so that they can withstand this pressure.

A **capillary** is a tiny, thin-walled blood vessel that allows an exchange of gases between the blood and cells. Capillaries lead to veins. **Veins** are blood vessels that carry blood back to the heart. When

NOTE

Be sure you know the donors and recipients for the different blood types.

the blood reaches the veins, it is not under the same high pressure as it was when it flowed from the heart into the arteries. Therefore, veins are thin-walled and do not have a lining of muscle. The contraction of skeletal muscles surrounding the veins enable the blood to move through the veins and back to the heart. There are valves in the veins that keep the blood from flowing backward.

The path of blood flow through the heart, the body, and then back to the heart is demonstrated in the following eight steps.

1. Oxygen-rich blood leaves the left ventricle and enters the aorta, which is the largest blood vessel in the body.

2. Blood travels through the aorta into the systemic circulatory system, which is made up of smaller arteries, arterioles, and capillaries.

3. The gas-and-nutrient exchange takes place between the blood and tissue through the capillary walls by the mechanisms of diffusion and osmosis. Oxygen and glucose are delivered to cells. The cells use oxygen and glucose to make ATP, which provides energy for the cell. Carbon dioxide, water, and other waste products are delivered to the blood to be carried away from the cells.

4. This oxygen-poor blood passes from capillaries to venules to veins. From the veins, blood flows to the superior or inferior vena cava, the largest veins in the body. Blood is returned to the heart through the veins by a passive mechanism of pushing from behind and a squeezing of the veins by skeletal muscles and gravity. The walls of veins do not contain muscle fibers like the walls of arteries.

5. The vena cava deliver the oxygen-poor blood to the right atrium of the heart. The blood passes through the tricuspid valve into the right ventricle.

6. The right ventricle sends the blood through the right and left pulmonary arteries to the lungs. In the lungs, the blood becomes oxygen-rich. The pulmonary arteries branch off into pulmonary capillaries. Carbon dioxide and water are exchanged for oxygen.

7. The pulmonary veins carry oxygenated blood to the left atrium of the heart. Blood passes from the left atrium through the bicuspid valve into the left ventricle.

8. The left ventricle pumps the blood back out to the body through the aorta.

The stimulation of the heart comes from within the heart muscle, but the rate of the heartbeat, or muscle contractions, is modified by chemicals such as hormones and nerve transmissions from the brain. The rate and volume of blood flowing through the vessels are directly proportional to the blood pressure and is partially maintained by the closed nature of the circulatory system. Arteries are able to alter their internal diameter through the processes of constriction and dilation, and blood pressure is inversely proportional to the diameter of the arteries. It is important to remember that arteries have high pressure, muscular walls, and can regulate the rate of blood flow. Arteries do not have valves. Veins, on the other hand, have low pressure, no muscle, and are passive receivers of blood. Veins have an internal, one-way valve leading to the heart to prevent the backflow of blood.

The Lymphatic System

The **lymphatic system** is a group of tissue and organs that collect fluid that leaks from the blood and returns it to the bloodstream so that it can be expelled. The fluid that leaks out of the blood is called **lymph**, which flows toward the heart. The lymphatic system—unlike the cardiovascular system—is an open circulatory system. As a result, lymph can move in and out of vessels. The lymphatic system together with the immune system helps the body to fight disease and pathogens. Other lymph vessels in the body move fats from the intestine into the blood so they can be carried to cells.

Every time the heart pumps blood at high pressure, a small amount of fluid is forced out of the capillary walls. Most of this fluid is reabsorbed by the capillaries, and the remaining fluid is collected by lymph capillaries, which are permeable, so fluids can pass into and out of them, and they can pick up interstitial fluids. Lymph capillaries absorb fluids, dead cell particles, pathogens, and toxic substances. Lymph capillaries carry lymph to larger lymph vessels. The lymph vessels return the fluid to the cardiovascular system when the fluid drains into blood vessels at the base of the neck. White blood cells mature in the lymphatic system and can then attack pathogens picked up by the lymph. There are also organs and tissue associated with the lymph system.

- **Lymph nodes:** Lymph nodes are small, bean-shaped organs that remove pathogens and dead cell material from the lymph. Lymph nodes are concentrated in the neck, armpits, and groin areas of the body. Infection-fighting white blood cells called **B-lymphocytes** are found in lymph nodes. When bacteria or other pathogens cause an infection, the number of B-lymphocytes increases. As lymph nodes fill with B-lymphocytes, they may become swollen and tender to the touch. Thus, swollen lymph nodes are a good indicator of infection in the body.

- **Bones:** Bone, in particular bone marrow, is another important part of the lymphatic system. **Bone marrow** is the soft tissue in the center of a bone where blood cells are produced. Bone marrow produces the white blood cells of the lymphatic system.

- **Tonsils:** Tonsils are small lymphatic organs at the back of the throat that help to defend against infection. White blood cells in the tonsils help to trap pathogens from entering the body cavity. When tonsils take up pathogens, they become swollen and sore.

- **Thymus:** The thymus is an organ found in the chest region that is part of the lymphatic system. Some of the white blood cells that are produced in bone marrow are processed and developed in the thymus. White blood cells leave the thymus and travel through the lymphatic system to lymph nodes and other areas of the body. The thymus shrinks as a person ages.

- **Spleen:** The spleen is the largest lymphatic organ in the body. It stores white blood cells and allows them to mature. As blood flows through the spleen, white blood cells attack or mark any pathogens that might be in the blood. If pathogens cause an infection in another area of the body, the spleen can release white blood cells into the bloodstream as it passes through.

The Immune System

The immune system helps to keep the body healthy and free from disease. There are a series of processes that are carried out by the immune system to help prevent the spread of disease through the body. Several types of cells play a role in the immune system:

- **Phagocyte cells:** Phagocyte cells are activated and float around the body. This type of cell includes neutrophils, monocytes, and macrophages. They seek out and "eat," or engulf, foreign antigens from pathogens or diseased cells.

- **Basophils and eosinophils:** These types of cells release chemicals that respond to inflammation due to infection.

- **Natural killer cells (NKCs):** These cells are released to attack foreign antigens.

- **Cytokines and interferons:** These are chemicals in the immune system that are released to block viruses from replicating and activate surrounding cells that have antiviral functions.

- **B-cells:** B-cells or B-lymphocytes produce antibodies against disease-specific antigens. Some B-cells can become memory B-cells that produce plasma cells after an infection has been overcome by the immune system. These plasma cells produce antibodies that help with long-term immunity to a specific virus or bacteria.

- **T-cells:** When T-cells encounter infected cells, they are activated and multiply. Some T-cells become memory T-cells, and others become helper T-cells. Memory T-cells recognize a bacteria or virus that has previously infected the body. These cells help with long-term immunity. Helper T-cells activate B-lymphocytes and other T-cells. Other T-cells, called **cytotoxic T-cells**, recognize and kill infected cells.

Active immunity occurs when the immune system is exposed to an antigen of a particular virus or pathogen. Antibodies are created and stored permanently in the immune system to prevent a future infection by the same virus or pathogen. Artificial active immunity can be obtained through immunization. This type of immunization involves the injection of a specific antigen so that the immune system can build up antibodies against it. Immunization in which a body is injected with antibodies to fight against specific infections is called **passive immunity**. This type of immunity is immediate, but short-lived.

The Digestive System

The digestive system breaks down the food that is consumed into nutrients that the body can use for growth and energy. The digestive system interacts with other body systems to utilize the energy obtained from food consumed. Blood transports nutrients through the circulatory system once food has been digested. The respiratory system provides oxygen to cells so that they can produce energy from the nutrients that travel through the circulatory system to the cells. In addition, the nervous system controls and regulates the functioning of the digestive system. The rate of digestion is directly proportional to the type and quantity of food ingested.

The human digestive process occurs in five steps: ingestion, digestion, secretion, absorption, and defecation. The digestive system consists of the following:

- **Alimentary canal:** The alimentary canal is a long muscular tube that starts at the mouth and ends at the anus. Digestion begins in the mouth through the process of mechanical and chemical digestion. Teeth break down and crush the food ingested. Saliva is secreted from glands in the mouth. The saliva contains many substances, including many enzymes that begin the chemical digestion of food. The alimentary canal is called the **gastrointestinal (GI) tract** and consists of the mouth, pharynx, esophagus, stomach, small intestine, and large intestine. The lining of the GI tract secretes mucus to lubricate the passage of food and to protect the lining of the tract from enzymes or acids. The associated organs of the digestive system aid the GI tract either by providing secretions or helping to break down food.

- **Esophagus:** As food is swallowed, it moves through the throat (pharynx) and into the esophagus. The esophagus is a long tube that moves the food through a wave of muscle contractions called **peristalsis**.

- **Stomach:** Both mechanical and chemical digestion take place in the stomach. The stomach is a muscular bag that contracts to crush and mix up food with acids and enzymes. The acids and the enzymes form what is called **gastric juice**. Acids act to kill some bacteria that may be swallowed with food, and enzymes break down proteins. A thick layer of mucus protects the lining of the stomach from the acidic gastric juice.

- **Small intestine:** After digestion in the stomach, food is reduced to a soupy mixture called **chyme**. Chyme leaves the stomach and moves to the small intestine. The small intestine is a long, muscular tube of narrow diameter where most chemical digestion takes place and most nutrients are absorbed. After nutrients are broken down, they are absorbed into the bloodstream.

- **Large intestine:** After food moves through the small intestine and some nutrients from the food are absorbed, food moves into the large intestine. In the large intestine, water and vitamins are absorbed. The solid material remaining in the large intestine is waste, which is compacted and stored in the rectum and eventually eliminated through the anus.

- **Accessory organs:** The digestion of nutrients in the small intestine takes place with the aid of three other organs: the pancreas, the liver, and the gall bladder. The pancreas produces fluids that break down proteins, carbohydrates, fats, and nucleic acids. The liver makes and releases a mixture called **bile**. Bile is stored in the gall bladder. The bile breaks down fats into small droplets.

There are several processes that occur in the digestive system:

1. **Ingestion:** Food is taken into the body through the mouth.
2. **Propulsion:** The tongue pushes food into the pharynx and triggers a swallowing reflex. Once food enters the pharynx, it is propelled through the GI tract by peristalsis. Peristalsis involves alternating involuntary waves of constriction and relaxation that move the food along the tract.

3. **Mechanical digestion:** Mechanical digestion involves the chewing of food, the churning and mixing of the food in the stomach, and the breaking down of food in the small intestine.

4. **Chemical digestion:** Chemical digestion takes place along the digestive tract between the mouth and the small intestine. Chemicals and enzymes break down food. Gastric juices in the stomach include stomach acids, mucus, and enzymes. Digestion of food begins in the stomach and continues in the small intestine. The liver and the pancreas aid in the digestion process that occurs in the small intestine. The liver produces bile that helps in the digestion of fats, and the pancreas produces pancreatic juice, which is a mixture of digestive enzymes and alkaline solution. All four types of molecules—carbohydrates, proteins, fats, and nucleic acids—are digested in the small intestine by enzymes that are specific to each type of molecule. The digestion of carbohydrates begins in the oral cavity and is completed in the small intestine. The digestion of proteins begins in the stomach and is completed in the small intestine. Pancreatic juice released into the small intestine contains nucleases (pancreatic ribonuclease and deoxyribonuclease) to hydrolyze ingested nucleic acids. Nucleosidases and phosphatases continue to break down the nucleic acids in the small intestine. Fats remain undigested until they reach the duodenum of the small intestine.

5. **Absorption:** The absorption of nutrients from food into the bloodstream occurs mostly in the small intestine. Some nutrients are absorbed by diffusion and others are pumped across a concentration gradient into cells. Large vessels transport nutrients from the intestine directly into the liver. The liver is involved in body metabolism by regulating the amount of glycogen it stores and the amount of glucose that is released into the bloodstream. Water is also absorbed by the large intestine and reabsorbed back into the bloodstream.

6. **Defecation:** Defecation includes ridding the body of waste material in the form of feces. This occurs through the large intestine, or colon. Waste products consist mostly of indigestible plant fibers and bacteria.

The Excretory System

As your cells perform the chemical activities to keep the body functioning, waste products such as carbon dioxide and ammonia are produced. These waste products are toxic to cells and must be removed in order to keep cells and the body healthy. The excretory system eliminates cellular wastes from the body through the lungs, skin, kidneys, and the digestive system and regulates the chemical composition, pH, and water balance of the blood.

Waste products are filtered through the blood by the kidneys and eliminated in urine. Urine is made by three processes: filtration, reabsorption, and secretion.

The kidneys are able to absorb wastes and excess substances from the blood selectively and pass them to urine. The kidneys then reabsorb any necessary nutrients needed by the body and return them to the blood. A huge volume of blood passes through the kidneys to extract a liquid filtrate containing water, urea, glucose, amino acids, ions, and vitamins. The body requires many of these nutrients, and the kidneys concentrate the urea to pass in urine and return most of the water and nutrients to the bloodstream. This selective reabsorption conserves water and electrolytes in the body and balances their concentration in the blood and body tissues. The circulating volume of blood has a direct effect on kidney activity.

Urine is made up of urea, uric acid, and creatinine. Urea is a waste product formed from the breakdown of amino acids (proteins). Uric acid is a waste product from the breakdown of nucleic acids (DNA, RNA), and creatinine is a waste product formed by muscle metabolism.

The excretory system that makes up the urinary system is composed of the following structures:

- **Kidneys:** The kidneys are a pair of organs that act to remove waste product from blood. Urine is produced in the renal cortex of the kidneys. Microscopic structures called **nephrons** fill the inside of the kidneys. The nephrons are the functional units of the kidneys, and the human body has millions of nephrons. Fluids and waste product are filtered through the blood into the nephron through a structure called the **glomerulus**, a mass of capillaries lying in Bowman's capsule, a component of the nephron. Filtered blood leaves the glomerulus and circulates around the nephrons. Valuable salts and ions are returned to the blood, and another tube in the kidneys called the **collecting duct** collects the waste from the nephrons. Concentrated fluid (urine) in the collecting ducts then moves from the kidneys into the ureters.

- **Ureters:** Urine that leaves the kidneys flows into the ureters. These are the tubes that connect the kidneys to the bladder.

- **Bladder:** The bladder is a sac-like organ in the body that functions to store urine. As the bladder fills with urine, it is able to stretch. This stretching stimulates neurons in the bladder wall that send a message to the brain that gives an individual the urge to urinate, or void. Voluntary muscles in the bladder hold the urine inside until it is ready to be released. At that time, muscles contract and squeeze urine out of the bladder.

- **Urethra:** Urine exits the body by traveling through a narrow tube called the **urethra**.

Other waste products such as excess salts and water are released from the body through the pores in the skin. Carbon dioxide is a waste product of the respiratory system, and lungs release water and carbon dioxide during exhalation.

The Integumentary System

The integumentary system is composed of skin, hair, nails, and sweat and sebaceous glands. It functions to protect the body from injury and dehydration, to maintain a constant temperature in the body, to produce vitamin D, to excrete waste materials and toxins, and to react to microorganisms and chemicals.

The skin and all its associated structures, such as hair, nails, sweat and oil glands, and sensory receptors, make up the largest organ of the body. The skin is the body's first line of defense against infection or injury, heat and water loss, and UV radiation. It also assists with vitamin D production and sensory input.

The skin is composed of three layers of tissue:

1. **Epidermis:** The epidermis is a thin layer of cells on the body's outer surface. The epidermis has the fibrous protein keratin that helps keep water from entering or exiting the skin layers. Another layer of the epidermis is thin and clear and made up mostly of dead skin cells. It is found on the palms of hands and the soles of feet. Below this layer is the epidermis layer that will form scabs when the skin is wounded. This layer has special cells that contain granules in the cytoplasm. Below this layer is a layer of the epidermis that serves as a protective skin layer. The innermost layer of the epidermis is a single layer of melanocytes, or cells that contain melanin. Melanin protects the body from harmful UV rays and gives skin its pigment, or color. This is the layer of the epidermis in which mitosis (cell division) takes place and epidermis cells are replaced.

2. **Dermis:** The dermis is a thick layer of dense connective tissue that lies beneath the epidermis layer. The connective tissue is made up of collagen fibers. This is the region of the skin where nerve endings are located. Therefore, this is the skin layer that is sensitive to touch, heat, and pain. The dermis layer also contains hair follicles, sweat glands, and blood vessels. The upper layer of the dermis is called the **papillary layer.** This is the layer of skin that, on your fingers, is textured with fingerprint markings. Fibers from the dermis layer extend deep into skin tissue to help anchor the skin to the body.

3. **Hypodermis:** The hypodermis is a deep layer of fat that helps to protect and insulate the body.

The Musculoskeletal System

The muscular and skeletal systems are tightly linked together and function to supply structure and movement for the body. The skeletal system gives shape and support to the body and helps to prevent injury to internal organs. The rib cage protects the heart and lungs, the vertebrae protect the spinal cord, and the skull protects the brain. Bones also function to store important minerals such as calcium in their hard outer layer and produce red blood cells in their spongy center. Muscles contract to provide movement, and the bones act as levers for this movement. Muscle tissue is made of special proteins called **microfilaments** that shorten and lengthen to provide movement.

Bones and muscles are combined into individual systems resembling levers. This lever system consists of a muscle that provides force to the system, a joint that acts as the fulcrum, and a bone that acts like a lever. This arrangement allows for movement with a minimal expenditure of energy. A longer axis of the lever, or the bone, produces a greater extent of the movement of the body.

The Skeletal System

The skeletal system is composed of bones, cartilage, and ligaments. There are two parts to the skeletal system: the **axial skeleton** and the **appendicular skeleton**. The axial skeleton consists of the skull, the vertebrae, and the ribs. This system provides protection to organs and supports body weight. The appendicular skeletal system is composed of the arms, legs, shoulders, and pelvis. This system allows for movement of the body.

- **Bones:** Bones are hard organs made of minerals and connective tissue. They can be short, long, flat, or irregularly shaped, and contain nerves and blood vessels. Calcium is the most abundant mineral in bone tissue. The minerals in bones are continually deposited by bone cells called **osteoblasts**. Bone is deposited in proportion to the compressional load, or weight, that the bone must support. Bone tissue containing calcium and phosphorus is also continually absorbed by other cells called **osteoclasts**. Connective tissue in bone is made mostly of the fibrous protein collagen. Collagen allows bones to be flexible so that they don't break every time they are struck or bumped.

  Compact bone tissue is dense, is what makes bones hard and rigid, and is the outer layer of bones. Tiny channels in the compact bone contain blood capillaries. Spongy bone tissue has many open spaces, and it provides strength and support for the bone; it is found in the midsection of the bone. In long bones, such as those in the arm or leg, an outer layer of compact bone surrounds a layer of spongy bone. Inside the spongy bone is the marrow. There are two types of bone marrow: red marrow and yellow marrow. Red marrow is the site of red and white blood cell production. Red marrow is found in the center of flat bones such as the ribs. Yellow marrow is found in the center of long bones, and it stores fat cells.

- **Ligaments:** Ligaments are tough, flexible strands of connective tissue that connect bones to one another. Ligaments hold together joints between bones. They allow for the movement and flexibility of the body. Some ligaments such as those along the vertebrae prevent too much movement of the bones.

- **Joints:** Joints are the places where bones connect. Joints can be fixed to restrict movement or movable to allow bones to move independently of each other. Examples of movable joints include hinge joints and ball-and-socket joints.

- **Cartilage:** Cartilage is a strong, flexible, smooth connective tissue that is found at the ends of bones; it does not contain any blood vessels. It allows for bones to move smoothly across each other. Cartilage like that found at the tip of the nose and the ears is soft and bendable. Growth plates are areas of cartilage at the ends of bones that continue to make new bone tissue as the body grows. Osteoclasts move into the cartilage and harden it, turning it into bone tissue. Most bones harden completely after they stop growing, but osteoclasts are still present to repair bone if it breaks. Cartilage is found in developing embryos to a greater extent than it is found in a fully developed human.

The Muscular System

The muscular system is mostly composed of muscles that allow the body to move and function. Muscles pump blood through the body, cause the lungs to expand and relax, hold the body upright, and allow for mobility. A change in body position is produced by a shift in weight, which is accomplished by muscular force. The use of muscular force utilizes a large amount of energy and results in waste given off as thermal energy. The release of thermal energy during the application of muscular force helps to maintain a constant body temperature.

Muscle tissue is made up of muscle cells, and there are three types of muscle tissue in the body:

1. **Skeletal muscle:** Skeletal muscles allow for voluntary movement of the body and are attached to bones by tendons. Skeletal muscle may be striated (striped). The functional unit of the muscle cell is the **sarcomere**, which is composed of microfilaments called **actin** (thin filaments) and **myosin** (thick filaments). These microfilaments slide past each other as muscles contract to provide movement. As a muscle contracts, or shortens, the attached bones are pulled closer to one another and this allows for movement. Most skeletal muscles work in pairs around a joint. One muscle in the pair is called the **flexor**, and it bends a joint. The other is the **extensor**, and it straightens the joint. When one muscle in the pair contracts, the other relaxes to allow movement.

2. **Cardiac muscle:** Cardiac muscle is the tissue that makes up the heart. The movement of cardiac muscle is involuntary, so that the heart contracts and relaxes without humans being conscious of it. Blood is continually pumped through the body, and in order to continually contract and relax the heart, muscle tissue requires a great amount of energy. In order to supply so much energy, cardiac muscle cells have a huge number of ATP-producing mitochondria.

3. **Smooth muscle:** Smooth muscle is found lining the walls of organs such as the stomach, blood vessels, intestines, and bladder. Smooth muscle functions to help move materials such as blood and food through the body. Like cardiac muscle, it is involuntary; that is, the body is not capable of conscious movement of smooth muscle.

Muscles contract in the following manner:

1. A nerve impulse is sent to a skeletal muscle.

2. The neuron sending the impulse releases neurotransmitters onto the muscle cell.

3. The muscle depolarizes.

4. Depolarization of the muscle causes the sarcoplasmic reticulum to release calcium ions.

5. The released calcium ions cause the actin and myosin filaments in the striated muscle to slide past one another.

6. The sliding movement causes the muscle to contract, a motion driven by ATP. Muscle contractions cause movement of the body.

7. As the muscle relaxes, the filaments slide back to their original positions, and the muscle lengthens again.

The Nervous System

The nervous system is made of structures, cells, and organs that control the actions and reactions of the body in response to stimuli either from the environment or from inside the body. A response to a stimulus involves the reception of the stimulus (sensory input), transmission of an impulse (integration), and a reaction to a stimulus (motor output). The nervous system is made up of two parts: the central nervous system and the peripheral nervous system.

The Central Nervous System

The **central nervous system (CNS)** is composed of the brain and the spinal cord, along with the cranial nerves. The brain is the central command organ of the nervous system. It is made up of several parts: the cerebrum (cerebral cortex), cerebellum, midbrain, hypothalamus, and pons. The cerebrum is divided into right and left hemispheres and consists of gray matter and white matter. It is the area of the brain in which sensory information is processed, and it controls voluntary movement. The cerebellum processes information that comes from inside the body. This allows the brain to keep track of body movements and position.

The rest of the brain makes up what is called the **brain stem**. The brain stem connects the brain to the spinal cord. The medulla in the brain stem controls involuntary processes, such as blood pressure, body temperature, heart rate, and breathing. The spinal cord allows the brain to communicate with the rest of the body. The spinal cord is composed of a bundle of nerves and is surrounded by protective vertebrae. Sensory information travels to the spinal cord, and the spinal cord sends impulses to the brain.

The Peripheral Nervous System

The **peripheral nervous system (PNS)** connects the CNS to the rest of the body. The PNS has two main components: sensory neurons and motor neurons. **Neurons** are the smallest functional units of the nervous system. They are excitable cells that conduct and transmit electrical signals that send sensory information to and from the brain. Neurons are composed of a **soma**, the cell body; **dendrites**, finger-like projections extending from the soma toward other neurons that allow the neuron to receive signals from other cells; and a single, long **axon**, along which the electrical signal travels to other neurons. At the end of each axon is an **axon terminal**. At the axon terminal, the electrical signal is converted to a chemical signal. This chemical signal is called a **neurotransmitter**, and it is released into the gap between two neurons called a **synaptic cleft**. The neurotransmitter crosses the synaptic cleft to the dendrites of another neuron.

Neurons are classified into three categories:

1. **Sensory neurons:** Sensory, or afferent, neurons receive impulses from the environment or inside the body and send them to the CNS.

2. **Motor neurons:** Motor, or efferent, neurons transmit nerve signals from the CNS to muscles or glands to produce a response to the initial stimulus. This causes a contraction of muscles or a secretion of hormones.

3. **Interneurons**: Interneurons, or association neurons, are neurons that link sensory neurons to motor neurons. They are found in the brain and the spinal cord.

In higher animals such as humans, well-developed sensory organs are involved in the reception of a stimulus. **External sensory organs** include the skin, eyes, ears, and nose. More primitive sense organs can be seen in some species, and other animals have well-developed sensory organs. Single-cell organisms such as *Euglena* have a primitive sensory organ called an eyespot.

Internal sensory information such as blood pressure, blood CO_2 level, muscle tension, and pain are received by internal sensory neurons.

Signals move through the CNS and the PNS with the help of special cells called **glial cells**. Glial cells act to protect and support neurons.

Some actions of the nervous system are involuntary. This means that these actions occur without a conscious decision. There is no control over the body to perform these actions. Actions that can be consciously controlled by the brain are called **voluntary actions**.

Transmission

The transmission of nerve impulses is electrical in nature and involves a difference in the concentration of certain ions, in particular, sodium (Na^+) and potassium (K^+). The difference in concentration forms a gradient along the nerve fibers. The electrical potential difference generated by the ion gradient between the inside of a neuron and the outside is called the **membrane potential**. A neuron that is not transmitting a signal is at its resting membrane potential. The threshold potential in a neuron that is transmitting a signal is called an **action potential**.

Nerve impulses are transmitted from one neuron to another across a tiny gap between the cells called a **synapse**. Most synapses are chemical synapses, which involve the release of chemicals called **neurotransmitters** by the presynaptic neuron (the neuron that is transmitting the nerve impulse). Presynaptic neurons synthesize neurotransmitters and package them into **synaptic vesicles**. The vesicles are stored in the neuron's synaptic terminals. The release of a neurotransmitter into the synaptic space between two neurons either stimulates or blocks the generation of a nerve impulse in the postsynaptic neuron (the neuron that is receiving the nerve impulse). This mechanism allows the synapse to function as a point of control in a neural pathway.

Reaction

A reaction to a stimulus may involve a change in position, movement, or secretory activity. Several biological systems may be involved in the motor output, or reaction, to stimuli. These systems include the skeletal and muscular systems, the endocrine system, and the digestive system. Other systems more indirectly involved in the reaction to stimuli are the circulatory system, the respiratory system, and the excretory system. The motor output response leaves the central nervous system through motor neurons, which communicate with effector cells such as muscle or endocrine cells.

The Endocrine System

The endocrine system controls body functions and helps to maintain homeostasis through the use of hormones. Hormones are chemical messengers that are made in a specific organ called an **endocrine gland** and can cause a change in another cell or tissue in a different part of the body. Signals sent by endocrine glands are indirect because they cycle through the whole body.

Hormones have multiple functions, including regulating growth, behavior, development, digestion, metabolism, heart rate and reproduction. Hormones travel through the bloodstream and can only affect specific cells that have receptors for a given hormone. Cells that have receptors for a hormone are called **target cells**. The hormones bind to the receptors on the target cells and carry out their function.

The endocrine glands in the human body include the following:

- **Pituitary gland:** The pituitary gland secretes hormones that affect all other glands. Therefore, it is called the **master gland**. It also stimulates growth and sexual development. The pituitary gland sits at the base of the hypothalamus. One lobe of the pituitary gland secretes hormones made in the hypothalamus, including oxytocin and antidiuretic hormone (ADH). The other lobe of the pituitary gland makes and secretes hormones into the bloodstream.

- **Hypothalamus:** The hypothalamus gland controls the release of hormones found in the pituitary gland. Located at the base of the brain, it receives information from nerves about internal and external body conditions and responds by sending out the appropriate neural, or endocrine, signal.

- **Thyroid gland:** The thyroid gland is located in the neck. Hormones secreted from the thyroid affect almost every tissue type in the body. It secretes two hormones, thyroxine (T4) and triiodothyronine (T3), which control the metabolism in the body and control blood calcium levels by removing calcium from the bloodstream and depositing it back into bone tissue. An excess of T3 and T4 can cause hyperthyroidism, and a deficit of these hormones can cause hypothyroidism.

- **Parathyroid gland:** There are four parathyroid glands, and all are located on the surface of the thyroid. The parathyroid glands secrete calcitonin, which lowers blood calcium levels, and parathyroid hormone, which raises blood calcium levels. The action of these two hormones maintains calcium homeostasis in the body.

- **Pineal gland:** The pineal gland is in the brain stem and produces hormones that are essential for the control of sleep, aging, reproduction, and body temperature. It synthesizes and secretes melatonin, which links biorhythms with environmental light (daily and seasonal).

- **Adrenal glands:** Adrenal glands are located above the kidneys and secrete hormones in response to stress on the body. Two of the hormones secreted are epinephrine and norepinephrine; they increase blood glucose and increase metabolic activity while constricting certain blood vessels. These hormones trigger a "fight-or-flight" response. Adrenal glands also secrete glucocorticoids such as cortisol (which increases blood glucose) and mineral corticoids (which promote reabsorption of Na^+ and excretion of K^- in the kidneys); these hormones provide a slower, longer-lasting response to stress in the body.

- **Pancreas:** The pancreas helps to regulate blood sugar (glucose) levels in the body. The pancreas produces two hormones that play a role in maintaining the body's energy supply: insulin, which lowers blood glucose, and glucagon, which raises blood glucose.

- **Gonads:** The testes and ovaries are gonads, or sex glands, that secrete sex hormones and produce gametes (sperm and ova). The testes produce hormones called **androgens** (including testosterone) that support sperm formation and promote development and maintenance of male secondary sex characteristics. The ovaries produce hormones called **estrogen** and **progesterone**. Estrogen stimulates growth of the uterine lining and promotes the development and maintenance of female secondary sex characteristics. Progesterone promotes growth of the uterine lining so that it can support an embryo during pregnancy.

- **Thymus gland:** The thymus gland secretes the hormone thymosin, which stimulates T-cell production for the immune system. It is located behind the sternum and between the lungs; the thymus is active only until puberty, after which it starts to shrink and is replaced by fat. The mechanism of hormone activity depends upon whether the hormone is a steroid hormone or a protein hormone. A steroid hormone can diffuse across the membrane of a target cell where it binds to a receptor protein in the cell nucleus. In the nucleus, the hormone will activate specific genes in the cell's DNA. If the hormone is a protein, it must bind to a receptor on the surface of the target cell. This triggers the production of a second messenger called **cyclic AMP** (cAMP). The cAMP activates enzymes in cells to initiate changes.

The endocrine system helps to keep the body in homeostasis by increasing or decreasing the amount of hormones found in the bloodstream. This process is a feedback mechanism. Information from one action controls or affects another action or process.

The Reproductive System

Sexual reproduction in humans involves the creation of offspring by the fusion of a male and female sex cell, or gamete. The male gamete is the sperm, and the female gamete is the ovum (egg). Sex cells contain half the number of chromosomes (23) as other cells in the body, and when the sperm and ovum fuse during the process of fertilization, their chromosomes combine to form a fertilized egg (zygote) with the normal number of chromosomes (46). The male and female reproductive systems have distinctly different components.

The Male Reproductive System

The male reproductive system functions to produce sperm and deliver them to the female reproductive system. Sperm are male sex cells, or gametes, and each sperm contains 23 chromosomes, which is half the number of other types of cells in the body. The male reproductive system also produces hormones involved in growth and development of males and gamete production. Male hormones are continually secreted throughout the life of a male.

There are several organs and structures in the male reproductive system.

- **Testes:** Testes are the main organ of the male reproductive system. They produce testosterone, which is the male sex hormone. Testosterone is the hormone responsible for many male traits, including facial and body hair and a deep voice. These traits are known as **secondary sex characteristics**. The testes are also the site of sperm production. Immature sperm cells are called **spermatids**. Testes are located within the scrotum, which are saclike structures that keep the testes outside the body so that they remain slightly cooler than body temperature.

- **Epididymis:** The epididymis is where sperm are stored after they have matured. The spermatids travel to the epididymis and mature into sperm cells.

- **Vas deferens:** When sperm leave the epididymis, they enter a tube called the **vas deferens.** In the vas deferens, sperm mix with fluid that comes from seminal vesicles and the prostate gland. The seminal vesicles provide sperm with fructose (sugar) and nutrients, and the prostate gland secretes a watery and alkaline fluid. The mixture of sperm and fluid is called **semen.** Semen acts to neutralize the acidic vaginal fluids during fertilization.

- **Urethra:** In leaving the body, sperm pass through a narrow tube called the **urethra.** Urine also passes through this tube.

- **Penis:** The penis is the organ that delivers semen into the female reproductive system.

The Female Reproductive System

The female reproductive system produces ova, or eggs, and hormones. It also provides a protective environment to nourish a developing fetus. The ovum, or egg, is the female gamete, and, therefore, like sperm, it only contains 23 chromosomes, or half the number of chromosomes of other cells in the body. The hormones secreted in the female reproductive system are estrogen and progesterone. These hormones control the development of female sex characteristics such as breasts and wide hips. They are also responsible for the development and release of eggs in a regulated cycle called the **menstrual cycle** and the preparation of the reproductive system for pregnancy.

There are several organs and structures in the female reproductive system.

- **Ovaries:** The ovaries are the reproductive organs in which eggs are produced. At sexual maturity, females have thousands of immature eggs (follicles) in the ovaries. During a lifetime, about 400 eggs will be released during the menstrual cycle of a female. The rest of the follicles will not leave the ovaries. Eggs are released about midway through the menstrual cycle, and a typical cycle lasts 28 days.

- **Fallopian tubes:** When eggs are released from the ovaries during a process called **ovulation,** they travel through the fallopian tubes. These are tubes that connect the ovaries to the uterus. Fertilization of an egg occurs in the upper third of the fallopian tube. During intercourse, a few hundred sperm travel up into the fallopian tubes. The sperm release an enzyme that helps to dissolve the outer covering of eggs. When one sperm enters the egg, the membrane is altered so that no other sperm can enter, and the process of embryo formation begins. The egg and sperm combine to form one cell (now with 46 chromosomes), and this cell divides to form an embryo. The genetic material from the sperm and the egg combine, and a unique individual develops.

- **Uterus:** The egg travels through the fallopian tube and into the uterus. This process takes about five to six days. A fertilized egg will implant itself in the thickened lining of the uterus and develop into an embryo and then a fetus. A developing fetus will release a hormone called **human chorionic gonadotropin** (HCG) that helps to maintain the protective uterine lining throughout pregnancy. A fetus matures and develops for about 38 weeks in the uterus.

An unfertilized ovum will not be implanted into the uterine lining and will be released from the uterus during a process of menstruation. During menstruation, the uterine lining is shed from the body. When menstruation ends, the lining of the uterus thickens, and the cycle begins again. Rising estrogen levels stimulate the development of a new lining in the uterus. Other hormones called **follicle stimulating hormone (FSH)** and **luteinizing hormone** (**LH**) also play a role in the menstrual cycle. FSH stimulates activity in the ovaries (and in the testes of males), and LH stimulates the release of an ovum (and the production of testosterone in males).

- **Vagina:** When a fetus is fully developed, it passes through the vagina during birth. The vagina is the canal between the uterus and outside the body. It is sometimes referred to as the **birth canal**.

The Stages of Fetal Development

A normal pregnancy spans about nine months. This time is measured from the date of the last start of menstruation to the birth of a fully developed baby. These nine months are broken down into three segments called **trimesters**. Each trimester spans a three-month period.

1. **First trimester:** The first trimester spans the first three months of development. The embryo implants in the first trimester. Soon after the first trimester begins, the placenta begins to grow. The placenta is a network of blood vessels that provides the embryo with oxygen and nutrients from the mother's blood. The placenta also carries waste away from the developing embryo. During the first trimester, the embryo becomes surrounded by amnion, a sac filled with fluid (amniotic fluid) that protects the embryo. The embryo is connected to the placenta through the umbilical cord. After ten weeks of development, the embryo becomes a fetus. During the first trimester, many organs such as the heart, liver, and brain form. Arms, legs, fingers, and toes also begin to develop.

2. **Second trimester:** The second trimester spans months four through six of development. During the second trimester, bones and joints begin to form. Muscles develop, and the fetus becomes stronger. It is during this trimester that fetal movement is detected. The fetus triples in size, and its brain rapidly develops and grows. Eventually, the fetus can make facial expressions. The fetus has the ability to hear, and it can make breathing movements and swallow. A protective coating called **vernix** forms on the skin.

3. **Third trimester:** The third trimester spans months seven through nine. During this trimester, the senses of sight, sound, taste, and touch are developed. The eyes can open and close, and the suck-swallow coordination is developed. The brain develops further, and organs become fully functional. Bones grow and harden, and the lungs completely develop. The skin thickens with brown fat that provides nutrition and insulation, helping to regulate body temperature in newborns. Amniotic fluid is absorbed during the eighth month. Antibodies from the mother are transferred to the baby. Eventually, the fetus is fully developed and ready to be born.

THE PRINCIPLES OF NUTRITION

Humans and other animals have three basic nutritional needs.

1. **Fuel** is required for all body activities.

2. **Organic molecules** are required to build molecules that are essential for proper body functions.

3. All animals must obtain **essential nutrients**, or substances that are not produced in the body, from foods.

Digestion breaks down the larger molecules of food into essential molecules of proteins, carbohydrates, and lipids (fats). Cells can then oxidize these smaller molecules for energy or assemble the smaller molecules into other proteins, carbohydrates, lipids, or nucleic acids that are essential to maintain cell structure and function. Eating too much or too little food, or the wrong kinds of food, can endanger our health.

Chemical Energy

Chemical energy obtained from food is used to power the body. Every activity that the body performs requires fuel in the form of chemical energy. The process of cellular metabolism produces ATP, which is a usable form of energy for all of the body's cells. The process of cellular metabolism involves the breakdown, or oxidizing, of large molecules (macromolecules) found in food, such as carbohydrates, lipids, and proteins. Usually, cells rely on carbohydrates and fats (lipids) as a source of readily usable fuel. If these molecules are in short supply, then proteins can be used as an energy source. Fats are the macromolecules that are the most energy-rich. One gram of fat gives off twice as much energy when it is oxidized than one gram of carbohydrate or protein.

The energy content of food is given in units of kilocalories. One kilocalorie is equal to 1,000 calories. In fact, the amount of calories listed on food labels is actually kilocalories, but is written as Calories (with a capital C).

The rate of energy consumption by the body is called its metabolic rate. The metabolic rate is equal to the sum of all of the energy-requiring reactions over a given period of time. The process of cellular metabolism must constantly drive chemical reactions in the cell in order for an organism to stay alive and for all body systems to function properly. The number of kilocalories that a resting body requires to maintain these functions—such as cellular maintenance, breathing, heartbeat, and regulation of body temperature—is called the basal metabolic rate (BMR). The BMR for healthy adult females is about 1,300 to 1,500 kcal per day, and about 1,600 to 1,800 kcal per day for a healthy adult male. Any activity performed beyond those activities essential to sustain bodily functions consumes more kilocalories of energy. The more strenuous the activity, the greater the energy demand. For example, running uses up more energy than walking.

If more energy is taken in, in the form of food, than the body requires to maintain its activity level, the energy is stored in various forms. The liver and muscles store energy in the form of glycogen. Most healthy bodies have enough glycogen stored to perform a day's worth of basic activities. Cells store extra energy as fat. The liver can convert carbohydrates and proteins to fat for storage. Most healthy humans have enough fats stored to provide energy to the body for several weeks without food. Undernourishment is a condition that results in a diet that is too low in calories.

Essential Nutrients

In addition to providing fuel in the form of carbohydrates, fats, and proteins, food must also provide essential nutrients for the body. Animal cells cannot produce nutrients from raw material, so they must be ingested in their complete form. Malnourishment is the result of a long-term deficiency of essential nutrients in the diet. There are four types of essential nutrients.

1. **Essential fatty acids:** Essential fatty acids include omega-3 and omega-6 fatty acids as well as linoleic acid. Linoleic acid is important because it is needed by cells to make the phospholipids of the cell membrane. Most balanced diets provide a sufficient amount of essential fatty acids.

2. **Essential amino acids:** Twenty amino acids are required to make proteins, and there are eight amino acids that the human body cannot synthesize. These eight amino acids are known as essential amino acids and must be taken into the body through the foods we eat. The body cannot store excess amino acids, so a deficiency of a single amino acid limits the use of other amino acids, disrupts protein synthesis, and can lead to protein deficiency in the body. Protein deficiency is the most common form of malnutrition seen in humans. All essential amino acids can be provided by eating meat, eggs, milk, and cheese. Vegetarians and vegans must be especially careful to obtain all eight essential amino acids. The key is to eat a variety of plant foods that supply sufficient quantities of amino acids. A combination of beans and corn can provide all eight essential amino acids.

3. **Vitamins:** A vitamin is an essential nutrient that is required by the body in very small amounts. There are thirteen essential vitamins: vitamin B_1, vitamin B_2, niacin (B_3), pantothenic acid (B_5), vitamin B_6, folic acid (B_9), vitamin B_{12}, biotin, vitamin C, vitamin A, vitamin D, vitamin E (tocopherol), and vitamin K. These vitamins can be obtained from a variety of foods, and all have essential functions in the body. For example, the B vitamins can function as coenzymes in the body during metabolic reactions, and vitamin C is required to produce connective tissue. Even though only a small amount is required, these vitamins are essential to good health. However, an excess of these vitamins can be harmful.

4. **Minerals:** Minerals are simple inorganic nutrients that are required by the body. Minerals like calcium and phosphorous are needed in relatively large amounts in order to construct and maintain healthy bone tissue. Calcium is also necessary for proper nerve and muscle function. Phosphorus is an essential component in ATP, DNA, and RNA. Iodine is required to make hormones produced in the thyroid that regulate the metabolic rate of the body. Sodium, potassium, and chloride are essential for nerve function and help to maintain the right amount of water in cells. Other essential minerals are magnesium, iron, fluorine, zinc, copper, manganese, cobalt, selenium, chromium, and molybdenum. Dietary source of minerals include dark green vegetables, legumes, proteins, and dairy products.

A normal and varied diet generally contains enough essential vitamins and minerals and is the best source of these nutrients. Certain people, however, can benefit from vitamin and mineral supplements. However, there is a concern that massive doses of certain vitamins can be harmful instead of beneficial and should therefore be avoided. An excess of fat-soluble vitamins (vitamins A, D, E, and K) can accumulate in the body to toxic levels, but an excess of water-soluble vitamins will be excreted in urine.

Food Labels

The Food and Drug Administration (FDA) requires that certain information be included on labels of packaged foods. Food labels include a list of ingredients listed in order from those used in the greatest amount to those used in the smallest amount.

Food labels also include nutrition facts. The serving size for the product is listed at the top of the label and is defined according to standards set by the FDA. The energy content of a single serving of the food product is listed in units of Calories (remember, this is actually in units of kilocalories).

Nutrients that are contained within one serving of the food product are listed as a percentage of the daily recommended amount based on a diet of 2,000 kcal per day. Emphasis is placed on informing consumers about nutrients that are linked to the risk of disease. These nutrients include fats (especially saturated and trans fats), cholesterol, and sodium. Other nutrients listed focus on those associated with a healthy diet, such as dietary fiber, protein, and certain vitamins and minerals (calcium, iron, vitamin A, B vitamins, and vitamin C).

Food labels allow consumers to compare nutrition facts of different brands and types of food choices. In this way, we can choose foods that will give us a balance of all the daily nutrition requirements. In a 2,000-kcal/day diet, it is recommended that an adult consume less than 65 g of fat, less than 20 g of saturated fats, less than 300 mg cholesterol, less than 2,400 mg sodium, 300 g of carbohydrates, and 25 g of dietary fiber.

Obesity and Weight Loss

Overnourishment, or consuming more food than is required to maintain all body functions and activities, leads to obesity. Obesity is the excessive accumulation of fat in cells, and it is now recognized by the World Health Organization (WHO) as a major global health problem.

Obesity can be brought on by a sedentary lifestyle, an increase in the availability of fattening foods, and oversized portions of certain foods. Over 30 percent of adults in the United States are considered obese, and another 35 percent are considered overweight. In addition, about 15 percent of all children and adolescents in the United States are overweight.

Obesity can contribute to many health problems, including diabetes, colon cancer, breast cancer, and cardiovascular disease. Some obese individuals may be predisposed to their overweight condition due to certain inherited factors. Scientists have isolated dozens of genes that are specific for weight-regulating hormones. For example, the hormone leptin is produced in adipose (fat) cells. As the amount of adipose tissue increases, leptin levels in the blood rise. This increase in leptin normally signals the brain to suppress appetite. Studies have shown that mice that inherit a defect in the gene for leptin become very obese because leptin does not accumulate in their bodies and signal the brain to stop eating.

Other research has been conducted to study the signaling pathways involved in regulating both long- and short-term appetite and the body's storage of fat. It is possible in the future that individuals with inheritable traits leading to obesity may be able to control the problem with effective and safe drugs.

Weight loss plans fall into several categories:

- **Low-carbohydrate diets:** Some low-carbohydrate diets promote eating high-protein, high-fat, and low-carbohydrate food. Others encourage dieters to eat high-fiber fruits, vegetables, and beans and grains and to get about 40 percent of daily calories from carbohydrates. The danger in these diets is that too much fat is consumed, which can contribute to heart and kidney disease.

- **Low-fat diets:** Low-fat diets suggest taking in less than 10 percent of daily calories from fat. The focus is on an increase in vegetables, high-fiber fruits, and grains. These diets can lack sufficient amounts of fatty acids and protein that may make it difficult for the body to absorb fat-soluble vitamins.

- **Glycemic index diets:** These diets focus on eating carbohydrates with a low glycemic index in order to lower blood sugar levels.

- **Formula diets:** A formula diet is based on eating packaged products of a set number of calories, proteins, fats, and carbohydrates. These diets often involve consuming special nutritionally sound shakes or bars and can be expensive to follow.

- **Group-approach diets:** The group-approach diet involves group meetings, diet plans, exercise plans, and group support.

Scientific studies seem to indicate that an increase in exercise along with a restricted, but balanced diet that provides all essential nutrients and at least 1,200-kcal per day is the healthiest way to approach weight loss. However, rather than on-again-off-again dieting, a change in eating habits and lifestyle to take weight off and keep it off is the better approach.

Diet and Disease Prevention

Diet, that is, what people eat, plays an important role in an individual's risk for developing certain diseases, including cardiovascular disease and cancer. Inheritable traits that predispose an individual to a certain disease are unavoidable, but diet is a controllable factor that can actually function to help prevent disease in some cases.

For example, high levels of low-density lipoproteins, or LDL cholesterol, generally correlate with blocked blood vessels (clogged arteries), high blood pressure, and subsequent heart attacks. In contrast, high-density lipoproteins (HDL cholesterol) may actually decrease the risk of blocked blood vessels because HDLs bring cholesterol to the liver, where it is broken down.

Diet seems to be linked to some forms of cancer. Some research suggests a link between diets high in carbohydrates and fats and an increase in the incidence of breast cancer. In addition, the incidence of colon and prostate cancer may be linked to diets rich in saturated fats or red meat. Some fruits and vegetable are rich in antioxidants that protect cells from damaging molecules called free radicals. Antioxidants may play a role in preventing cancer. As precautions to help lower the risk of cancer, the American Cancer Society recommends dietary guidelines that include eating five or more servings of fruits and vegetables a day, eating whole grains, limiting the consumption of red meats and alcoholic beverages, and increasing physical activity.

FACTORS AFFECTING HEALTH

Some aspects of health are uncontrollable. For example, age, gender, and genetic makeup are not something that an individual can change. Wellness, however, can be affected by several factors that are controllable, such as diet, exercise, and personal relationships. Individuals can affect their own health by lifestyle choices that they make. Physical activity and a healthy, well-balanced diet can have a positive effect on health. Adequate sleep and preventative health care also have a positive effect on health. Other factors, such as obesity and alcohol and tobacco consumption, can have a negative effect on health. In fact, these three factors are some of the leading causes of death in the United States.

Wellness

A healthy lifestyle can be obtained by taking a holistic approach to health. A holistic approach includes understanding the importance of the following six dimensions of wellness: physical, emotional, spiritual, intellectual, interpersonal, and environmental.

1. **Physical wellness:** Physical wellness is determined by coordination, strength, and the command of the five senses (sight, hearing, taste, smell, and touch).

2. **Emotional wellness:** Emotional wellness reflects an individual's ability to understand and cope with various feelings and emotions in a healthy and positive way.

3. **Spiritual wellness:** Spiritual wellness involves developing a set of guided beliefs, principles, or values that give one's life meaning and purpose.

4. **Intellectual wellness:** Intellectual wellness involves engaging in pursuits that will continually challenge the mind and keep it active, including creative pursuits, problem solving, and processing information.

5. **Interpersonal wellness:** Interpersonal wellness involves the maintenance of healthy, supportive, and satisfying relationships with others.

6. **Environmental wellness:** Environmental wellness involves positive input from one's environment. A clean, safe environment contributes to wellness.

Stress

Another factor that can affect health is stress. Stress refers to both the stressor and the stress response. A **stressor** is the situation that triggers an emotional or physical reaction. The physical and emotional reactions that one exhibits are called the **stress response**. Stress responses are controlled by the nervous system and the endocrine system. The sympathetic division of the nervous system, which activates the "fight-or-flight" response, triggers signals that tell the body to stop storing energy and use it in response to a crisis. The nervous system triggers the endocrine system, which releases hormones and other chemical signals to the bloodstream. Some key hormones released in response to stress are cortisol and epinephrine. Stress can be managed by developing a healthy lifestyle, improving time management, learning to identify stressors, and changing unhealthy thought patterns. Relaxation is another method that is effective in dealing with stress.

Aging

In midlife, individuals may see a decline in health in terms of loss of bone mass, compression of vertebrae, loss of lean body mass, vision loss, hearing loss, fertility loss, and a loss of or decrease in sexual function. Women in particular experience loss of calcium in bones, a condition called **osteoporosis**, and a decline in their reproductive cycle (menopause). Both men and women can suffer from osteoarthritis due to the wearing down of joint tissue.

Through good health habits, it is possible to delay, lessen, prevent, and sometimes reverse changes in health associated with aging. Some of these habits include challenging the mind, developing a physical fitness regimen, establishing healthy eating habits, maintaining a healthy weight, controlling alcohol consumption and dependence on medication, refraining from smoking, and keeping up to date with preventative medical care. Physical examinations should include detection of treatable diseases or conditions.

Physical Fitness

The level of physical fitness practiced by an individual affects overall health. There are five basic components to physical fitness:

1. **Cardiorespiratory endurance:** Cardiorespiratory endurance is the ability to perform long, large-muscle, dynamic exercises at a moderate- to high-intensity level. This type of training increases the strength of the heart and positively affects other related body functions, such as heart rate, blood pressure, metabolism, and certain chemical systems in the body.

2. **Muscular strength:** Strength training improves physical fitness and increases muscle mass. An increase in muscle mass means the body requires more energy to carry out life functions.

3. **Muscular endurance:** The development of muscular endurance involves developing the ability to contract a specific muscle group for a long period of time or to continually contract a muscle group for a long period of time.

4. **Flexibility:** Flexibility is the ability to move a joint through its full range of motion. Flexibility depends on the structure of a particular joint, the length and elasticity of the connective tissue, and the nervous system activity around the joint. Flexible and pain-free joints are an important part of maintaining good health. Stretching is a good way to improve and maintain flexibility.

5. **Body composition:** A healthy body composition includes a higher proportion of nonfat body mass than fat mass. This proportion varies by sex and age. Too high a concentration of body fat, especially in the abdominal region, can lead to issues such as high blood pressure, heart disease, stroke, joint problems, gallbladder disease, back pain, diabetes, and cancer.

For optimal fitness and health, 20–60 minutes of endurance exercise three to five times a week and strength training twice a week is recommended. Exercise lowers the risk of cardiovascular disease by lowering blood fat levels, reducing high blood pressure, and preventing the blocking of arteries. Exercise can also reduce the risk of some cancers, osteoporosis, and diabetes. Other benefits of exercise include an enhanced immune system, improved psychological health, and the prevention of injury and low back pain.

Nutrition

The body requires about 45 essential nutrients to maintain a maximum level of health. Most foods provide one or more essential nutrients and act as fuel for the body.

In addition to essential nutrients, water is required for the body in order to digest and absorb food, transport substances to different regions of the body, and maintain cellular health and overall wellbeing.

Risk Factors, Disease, and Disease Prevention

A disease can be bacterial, viral, or fungal and can enter the body through the transfer of bodily fluids (saliva, semen, and blood), airborne droplets, or fecal materials. Other organisms, such as mosquitoes or fleas, can indirectly transfer disease from one host organism to another. A full-blown infection occurs when there is an environment in the body for the disease to "live" or reproduce. Infectious diseases also need an exit point in the body, so that they can leave and spread the infection to another host. Viral particles can leave the body through the nose via a sneeze or through the mouth via a cough and enter a second host. Some common infectious diseases include influenza, rhinitis (the common cold), pneumonia, tuberculosis, mononucleosis, Lyme disease, streptococcal infections, measles, mumps, rubella, pertussis, chicken pox, and herpes viruses.

Bacterial infections can be treated with oral antibiotics that act to kill the bacteria cells. The body can build up a defense against viral infections through the administration of vaccines. A vaccine will manipulate the immune system and cause the body to develop immunity to a specific viral disease agent. Vaccines protect against future infection from a specific virus, and they are administered through injection, oral medication, or a nasal spray.

Sexually Transmitted Diseases

There are seven sexually transmitted diseases (STDs) that can have a major affect on one's health. **Acquired Immune Deficiency Syndrome (AIDS)** is the most serious and life-threatening sexually transmitted disease. It is caused by the **Human Immunodeficiency Virus (HIV)** and compromises the immune system of an infected individual. **Chlamydia** is an STD that causes painful urination. It can lead to another disorder called **pelvic inflammatory disease (PID)** if it is left untreated. PID can lead to an increased risk of infertility in men and women, ectopic pregnancies in women, and inflammation of sperm-carrying ducts in men.

Gonorrhea causes urinary discomfort in men and a yellowish green discharge. Women infected with gonorrhea usually have no symptoms, but can experience painful urination, vaginal discharge, and severe cramps. Gonorrhea can also lead to PID and potential infertility in both women and men. Antibiotics are used to treat gonorrhea. Left untreated, gonorrhea can spread to the blood, resulting in a life-threatening condition called **disseminated gonococcal infection (DGI)**. **Human papilloma virus (HPV)** causes genital warts, genital cancers, cervical cancer, penile cancer, and some forms of rectal cancers. A new vaccine has been developed to prevent the spread of HPV. **Hepatitis B** causes inflammation of the liver and can cause serious and permanent damage. There is a vaccine against this disease as well. **Syphilis** is caused by a bacterial infection and is treated with antibiotics. It causes ulcers, sore throat, and hair loss in its early stages; late stages of infection can cause permanent damage and death.

Cardiovascular Disease

There are six major preventable risk factors for cardiovascular disease (disease affecting the cardio-vascular system). These risk factors include smoking, high blood pressure, high LDL/low HDL cholesterol levels, physical inactivity, obesity, and diabetes. Smoking lowers HDL levels, increases blood pressure and heart rate, and increases plaque formation and the chance of a blood clot. High blood pressure leads to hypertension, and high LDL levels contribute to clogged arteries. All of these risk factors can be reduced by good overall health and nutrition and exercise practices. Unavoidable risk factors are age, race, and family history.

Some common cardiovascular diseases include atherosclerosis (hardening of the arteries), heart attack, stroke, congestive heart failure, peripheral arterial disease (PAD), congenital heart disease, rheumatic heart disease, and heart valve malfunctions.

Cancer

Cancer can be found in all areas of the body, and treatment depends on the location of the tumor or tumors. The spreading of cancer cells from one area of the body to another is called **metastasis**. Cancer is caused by an uncontrolled growth of cells that cause an outgrowth, or tumor, of abnormal cell types. This uncontrolled growth can be due to genetics, exposure to agents that cause mutations in DNA (mutagens), viral infection, and chemical substances in food or the atmosphere. Cancer is categorized into five progressive stages (stage 0 to IV).

Some types of cancer are lung cancer, oral cancer, colon cancer, rectal cancer, skin cancer, prostate cancer, breast cancer, ovarian cancer, cervical cancer, uterine cancer, and testicular cancer. Tumors are classified according to the type of cells they have. **Carcinomas** form from epithelial cells, **sarcomas** are found in connective tissue, **melanoma** are found in skin cells, **lymphomas** are cancers of the lymph nodes, **neuroblastomas** occur in immature CNS cells, **hepatomas** are found in liver cells, and **adenocarcinomas** are found in endocrine glands.

Strategies for preventing cancer can include avoiding tobacco, eating a healthy and well-balanced diet, controlling weight, exercising, avoiding exposure to the sun, avoiding exposure to hazardous materials, and having routine cancer screening tests.

Immune Disorders

Immune disorders occur when the body comes under attack by its own cells. Often, the immune system can detect attacking cells such as cancer cells, and it is capable of destroying these harmful cells. If the immune system breaks down, due to infections such as HIV, age, chemotherapy, and other immune disorders, harmful cells can grow uncontrollably before the immune system is able to detect any danger.

In addition, some immune disorders cause the immune system to confuse its own cells with foreign organisms. Autoimmune diseases in which the immune system attacks the body's own cells include rheumatoid arthritis and lupus erythematosus.

Diabetes

Diabetes is a disease in which the pancreas does not produce insulin normally. There are three types of diabetes.

1. Type I diabetes is an autoimmune disease that occurs when the pancreas produces little to no insulin. Type I diabetes is usually diagnosed in childhood and requires insulin injections to help the pancreas function.

2. Type II diabetes occurs when the pancreas stops producing enough insulin or the body becomes resistant to insulin. Type II diabetes can often be controlled by diet and exercise.

3. Gestational diabetes is brought on during pregnancy and is a temporary condition that generally disappears at the end of pregnancy.

Other Factors Affecting Health

Asthma is caused by the inflammation of airways and a spasm of the muscles surrounding the airways. It can be linked to both biological and environmental factors. Asthma can be brought on by seasonal allergies, exercise, and occupational hazards. Anti-inflammatory drugs and muscle-relaxing medication can help relieve asthma symptoms.

Osteoarthritis is caused by the wear and tear of joints and is most common in older people. There is no cure for arthritis, but pain medication can help manage the symptoms.

Genetic disorders are inherited from biological parents. Parents pass one or two copies of a gene for an inheritable disease to an offspring. Some common inheritable, or genetic, diseases are hemophilia (blood disease), retinitis pitmentosa (eye disease), color blindness (eye disease), cystic fibrosis (lung disease), thalassemias (blood disorders), polydactyl (extra fingers or toes), achondroplasia (dwarfism), and polycystic kidney disease.

Some **neurological disorders** can also negatively affect health. Rett syndrome is a neurological disorder that affects brain development. It is similar to autism. Huntington's disease is characterized by the degeneration of brain cells in areas affecting intellect, emotional control, and muscle control.

Safety

Many injuries are caused by the interaction of humans with environmental factors or with other humans. Personal safety is necessary to protect oneself from harm or injury. It is necessary to be aware of one's surroundings and avoid atypical patterns in order to maintain safety. **Residential safety**, **recreational safety**, and **motor vehicle safety** are all ways to prevent injury.

Violence is defined as the intent to inflict harm on another person through physical force. Types of violence and intentional injury include assault, homicide, child abuse, sexual abuse, rape, gang-related violence, bullying, and terrorism. Alcohol and drug use often contribute to violence. Strategies for reducing violence include conflict resolution, developing social skills, and educational programs for victims and offenders.

Consumer awareness involves gathering information on health-related issues. As a nurse, you can provide materials for patient education, such as health reference publications and informational packets. In general, a patient should seek the help of a healthcare professional for symptoms that are severe, unusual, persistent, or recurrent.

Environmental health concerns include concern for air quality, global warming, various forms of pollution, and infectious diseases. Concern for water quality focuses on pathogenic organisms that can live in water, chemicals and hazardous waste that may contaminate a water supply, and water shortages (drought). Water can be polluted by animal waste, biological imbalance, pesticides, toxins, and other chemical waste that can cause mutations in DNA, cancer in certain cells, or birth defects in unborn offspring. Sewage and water treatment helps to prevent pathogens from polluting drinking water.

Land pollution is caused by landfills that release chemicals into the ground, pesticides, automobiles, radiation, and accidental chemical or hazardous waste spills. Land pollution can be prevented by conservation efforts in an effort to prevent cancers and other related health problems.

HEALTH GLOSSARY

A

abductor
A muscle that draws a part of the body away from the median line or normal position.

acetabulum
The socket of the hip bone.

adductor
A muscle that pulls a part of the body toward the median line.

adrenal glands
The two small glands that are on the upper part of the kidneys.

adrenalin
A hormone produced by the adrenal glands; a drug containing this hormone used to raise blood pressure.

alimentary canal
The passageway in the body extending from the mouth to the anus.

alveolus
An air cell of a lung; a tooth socket.

anatomy
The science of the structure of plants and animals.

aorta
The main artery of the body.

artery
A blood vessel carrying blood away from the heart to all parts of the body.

atrium
A chamber of the heart.

atrophy
A wasting away or failure of an organ to grow.

auditory
A term referring to the sense of hearing.

axilla
The armpit.

B

backbone
The column of bones (vertebrae) along the center of the back.

bile
A substance produced by the liver and stored in the gallbladder.

brachial
A term referring to the upper part of the forelimb of the vertebrae.

bronchus
Either of the two main branches or tubes extending from the trachea (windpipe).

bursa
A sac or cavity, especially between joints.

C

cardiac
Of or near the heart.

caudal
Near the tail.

cell
The basic unit of protoplasm.

cephalic
Of the head, skull, or cranium.

clavicle
The collarbone.

clonus
A series of muscle spasms.

colon
The part of the large intestine extending from the cecum to the rectum.

conjunctiva
The mucous membrane lining the inner surface of the eyelids and covering the front part of the eyeball.

cornea
The transparent outer coating of the eyeball.

cranium

The skull, especially that part containing the brain.

cutaneous

Of or on the skin; affecting the skin.

D

dactyl

A finger or toe.

dermis

The layer of skin just below the epidermis.

digit

A finger or toe.

duct

A tube through which secretions or excretions pass through the body.

duodenum

The first section of the small intestine below the stomach.

E

enamel

The hard, white coating of the crowns of teeth.

endothelium

A membrane that lines the heart, blood vessels, and lymphatic vessels.

epidermis

The outermost layer of the skin.

esophagus

The passage for food from the pharynx to the stomach; gullet.

eviscerate

To remove the entrails from; disembowel.

extensor

A muscle that straightens some part of the body.

F

fascia

A thin layer of connective tissue.

femur

The thigh bone.

fibrin
A protein formed in the clotting of blood.

flexor
A muscle that bends a part of the body.

foramen
A small opening.

G

ganglion
A mass of nerve cells serving as a center from which nerve impulses are transmitted.

gastric
In or near the stomach.

genitals
The sexual organs.

glottis
The opening between the vocal cords in the larynx.

gullet
The esophagus.

H

hemoglobin
The red coloring matter of the red blood cells.

humerus
The bone of the upper arm or forelimb, extending from the shoulder to the elbow.

hyoid
A U-shaped bone at the base of the tongue.

hypophysis
The pituitary gland.

I

ileum
The lowest part of the small intestine.

ilium
The uppermost part of the three sections of the hipbone.

insulin
A secretion of the pancreas that helps the body use sugar.

intestines
The lower part of the alimentary canal, extending from the stomach to the anus.

J

jejunum
The middle part of the small intestine.

jugular
Two large veins in the neck carrying blood from the head to the heart.

K

kidney
Either of a pair of organs that separate water and products from the blood and excrete them as urine through the bladder.

L

lacrimal
Of, for, or producing tears.

larynx
A structure serving as an organ of the voice.

ligament
A band of tough tissue connecting bones or holding organs in place.

lumbar
Pertaining to the small of the back.

lymph
A clear, yellowish fluid found in the lymphatic system of the body.

lymphatic system
A system of vessels and nodes that leads from the tissue spaces to large veins entering the heart.

M

mastication
The act of chewing.

maxilla
The upper jawbone.

membrane
A thin, soft layer of tissue that covers or lines an organ or part.

meninges
The three membranes that enclose the brain and spinal cord.

meningitis
Inflammation of the meninges.

metacarpals

The bones in the hand between the wrist and the fingers.

metatarsals

The bones in the foot between the ankle and toes.

mucous membrane

A membrane lining cavities leading to the outside of the body, such as to the mouth, nose, lungs, and anus; mucosa.

mucus

The slimy secretion that moistens and protects the mucous membrane.

N

neural

Pertaining to the nerves or the nervous system.

nutrition

The series or processes by which an organism takes in and assimilates food for promoting growth and repairing tissues.

O

occiput

The back of the skull or head.

ocular

Pertaining to the eye.

olfactory

A term referring to the sense of smell.

ophthalmic

Of or connected with the eyes.

optic nerve

The nerve running from the brain to the eye.

orbit

The eye socket.

osteology

The study of bones.

P

pancreas

The gland that secretes insulin and other digestive juices.

parathyroid

Four small glands embedded in the thyroid gland; their secretions increase the calcium content in the blood.

pathogenic

Disease-producing.

pepsin

An enzyme secreted in the stomach, aiding in the digestion of proteins.

pharynx

The cavity extending from the mouth and nasal passages to the larynx and esophagus; throat.

placenta

The structure through which the fetus is nourished.

protoplasm

The essential living matter of animal and plant cells.

protozoa

A one-celled microscopic organism.

pubis

The bone that makes up the front part of the pelvis.

Q

quadrant

A term referring to four or part of four.

quadruped

A mammal or animal with four feet.

R

radius

The bone of the forearm on the same side as the thumb.

rectum

The lowest segment of the large intestine, ending at the anus.

retina

The innermost coating of the back part of the eyeball.

riboflavin

A factor of the vitamin B complex, found in milk, eggs, liver, fruits, leafy vegetables, etc.

S

scapula

The shoulder blade.

semen
The sperm-containing fluid secreted by the male reproductive organs.

sphincter
A round muscle that can open or close a natural opening in the body by expanding and contracting.

sternum
The breastbone.

striated
Streaked with fine lines; striped.

T

tarsals
The bones of the ankle.

tendons
The connective tissue that joins muscles to bones.

thrombin
A substance that aids in the clotting of blood.

thyroid gland
A large ductless gland near the trachea that produces thyroxine, which regulates metabolism.

tibia
The inner bone of the leg below the knee; shinbone.

trachea
The windpipe; the tube that conveys air from the larynx to the bronchi.

U

ulna
The bone of the forearm on the side opposite the thumb.

urea
A soluble, crystalline solid, found in urine.

urine
A yellowish fluid in mammals, containing urea and other waste products.

V

vagina
In female mammals, the canal leading from the vulva to the uterus.

vermiform
A small saclike appendage of the large intestine.

viscera

The internal organs of the body, such as the heart, lungs, stomach, etc.

vomer

A bone forming part of the nasal septum.

Z

zoology

The branch of biology dealing with the classification of animals and the study of animal life.

SCIENCE ANSWER SHEET

Test 1: Human Anatomy and Physiology

1. Ⓐ Ⓑ Ⓒ Ⓓ	11. Ⓐ Ⓑ Ⓒ Ⓓ	21. Ⓐ Ⓑ Ⓒ Ⓓ	31. Ⓐ Ⓑ Ⓒ Ⓓ	41. Ⓐ Ⓑ Ⓒ Ⓓ
2. Ⓐ Ⓑ Ⓒ Ⓓ	12. Ⓐ Ⓑ Ⓒ Ⓓ	22. Ⓐ Ⓑ Ⓒ Ⓓ	32. Ⓐ Ⓑ Ⓒ Ⓓ	42. Ⓐ Ⓑ Ⓒ Ⓓ
3. Ⓐ Ⓑ Ⓒ Ⓓ	13. Ⓐ Ⓑ Ⓒ Ⓓ	23. Ⓐ Ⓑ Ⓒ Ⓓ	33. Ⓐ Ⓑ Ⓒ Ⓓ	43. Ⓐ Ⓑ Ⓒ Ⓓ
4. Ⓐ Ⓑ Ⓒ Ⓓ	14. Ⓐ Ⓑ Ⓒ Ⓓ	24. Ⓐ Ⓑ Ⓒ Ⓓ	34. Ⓐ Ⓑ Ⓒ Ⓓ	44. Ⓐ Ⓑ Ⓒ Ⓓ
5. Ⓐ Ⓑ Ⓒ Ⓓ	15. Ⓐ Ⓑ Ⓒ Ⓓ	25. Ⓐ Ⓑ Ⓒ Ⓓ	35. Ⓐ Ⓑ Ⓒ Ⓓ	45. Ⓐ Ⓑ Ⓒ Ⓓ
6. Ⓐ Ⓑ Ⓒ Ⓓ	16. Ⓐ Ⓑ Ⓒ Ⓓ	26. Ⓐ Ⓑ Ⓒ Ⓓ	36. Ⓐ Ⓑ Ⓒ Ⓓ	46. Ⓐ Ⓑ Ⓒ Ⓓ
7. Ⓐ Ⓑ Ⓒ Ⓓ	17. Ⓐ Ⓑ Ⓒ Ⓓ	27. Ⓐ Ⓑ Ⓒ Ⓓ	37. Ⓐ Ⓑ Ⓒ Ⓓ	47. Ⓐ Ⓑ Ⓒ Ⓓ
8. Ⓐ Ⓑ Ⓒ Ⓓ	18. Ⓐ Ⓑ Ⓒ Ⓓ	28. Ⓐ Ⓑ Ⓒ Ⓓ	38. Ⓐ Ⓑ Ⓒ Ⓓ	48. Ⓐ Ⓑ Ⓒ Ⓓ
9. Ⓐ Ⓑ Ⓒ Ⓓ	19. Ⓐ Ⓑ Ⓒ Ⓓ	29. Ⓐ Ⓑ Ⓒ Ⓓ	39. Ⓐ Ⓑ Ⓒ Ⓓ	49. Ⓐ Ⓑ Ⓒ Ⓓ
10. Ⓐ Ⓑ Ⓒ Ⓓ	20. Ⓐ Ⓑ Ⓒ Ⓓ	30. Ⓐ Ⓑ Ⓒ Ⓓ	40. Ⓐ Ⓑ Ⓒ Ⓓ	50. Ⓐ Ⓑ Ⓒ Ⓓ

Test 2: Human Anatomy and Physiology

1. Ⓐ Ⓑ Ⓒ Ⓓ	11. Ⓐ Ⓑ Ⓒ Ⓓ	21. Ⓐ Ⓑ Ⓒ Ⓓ	31. Ⓐ Ⓑ Ⓒ Ⓓ	41. Ⓐ Ⓑ Ⓒ Ⓓ
2. Ⓐ Ⓑ Ⓒ Ⓓ	12. Ⓐ Ⓑ Ⓒ Ⓓ	22. Ⓐ Ⓑ Ⓒ Ⓓ	32. Ⓐ Ⓑ Ⓒ Ⓓ	42. Ⓐ Ⓑ Ⓒ Ⓓ
3. Ⓐ Ⓑ Ⓒ Ⓓ	13. Ⓐ Ⓑ Ⓒ Ⓓ	23. Ⓐ Ⓑ Ⓒ Ⓓ	33. Ⓐ Ⓑ Ⓒ Ⓓ	43. Ⓐ Ⓑ Ⓒ Ⓓ
4. Ⓐ Ⓑ Ⓒ Ⓓ	14. Ⓐ Ⓑ Ⓒ Ⓓ	24. Ⓐ Ⓑ Ⓒ Ⓓ	34. Ⓐ Ⓑ Ⓒ Ⓓ	44. Ⓐ Ⓑ Ⓒ Ⓓ
5. Ⓐ Ⓑ Ⓒ Ⓓ	15. Ⓐ Ⓑ Ⓒ Ⓓ	25. Ⓐ Ⓑ Ⓒ Ⓓ	35. Ⓐ Ⓑ Ⓒ Ⓓ	45. Ⓐ Ⓑ Ⓒ Ⓓ
6. Ⓐ Ⓑ Ⓒ Ⓓ	16. Ⓐ Ⓑ Ⓒ Ⓓ	26. Ⓐ Ⓑ Ⓒ Ⓓ	36. Ⓐ Ⓑ Ⓒ Ⓓ	46. Ⓐ Ⓑ Ⓒ Ⓓ
7. Ⓐ Ⓑ Ⓒ Ⓓ	17. Ⓐ Ⓑ Ⓒ Ⓓ	27. Ⓐ Ⓑ Ⓒ Ⓓ	37. Ⓐ Ⓑ Ⓒ Ⓓ	47. Ⓐ Ⓑ Ⓒ Ⓓ
8. Ⓐ Ⓑ Ⓒ Ⓓ	18. Ⓐ Ⓑ Ⓒ Ⓓ	28. Ⓐ Ⓑ Ⓒ Ⓓ	38. Ⓐ Ⓑ Ⓒ Ⓓ	48. Ⓐ Ⓑ Ⓒ Ⓓ
9. Ⓐ Ⓑ Ⓒ Ⓓ	19. Ⓐ Ⓑ Ⓒ Ⓓ	29. Ⓐ Ⓑ Ⓒ Ⓓ	39. Ⓐ Ⓑ Ⓒ Ⓓ	49. Ⓐ Ⓑ Ⓒ Ⓓ
10. Ⓐ Ⓑ Ⓒ Ⓓ	20. Ⓐ Ⓑ Ⓒ Ⓓ	30. Ⓐ Ⓑ Ⓒ Ⓓ	40. Ⓐ Ⓑ Ⓒ Ⓓ	50. Ⓐ Ⓑ Ⓒ Ⓓ

answer sheet

Test 3: Human Anatomy and Physiology

1. Ⓐ Ⓑ Ⓒ Ⓓ   21. Ⓐ Ⓑ Ⓒ Ⓓ   41. Ⓐ Ⓑ Ⓒ Ⓓ   61. Ⓐ Ⓑ Ⓒ Ⓓ   81. Ⓐ Ⓑ Ⓒ Ⓓ
2. Ⓐ Ⓑ Ⓒ Ⓓ   22. Ⓐ Ⓑ Ⓒ Ⓓ   42. Ⓐ Ⓑ Ⓒ Ⓓ   62. Ⓐ Ⓑ Ⓒ Ⓓ   82. Ⓐ Ⓑ Ⓒ Ⓓ
3. Ⓐ Ⓑ Ⓒ Ⓓ   23. Ⓐ Ⓑ Ⓒ Ⓓ   43. Ⓐ Ⓑ Ⓒ Ⓓ   63. Ⓐ Ⓑ Ⓒ Ⓓ   83. Ⓐ Ⓑ Ⓒ Ⓓ
4. Ⓐ Ⓑ Ⓒ Ⓓ   24. Ⓐ Ⓑ Ⓒ Ⓓ   44. Ⓐ Ⓑ Ⓒ Ⓓ   64. Ⓐ Ⓑ Ⓒ Ⓓ   84. Ⓐ Ⓑ Ⓒ Ⓓ
5. Ⓐ Ⓑ Ⓒ Ⓓ   25. Ⓐ Ⓑ Ⓒ Ⓓ   45. Ⓐ Ⓑ Ⓒ Ⓓ   65. Ⓐ Ⓑ Ⓒ Ⓓ   85. Ⓐ Ⓑ Ⓒ Ⓓ
6. Ⓐ Ⓑ Ⓒ Ⓓ   26. Ⓐ Ⓑ Ⓒ Ⓓ   46. Ⓐ Ⓑ Ⓒ Ⓓ   66. Ⓐ Ⓑ Ⓒ Ⓓ   86. Ⓐ Ⓑ Ⓒ Ⓓ
7. Ⓐ Ⓑ Ⓒ Ⓓ   27. Ⓐ Ⓑ Ⓒ Ⓓ   47. Ⓐ Ⓑ Ⓒ Ⓓ   67. Ⓐ Ⓑ Ⓒ Ⓓ   87. Ⓐ Ⓑ Ⓒ Ⓓ
8. Ⓐ Ⓑ Ⓒ Ⓓ   28. Ⓐ Ⓑ Ⓒ Ⓓ   48. Ⓐ Ⓑ Ⓒ Ⓓ   68. Ⓐ Ⓑ Ⓒ Ⓓ   88. Ⓐ Ⓑ Ⓒ Ⓓ
9. Ⓐ Ⓑ Ⓒ Ⓓ   29. Ⓐ Ⓑ Ⓒ Ⓓ   49. Ⓐ Ⓑ Ⓒ Ⓓ   69. Ⓐ Ⓑ Ⓒ Ⓓ   89. Ⓐ Ⓑ Ⓒ Ⓓ
10. Ⓐ Ⓑ Ⓒ Ⓓ   30. Ⓐ Ⓑ Ⓒ Ⓓ   50. Ⓐ Ⓑ Ⓒ Ⓓ   70. Ⓐ Ⓑ Ⓒ Ⓓ   90. Ⓐ Ⓑ Ⓒ Ⓓ
11. Ⓐ Ⓑ Ⓒ Ⓓ   31. Ⓐ Ⓑ Ⓒ Ⓓ   51. Ⓐ Ⓑ Ⓒ Ⓓ   71. Ⓐ Ⓑ Ⓒ Ⓓ   91. Ⓐ Ⓑ Ⓒ Ⓓ
12. Ⓐ Ⓑ Ⓒ Ⓓ   32. Ⓐ Ⓑ Ⓒ Ⓓ   52. Ⓐ Ⓑ Ⓒ Ⓓ   72. Ⓐ Ⓑ Ⓒ Ⓓ   92. Ⓐ Ⓑ Ⓒ Ⓓ
13. Ⓐ Ⓑ Ⓒ Ⓓ   33. Ⓐ Ⓑ Ⓒ Ⓓ   53. Ⓐ Ⓑ Ⓒ Ⓓ   73. Ⓐ Ⓑ Ⓒ Ⓓ   93. Ⓐ Ⓑ Ⓒ Ⓓ
14. Ⓐ Ⓑ Ⓒ Ⓓ   34. Ⓐ Ⓑ Ⓒ Ⓓ   54. Ⓐ Ⓑ Ⓒ Ⓓ   74. Ⓐ Ⓑ Ⓒ Ⓓ   94. Ⓐ Ⓑ Ⓒ Ⓓ
15. Ⓐ Ⓑ Ⓒ Ⓓ   35. Ⓐ Ⓑ Ⓒ Ⓓ   55. Ⓐ Ⓑ Ⓒ Ⓓ   75. Ⓐ Ⓑ Ⓒ Ⓓ   95. Ⓐ Ⓑ Ⓒ Ⓓ
16. Ⓐ Ⓑ Ⓒ Ⓓ   36. Ⓐ Ⓑ Ⓒ Ⓓ   56. Ⓐ Ⓑ Ⓒ Ⓓ   76. Ⓐ Ⓑ Ⓒ Ⓓ   96. Ⓐ Ⓑ Ⓒ Ⓓ
17. Ⓐ Ⓑ Ⓒ Ⓓ   37. Ⓐ Ⓑ Ⓒ Ⓓ   57. Ⓐ Ⓑ Ⓒ Ⓓ   77. Ⓐ Ⓑ Ⓒ Ⓓ   97. Ⓐ Ⓑ Ⓒ Ⓓ
18. Ⓐ Ⓑ Ⓒ Ⓓ   38. Ⓐ Ⓑ Ⓒ Ⓓ   58. Ⓐ Ⓑ Ⓒ Ⓓ   78. Ⓐ Ⓑ Ⓒ Ⓓ   98. Ⓐ Ⓑ Ⓒ Ⓓ
19. Ⓐ Ⓑ Ⓒ Ⓓ   39. Ⓐ Ⓑ Ⓒ Ⓓ   59. Ⓐ Ⓑ Ⓒ Ⓓ   79. Ⓐ Ⓑ Ⓒ Ⓓ   99. Ⓐ Ⓑ Ⓒ Ⓓ
20. Ⓐ Ⓑ Ⓒ Ⓓ   40. Ⓐ Ⓑ Ⓒ Ⓓ   60. Ⓐ Ⓑ Ⓒ Ⓓ   80. Ⓐ Ⓑ Ⓒ Ⓓ   100. Ⓐ Ⓑ Ⓒ Ⓓ

Test 4: Anatomy, Physiology, and Health Science

1. Ⓐ Ⓑ Ⓒ Ⓓ   9. Ⓐ Ⓑ Ⓒ Ⓓ   17. Ⓐ Ⓑ Ⓒ Ⓓ   25. Ⓐ Ⓑ Ⓒ Ⓓ   33. Ⓐ Ⓑ Ⓒ Ⓓ
2. Ⓐ Ⓑ Ⓒ Ⓓ   10. Ⓐ Ⓑ Ⓒ Ⓓ   18. Ⓐ Ⓑ Ⓒ Ⓓ   26. Ⓐ Ⓑ Ⓒ Ⓓ   34. Ⓐ Ⓑ Ⓒ Ⓓ
3. Ⓐ Ⓑ Ⓒ Ⓓ   11. Ⓐ Ⓑ Ⓒ Ⓓ   19. Ⓐ Ⓑ Ⓒ Ⓓ   27. Ⓐ Ⓑ Ⓒ Ⓓ   35. Ⓐ Ⓑ Ⓒ Ⓓ
4. Ⓐ Ⓑ Ⓒ Ⓓ   12. Ⓐ Ⓑ Ⓒ Ⓓ   20. Ⓐ Ⓑ Ⓒ Ⓓ   28. Ⓐ Ⓑ Ⓒ Ⓓ   36. Ⓐ Ⓑ Ⓒ Ⓓ
5. Ⓐ Ⓑ Ⓒ Ⓓ   13. Ⓐ Ⓑ Ⓒ Ⓓ   21. Ⓐ Ⓑ Ⓒ Ⓓ   29. Ⓐ Ⓑ Ⓒ Ⓓ   37. Ⓐ Ⓑ Ⓒ Ⓓ
6. Ⓐ Ⓑ Ⓒ Ⓓ   14. Ⓐ Ⓑ Ⓒ Ⓓ   22. Ⓐ Ⓑ Ⓒ Ⓓ   30. Ⓐ Ⓑ Ⓒ Ⓓ   38. Ⓐ Ⓑ Ⓒ Ⓓ
7. Ⓐ Ⓑ Ⓒ Ⓓ   15. Ⓐ Ⓑ Ⓒ Ⓓ   23. Ⓐ Ⓑ Ⓒ Ⓓ   31. Ⓐ Ⓑ Ⓒ Ⓓ   39. Ⓐ Ⓑ Ⓒ Ⓓ
8. Ⓐ Ⓑ Ⓒ Ⓓ   16. Ⓐ Ⓑ Ⓒ Ⓓ   24. Ⓐ Ⓑ Ⓒ Ⓓ   32. Ⓐ Ⓑ Ⓒ Ⓓ   40. Ⓐ Ⓑ Ⓒ Ⓓ

Test 5: Anatomy, Physiology, and Health Science

1. Ⓐ Ⓑ Ⓒ Ⓓ	7. Ⓐ Ⓑ Ⓒ Ⓓ	13. Ⓐ Ⓑ Ⓒ Ⓓ	19. Ⓐ Ⓑ Ⓒ Ⓓ	25. Ⓐ Ⓑ Ⓒ Ⓓ
2. Ⓐ Ⓑ Ⓒ Ⓓ	8. Ⓐ Ⓑ Ⓒ Ⓓ	14. Ⓐ Ⓑ Ⓒ Ⓓ	20. Ⓐ Ⓑ Ⓒ Ⓓ	26. Ⓐ Ⓑ Ⓒ Ⓓ
3. Ⓐ Ⓑ Ⓒ Ⓓ	9. Ⓐ Ⓑ Ⓒ Ⓓ	15. Ⓐ Ⓑ Ⓒ Ⓓ	21. Ⓐ Ⓑ Ⓒ Ⓓ	27. Ⓐ Ⓑ Ⓒ Ⓓ
4. Ⓐ Ⓑ Ⓒ Ⓓ	10. Ⓐ Ⓑ Ⓒ Ⓓ	16. Ⓐ Ⓑ Ⓒ Ⓓ	22. Ⓐ Ⓑ Ⓒ Ⓓ	28. Ⓐ Ⓑ Ⓒ Ⓓ
5. Ⓐ Ⓑ Ⓒ Ⓓ	11. Ⓐ Ⓑ Ⓒ Ⓓ	17. Ⓐ Ⓑ Ⓒ Ⓓ	23. Ⓐ Ⓑ Ⓒ Ⓓ	29. Ⓐ Ⓑ Ⓒ Ⓓ
6. Ⓐ Ⓑ Ⓒ Ⓓ	12. Ⓐ Ⓑ Ⓒ Ⓓ	18. Ⓐ Ⓑ Ⓒ Ⓓ	24. Ⓐ Ⓑ Ⓒ Ⓓ	30. Ⓐ Ⓑ Ⓒ Ⓓ

Test 6: Body Structure and Function

1. Ⓐ Ⓑ Ⓒ Ⓓ	7. Ⓐ Ⓑ Ⓒ Ⓓ	13. Ⓐ Ⓑ Ⓒ Ⓓ	19. Ⓐ Ⓔ Ⓒ Ⓓ	25. Ⓐ Ⓑ Ⓒ Ⓓ
2. Ⓐ Ⓑ Ⓒ Ⓓ	8. Ⓐ Ⓑ Ⓒ Ⓓ	14. Ⓐ Ⓑ Ⓒ Ⓓ	20. Ⓐ Ⓔ Ⓒ Ⓓ	26. Ⓐ Ⓑ Ⓒ Ⓓ
3. Ⓐ Ⓑ Ⓒ Ⓓ	9. Ⓐ Ⓑ Ⓒ Ⓓ	15. Ⓐ Ⓑ Ⓒ Ⓓ	21. Ⓐ Ⓔ Ⓒ Ⓓ	27. Ⓐ Ⓑ Ⓒ Ⓓ
4. Ⓐ Ⓑ Ⓒ Ⓓ	10. Ⓐ Ⓑ Ⓒ Ⓓ	16. Ⓐ Ⓑ Ⓒ Ⓓ	22. Ⓐ Ⓔ Ⓒ Ⓓ	28. Ⓐ Ⓑ Ⓒ Ⓓ
5. Ⓐ Ⓑ Ⓒ Ⓓ	11. Ⓐ Ⓑ Ⓒ Ⓓ	17. Ⓐ Ⓑ Ⓒ Ⓓ	23. Ⓐ Ⓔ Ⓒ Ⓓ	29. Ⓐ Ⓑ Ⓒ Ⓓ
6. Ⓐ Ⓑ Ⓒ Ⓓ	12. Ⓐ Ⓑ Ⓒ Ⓓ	18. Ⓐ Ⓑ Ⓒ Ⓓ	24. Ⓐ Ⓔ Ⓒ Ⓓ	30. Ⓐ Ⓑ Ⓒ Ⓓ

Test 7: Physiology and Health Science

1. Ⓐ Ⓑ Ⓒ Ⓓ	15. Ⓐ Ⓑ Ⓒ Ⓓ	29. Ⓐ Ⓑ Ⓒ Ⓓ	43. Ⓐ Ⓑ Ⓒ Ⓓ	57. Ⓐ Ⓑ Ⓒ Ⓓ
2. Ⓐ Ⓑ Ⓒ Ⓓ	16. Ⓐ Ⓑ Ⓒ Ⓓ	30. Ⓐ Ⓑ Ⓒ Ⓓ	44. Ⓐ Ⓑ Ⓒ Ⓓ	58. Ⓐ Ⓑ Ⓒ Ⓓ
3. Ⓐ Ⓑ Ⓒ Ⓓ	17. Ⓐ Ⓑ Ⓒ Ⓓ	31. Ⓐ Ⓑ Ⓒ Ⓓ	45. Ⓐ Ⓑ Ⓒ Ⓓ	59. Ⓐ Ⓑ Ⓒ Ⓓ
4. Ⓐ Ⓑ Ⓒ Ⓓ	18. Ⓐ Ⓑ Ⓒ Ⓓ	32. Ⓐ Ⓑ Ⓒ Ⓓ	46. Ⓐ Ⓑ Ⓒ Ⓓ	60. Ⓐ Ⓑ Ⓒ Ⓓ
5. Ⓐ Ⓑ Ⓒ Ⓓ	19. Ⓐ Ⓑ Ⓒ Ⓓ	33. Ⓐ Ⓑ Ⓒ Ⓓ	47. Ⓐ Ⓑ Ⓒ Ⓓ	61. Ⓐ Ⓑ Ⓒ Ⓓ
6. Ⓐ Ⓑ Ⓒ Ⓓ	20. Ⓐ Ⓑ Ⓒ Ⓓ	34. Ⓐ Ⓑ Ⓒ Ⓓ	48. Ⓐ Ⓑ Ⓒ Ⓓ	62. Ⓐ Ⓑ Ⓒ Ⓓ
7. Ⓐ Ⓑ Ⓒ Ⓓ	21. Ⓐ Ⓑ Ⓒ Ⓓ	35. Ⓐ Ⓑ Ⓒ Ⓓ	49. Ⓐ Ⓑ Ⓒ Ⓓ	63. Ⓐ Ⓑ Ⓒ Ⓓ
8. Ⓐ Ⓑ Ⓒ Ⓓ	22. Ⓐ Ⓑ Ⓒ Ⓓ	36. Ⓐ Ⓑ Ⓒ Ⓓ	50. Ⓐ Ⓑ Ⓒ Ⓓ	64. Ⓐ Ⓑ Ⓒ Ⓓ
9. Ⓐ Ⓑ Ⓒ Ⓓ	23. Ⓐ Ⓑ Ⓒ Ⓓ	37. Ⓐ Ⓑ Ⓒ Ⓓ	51. Ⓐ Ⓑ Ⓒ Ⓓ	65. Ⓐ Ⓑ Ⓒ Ⓓ
10. Ⓐ Ⓑ Ⓒ Ⓓ	24. Ⓐ Ⓑ Ⓒ Ⓓ	38. Ⓐ Ⓑ Ⓒ Ⓓ	52. Ⓐ Ⓑ Ⓒ Ⓓ	66. Ⓐ Ⓑ Ⓒ Ⓓ
11. Ⓐ Ⓑ Ⓒ Ⓓ	25. Ⓐ Ⓑ Ⓒ Ⓓ	39. Ⓐ Ⓑ Ⓒ Ⓓ	53. Ⓐ Ⓑ Ⓒ Ⓓ	67. Ⓐ Ⓑ Ⓒ Ⓓ
12. Ⓐ Ⓑ Ⓒ Ⓓ	26. Ⓐ Ⓑ Ⓒ Ⓓ	40. Ⓐ Ⓑ Ⓒ Ⓓ	54. Ⓐ Ⓑ Ⓒ Ⓓ	68. Ⓐ Ⓑ Ⓒ Ⓓ
13. Ⓐ Ⓑ Ⓒ Ⓓ	27. Ⓐ Ⓑ Ⓒ Ⓓ	41. Ⓐ Ⓑ Ⓒ Ⓓ	55. Ⓐ Ⓑ Ⓒ Ⓓ	69. Ⓐ Ⓑ Ⓒ Ⓓ
14. Ⓐ Ⓑ Ⓒ Ⓓ	28. Ⓐ Ⓑ Ⓒ Ⓓ	42. Ⓐ Ⓑ Ⓒ Ⓓ	56. Ⓐ Ⓑ Ⓒ Ⓓ	70. Ⓐ Ⓑ Ⓒ Ⓓ

TEST 1: HUMAN ANATOMY AND PHYSIOLOGY

50 Questions • 45 Minutes

Directions: Read each question carefully and consider all possible answers. When you have decided which choice is best, blacken the corresponding space on your answer sheet. There is only one best answer for each question.

Cells and Tissues

1. Cholesterol, in spite of its bad reputation, is an essential component of
   A. microtubules.
   B. the cell membrane.
   C. ribosomes.
   D. cytosol.

2. Synthesis of phospholipids, steroid hormones, and glycogen occurs within the
   A. rough endoplasmic reticulum.
   B. mitochondria.
   C. smooth endoplasmic reticulum.
   D. Golgi apparatus.

3. Following synthesis at the rough endoplasmic reticulum, new proteins are stored and "packaged" by
   A. the smooth endoplasmic reticulum.
   B. the cell membrane.
   C. the Golgi apparatus.
   D. lysosomes.

4. Cell membranes control the movement of substances into and out of the cell and are best described as
   A. selectively permeable.
   B. freely permeable.
   C. impermeable.
   D. totally permeable.

5. Mammalian cells suspended within a hypertonic solution will
   A. swell and possibly rupture.
   B. lose water by osmosis.
   C. take on water by osmosis.
   D. remain unchanged since intracellular fluid is also hypertonic.

6. Glucose, a primary energy source for skeletal muscle, is insoluble in lipids and is too large to pass through membrane channels. Movement of glucose into skeletal muscle cells occurs via
   A. active transport.
   B. exocytosis.
   C. diffusion.
   D. facilitated diffusion.

7. The _____ are the control centers of cellular operations and usually contain nucleoli.
   A. nuclei
   B. mitochondria
   C. ribosomes
   D. lysosomes

8. _____, a multifunctional tissue, is comprised of layers of cells that cover both internal and external structures, including all exposed body surfaces. Although avascular, it is characterized by a high level of regeneration.

   A. Muscle tissue
   B. Neural tissue
   C. Epithelia
   D. Connective tissue

9. Connection of skeletal muscle to bones is made by tendons, which consist primarily of _____ fibers.

   A. collagen
   B. elastic
   C. reticular
   D. nerve

10. Joint cavities are found at articulations, are fluid-filled, and are lined by _____ membranes.

   A. mucus
   B. serous
   C. cutaneous
   D. synovial

Integumentary System

11. Protection of the skin from the harmful effects of ultraviolet light is provided by the pigment _____, which is produced by specialized cells within the stratum germinativum.

   A. carotene
   B. melanin
   C. keratin
   D. hemoglobin

12. Lines of cleavage result from the parallel arrangements of _____ within the skin. They are significant in that incisions made parallel to a cleavage line tend to remain closed, whereas incisions crossing lines of cleavage tend to pull open.

   A. sebaceous glands
   B. smooth muscle
   C. blood vessels
   D. collagen

13. The ear canal is protected against the invasion of foreign particles by a material produced by _____ glands.

   A. ceruminous
   B. sebaceous
   C. apocrine
   D. merocrine

14. _____ sweat glands become functional at puberty. Its product supports bacterial growth, which intensifies its odor.

   A. Merocrine
   B. Apocrine
   C. Sebaceous
   D. Ceruminous

15. Merkel discs and Meisnner corpuscles in the skin are functionally involved in

   A. sweat production.
   B. transport of blood.
   C. sensation.
   D. oil production.

Skeletal System

16. New bone matrix accompanied by increased strength and mass results from the activity of

   A. osteoblasts.
   B. osteoclasts.
   C. osteocytes.
   D. lacunae.

17. Blood cell formation in adults is a function of red bone marrow primarily located within
- **A.** the periosteum.
- **B.** the endosteum.
- **C.** compact bone.
- **D.** spongy bone.

18. When blood calcium levels fall to below normal levels, osteoclast activity is stimulated, and calcium excretion is decreased under the influence of elevated levels of
- **A.** calcitonin.
- **B.** parathyroid hormone.
- **C.** calcitriol.
- **D.** thyroxine.

19. The fetal skeleton begins as a model formed by cartilage. Replacement of cartilage by bone is the process of
- **A.** intramembranous ossification.
- **B.** endochondral ossification.
- **C.** osteoclast activation.
- **D.** osteoblast inhibition.

20. A freely moveable joint, such as those found at the elbow and ankle, is functionally categorized as a(n)
- **A.** synarthrosis.
- **B.** amphiarthrosis.
- **C.** diarthrosis.
- **D.** arthritis.

21. Movement at a joint that takes a body part away from the long axis of the body is
- **A.** flexion.
- **B.** extension.
- **C.** abduction.
- **D.** adduction.

Muscle

22. Following the release of a transmitter substance at the neuromuscular junction, the action of that transmitter is terminated by
- **A.** acetylcholine.
- **B.** acetylcholinesterase.
- **C.** epinephrine.
- **D.** monoamine oxidase.

23. Following production of an action potential at the end plate, that electrical activity is conducted to the interior of the cell via the
- **A.** motor neuron.
- **B.** muscle capillaries.
- **C.** epimysium.
- **D.** transverse tubules.

24. Skeletal muscle contraction, resulting from the interaction of myosin and actin, is a consequence of the release of calcium ions from the
- **A.** motor neuron.
- **B.** end plate.
- **C.** mitochondria.
- **D.** sarcoplasmic reticulum.

25. Relaxed muscles produce more energy than is required for resting metabolism. That energy is stored in the form of
- **A.** ATP.
- **B.** ADP.
- **C.** creatine.
- **D.** creatine phosphate.

26. Lifting progressively heavier weight requires the activation of an increased number of motor units, which is
- **A.** complete tetanus.
- **B.** recruitment.
- **C.** muscle tone.
- **D.** a twitch.

27. Slow muscle fibers are particularly resistant to fatigue, a property due in part to the presence of _____, a protein that reversibly binds oxygen.
    A. hemoglobin
    B. myoglobin
    C. ATP
    D. ADP

28. Intercalated discs form connections between adjacent _____ muscle cells and play a major role in the function of that type of muscle.
    A. striated
    B. voluntary
    C. cardiac
    D. smooth

29. Individual muscle fibers and motor units either produce maximal tension in response to a stimulus or develop no tension at all. This is referred to as the _____ principle.
    A. muscle tone
    B. tetanus
    C. twitch
    D. all-or-none

30. _____ are glial cells within the central nervous system that play a role in maintaining the blood-brain barrier.
    A. Ependymal cells
    B. Microglia
    C. Astrocytes
    D. Oligodendrocytes

31. Following an action potential, sodium is returned to the extracellular space through the process of
    A. diffusion.
    B. filtration.
    C. osmosis.
    D. active transport.

32. Spinal cord transection will result in a loss of respiration if the trauma is at upper _____ levels interrupting outflow of the phrenic nerve.
    A. cervical
    B. thoracic
    C. lumbar
    D. sacral

33. Sensitivity of muscle spindles is controlled by the central nervous system through its ability to activate
    A. alpha motor neurons.
    B. gamma motor neurons.
    C. large diameter afferent axons.
    D. the neuromuscular junction.

34. Damage to the _____ lobe of the cerebral cortex may result in deficits in conscious perception of auditory stimuli.
    A. frontal
    B. parietal
    C. occipital
    D. temporal

35. Sensory and motor innervation of the face is the domain of the ophthalmic, maxillary, and mandibular branches of the _____ nerve.
    A. trochlear
    B. trigeminal
    C. facial
    D. vestibulocochlear

36. Information regarding fine touch to the body surface ascends the spinal cord within the
    A. spinothalamic tracts.
    B. lateral corticospinal tracts.
    C. posterior (dorsal) columns.
    D. spinocerebellar tracts.

37. Active dreaming and autonomic altera-
tions of blood pressure along with EEG
tracings resembling the awake state are
characteristic of
   A. slow wave sleep.
   B. rapid eye movement (REM) sleep.
   C. coma.
   D. arousal.

38. Parasympathetic autonomic outflow to
the heart, lungs, and digestive system is a
primary function of cranial nerve number
   A. I.
   B. II.
   C. X.
   D. XII.

Endocrinology and Reproduction

39. Release of thyroid hormones is triggered
by _____ from the anterior pituitary
gland.
   A. thyrotropin releasing hormone
   B. thyrotropin
   C. thyroxine
   D. iodide

40. In response to the release of _____
by the adenohypophysis, levels of gluco-
corticoids are elevated.
   A. corticotropin releasing hormone
   B. cortisol
   C. aldosterone
   D. adrenocorticotropic hormone

41. _____ stimulates the smooth muscle
of the uterine wall during the labor and
delivery process. After delivery, it promotes
the ejection of milk.
   A. Oxytocin
   B. Vasopressin
   C. Somatotropin
   D. Prolactin

42. In females, _____ promotes estrogen
secretion from cells within the ovaries,
while in males, it stimulates sperm pro-
duction within the testes.
   A. testosterone
   B. melanotropin
   C. follicle stimulating hormone
   D. luteinizing hormone

43. Pancreatic beta cells produce the hormone
_____, which lowers blood glucose
levels by promoting glucose uptake and
utilization.
   A. glucagon
   B. insulin
   C. epinephrine
   D. renin

44. An individual with an abnormally high
basal metabolic rate accompanied by
weight loss and unusual temperature sensi-
tivity is probably suffering from
   A. high levels of growth hormone.
   B. low levels of growth hormone.
   C. high levels of thyroid hormones.
   D. low levels of thyroid hormones.

45. Insulin is released by the beta cells of the
pancreas in response to
   A. low blood glucose levels.
   B. high blood glucose levels.
   C. high prolactin levels.
   D. high growth hormone levels.

46. The mineralocorticoid _____ is a
product of the adrenal cortex.
   A. epinephrine
   B. norepinephrine
   C. ACTH
   D. aldosterone

47. Abnormally low levels of parathyroid hormone could result in
    A. convulsions.
    B. hyperglycemia.
    C. hypoglycemia.
    D. excess water loss via the kidneys.

48. Of the following glands, the one that regulates the metabolic rate is the
    A. adrenal gland.
    B. salivary gland.
    C. thyroid.
    D. thymus.

49. The functional unit (or nephron) of the human kidney consists of
    A. Bowman's capsule and veins.
    B. Bowman's capsule, the glomerulus, and renal tubule.
    C. the ureter and renal tubule.
    D. the ureter, urethra, and renal tubule.

50. An organ that functions both as an endocrine and an exocrine gland is the
    A. salivary gland.
    B. gallbladder.
    C. thyroid gland.
    D. pancreas.

TEST 2: HUMAN ANATOMY AND PHYSIOLOGY

50 Questions • 50 Minutes

Directions: Read each question carefully and consider all possible answers. When you have decided which choice is best, blacken the corresponding space on your answer sheet. There is only one best answer for each question.

Blood

1. Maintenance of the osmotic pressure of plasma is a major role of
   A. albumin.
   B. globulins.
   C. fibrinogen.
   D. platelets.

2. Anemia is a condition resulting from abnormally low levels of
   A. platelets.
   B. plasma proteins.
   C. leukocytes.
   D. erythrocytes or hemoglobin.

3. Production of red blood cells is stimulated by the release of _____ from specialized cells of the kidneys in response to hypoxia (low oxygen levels).
   A. platelets
   B. erythrocytes
   C. erythropoietin
   D. leukocytes

4. Blood typing is a classification determined by the identification of
   A. erythrocyte surface antigens.
   B. erythrocyte surface antibodies.
   C. plasma antigens.
   D. plasma antibodies.

5. Rh-positive blood indicates the presence of the
   A. Rh antigen in plasma.
   B. Rh antigen on the surfaces of erythrocytes.
   C. Rh antibody on erythrocyte surfaces.
   D. Rh antibody in plasma.

6. Transfusion of blood from a Type A donor to a Type B recipient will result in
   A. agglutination.
   B. blood vessel spasm.
   C. platelet plug formation.
   D. slowly progressive anemia.

7. The most numerous leukocytes are _____. They are granulocytes and represent one of the earliest defenses against infection.
   A. lymphocytes
   B. monocytes
   C. basophils
   D. neutrophils

8. T-cells, B-cells, and NK-cells are classes of _____, agranulocytes involved in immunity processes.
   A. monocytes
   B. lymphocytes
   C. neutrophils
   D. eosinophils

9. Release of ADP, thromboxane A$_2$, and serotonin are events associated with the _____ phase of hemostasis.

    A. vascular

    B. platelet

    C. coagulation

    D. inflammation

10. The last step in the final common pathway of coagulation involves the production of insoluble strands of the protein

    A. prothrombin.

    B. thrombin.

    C. fibrinogen.

    D. fibrin.

11. Of the following, the only safe blood transfusion would be

    A. group A blood into a group O person.

    B. group B blood into a group A person.

    C. group O blood into a group AB person.

    D. group AB blood into a group B person.

Cardiovascular

12. Action potentials in cardiac cells are longer in duration than those in skeletal muscle. The long plateau seen in cardiac action potentials is primarily due to

    A. calcium entry into the cell.

    B. calcium exit from the cell.

    C. sodium entry into the cell.

    D. sodium exit from the cell.

13. Conducting cells of the heart do not maintain a stable resting membrane potential. The rate of spontaneous depolarizations is greatest within

    A. the AV node.

    B. the SA node.

    C. bundle branch fibers.

    D. purkinje fibers.

14. Depolarization of the ventricles is reflected in the _____ of the electrocardiogram.

    A. P wave

    B. QRS complex

    C. T wave

    D. P-R segment

15. The maximum ventricular volume within a cardiac cycle is expressed as the

    A. stroke volume.

    B. ejection fraction.

    C. end-systolic volume.

    D. end-diastolic volume.

16. The amount of tension the ventricles must produce in order to open semilunar valves and eject blood is the

    A. preload.

    B. afterload.

    C. cardiac output.

    D. stroke volume.

17. Norepinephrine acts at _____ receptors of the heart, resulting in an increase in heart rate.

    A. alpha 1

    B. alpha 2

    C. beta 1

    D. beta 2

18. Exchange of materials from the vascular system to surrounding interstitial fluids is a property of

    A. arteries.

    B. arterioles.

    C. capillaries.

    D. veins.

19. Pressure in veins is low and significantly influenced by the force of gravity. In the extremities, unidirectional blood flow is maintained by
    A. venous valves.
    B. venous smooth muscle.
    C. precapillary sphincters.
    D. semilunar valves.

20. Pulse pressure, the difference between systolic and diastolic pressure, is greatest within
    A. arteries.
    B. arterioles.
    C. capillaries.
    D. veins.

21. The primary responsibility for rapid correction of blood pressure alterations involves
    A. angiotensin.
    B. antidiuretic hormone.
    C. chemoreceptors.
    D. baroreceptor reflexes.

Respiration

22. During the act of swallowing, entry of liquids and solid materials into the respiratory tract is prevented by the
    A. glottis.
    B. epiglottis.
    C. pharynx.
    D. hard palate.

23. _____ is the volume of air moved into or out of the respiratory system during a single respiratory cycle.
    A. Tidal volume
    B. Minute volume
    C. Residual volume
    D. Inspiratory reserve volume

24. The volume of air in the respiratory conduction passages that does NOT participate in gas exchange is the
    A. vital capacity.
    B. expiratory reserve volume.
    C. anatomical dead space.
    D. total lung capacity.

25. Movement of respiratory gases is primarily dependent upon the presence of a(n) _____ gradient.
    A. concentration
    B. osmotic
    C. partial pressure
    D. temperature

26. Contraction of the diaphragm results in inspiration as a result of
    A. increased thoracic cavity volume.
    B. decreased thoracic cavity volume.
    C. increased abdominal cavity volume.
    D. decreased abdominal cavity volume.

27. Oxygen unloading at the tissue level is accelerated by
    A. elevated blood pressure.
    B. lowered blood pressure.
    C. elevated pH.
    D. decreased pH.

28. Although most carbon dioxide is transported as bicarbonate, and some is dissolved in plasma, about 20% is carried
    A. by leukocytes.
    B. by plasma proteins.
    C. as carbaminohemoglobin.
    D. on the surface of erythrocytes.

29. The reaction of carbon dioxide and water leading to the formation of carbonic acid is catalyzed by
    A. antigens on the surface of erythrocytes.
    B. antibodies within plasma.
    C. enzymes in plasma.
    D. carbonic anhydrase within erythrocytes.

30. Length of inspiration is shortened by inhibitory impulses originating within the
    A. apneustic center.
    B. pneumotaxic center.
    C. inspiratory center.
    D. precentral gyrus.

Renal

31. Decline in systemic blood pressure leads to the release of renin, which results in the production of
    A. angiotensinogen.
    B. angiotensin I.
    C. angiotensin II.
    D. carbonic anhydrase.

32. Angiotensin II has multiple direct and indirect effects, including
    A. vasoconstriction.
    B. vasodilation.
    C. inhibition of aldosterone release.
    D. increased urine output.

33. _____ are examples of substances that are NOT significantly reabsorbed by the kidneys and are therefore excreted.
    A. Amino acids
    B. Vitamins
    C. Nitrogenous by-products of protein catabolism
    D. Water and electrolytes

34. Glucose and most other nutrients, such as amino acids and vitamins, are reabsorbed within the _____ of the nephron.
    A. collecting duct
    B. proximal convoluted tubule
    C. loop of Henle
    D. distal convoluted tubule

35. The movement of urine from the kidneys to the bladder is driven by
    A. gravity.
    B. peristalsis.
    C. bladder pressure.
    D. blood pressure.

36. Urinary continence is maintained by contraction of the external urethral sphincter, which is innervated by the
    A. sympathetic division of the ANS.
    B. parasympathetic division of the ANS.
    C. phrenic nerve.
    D. pudendal nerve.

37. The cation in the highest concentration within extracellular fluid that plays a major role in water distribution is
    A. sodium.
    B. potassium.
    C. calcium.
    D. magnesium.

38. The hormone most responsible for the renal regulation of sodium is
    A. thyroxine.
    B. insulin.
    C. glucagon.
    D. aldosterone.

39. Acid-base regulation is most powerful and most complete by

A. buffers.

B. respiratory mechanisms.

C. renal mechanisms.

D. urinary bladder activity.

40. Uncontrolled diabetes mellitus results in

A. respiratory acidosis.

B. respiratory alkalosis.

C. metabolic acidosis.

D. metabolic alkalosis.

Digestion

41. Absorption of vitamin B_{12} (required for erythrocyte production) is promoted by intrinsic factor—a product of cells found within the

A. small intestine.

B. stomach.

C. pancreas.

D. large intestine.

42. Bile that is NOT immediately needed for digestion is stored and concentrated within the

A. liver.

B. gallbladder.

C. pancreas.

D. ileum.

43. Secretion of pancreatic juice is stimulated by _____, released in response to proteins and fats within the small intestine.

A. secretin

B. cholecystokinin

C. insulin

D. aldosterone

44. Diarrhea and constipation result primarily from altered motility of the

A. stomach.

B. small intestine.

C. liver.

D. large intestine.

45. In order to be absorbed, carbohydrates must be reduced to the form of

A. monosaccharides.

B. disaccharides.

C. polysaccharides.

D. oligosaccharides.

46. Protein digestion begins in the stomach by a group of proteolytic enzymes referred to as

A. lipase.

B. sucrase.

C. pepsin.

D. amylase.

47. Vitamin _____ is water-soluble and readily absorbed from the intestine by diffusion.

A. A

B. D

C. E

D. C

48. Gastric ulcers occur when the protective inner layer of the stomach is damaged and the _____ layer, with its blood vessels and nerve cells, is exposed to acid.

A. serosal

B. mucosal

C. submucosal

D. muscular

49. Saliva contains mucus, water, and
_____, which partially digests
polysaccharides.
   A. lipase
   B. amylase
   C. pepsin
   D. insulin

50. Smooth muscle activity of the digestive
system is stimulated by increased levels of
_____ activity.
   A. parasympathetic autonomic
   B. sympathetic autonomic
   C. thyroid gland
   D. aldosterone

TEST 3: HUMAN ANATOMY AND PHYSIOLOGY

100 Questions • 100 Minutes

Directions: Read each question carefully and consider all possible answers. When you have decided which choice is best, blacken the corresponding space on your answer sheet. There is only one best answer for each question.

1. The _____ system picks up fluid leaked from blood vessels, houses white blood cells, and is highly involved in mechanisms of immunity.
   A. urinary
   B. endocrine
   C. integumentary
   D. lymphatic

2. The major muscle component of inspiration is the
   A. diaphragm.
   B. external intercostal muscles.
   C. internal intercostal muscles.
   D. abdominal muscles.

3. Skin, nails, and hair are components of the _____ system.
   A. integumentary
   B. lymphatic
   C. skeletal
   D. endocrine

4. Water reabsorption in the collecting duct of the kidneys is controlled by _____ from the posterior pituitary.
   A. oxytocin
   B. ADH
   C. epinephrine
   D. aldosterone

5. Most homeostatic control mechanisms are
   A. positive feedback mechanisms.
   B. negative feedback mechanisms.
   C. neural mechanisms.
   D. endocrine mechanisms.

6. The most important structure(s) in the routine control of respiration is (are) the
   A. trachea.
   B. irritant receptors.
   C. peripheral chemoreceptors.
   D. central chemoreceptors.

7. A _____ plane is a vertical plane that divides the body into left and right parts.
   A. frontal
   B. transverse
   C. sagittal
   D. coronal

8. Cardiac output is equal to
   A. heart rate.
   B. stroke volume.
   C. the product of stroke volume and heart rate.
   D. stroke volume divided by heart rate.

9. If both parents have blood type AB, what will be the blood types of offspring?
   A. A
   B. AB
   C. A, AB, and B
   D. O

10. The right ventricle pumps blood through the _____ valve into the _____.
    A. atrioventricular; pulmonary veins
    B. pulmonary semilunar; pulmonary veins
    C. atrioventricular; pulmonary arteries
    D. pulmonary semilunar; pulmonary arteries

11. The primary Beta-2 catechol amine agonist is
    A. acetylcholine.
    B. epinephrine.
    C. norepinephrine.
    D. nicotine.

12. Action potentials result from an increased membrane permeability to
    A. calcium.
    B. sodium.
    C. potassium.
    D. chloride.

13. Food is prevented from entering the trachea during swallowing by the
    A. glottis.
    B. esophageal sphincter.
    C. cardiac sphincter.
    D. epiglottis.

14. Oxygen transported in blood is mainly
    A. dissolved in plasma.
    B. combined with hemoglobin.
    C. CO_2.
    D. carried as bicarbonate.

15. Pyramidal tract fibers originate in the
    A. precentral gyrus.
    B. postcentral gyrus.
    C. thalamus.
    D. spinal cord.

16. The transmitter substance at the neuro-muscular junction is
    A. acetylcholinesterase.
    B. norepinephrine.
    C. acetylcholine.
    D. epinephrine.

17. _____ dilate or constrict to control the flow of blood into a particular capillary bed.
    A. Arteries
    B. Arterioles
    C. Capillaries
    D. Veins

18. Hormone secretion and neurotransmitter release use the process of _____ to move substances from the cell interior into the extracellular space.
    A. phagocytosis
    B. endocytosis
    C. exocytosis
    D. pinocytosis

19. The area innervated by all the axons in a single dorsal root is a
    A. receptive field.
    B. dermatome.
    C. sensory unit.
    D. motor unit.

20. Stratified squamous anatomically describes a form of _____ tissue.
    A. muscle
    B. nerve
    C. connective
    D. epithelial

21. _____ forms most of the embryonic skeleton, connects the ribs of the sternum, and comprises the solid supportive structures of the nose and trachea.
    A. Bone
    B. Areolar connective tissue
    C. Adipose tissue
    D. Cartilage

22. _____ is the fibrous protein found in the stratum corneum that helps give the epidermis its protective properties.
   A. Keratin
   B. Melanin
   C. Carotene
   D. Hemoglobin

23. Pain information is carried by _____ afferents.
   A. A Delta
   B. C
   C. A Alpha
   D. A Delta and C

24. Increased parasympathetic activity will result in
   A. increased heart rate.
   B. increased cardiac output.
   C. vasoconstriction.
   D. decreased heart rate.

25. The receptor for the stretch reflex is the
   A. Golgi tendon organ.
   B. free nerve ending.
   C. hair cell.
   D. muscle spindle.

26. The glomerular membrane is
   A. more permeable than most other capillaries.
   B. less permeable than most other capillaries.
   C. highly permeable to proteins.
   D. highly permeable to erythrocytes.

27. CO_2 in blood is mainly
   A. dissolved in plasma.
   B. carried as bicarbonate.
   C. dissolved in RBCs.
   D. combined with hemoglobin.

28. Glucose is returned in blood in the kidneys by
   A. glomerular filtration.
   B. tubular reabsorption.
   C. tubular secretion.
   D. reabsorption in the collection duct.

29. The outer surface of the diaphysis of a long bone is covered with a double-layered membrane called the _____. The inner layer of that membrane contains bone-forming cells called _____.
   A. endosteum; osteoblasts
   B. endosteum; osteoclasts
   C. periosteum; osteoclasts
   D. periosteum; osteoblasts

30. Atrial contraction is
   A. initiated by the AV node.
   B. most important in a resting subject.
   C. initiated by the SA node.
   D. responsible for most of the ventricular filling.

31. The first heart sound is a result of
   A. closing of the pulmonary valve.
   B. closing of the AV valves.
   C. closing of the aortic valve.
   D. contraction of the atria.

32. The portion of the skull overlying the region of the cerebral cortex primarily involved with visual process is the _____ bone.
   A. frontal
   B. parietal
   C. occipital
   D. temporal

33. Normally, most of the body's total blood is found in the
   A. veins.
   B. arteries.
   C. capillaries.
   D. heart.

34. The kneecap, or patella, is an example of a(n) _____ bone.
   A. long
   B. short
   C. flat
   D. irregular

35. The normal pacemaker of the heart is the
   A. SA node.
   B. AV node.
   C. atria.
   D. ventricle.

36. Blood pressure is highest in
   A. arteries.
   B. arterioles.
   C. capillaries.
   D. veins.

37. Water permeability is greatest in the _____ of the nephron.
   A. collecting duct
   B. distal convoluted tubule
   C. loop of Henle
   D. proximal convoluted tubule

38. Type I diabetes mellitus is characterized by
   A. high insulin levels.
   B. ineffective insulin receptors.
   C. low blood glucose levels.
   D. decreased insulin production.

39. The division of the autonomic nervous system that functions during emergencies is the
   A. sympathetic.
   B. parasympathetic.
   C. craniosacral.
   D. somatic.

40. Sympathetic preganglionic neurons originate in the
   A. cervical spinal cord.
   B. thoracic spinal cord.
   C. sacral spinal cord.
   D. coccygeal spinal cord.

41. Cellular energy production takes place within
   A. rough endoplasmic reticulum.
   B. smooth endoplasmic reticulum.
   C. mitochondria.
   D. Golgi apparatus.

42. _____ is a bending movement that decreases the angle of a joint and brings two articulating bones closer together.
   A. Retraction
   B. Flexion
   C. Extension
   D. Rotation

43. New epidermal cells are formed in the stratum
   A. germinativum.
   B. corneum.
   C. spinosum.
   D. lucidum.

44. Women have a larger percentage of adipose tissue than men; this tissue is mainly found in the
   A. epidermis.
   B. dermis.
   C. subcutaneous layer.
   D. muscle.

45. Membranes that line body cavities that open to the outside are
   A. mucosal.
   B. serous.
   C. synovial.
   D. cutaneous.

46. Epidermal cells are supplied with nutrition from blood vessels located within the
   A. epidermis.
   B. dermis.
   C. subcutaneous layer.
   D. All of the above

47. The terms *visceral, nonstriated,* and *involuntary* are descriptive of _____ muscle.
   A. skeletal
   B. smooth
   C. cardiac
   D. postural

48. Blood cell formation is a function of the _____ system.
   A. circulatory
   B. skeletal
   C. endocrine
   D. muscular

49. Blood calcium is elevated by
   A. calcitonin.
   B. parathyroid hormone.
   C. growth hormone.
   D. thyroxine.

50. A 7-year-old patient is perspiring freely on the forehead, palms, and soles, indicating activity of the
   A. eccrine glands.
   B. apocrine glands.
   C. sebaceous glands.
   D. ceruminous glands.

51. Flexion of the elbow results from contraction of the _____ muscle, and flexion of the knee involves contraction of the _____ muscle.
   A. triceps brachii; biceps femoris
   B. biceps brachii; triceps femoris
   C. biceps femoris; biceps brachii
   D. triceps femoris; triceps brachii

52. Sweat glands that become functional at puberty are
   A. apocrine.
   B. eccrine.
   C. sebaceous.
   D. ceruminous.

53. An individual with higher than normal blood calcium (hypercalcemia) will compensate by elevating levels of
   A. parathyroid hormone.
   B. calcitonin.
   C. Both A and B
   D. Neither A nor B

54. The _____ system carries hormones to their sites of action.
   A. endocrine
   B. cardiovascular
   C. respiratory
   D. skeletal

55. The most rapidly conducting axons within the human nervous system are _____ and_____.
   A. unmyelinated; small diameter
   B. unmyelinated; large diameter
   C. myelinated; small diameter
   D. myelinated; large diameter

56. The basic unit of structure and function within the kidneys is the
    A. glomerulus.
    B. nephron.
    C. ureter.
    D. urethra.

57. The esophagus enters the stomach at the _____ region.
    A. fundus
    B. cardiac
    C. body
    D. pyloric

58. Release of _____ by the posterior pituitary will lead to contractions of the smooth muscle of the uterus.
    A. ADH
    B. ACTH
    C. oxytocin
    D. prolactin

59. Inhibition of ADH release will result in
    A. high blood pressure.
    B. increased urine output.
    C. uterine contractions.
    D. decreased urine output.

60. Ovulation occurs in response to
    A. FSH.
    B. ADH.
    C. prolactin.
    D. LH.

61. Heartburn results from reflux of gastric fluids into the esophagus. The structure that normally prevents this is the
    A. pyloric sphincter.
    B. cardiac sphincter.
    C. ileocecal valve.
    D. epiglottis.

62. Fat is broken down in the duodenum by _____ from the gallbladder.
    A. lipase
    B. amylase
    C. bile
    D. HCl

63. Most digestion takes place in the
    A. stomach.
    B. duodenum.
    C. ileum.
    D. jejunum.

64. Visual receptors are located on the
    A. lens.
    B. cornea.
    C. retina.
    D. optic tract.

65. Most food absorption takes place in the
    A. duodenum.
    B. colon.
    C. ileum.
    D. stomach.

66. Centers for cardiovascular and respiratory control, vomiting, and coughing are found within the _____, the most inferior part of the brain stem.
    A. midbrain
    B. pons
    C. medulla
    D. thalamus

67. Bile is manufactured in the
    A. duodenum.
    B. liver.
    C. gallbladder.
    D. pancreas.

68. A patient who is abnormally short and developmentally disabled suggests that the patient
    A. had hyperthyroidism as an infant.
    B. had hypothyroidism as an infant.
    C. has adult hyperthyroidism.
    D. has adult hypothyroidism.

69. Receptors used for color vision are
    A. hair cells.
    B. rods.
    C. cones.
    D. retinae.

70. The inner lining of the digestive system is the _____ layer.
    A. mucosal
    B. submucosal
    C. muscular
    D. serosal

71. The _____ has both endocrine and exocrine functions.
    A. adrenal cortex
    B. pancreas
    C. parathyroid
    D. thyroid

72. Lacrimation refers to the production of
    A. salvia.
    B. mucous.
    C. tears.
    D. urine.

73. The sense of smell travels over cranial nerve number
    A. I.
    B. II.
    C. III.
    D. IV.

74. The gland adjacent to the urethra that enlarges in older males is the
    A. testes.
    B. seminal vesicle.
    C. bulbourethral gland.
    D. prostate.

75. Linear acceleration of the head is detected by receptors within the
    A. semicircular canals.
    B. utricles and saccules.
    C. cochlea.
    D. middle ear.

76. The most abundant protein in blood is
    A. alpha globulin.
    B. albumin.
    C. gamma globulin.
    D. fibrin.

77. Fertilization normally occurs within the
    A. fallopian tube.
    B. ovary.
    C. uterus.
    D. vagina.

78. Depression is characterized by
    A. high levels of norepinephrine.
    B. low levels of serotonin.
    C. high levels of serotonin.
    D. low levels of norepinephrine.

79. Lymphatic vessels originate at
    A. vascular capillaries.
    B. lymphatic capillaries.
    C. lymph nodes.
    D. lymphocytes.

80. Human chorionic gonadotropin (HCG) is responsible for
    A. maintaining the corpus luteum.
    B. lowering estrogen levels.
    C. lowering progesterone levels.
    D. initiating menstruation.

81. Loss of the sense of sweet and sour tastes from the tongue indicates damage to the _____ nerve.
    A. first
    B. fifth
    C. seventh
    D. tenth

82. Salivation, lacrimation, urination, and defecation are primarily under control of the _____ division of the autonomic nervous system.
    A. sympathetic
    B. parasympathetic
    C. somatic
    D. voluntary

83. Sperm cells are stored in the _____ after leaving the seminiferous tubules.
    A. epididymis
    B. vas deferens
    C. seminal vesicle
    D. prostate

84. The hormone from the pancreas that is responsible for elevating blood glucose levels between meals is
    A. insulin.
    B. glucagon.
    C. somatostatin.
    D. epinephrine.

85. The most abundantly formed elements in blood are
    A. white blood cells.
    B. red blood cells.
    C. globulins.
    D. albumins.

86. The most rapid mechanism of pH adjustment involves
    A. buffers.
    B. the respiratory system.
    C. the kidneys.
    D. the liver.

87. Normal pH of blood is
    A. 6
    B. 7.4
    C. 8
    D. 1.0

88. Hematocrit is a measure of _____ levels.
    A. white cell
    B. plasma
    C. blood
    D. erythrocyte

89. Cardiac muscle, because of its constant activity, has a high oxygen demand, which must be met without interruption. Oxygen is supplied to cardiac muscle by
    A. the blood being pumped through the chambers of the heart.
    B. coronary arteries.
    C. coronary veins.
    D. pulmonary arteries.

90. Auditory receptors are
    A. rods.
    B. hair cells.
    C. cones.
    D. muscle spindles.

91. Blood containing the A antigen and the B antibody is type
    A. A
    B. B
    C. AB
    D. O

92. Hemoglobin forms abnormal long chains in
    A. pernicious anemia.
    B. iron deficiency anemia.
    C. aplastic anemia.
    D. sickle cell anemia.

93. Auditory receptors are found within the
    A. outer ear.
    B. middle ear.
    C. auditory ossicles.
    D. cochlea.

94. Female menopause is characterized by low levels of
    A. GnRH.
    B. LH.
    C. FSH.
    D. estrogen.

95. Hyperventilation resulting from hysteria may cause
    A. respiratory acidosis.
    B. respiratory alkalosis.
    C. metabolic acidosis.
    D. metabolic alkalosis.

96. The major component of plasma is
    A. ions.
    B. proteins.
    C. water.
    D. gases.

97. _____ acts as a contraceptive agent by inhibiting release of GnRH.
    A. Sperm
    B. Estrogen
    C. Testosterone
    D. LH

98. Coagulation is inhibited by
    A. fibrin.
    B. calcium.
    C. thrombin.
    D. heparin.

99. Ovulation is triggered by the release of
    A. FSH.
    B. LH.
    C. GnRH.
    D. estrogen.

100. Testosterone is produced by _____ cells.
    A. prostate
    B. seminiferous
    C. epididymis
    D. interstitial

TEST 4: ANATOMY, PHYSIOLOGY, AND HEALTH SCIENCE

40 Questions • 35 Minutes

> **Directions:** Each question or incomplete statement below is followed by four suggested answers or completions. For each question, select the best choice and fill in the corresponding space on your answer sheet.

1. Muscles whose functions are to close off body openings are
   A. flexors.
   B. sphincters.
   C. extensors.
   D. adductors.

2. Bile aids in the digestion of
   A. amino acids.
   B. fats.
   C. starches.
   D. carbohydrates.

3. Urea is removed from the blood as it goes through the
   A. bladder.
   B. pancreas.
   C. spleen.
   D. kidney.

4. The blood group of a universal recipient is
   A. AB
   B. B
   C. O
   D. A

5. The stimulant in coffee is
   A. tannic acid.
   B. theobromine.
   C. theophylline.
   D. caffeine.

6. Which of the following foods is the most economical source of proteins?
   A. Dried milk
   B. Green leafy vegetables
   C. Meats
   D. Eggs

7. Connective tissue that attaches muscles to the bones is called
   A. a tendon.
   B. a ligament.
   C. cartilage.
   D. osseous.

8. The hormone produced by the testes is
   A. progesterone.
   B. estrogen.
   C. testosterone.
   D. aldosterone.

9. The elbow joint is an example of
   A. ball-and-socket joint.
   B. hinge joint.
   C. pivot joint.
   D. saddle joint.

10. The movement that propels food down the digestive tract is called
    A. pyloraspasm.
    B. rugae.
    C. mastication.
    D. peristalsis.

11. In mumps, the gland affected is the
    A. parathyroid.
    B. pituitary.
    C. parotid.
    D. pineal.

12. The negatively charged particle found within the atom is the
    A. proton.
    B. electron.
    C. nucleus.
    D. neutron.

13. The exchange of nutrients and waste products occurs in the
    A. venules.
    B. capillaries.
    C. arterioles.
    D. arteries.

14. Hemoglobin is found in
    A. basophils.
    B. neutrophils.
    C. monocytes.
    D. erythrocytes.

15. Organic substances made up of several amino acids bound together are
    A. carbohydrates.
    B. fats.
    C. proteins.
    D. fatty acids.

16. The exchange of carbon dioxide and oxygen in the lungs occurs in the
    A. venules.
    B. alveoli.
    C. bronchi.
    D. bronchioles.

17. The pacemaker of the heart is the
    A. Bundle of His.
    B. AV node.
    C. purkinje fibers.
    D. SA node.

18. Mitral stenosis involves the
    A. aortic valve.
    B. pulmonary valve.
    C. bicuspid valve.
    D. tricuspid valve.

19. The smallest known microorganisms are
    A. bacteria.
    B. viruses.
    C. fungi.
    D. protozoa.

20. Which one of the following arteries carries deoxygenated blood?
    A. Pulmonary
    B. Coronary
    C. Vena cava
    D. Aorta

21. Electrolyte balance is maintained primarily by the action of the
    A. testes.
    B. kidney.
    C. bladder.
    D. liver.

22. The mineral that is necessary for the proper functioning of the thyroid gland is
    A. sodium.
    B. iodine.
    C. calcium.
    D. iron.

23. Vitamin C prevents
    A. beriberi.
    B. rickets.
    C. pellagra.
    D. scurvy.

24. The function of leukocytes is to
    A. carry oxygen.
    B. destroy bacteria.
    C. carry food.
    D. regulate metabolism.

25. Insulin is produced in the
    A. pituitary gland.
    B. thymus.
    C. pancreas.
    D. pineal gland.

26. The end product of protein metabolism is
    A. amino acids.
    B. glucose.
    C. glycogen.
    D. fatty acids.

27. Carbohydrates are absorbed into the blood as
    A. glycogen.
    B. amino acids.
    C. glucose.
    D. fatty acids.

28. When one muscle of a pair contracts, the opposing muscle must
    A. also contract.
    B. relax.
    C. produce more energy.
    D. remain in the same position.

29. The respiratory center is located in the part of the brain known as the
    A. thalamus.
    B. cerebrum.
    C. pons.
    D. medulla oblongata.

30. Rays pass through various parts of the eye in a process of bending called
    A. refraction.
    B. reflexion.
    C. retraction.
    D. retroversion.

31. The part of the eye commonly called the "window" is the
    A. retina.
    B. cornea.
    C. lens.
    D. pupil.

32. A calorie is a form of
    A. light.
    B. heat.
    C. darkness.
    D. sound.

33. The vitamin known as the "sunshine" vitamin is
    A. vitamin E.
    B. vitamin B.
    C. vitamin K.
    D. vitamin D.

34. The process by which the body changes food into substances that can be readily used by the body is
    A. digestion.
    B. deglutition.
    C. micturition.
    D. absorption.

35. The thyroid gland cannot function properly without
    A. chloride.
    B. iodine.
    C. phosphorous.
    D. iron.

36. The vitamin that is necessary for coagulation of the blood is
    A. vitamin K.
    B. vitamin C.
    C. vitamin A.
    D. vitamin E.

37. Another name for vitamin B_1 is
    A. niacin.
    B. thiamin.
    C. riboflavin.
    D. pyridoxine.

38. Food is moved through the alimentary canal by wave-like motions called
    A. excretions.
    B. mastication.
    C. contractions.
    D. peristalsis.

39. The femur is a bone located in the
    A. forearm.
    B. upper arm.
    C. thigh.
    D. lower leg.

40. The liquid portion of the blood is called
    A. serum.
    B. gamma globulin.
    C. plasma.
    D. lymph.

STOP

IF YOU FINISH BEFORE TIME IS CALLED, YOU MAY CHECK YOUR WORK ON THIS SECTION ONLY. DO NOT TURN TO ANY OTHER SECTION IN THE TEST.

TEST 5: ANATOMY, PHYSIOLOGY, AND HEALTH SCIENCE

30 Questions • 25 Minutes

> **Directions:** For each question, choose the answer that you consider correct or most nearly correct. Fill in the corresponding space on your answer sheet.

1. The force of the blood exerted against the wall of the blood vessel is called
   A. pulse deficit.
   B. apical pulse.
   C. blood pressure.
   D. pulse pressure.

2. The relative amount of moisture in the air is the
   A. evaporation factor.
   B. temperature.
   C. dew.
   D. humidity.

3. A laboratory sample is called a(n)
   A. collection.
   B. agar.
   C. specimen.
   D. symptom.

4. *Defecation* means
   A. swallowing.
   B. eliminating solid waste.
   C. irrigating the colon.
   D. relieving flatus.

5. An object completely free of all micro-organisms is
   A. sterile.
   B. clean.
   C. septic.
   D. contaminated.

6. Carbon dioxide is a
   A. respiratory depressant.
   B. circulatory stimulant.
   C. respiratory stimulant.
   D. circulatory depressant.

7. The presence of protein in the urine is called
   A. polyuria.
   B. anuria.
   C. albuminuria.
   D. hematuria.

8. The substance basic to life is
   A. carbohydrates.
   B. proteins.
   C. starches.
   D. fats.

9. In diseases of the gallbladder, which of the following nutrients is limited?
   A. Starches
   B. Proteins
   C. Fats
   D. Carbohydrates

10. Water-soluble vitamins include
    A. vitamin A.
    B. vitamin C.
    C. vitamin D.
    D. vitamin K.

11. Diets in the United States are most often deficient in
   A. iron and calcium.
   B. calcium and potassium.
   C. iodine and sodium.
   D. phosphorous and iron.

12. Tetany may be corrected by increasing the amount of
   A. iron.
   B. iodine.
   C. calcium.
   D. thiamine.

13. Which helps conserve body heat?
   A. Increased sweat production
   B. Increased respiratory activity
   C. Dilation of the capillaries of the skin
   D. Constriction of the capillaries of the skin

14. Milk is not a "perfect food" because it lacks
   A. iron.
   B. calcium.
   C. phosphorous.
   D. carbohydrates.

15. The body obtains most of its nitrogen from
   A. carbohydrates.
   B. proteins.
   C. fats.
   D. cellulose.

16. An ion is
   A. one molecule of water.
   B. one particle of hydrogen.
   C. the same as a neutron.
   D. an atom with an electric charge.

17. The basic unit of the living organism is
   A. the brain.
   B. the cell.
   C. a tissue.
   D. the nervous system.

18. The diffusion of water through a semi-permeable membrane is known as
   A. anabolism.
   B. synthesis.
   C. mitosis.
   D. osmosis.

19. A physician who specializes in diseases of the heart is known as a
   A. dermatologist.
   B. cardiologist.
   C. pediatrician.
   D. neurologist.

20. A fracture that occurs without completely separating the bone is called
   A. complex.
   B. compound.
   C. greenstick.
   D. comminuted.

21. Smoking and pollution, which have a deadly effect upon the lungs and pulmonary function, are classified as
   A. environmental factors.
   B. biological factors.
   C. sociological factors.
   D. physiological factors.

22. In the digestive process, almost all of the water is reabsorbed by the
   A. sigmoid.
   B. cecum.
   C. colon.
   D. rectum.

23. In what structure does fertilization normally occur?

    A. Vagina

    B. Cervix

    C. Ovary

    D. Fallopian tube

24. The process in which carbon dioxide and water are combined under the influence of light in green plants is called

    A. respiration.

    B. fermentation.

    C. assimilation.

    D. photosynthesis.

25. The most abundant gas in the atmosphere is

    A. oxygen.

    B. nitrogen.

    C. carbon dioxide.

    D. chlorine.

26. A protein substance that initiates and accelerates a chemical reaction is called a(n)

    A. gene.

    B. enzyme.

    C. hormone.

    D. base.

27. Amino acids that CANNOT be manufactured by the body are called

    A. essential amino acids.

    B. synthetic amino acids.

    C. basic amino acids.

    D. dependent amino acids.

28. The instrument used to measure air pressure is called a

    A. thermometer.

    B. hydrometer.

    C. barometer.

    D. sphygmomanometer.

29. An elevation above normal body temperature is called

    A. hypothermia.

    B. pyrexia.

    C. intermittent.

    D. remittent.

30. The instrument used to examine the ears is called a(n)

    A. ophthalmoscope.

    B. stethoscope.

    C. cystoscope.

    D. otoscope.

STOP

IF YOU FINISH BEFORE TIME IS CALLED, YOU MAY CHECK YOUR WORK ON THIS SECTION ONLY. DO NOT TURN TO ANY OTHER SECTION IN THE TEST.

TEST 6: BODY STRUCTURE AND FUNCTION

30 Questions • 25 Minutes

> **Directions:** For each question, choose the answer that you consider correct. Fill in the corresponding space on your answer sheet.

1. The body's continuous response to changes in the external and internal environment is called
   - A. homeostasis.
   - B. diffusion.
   - C. osmosis.
   - D. filtration.

2. The ability of a cell to reproduce is called
   - A. osmosis.
   - B. crenation.
   - C. lysis.
   - D. mitosis.

3. The immunity that occurs when a person is given a substance containing antibodies or antitoxins is called
   - A. active.
   - B. autoimmune.
   - C. passive.
   - D. permanent.

4. The part of the cell necessary for reproduction is the
   - A. cytoplasm.
   - B. nucleus.
   - C. protoplasm.
   - D. cytoplasmic membrane.

5. The hormone that regulates the metabolic rate of the body cells is
   - A. oxytocin.
   - B. aldosterone.
   - C. thyroxin.
   - D. cortisone.

6. The sudoriferous glands secrete
   - A. sebum.
   - B. perspiration.
   - C. hormones.
   - D. synovial fluid.

7. Tanning of the skin is due to
   - A. keratin.
   - B. sebum.
   - C. sweat.
   - D. melanin.

8. The ovaries produce the hormones
   - A. estrogen and testosterone.
   - B. progesterone and testosterone.
   - C. estrogen and progesterone.
   - D. progesterone and prolactin.

9. The tissue that forms a protective covering for the body and lines the intestinal and respiratory tract is called the
   - A. periosteum.
   - B. pericardium.
   - C. epithelium.
   - D. connective tissue.

10. The hip joint is an example of a
    - A. ball and socket joint.
    - B. hinge joint.
    - C. pivot joint.
    - D. saddle joint.

11. The endocrine gland that prepares the body for the "fight or flight" response is the
   A. adrenal cortex.
   B. adrenal medulla.
   C. pituitary.
   D. thyroid.

12. Tears drain into the nose through the
   A. ciliary body.
   B. lacrimal gland.
   C. eustachian tube.
   D. nasolacrimal duct.

13. Respiration and heart rate are controlled by the
   A. cerebellum.
   B. cerebrum.
   C. medulla oblongota.
   D. pons.

14. The main function of the large intestine is to
   A. absorb digested food.
   B. absorb water from waste materials.
   C. produce digestive enzymes.
   D. secrete digestive enzymes.

15. The hormone produced by the adrenal glands is
   A. progesterone.
   B. estrogen.
   C. testosterone.
   D. aldosterone.

16. The sloughing off of the endometrium is called
   A. menarche.
   B. menopause.
   C. menstruation.
   D. myometritis.

17. The dorsal cavity has two subdivisions, namely
   A. thoracic and abdominopelvic.
   B. cranial and spinal.
   C. thoracic and spinal.
   D. medial and lateral.

18. The chamber of the heart that receives venous blood from body tissue is the
   A. right atrium.
   B. left atrium.
   C. right ventricle.
   D. left ventricle.

19. The major work of the heart is completed by the
   A. right ventricle.
   B. left ventricle.
   C. right atrium.
   D. left atrium.

20. The shape of the eyeball is maintained by the
   A. aqueous humor.
   B. vitreous humor.
   C. eye muscles.
   D. eyelid.

21. The inner lining of the heart is the
   A. endocardium.
   B. myocardium.
   C. pericardium.
   D. pleura.

22. The muscular structure that forms the floor of the pelvis is the
   A. peritoneum.
   B. perineum.
   C. mons pubis.
   D. rectus abdominis.

23. The large, round portion at the upper and lateral portion of the femur most often involved in hip fractures is the
    A. acetabulum.
    B. acromiom.
    C. greater trochanter.
    D. tricuspid valve.

24. One of the large muscles that is used in climbing stairs and that forms most of the buttocks is the
    A. gluteus maximus.
    B. gluteus medius.
    C. vastus lateralis.
    D. vastus medialis.

25. The basic unit of function of the kidney is the
    A. medulla.
    B. hilus.
    C. nephron.
    D. cortex.

26. Which of the following is abnormal for urine?
    A. Clear, amber liquid
    B. Nitrogenous waste products
    C. Slightly aromatic
    D. High specific gravity

27. The hormone that regulates blood composition and blood volume by acting on the kidney is
    A. antidiuretic (ADH).
    B. aldosterone.
    C. parathormone.
    D. oxytocin.

28. Composition of urine normally includes
    A. creatinine, urea, and water.
    B. creatinine, ammonia, and sugar.
    C. nitrogen wastes, sugar, and hormones.
    D. nitrogen wastes, water, and pus cells.

29. An injury to the left motor area of the cerebrum would cause paralysis of
    A. the right side of the body.
    B. the left side of the body.
    C. both arms and legs.
    D. both arms.

30. Electrolyte balance is maintained chiefly by the action of the
    A. bladder.
    B. kidney.
    C. islets of Langerhans.
    D. gonads.

STOP

IF YOU FINISH BEFORE TIME IS CALLED, YOU MAY CHECK YOUR WORK ON THIS SECTION ONLY. DO NOT TURN TO ANY OTHER SECTION IN THE TEST.

TEST 7: PHYSIOLOGY AND HEALTH SCIENCE

70 Questions • 70 Minutes

Directions: Read each question carefully and consider all possible answers. When you have decided which choice is best, fill in the corresponding space on your answer sheet. There is only one best answer for each question.

1. Diabetes mellitus initially results from
   A. oversecretion of pancreatin.
   B. undersecretion of insulin.
   C. excessive intake of sugar.
   D. inadequate intake of fats.

2. The so-called "bag of water," which breaks during labor in the pregnant female, is the
   A. amniotic sac.
   B. yolk sac.
   C. placenta.
   D. chorionic membrane.

3. Sebaceous glands are most numerous in areas where
   A. there are small amounts of hair.
   B. there are large amounts of hair.
   C. the skin is thin.
   D. sweat glands are located.

4. Hereditary determiners are found in
   A. PKU.
   B. RNA.
   C. DNA.
   D. SMA.

5. Skin color varies with the amount of
   A. melanin.
   B. matrix.
   C. hair.
   D. keratin.

6. The deciduous teeth contain no
   A. cuspids.
   B. bicuspids.
   C. canines.
   D. incisors.

7. The material covering the surface of the tooth below the gum line is
   A. cementum.
   B. dentine.
   C. enamel.
   D. pulp.

8. Hemoglobin is a molecule composed principally of
   A. ferritin.
   B. amino acids.
   C. iron.
   D. myosin.

9. The sex of a new individual is determined by
   A. the female.
   B. the male.
   C. either the female or the male.
   D. neither the female nor the male.

10. The umbilical cord is cut immediately after a baby is born because
    A. of the need to stop circulation between the fetus and the placenta.
    B. the mother's blood will contaminate the baby's blood.
    C. the baby has less need for blood.
    D. the mother will hemorrhage.

11. The major difference between plasma and blood is
    A. cellular content.
    B. acid-base balance.
    C. anion-cation placement.
    D. solute-solvent concentrations.

12. The blood cells that cause blood clotting are called
    A. leucocytes.
    B. erythrocytes.
    C. thrombocytes.
    D. lymphocytes.

13. The longest, strongest, and heaviest bone in the body is the
    A. tibia.
    B. spinal column.
    C. femur.
    D. radius.

14. Iron is needed for
    A. development of nervous tissue.
    B. formation of red blood cells.
    C. growth of hair and nails.
    D. utilization of vitamins.

15. Which of the following is necessary for digestion?
    A. Transamination
    B. Glucogenolysis
    C. Krebs cycle
    D. Peristalsis

16. Which of the following organs is vital to life?
    A. Adrenal glands
    B. Thymus
    C. Liver
    D. Spleen

17. Gram-negative bacterial pathogens are generally more difficult to treat clinically than grampositive due to differences in
    A. cell wall compositions.
    B. ribosomes.
    C. nucleon regions.
    D. mesosomes.

18. Three-dimensional vision is related to which of the following structures?
    A. Iris
    B. Pupil
    C. Optic chiasma
    D. Retina

19. Urea formation is the human body's method of eliminating excess
    A. carbon.
    B. hydrogen.
    C. nitrogen.
    D. phosphorus.

20. Which of the following hormones is predominant in females?
    A. Androgen
    B. Testosterone
    C. Gonadotrophin
    D. Estrogen

21. Proteins are polymers of
    A. hydrocarbons.
    B. amino acids.
    C. heterocyclics.
    D. alcohols.

22. Which one of the following statements is true?

    A. Bone marrow produces red blood cells in the adult.

    B. The spleen synthesizes vitamins in the child.

    C. The liver manufactures glucose and stores bile.

    D. The lymphatic system refines fats and stores water.

23. The most widely distributed of all tissues is

    A. epithelial.

    B. muscle.

    C. connective.

    D. nervous.

24. The chemical reaction that supplies immediate energy for muscular contractions can be summarized as

    A. $ATP \rightarrow ADP + P$.

    B. lactic acid $\rightarrow CO_2 + H_2O$.

    C. lactic acid $\rightarrow$ glycogen.

    D. glycogen $\rightarrow ATP$.

25. The body's reaction to stress includes which of the following mechanisms?

    A. Conversion of carbohydrates into glycogen

    B. Decreased pumping action of the heart

    C. Secretion of adrenalin

    D. Pooling of blood in the veins

26. After rigorous exercise, the body is depleted of

    A. Na and H_2O.

    B. glucose and H_2O.

    C. H_2O and K.

    D. H_2O and colloids.

27. Which of the following is related to the cause of heart disease?

    A. Absence of serum transaminase

    B. Accumulation of urea nitrogen

    C. Decreased levels of bilirubin

    D. Increased levels of blood cholesterol

28. The endocrine glands in the body have the function of

    A. purifying the blood.

    B. regulating bodily activities.

    C. controlling the blood distribution.

    D. preventing antigenic action.

29. Persons with overactive thyroids have which of the following changes in body functions?

    A. Decrease in metabolic rate

    B. Increase in metabolic rate

    C. Loss of appetite

    D. Gain in weight

30. The basic unit of the lung tissue is

    A. lacuna.

    B. nephron.

    C. alveolus.

    D. cyton.

31. Hemorrhoids, commonly called piles, affect which of the following structures?

    A. Pyloric sphincter

    B. Rectal sphincter

    C. Urethral orifice

    D. Mitral orifice

32. Before amino acids can be metabolized to release energy, which of the following must occur?

    A. Fermentation

    B. Hydrolysis

    C. Deamination

    D. Anabolism

33. A biochemical reaction, common to the digestion of carbohydrates, lipids, and proteins, is enzymatic
   A. fermentation.
   B. deamination.
   C. glycogenolysis.
   D. hydrolysis.

34. Fats yield more calories per gram and oxidize slower than carbohydrates, proteins, and nucleic acids due to excess atoms of
   A. hydrogen.
   B. oxygen.
   C. nitrogen.
   D. phosphorus.

35. In the circulatory system, oxygenated blood is pumped out of the heart from the
   A. right ventricle.
   B. left ventricle.
   C. right atrium.
   D. left atrium.

36. A person who escapes major infections and accidental death has an enhanced probability of living to age 100 if his or her apolipoprotein (E) allelic gene combination is
   A. E-2/E-4
   B. E-3/E-4
   C. E-2/E-2
   D. E-4/E-4

37. Smooth muscle tissue is found in the
   A. heart.
   B. kidneys.
   C. intestines.
   D. skeletal muscles.

38. The exchange of gases between the respiratory system and the circulatory system is by means of the pulmonary
   A. arteries.
   B. veins.
   C. capillaries.
   D. venules.

39. In the production of monoclonal antibodies, antigens, and lymphocytes from an experimental animal are fused with myeloma tumor cells to form a cell-type known as which of the following?
   A. Hydroma.
   B. Polycloma.
   C. Hybridoma.
   D. None of the above

40. In systemic circulation, venous blood is different from arterial blood in that the
   A. CO_2 concentration is lower than the O_2 concentration.
   B. CO_2 concentration is higher than the O_2 concentration.
   C. overall concentration is high and the rate of flow is low.
   D. overall concentration is low and the rate of flow is high.

41. Sperm and egg cells have the haploid number of chromosomes as a result of
   A. meiosis.
   B. cleavage.
   C. mitosis.
   D. fertilization.

42. Fraternal twins develop from
   A. one fertilized egg.
   B. two fertilized eggs.
   C. one egg fertilized by two sperms.
   D. two eggs fertilized by the same sperm.

43. The term *restriction fragment length polymorphism (RFLP)* refers to differences in length between
   A. chromosome fragments.
   B. fragments of DNA.
   C. ribosomal fragments.
   D. fragments of protein molecules.

44. The "pacemaker" of the heart is located in the
   A. left atrium.
   B. left ventricle.
   C. right atrium.
   D. right ventricle.

45. Which generalization concerning sex determination is true?
   A. The female determines the sex of the offspring.
   B. The XY chromosomes are found in the male.
   C. The sex of the offspring is first determined during maturation.
   D. There is a greater chance of getting female offspring than male offspring.

46. A decrease in the number of red corpuscles would result in a corresponding decrease in the blood's ability to
   A. transport oxygen.
   B. destroy disease germs.
   C. form fibrinogen.
   D. absorb glucose.

47. Heat shock proteins (HSPs) may enable structural and functional proteins, under conditions of elevated temperatures, to
   A. expand their active sites.
   B. re-establish their molecular geometry.
   C. lower their optimal temperature.
   D. crystallize.

48. In the average person, the largest part of the central nervous system is the
   A. cerebrum.
   B. cerebellum.
   C. medulla.
   D. spinal cord.

49. Which one of the following terms is NOT directly associated with the same sense organ as the three others?
   A. Stapes
   B. Cochlea
   C. Tympanic membrane
   D. Cornea

50. Human activity on the earth's biodiversity has caused
   A. more species to occupy the total available space.
   B. a decrease in biodiversity.
   C. no change in overall space-species relationship.
   D. an increase in biodiversity.

51. If the order of strength of the following bases is: $HCO_3 > C_2H_3O_2 > HSO_4 > Cl$, the weakest acid is
   A. HC_1 ($H+ + C_1-$).
   B. $HC_2H_3O_2$ ($H+ + C_2H_3O_2-$).
   C. H_2SO_4 ($H+ + HSO_4$).
   D. H_2CO_3 ($H+ + HCO_3-$).

52. In a chemical reaction, [A] and [B] combine to form [C] and [D], as expressed by the reaction [A][B] = [C][D]. Select the statement that best describes the equilibrium condition.
   A. Reaction is shifted to the right.
   B. Concentrations of reactants and products are constant.
   C. Reaction is shifted to the left.
   D. Concentration of products is greater than the concentration reactants.

53. Down syndrome is a genetic disorder caused by
    A. an extra copy of chromosome 21.
    B. a defective gene on chromosome 21.
    C. fragmentation of one copy of chromosome 23.
    D. a missing copy of chromosome 23.

54. In cellular metabolism, glycolysis
    A. requires O_2.
    B. does not require O_2.
    C. occurs only in animal cells.
    D. produces $CO_2 + H_2O$.

55. If 5×10^5 lbs. of NaCl were dumped into a 0.5-acre pond, what would happen to the water concentration inside a frog's body cells?
    A. It would not change.
    B. It would increase.
    C. It would decrease.
    D. It would approach boiling.

56. An astronaut, without a pressurized suit and with a blood pressure of 120/70, is accidentally sucked out of a spacecraft, halfway between the Earth and the moon. He or she would
    A. experience a collapse of blood vessels.
    B. rapidly develop cancer.
    C. experience an expansion of blood vessels.
    D. experience no adverse medical effect.

57. Which of the following viruses have been associated with cancer in animals?
    A. Adenovirus
    B. Retrovirus
    C. Papovavirus
    D. All of the above

58. The major contributions of whole wheat or enriched bread or cereal to the diet are
    A. carbohydrate and vitamin B complex.
    B. protein and iron.
    C. calcium and riboflavin.
    D. protein and vitamin B complex.

59. A good label for canned goods always includes
    A. picture of product to give idea of color, size, and appearance.
    B. net contents, number of portions, and quality of product.
    C. brief but specific instructions or directions for use.
    D. brand name.

60. Caloric needs are highest during
    A. infancy.
    B. childhood.
    C. adulthood.
    D. middle age.

61. Isolated genes shown to initiate malignancies are known as
    A. carcinogens.
    B. oncogenes.
    C. prions.
    D. None of the above

62. One of the most contentious current problems relative to science ethics involves
    A. organ transplants.
    B. blood transfusion.
    C. human embryonic stem cell research.
    D. hospitalization time.

63. In the life cycle of the AIDS-causing virus (HIV), the pathogens bind to lymphocyte membrane receptors by their surface
    A. glycoproteins.
    B. capsids.
    C. reverse transcriptase molecules.
    D. prions.

64. After an AIDS virus enters a lymphocyte, it synthesizes viral DNA from a template composed of
   A. double-stranded DNA.
   B. double-stranded RNA.
   C. single-stranded DNA.
   D. single-stranded RNA.

65. In patients with cystic fibrosis, the accumulation of mucus around the membranes of cells in the lungs, liver, and pancreas has been shown to be caused by the blockage of ionic channels for
   A. CA++
   B. Cl–
   C. K+
   D. Na+

66. Choose the correct statement, relative to the distribution of sodium (Na^+) and potassium (K^+), on opposites of cell membranes.
   A. High Na+ outside
   B. High K+ outside
   C. Low Na+ outside
   D. Low K+ inside

67. Which of the following are requirements for cloning a gene?
   A. An enzyme to fragment DNA
   B. A vector (a bacterial plasmid or a virus)
   C. A host cell or organism
   D. All of the above

68. Small circular self-duplicating DNA molecules found in bacterial cells are
   A. microbodies.
   B. oligaproteins.
   C. plasmids.
   D. None of the above

69. Enzymes necessary for fragmenting genes to be cloned are
   A. restriction enzymes.
   B. splicing enzymes.
   C. recombinases.
   D. polymerases.

70. In the formation of recombinant DNA, the DNA from two different sources is spliced by an enzyme
   A. polymerase.
   B. DNA ligase.
   C. recombinant dehydrogenase.
   D. None of the above

STOP

IF YOU FINISH BEFORE TIME IS CALLED, YOU MAY CHECK YOUR WORK ON THIS SECTION ONLY. DO NOT TURN TO ANY OTHER SECTION IN THE TEST.

ANSWER KEYS AND EXPLANATIONS

Test 1: Human Anatomy and Physiology

1. B	11. B	21. C	31. D	41. A
2. C	12. D	22. B	32. A	42. C
3. C	13. A	23. D	33. B	43. B
4. A	14. B	24. D	34. D	44. C
5. B	15. C	25. D	35. B	45. B
6. D	16. A	26. B	36. C	46. D
7. A	17. D	27. B	37. B	47. A
8. C	18. B	28. C	38. C	48. C
9. A	19. B	29. D	39. B	49. B
10. D	20. C	30. C	40. D	50. D

1. **The correct answer is B.** Cholesterol is an essential component of cell membranes. Microtubules (choice A) are composed of proteins arranged in very small diameter tubes. Ribosomes (choice C) contain proteins and RNA. Cytosol (choice D) is the fluid component of cytoplasm.

2. **The correct answer is C.** The function of smooth endoplasmic reticulum is lipid and carbohydrate synthesis. Rough endoplasmic reticulum (choice A) is involved in the production of proteins. Mitochondria (choice B) are devoted to energy (ATP) production, and Golgi apparatus (choice D) function in the storage and packaging of cellular secretory products.

3. **The correct answer is C.** Golgi apparatus store or aid in the storage of secretory products and lysosomal enzymes. The function of smooth endoplasmic reticulum (choice A) is lipid and carbohydrate synthesis. Control of the entry and exit of materials is the primary function of the cell's membrane (choice B) and lysosomes (choice D) are responsible for the removal of unwanted intracellular items.

4. **The correct answer is A.** Cell membranes are selectively permeable and can determine which substances may cross and which may not. Freely permeable (choice B) and totally permeable (choice D) membranes would allow any substances to pass through, and an impermeable (choice C) membrane is one through which nothing can pass.

5. **The correct answer is B.** The cell will lose water by osmosis down water's concentration gradient, which is lower in a hypertonic solution. Cells will swell (choice A) when placed in a hypotonic solution. Osmosis (choice C) cannot move water from an area of low concentration (the hypertonic solution) into the cell interior with its higher water concentration. Intracellular fluid is not hypertonic (choice D).

6. **The correct answer is D.** Glucose enters skeletal muscle cells by facilitated diffusion via a carrier protein, which must be activated by insulin. Active transport (choice A) is not involved in glucose movement into muscle cells. Exocytosis (choice B) is a process of removing substances from the cell's interior. Glucose cannot enter these cells by simple diffusion (choice C) because of its lipophobic properties and its size.

7. **The correct answer is A.** The nucleus stores information to control protein synthesis and determines the structure and function of the cell. Mitochondria (choice B) are sites of energy production. Ribosomes (choice C) manufacture proteins intracellularly and lysosomes (choice D) are intracellular vesicles containing enzymes.

8. **The correct answer is C.** Epithelia line all body surfaces and perform many functions, including protection and control of permeability. Muscle (choice A) is primarily characterized by the ability to contract, and neural tissue (choice B) provides for the rapid conduction of action potentials. Connective tissues (choice D) are found throughout the body, but they are never exposed to the external environment.

9. **The correct answer is A.** Tendons consist primarily of collagen fibers, which are characterized by extreme flexibility and strength. Elastic fibers (choice B) return to their original length after stretching. Reticular fibers (choice C) provide the structural framework of organs, such as the spleen and liver. Nerve (choice D) tissue is not connective in function.

10. **The correct answer is D.** Synovial membranes surround the joint cavities, which are filled with synovial fluid. Mucous (choice A) membranes line cavities that communicate with the external environment, while serous (choice B) membranes line the components of the ventral body cavity and do not communicate with the external environment. The cutaneous (choice C) membrane is skin.

11. **The correct answer is B.** Melanin is the brown/black protective pigment produced by melanocytes within the deepest layer of the epidermis. Carotene (choice A) is an orange-yellow pigment most commonly found in the stratum corneum of light-skinned individuals. Keratin (choice C) is a protective protein that begins to appear in the middle layers of the epidermis. Hemoglobin (choice D) is the oxygen-carrying substance found within red blood cells.

12. **The correct answer is D.** Collagen and elastic fibers in the skin are arranged in parallel bundles orientated to resist applied forces. Smooth muscle (choice B) within the skin does not have a directional orientation. Sebaceous glands (choice A), or oil glands, produce sebum. Blood vessels (choice C) within the skin do not alter the opening properties of an incision and do not have a parallel pattern of organization.

13. **The correct answer is A.** Ceruminous glands produce cerumen (ear wax). Sebaceous (choice B) glands produce sebum, which protects and conditions hair shafts and skin. Apocrine and merocrine (choices C and D) glands are forms of sweat glands.

14. **The correct answer is B.** Apocrine glands do not become functional until puberty when sex hormone levels rise; merocrine (choice A) gland activity is lifelong. Sebaceous (choice C) glands produce sebum, and ceruminous (choice D) glands produce cerumen (ear wax).

15. **The correct answer is C.** Merkel discs and Meisnner corpuscles are sensory receptors found within cutaneous tissue. Sweat production (choice A) is provided by sudoriferous glands, and oil production (choice D) is provided by sebaceous glands. Blood transport (choice B) is provided by components of the vascular system.

16. **The correct answer is A.** Osteoblasts produce and release the components of bone matrix, leading to increased bone mass and strength. Osteoclasts (choice B) remove bone matrix, causing bone to

weaken. Osteocytes (choice C) are mature bone cells, which maintain and monitor protein and mineral content of bone. Lacunae (choice D) are fluid-filled pockets within which osteocytes are found.

17. **The correct answer is D.** Red bone marrow, found within the trabecular network of spongy bone, is a major site of blood cell formation in adults. The periosteum (choice A) is the membrane covering the outer surface of bone and endosteum (choice B) is the membranous lining of the medullary cavity. Compact bone (choice C) comprises the shafts of long bones and does not perform blood-forming functions.

18. **The correct answer is B.** Parathyroid hormone levels increase in response to hypocalcemia to promote bone resorption and reduce renal elimination of calcium. Calcitonin (choice A) lowers blood calcium by inhibiting osteoclast activity. Calcitriol (choice C) acts within the digestive tract to promote calcium absorption. Thyroxine (choice D) stimulates osteoblast activity and lowers blood calcium levels.

19. **The correct answer is B.** Endochondral ossification is the process of replacing hyaline cartilage with bone. Intramembranous ossification (choice A) is the formation of bone on or within loose fibrous connective tissue. Both osteoclast (choice C) activation and osteoblast (choice D) inhibition would slow the rate of bone formation.

20. **The correct answer is C.** Diarthrosis refers to a freely movable (synovial) joint. Synarthrosis (choice A) refers to an immovable joint such as a suture of the skull. Amphiarthrosis (choice B) is a slightly movable joint exemplified by the symphysis at the junction of the left or right pubic bones of the pelvis. Arthritis (choice D) refers to a group of pathologies of the joints.

21. **The correct answer is C.** Abduction is movement away from the axis and away from the anatomical position. Flexion (choice A) is movement of the anterior-posterior plane resulting in a decreased angle of the joint. Extension (choice B) increases the angle at a joint and returns the body to the anatomical position. Adduction (choice D) is movement toward the longitudinal axis and restoration of the anatomical position.

22. **The correct answer is B.** Acetylcholinesterase breaks down the transmitter substance, acetylcholine (choice A), into acetate and choline, which are inactive at the neuromuscular junction. Epinephrine (choice C) is not involved with the neuromuscular junction, and monoamine oxidase (choice D) is an enzyme that regulates levels of available catechol amines.

23. **The correct answer is D.** Electrical activity initiated on the muscle surface sweeps across the membrane and descends each transverse tubule into the muscle interior. Motor neurons (choice A) deliver action potential activity to the neuromuscular junction. Blood vessels such as muscle capillaries (choice B) are not involved in electrical activity propagation. Epimysium (choice C) is the connective tissue covering of an entire muscle.

24. **The correct answer is D.** Sarcoplasmic reticulum stores calcium ions released upon the arrival of action potential activity via the transverse tubules. The motor neuron (choice A) delivers action potentials to the end plate (choice B) on the surface of the muscle. Mitochondria (choice C) are involved in energy production and are not calcium storage sites.

25. The correct answer is D. Muscles at rest transfer high-energy phosphate groups from ATP to creatine (choice C), forming creatine phosphate and ADP. When needed, that energy is transferred back to ADP (choice B), resulting in production of ATP (choice A).

26. The correct answer is B. Recruitment is the process of activating additional motor units to meet the demand for increased contraction force. Complete tetanus (choice A) refers to muscle contraction in which there is no relaxation phase. Muscle tone (choice C) is the partial contracture of resting muscle. A twitch (choice D) is a single stimulus-contraction-relaxation sequence.

27. The correct answer is B. Myoglobin is a red pigment that reversibly binds oxygen in muscle. It is structurally related to hemoglobin (choice A), the oxygen-carrying pigment found in blood. ATP and ADP (choices C and D) are involved in phosphate energy group utilization.

28. The correct answer is C. Cardiac muscle cells influence the electrical activity of adjacent cells through intercalated discs. Striated and voluntary (choices A and B) are synonymous with skeletal muscle, which does not have intercalated discs. Smooth (choice D) muscle cells communicate through dense bodies.

29. The correct answer is D. The all-or-none principle states that a muscle fiber (or motor unit) is either maximally contracted or not contracted at all. Muscle tone (choice A) is the partial contracture present in a resting muscle. Tetanus (choice B) occurs when stimuli are produced so rapidly that there is no muscle relaxation. A twitch (choice C) is a single stimulus contraction-relaxation sequence.

30. The correct answer is C. Astrocytes interface with neurons and blood vessels, regulating movement of substances between those compartments. Ependymal cells (choice A) are involved in the production and circulation of cerebrospinal fluid. Microglia (choice B) function to remove unwanted materials from the brain and oligodendrocytes (choice D) myelinate CNS axons.

31. The correct answer is D. Following action potential activity, sodium and potassium are returned to their respective starting compartments by the active transport of the sodium-potassium pump. Since these movements are against concentration gradients, diffusion (choice A) would be ineffective. Filtration (choice B) is a process of capillaries, and osmosis (choice C) refers to the movement of water.

32. The correct answer is A. The phrenic nerve, which supplies the diaphragm, exits the spinal cord at upper cervical levels. While the outflow of lower spinal levels may influence respiration, they are unable to sustain adequate ventilation.

33. The correct answer is B. Gamma motor neurons (efferents), when activated, render the muscle spindles more sensitive to stretch. Alpha motor neurons (choice A) and large diameter afferents are axons (choice C) going away from muscle to the CNS. The neuromuscular junction (choice D) does not normally influence reflex activity.

34. The correct answer is D. The temporal lobe functions in the conscious perception of auditory and olfactory stimuli. The frontal lobe (choice A) contains centers for voluntary control of skeletal muscle and plays a role in emotion. Parietal lobe (choice B) function includes conscious perception of skin sensations such as touch, pain, and temperature. The occipital lobe (choice C) is involved in the conscious perception of visual stimuli.

35. **The correct answer is B.** The trigeminal nerve is the major component of sensory and motor innervation to the face. Trochlear (choice A) function involves control of eye movements. The facial (choice C) nerve subserves taste receptors from the anterior 23 of the tongue, and the vestibulocochlear (choice D) nerve functions in auditory and vestibular activities.

36. **The correct answer is C.** The posterior columns contain the ascending pathways for fine touch and pressure to the body surface. Spinothalamic tract (choice A) axons carry information about pain, temperature, and crude touch. The lateral corticospinal tract (choice B) is part of the motor system (descending), and the spinocerebellar tracts (choice D) subserve proprioception.

37. **The correct answer is B.** REM sleep is characterized by active, often visual dreaming, accompanied by changes in autonomic activity; the EEG shows a high frequency and resembles the awake EEG. The EEG in slow wave (choice A), or non-REM sleep, shows a characteristic low-frequency wave. Arousal (choice D) is the awakening from sleep, and dreaming is not a component of coma (choice D).

38. **The correct answer is C.** The tenth (vagus) nerve contains the primary autonomic outflow to the organs of the thoracic and abdominopelvic cavities. The first (olfactory) cranial nerve (choice A) functions in the sense of smell (olfaction). The second (optic) cranial nerve (choice B) subserves the sense of vision, while the twelfth (hypoglossal) nerve (choice D) controls the musculature of the tongue.

39. **The correct answer is B.** Thyrotropin from the anterior pituitary regulates the growth and development of the thyroid gland and controls its release of thyroid hormones. Thyrotropin releasing hormone (choice A), from the hypothalamus, promotes the release of thyrotropin. Thyroxine (choice C) is one of the hormones released by the thyroid gland. Iodide (choice D) is a constituent of thyroid hormones.

40. **The correct answer is D.** Adrenocorticotropic hormone (ACTH) from the adenohypophysis (anterior pituitary) stimulates the release of glucocorticoids, including cortisol (choice B), from the adrenal cortex. Corticotropin releasing hormone (CRH) (choice A) is produced by the hypothalamus and promotes the release of ACTH. Aldosterone (choice C) is a mineralocorticoid produced by the adrenal cortex.

41. **The correct answer is A.** Oxytocin promotes labor and delivery by inducing uterine smooth muscle contraction. Vasopressin (antidiuretic hormone—ADH) (choice B) promotes water reabsorption by the kidneys. Somatotropin (growth hormone) (choice C) stimulates cell growth by accelerating protein synthesis. Prolactin (choice D) participates in the stimulation of mammary gland development and promotes milk production.

42. **The correct answer is C.** Follicle stimulating hormone (FSH), a gonadotropin from the anterior pituitary, promotes follicle development and estrogen secretion in females, whereas in males it promotes sperm cell production. Testosterone (choice A) is an androgen with most of its effects seen in males. Melanotropin (choice B) activates melanocytes within the skin. Luteinizing hormone (choice D) is responsible for initiating ovulation.

43. **The correct answer is B.** Insulin is the hormone that lowers blood glucose levels through a number of mechanisms including activating receptors involved in the facilitated diffusion of glucose into muscle. Glucagon (choice A) is the pancreatic hormone responsible for elevating blood glucose levels; epinephrine (choice C) also elevates blood glucose. Renin (choice D), a hormone from the kidneys, initiates the renin-angiotensin system, which is involved in blood pressure control.

44. **The correct answer is C.** These symptoms suggest high levels of thyroid hormones (hyperthyroidism); opposite symptoms (i.e., low basal metabolic rate, weight gain, and sensitivity to cold) would be symptomatic of hypothyroidism. Neither high nor low levels of growth hormone would produce these symptoms.

45. **The correct answer is B.** Insulin is released by beta cells when blood glucose exceeds normal levels (70–110 mg/dL). Low blood glucose (choice A) triggers the release of glucagon from the pancreas. Prolactin (choice C) is not involved in the control of blood glucose. Elevated growth hormone levels (choice D) cause elevations of blood glucose.

46. **The correct answer is D.** Aldosterone is the hormone from the adrenal cortex that participates in the regulation of sodium and potassium levels. Epinephrine and norepinephrine (choices A and B) are products of the adrenal medulla. ACTH (choice C) is produced by the anterior pituitary.

47. **The correct answer is A.** Low parathyroid hormone levels would lead to hypocalcemia, which in turn could cause convulsions. Parathyroid hormone is not involved in the regulation of blood glucose levels, nor does it influence water retention/loss mechanisms in the kidneys.

48. **The correct answer is C.** The thyroid regulates metabolic rate under normal conditions. A deficiency of thyroid hormone will cause a low basal metabolism, while an excess of the hormone will increase the metabolic rate.

49. **The correct answer is B.** The kidney filters wastes from the blood. Each nephron performs this function; thus, it is the functional unit. Wastes and water are filtered out from the blood in the glomerulus, a mass of capillaries lying in Bowman's capsule; the water and wastes pass through the capsule wall into the renal tubule. Much of the water is reabsorbed into the bloodstream through the walls of the capillaries surrounding the loop of Henle of the renal tubule. The remaining liquid, or urine, passes into the renal pelvis, to the ureter and bladder, and is eventually eliminated through the urethra.

50. **The correct answer is D.** An endocrine (or ductless) gland secretes hormone(s) directly into the bloodstream. The hormone is transported by the blood and will affect only the target tissue. An exocrine gland passes its secretion through a duct to a specific site. The pancreatic islet cells secrete the hormone insulin; other cells of the pancreas secrete pancreatic juice, containing enzymes, through the pancreatic duct into the duodenum.

Test 2: Human Anatomy and Physiology

1. A	11. C	21. D	31. B	41. B
2. D	12. A	22. B	32. A	42. B
3. C	13. B	23. A	33. C	43. B
4. A	14. B	24. C	34. B	44. D
5. B	15. D	25. C	35. B	45. A
6. A	16. B	26. A	36. D	46. C
7. D	17. C	27. D	37. A	47. D
8. B	18. C	28. C	38. D	48. C
9. B	19. A	29. D	39. C	49. B
10. D	20. A	30. B	40. C	50. A

1. **The correct answer is A.** Albumin is the major plasma protein and is responsible for maintaining osmotic pressure and plasma volume. Globulins (choice B) function in the transport of materials and have immune functions. Fibrinogen (choice C) is a clotting factor. Platelets (choice D) do not significantly alter plasma osmotic pressure.

2. **The correct answer is D.** Anemia, a decrease in oxygen delivery, results from deficiencies in erythrocytes or hemoglobin within erythrocytes. Platelets, plasma proteins, and leukocytes (choices A, B, and C) do not participate in oxygen transport.

3. **The correct answer is C.** Erythropoietin is released by cells in the kidneys when they are faced with low oxygen levels; erythropoietin promotes erythropoiesis, red blood cell formation. Neither platelets nor leukocytes (choices A and D) are involved in oxygen delivery. Erythrocytes (choice B) are red blood cells.

4. **The correct answer is A.** Blood typing is based on the identification of antigens (agglutinogens) located on the surfaces of erythrocytes. Antibodies relevant to blood typing (agglutinins) are found in plasma, but blood type is based on red blood cell surface antigens.

5. **The correct answer is B.** Rh+ indicates the presence of the Rh D antigen on the surfaces of erythrocytes; Rh− indicates the absence of that antigen. Rh antigens are not found in plasma, nor are Rh antibodies. Rh antibodies are found in plasma.

6. **The correct answer is A.** The anti-A antibodies from the plasma of the Type B blood will attack the A-antigens of the Type A blood, leading to agglutination, the clumping and breakdown of erythrocytes. Blood vessel spasm (choice B) and platelet plug formation (choice C) are processes involved in hemostasis. The onset of decreased oxygen delivery would be very rapid.

7. **The correct answer is D.** Neutrophils are granulocytes and are usually the first white blood cells to arrive at an injury site or infection. Lymphocytes and monocytes (choices A and B) are agranulocytes. Basophils (choice C), accounting for less than 1% of the circulating leukocyte population, produce histamine and heparin.

8. **The correct answer is B.** T-cells, B-cells, and NK-cells are classes of lymphocytes (indistinguishable under the light microscope), which are involved in immune processes. Neutrophils and eosinophils (choices C and D) are granulocytes and are not involved in immunity.

9. **The correct answer is B.** During the platelet phase of hemostasis, platelets stick to damaged endothelium and become activated, releasing ADP, thromboxane A_2, and serotonin, substances that participate in the hemostasis process. The vascular (choice A) phase is characterized by contraction of the smooth muscle of the blood vessel wall. Coagulation (choice C) refers to blood clotting. There is no inflammation (choice D) phase of hemostasis.

10. **The correct answer is D.** The last step in the final common pathway produces insoluble strands of fibrin that form the matrix of the blood clot. The conversion of prothrombin to thrombin (choices A and B) is the initial step in the final common pathway. Fibrinogen (choice C), a plasma protein, is the precursor to fibrin.

11. **The correct answer is C.** Group O blood lacks antigen A and antigen B. Although it can form antibodies against both A and B, it cannot stimulate the formation of antibodies against A and B. Persons of group O are known as *universal donors*. Group AB blood has both antigens A and B but cannot form antibodies against either. Persons of group AB are known as *universal recipients*. Since group O has neither antigen, and AB cannot form either antibody, the only safe transfusion of those listed is choice C. Persons of group A contain antigen A and can form antibodies against antigen B; blood group B contains antigen B and can form antibodies against A.

12. **The correct answer is A.** Calcium entry into cardiac cells results in a plateau of about 175 m/sec. Calcium exit from the cell (choice B) would shorten the action potential. Sodium entry into the cell (choice C) leads to the rapid initial depolarization, and sodium exit (choice D) occurs after the action potential is completed.

13. **The correct answer is B.** Spontaneous depolarizations occur most rapidly within the SA node, and it is therefore the normal pacemaker of the heart. The AV node, bundle branch fibers, and purkinje fibers (choices A, C, and D) also depolarize spontaneously but at a slower rate than the SA cells.

14. **The correct answer is B.** The QRS complex results from ventricular depolarization. The P wave (choice A) reflects atrial depolarization and the T wave (choice C) relates to ventricular repolarization. The P-R segment (choice D) reflects the time between atrial and ventricular depolarization.

15. **The correct answer is D.** End-diastolic volume is the quantity of blood in the ventricles just before the initiation of ventricular contraction (systole). Stroke volume (choice A) is the quantity of blood ejected during ventricular contraction. Ejection fraction (choice B) evaluates the efficiency of ventricular emptying during systole. End-systolic volume (choice C) volume is the quantity of blood remaining within the ventricles after ventricular contraction.

16. **The correct answer is B.** Afterload reflects the forces that the ventricles must overcome in order to eject blood. Preload (choice A) is the degree of stretching during ventricular diastole and is directly proportional to the end-diastolic volume. Cardiac output (choice C) measures the volume of blood pumped by the ventricles in one minute. Stroke volume (choice D) is the quantity of blood ejected during ventricular contraction.

17. **The correct answer is C.** Beta 1 receptor activation by norepinephrine results in increased heart rate and increased force of contraction. Alpha 1 (choice A) receptor

activation leads to vasoconstriction. Alpha 2 (choice B) receptors in the CNS cause vasodilation. Beta 2 (choice D) receptors primarily influence bronchioles, producing bronchodilation.

18. **The correct answer is C.** Capillaries are the only blood vessels involved in exchange of materials. Arteries (choice A) carry blood from the heart under high pressure. Arterioles (choice B) control the flow of blood into capillary beds. Veins (choice D) return blood to the heart.

19. **The correct answer is A.** Venous valves prohibit backflow of blood toward the capillaries. Venous smooth muscle (choice B) in veins alters vessel diameter but does not impede backflow. Precapillary sphincters (choice C) control blood flow into capillary beds. Semilunar valves (choice D) are found within the heart.

20. **The correct answer is A.** Pulse pressure is much greater in arteries. Arterioles (choice B) have a small pulse pressure, while blood flow through capillaries and veins (choices C and D) is not pulsatile.

21. **The correct answer is D.** Baroreceptor reflexes are responsible for rapid adjustments of blood pressure. Chemoreceptors (choice C) are primarily concerned with control of respiration. Angiotensin II and antidiuretic hormone (choices A and B) are involved in long-term regulation of blood pressure.

22. **The correct answer is B.** During swallowing, material is kept out of the respiratory tract by the folding of the epiglottis over the glottis (choice A). The pharynx (choice C) is the chamber shared by the digestive and respiratory systems. The hard palate (choice D) forms the anterior roof of the mouth.

23. **The correct answer is A.** Tidal volume is the volume of a single breath. Minute volume (choice B) is the volume of air moved within one minute. Residual volume (choice C) is the amount of air remaining in the lungs after a maximal expiration. Inspiratory reserve volume (choice D) is the amount of air that can be inhaled in excess of a tidal inspiration.

24. **The correct answer is C.** Anatomical dead space never goes further than the conducting passages and is not involved in gas exchange. Vital capacity (choice A) is the maximal amount of air that an individual can move into or out of the lungs in a single respiratory cycle. Expiratory reserve volume (choice B) is the additional amount of air that can be expired from the lungs by determined effort after normal expiration. Total lung capacity (choice D) is the total volume of the lungs.

25. **The correct answer is C.** Gases diffuse down a partial pressure gradient, not a concentration (choice A) gradient. Osmotic (choice B) pressures and gradients refer to properties of fluids. Within normal limits, temperature (choice D) plays a minimal role in gas movement.

26. **The correct answer is A.** Increasing thoracic volume leads to decreased intrathoracic pressure and inspiration. Decreasing thoracic volume (choice B) increases intrathoracic pressure, leading to expiration. Changes in abdominal volumes (choices C and D) do not directly affect respiration except through their influences on thoracic volumes.

27. **The correct answer is D.** Declining blood pH weakens the hemoglobin-oxygen bond (the Bohr effect) and promotes oxygen release to tissues. Conversely, elevated pH (choice C) will strengthen the bond. Changes in blood pressure (choices A and B) do not appreciably affect oxygen unloading.

28. **The correct answer is C.** A significant portion of carbon dioxide is transported within erythrocytes as carbamino-hemoglobin. Blood gases are not transported by leukocytes or plasma proteins (choices A and B), nor are they transported on the surface of red blood cells (choice D).

29. **The correct answer is D.** Carbonic anhydrase within erythrocytes reversibly catalyzes the reaction of carbon dioxide and water, a reaction that is very slow in the absence of the enzyme. Antigens, antibodies, and plasma enzymes do not influence the reaction.

30. **The correct answer is B.** The pneumotaxic center of the pons sends inhibitory signals to the inspiratory center, resulting in shortened duration of inspiration.

31. **The correct answer is B.** Angiotensin I is the result of the action of renin on angiotensinogen (choice A). Angiotensin II (choice C) is subsequently formed from angiotensin I. Carbonic anhydrase (choice D) is the enzyme that catalyzes the reaction of carbon dioxide and water.

32. **The correct answer is A.** Angiotensin II is a potent vasoconstrictor and an important component in reversing a hypotensive condition; it is not a vasodilator. Angiotensin II promotes aldosterone release and acts to conserve water rather than eliminate water.

33. **The correct answer is C.** Nitrogenous byproducts of protein catabolism (including uric acid, creatinine, and urea) are not significantly reabsorbed and therefore appear in urine. Amino acids, vitamins, water, and electrolytes (choices A, B, and D) are all reabsorbed within the nephron.

34. **The correct answer is B.** Nutrients are reabsorbed from the proximal convoluted tubule. The other segments of the nephron are primarily involved in the regulation of the blood levels of electrolytes and of water.

35. **The correct answer is B.** Peristaltic waves of the smooth muscle of the ureters propel urine from the kidneys to the bladder; gravity (choice A) does not play a significant role. Bladder pressure (choice C) would not promote flow toward the bladder, and blood pressure (choice D) is not a factor in ureters' action.

36. **The correct answer is D.** The somatic motor fibers of the pudendal nerve regulate the contracture of the external sphincter. As a skeletal muscle structure, the external sphincter is not innervated by the autonomic nervous system. The phrenic nerve (choice C) innervates the diaphragm.

37. **The correct answer is A.** Sodium is the major positive-charged ion within extracellular fluid and is a primary controller of water distribution. Potassium and magnesium (choices B and D) are more concentrated within intracellular fluid. Calcium (choice C) does not play a major role in water distribution.

38. **The correct answer is D.** Aldosterone promotes the reabsorption of sodium within the kidneys. Thyroxine (choice A) is a thyroid hormone and is not involved with sodium levels. Insulin and glucagon (choices B and C) are involved in the control of blood glucose levels.

39. **The correct answer is C.** Although generally slower, the kidneys are the most powerful and complete correctors of pH imbalance. Buffers (choice A) are the most rapid but the weakest mechanisms. Although more powerful than buffers, respiratory mechanisms (choice B) rarely complete a correction of pH imbalance. The bladder (choice D) is not involved in acid-base balance.

40. **The correct answer is C.** Lack of insulin leads to the utilization of fats for energy. Byproducts include ketone bodies, which are acidic and responsible for the acidosis seen in these patients. Diabetic patients are not alkalotic, and diabetes does not result in acid production through actions on the respiratory system.

41. **The correct answer is B.** Intrinsic factor is produced by cells of the stomach and promotes the absorption of vitamin B_{12}. The small intestine (choice A) is the site of action of intrinsic factor but not the source. The pancreas (choice C) and large intestine (choice D) do not participate in vitamin B_{12} absorption.

42. **The correct answer is B.** The gallbladder stores bile and concentrates it up to tenfold. Bile is manufactured in the liver (choice A) but not stored there. Neither the pancreas nor the ileum (choices C and D) are involved in bile storage.

43. **The correct answer is B.** Cholecystokinin (CCK) is released from the intestine in response to the presence of proteins or fats. Secretin (choice A) is released in response to the presence of acid from the stomach. Neither insulin nor aldosterone (choices C and D) are released from intestinal tissues.

44. **The correct answer is D.** Because of its role in water reabsorption, excess motility of the large intestine may lead to diarrhea, while decreased motility may lead to constipation. The stomach, liver, and small intestine (choices A, B, and C) are not controllers of water reabsorption.

45. **The correct answer is A.** Carbohydrates must be reduced to monosaccharides in order for intestinal absorption to occur. Disaccharides (choice B) are enzymatically broken down in the small intestine, as are the polysaccharides glycogen and starch (choice C), which are broken down into oligosaccharides (choice D).

46. **The correct answer is C.** Pepsin results in the breakdown of proteins into polypeptides. Lipase (choice A) participates in fat digestion. Sucrase (choice B) breaks sucrose down into monosaccharides. Amylase (choice D) initiates the digestion of starch.

47. **The correct answer is D.** Vitamin C is a water-soluble vitamin. Vitamins A, D, E, and K are fat-soluble.

48. **The correct answer is C.** Pain and bleeding associated with gastric ulcers result from erosion of the mucosal layer, which exposes the vascular and highly innervated submucosal layer. The muscular layer and the outer (serosal) layer generally are not involved in ulcer production.

49. **The correct answer is B.** Amylase is an enzyme found in saliva, which begins the breakdown of starch. Lipase (choice A) is involved in fat digestion; pepsin (choice C) begins the digestion of proteins; and insulin (choice D) is involved in glucose processes.

50. **The correct answer is A.** Digestive smooth muscle is activated by the parasympathetic division of the autonomic nervous system. The sympathetic (choice B) division inhibits digestive activity. Neither the thyroid gland nor aldosterone (choices C and D) are involved in control of gastrointestinal smooth muscle.

Test 3: Human Anatomy and Physiology

1. D	21. D	41. C	61. B	81. C
2. A	22. A	42. B	62. C	82. B
3. A	23. D	43. A	63. B	83. A
4. B	24. D	44. C	64. C	84. B
5. B	25. D	45. A	65. C	85. B
6. D	26. A	46. B	66. C	86. A
7. C	27. B	47. B	67. B	87. B
8. C	28. B	48. B	68. B	88. B
9. C	29. D	49. B	69. C	89. B
10. D	30. C	50. A	70. A	90. B
11. B	31. B	51. B	71. B	91. A
12. B	32. C	52. A	72. C	92. D
13. D	33. A	53. B	73. A	93. D
14. B	34. B	54. B	74. D	94. D
15. A	35. A	55. D	75. B	95. B
16. C	36. A	56. B	76. B	96. C
17. B	37. D	57. B	77. A	97. B
18. C	38. D	58. C	78. B	98. D
19. B	39. A	59. B	79. B	99. B
20. D	40. B	60. D	80. A	100. D

1. **The correct answer is D.** Only the lymphatic system is involved in all three of these processes, although the urinary system does receive fluid from blood vessels.

2. **The correct answer is A.** Internal and abdominal muscles (choices C and D) aid expiration. The external intercostal muscles (choice B) aid inspiration, but the diaphragm (choice A) is the major muscle.

3. **The correct answer is A.** The integument is comprised of skin, hair, nails, and associated structures, such as sweat and sebaceous glands.

4. **The correct answer is B.** Oxytocin and antidiuretic hormone (ADH) are both products of the posterior pituitary. Oxytocin acts on uterine smooth muscle and mammary tissue, whereas ADH acts within the kidneys to promote water reabsorption. ADH is also a vasoconstrictor, and these two actions combine to elevate blood pressure.

5. **The correct answer is B.** Homeostasis, the tendency to maintain a constant internal environment, most commonly depends upon negative feedback processes, which tend to counter the effects of change. Positive feedback mechanisms enhance the effects of change, and they generally have a beneficial effect on homeostasis.

6. **The correct answer is D.** Central chemoreceptors respond to changes in CO_2, which is the most important factor in the control of minute-to-minute respiration.

7. **The correct answer is C.** Sagittal planes divide the body into left and right parts. Frontal (choice A), or coronal (choice D), planes vertically divide the body into anterior and posterior segments. A transverse (choice B) section divides the body into superior and inferior parts.

8. **The correct answer is C.** Cardiac output, the volume of blood pumped by the heart per minute, is equal to the product of stroke volume (mL/beat) and heart rate (bpm).

9. **The correct answer is C.** If both parents are AB, they can only produce two different kinds of gametes (sperm and eggs), A and B. So the blood types of children will be A, AB, and B.

10. **The correct answer is D.** Blood exits the right ventricle through the pulmonary semilunar (pulmonic) valve and enters the pulmonary arteries, which lead to the lungs. Atrioventricular valves (bicuspid and tricuspid) are situated between atria and ventricles. Pulmonary veins come from the lungs back to the heart.

11. **The correct answer is B.** While both norepinephrine (choice C) and epinephrine (choice B) act at Alpha and Beta-1 receptors, epinephrine is the primary agonist at the Beta-2 sites, where it leads to pronounced bronchodilation. Acetylcholine and nicotine (choices A and D) are not catechol amines.

12. **The correct answer is B.** The resting membrane is relatively impermeable to sodium, which is in a high concentration in the extracellular space relative to the intracellular space. An action potential results from the opening of sodium channels, allowing sodium to diffuse into the intracellular space and making that region positive relative to the outside of the cell.

13. **The correct answer is D.** During swallowing, the epiglottis covers the trachea to prevent ingested material from entering the respiratory tract.

14. **The correct answer is B.** The amount of dissolved oxygen in blood is minimal compared to the amount carried as oxyhemoglobin. Carbon dioxide (choice C) and bicarbonate (choice D) are not physiologic oxygen transporters.

15. **The correct answer is A.** Pyramidal tract fibers are motor in function and originate in the primary motor cortex, which is directly anterior to the central sulcus, the precentral gyrus. The postcentral gyms is part of the somatosensory system.

16. **The correct answer is C.** Epinephrine (choice D) and norepinephrine (choice B) are catechol amine transmitters in the autonomic and central nervous systems. Acetylcholinesterase (choice A) is the enzyme that metabolizes acetylcholine (choice C) at autonomic and neuromuscular sites.

17. **The correct answer is B.** Arterioles are located between arteries and capillaries. Dilation or constriction of arterioles regulates the flow of blood into capillary beds and provides adjustment of arterial blood pressure.

18. **The correct answer is C.** Exocytosis moves substances from the intracellular space into extracellular fluid. Endocytosis (choice B) is a mechanism for moving large particles into cells. Phagocytosis (choice A) is a type of endocytosis by which solid particles are engulfed. Pinocytosis (choice D) is endocytosis of fluids.

19. **The correct answer is B.** Dermatomes are body regions innervated by individual dorsal roots and can be related to segmental spinal levels. Receptive fields, sensory units, and motor units (choices A, C, and D) related to innervation are characteristics of individual neurons rather than nerve trunks.

20. **The correct answer is D.** Epithelial tissue is characterized by cell shape (squamous, cuboidal, columnar) and cell layering (simple or compound).

21. **The correct answer is D.** Cartilage forms the skeleton of the embryo and is subsequently converted to bone. Cartilage also forms the nasal septum and the rings of the trachea. Its flexibility makes it an appropriate material to join the ribs to the sternum.

22. **The correct answer is A.** Keratin is a protein that waterproofs and adds structural strength to skin. It is formed in the deepest layer of the epidermis and migrates to the surface with time. Melanin, carotene, and hemoglobin (choices B, C, and D) are pigments in the skin.

23. **The correct answer is D.** Sharp "pricking" pain information is carried over the small, slowly conducting myelinated A Delta fibers, while burning and aching pain information is transmitted over the even more slowly conducted unmyelinated C fibers. A Alpha fibers (choice C), with their high conduction velocity, are involved in other areas, such as proprioception.

24. **The correct answer is D.** Activation of the parasympathetic division will lead directly to a slowing of the heart through activity of the vagus nerve. Vasoconstriction (choice C), increased heart rate and cardiac output (choices A and B), and inhibition of digestion are within the domain of the sympathetic division.

25. **The correct answer is D.** Muscle spindles respond to moderate muscle stretch. The Golgi tendon organ (choice A) is the receptor for the inverse stretch reflex, free nerve endings (choice B) are involved in pain reception, and hair cells (choice C) are receptors within the auditory and vestibular systems.

26. **The correct answer is A.** Although the glomerulus is more permeable than most membranes, it still restricts the passage of proteins, blood cells, and other large particles. Damage to the glomerulus can produce filtration disorders such as glomerulonephritis, and substances such as blood and protein may appear in the urine.

27. **The correct answer is B.** Some CO_2 is carried in a dissolved form obeying Henry's Law, and some is carried by hemoglobin. Most CO_2, however, is carried as bicarbonate.

28. **The correct answer is B.** Tubular reabsorption is the process by which the kidneys return water and solutes, including glucose, vitamins, and amino acids, to blood. Filtration and secretion (choices A and C) involve movement of substances from blood into urine. Glucose is not reabsorbed from the collecting duct (choice D).

29. **The correct answer is D.** Periosteum covers the outer surface of long bones. It contains osteoblasts, cells that form new bone cells. Endosteum lines the hollow inner surface of a long bone. Osteoclasts break down bone cells.

30. **The correct answer is C.** Activity in the sinoatrial node is responsible for initiating the cardiac cycle, beginning with atrial depolarization and contraction. In a resting subject, the contribution of atrial contraction to ventricular filling is relatively minimal. The AV node is below the atria.

31. **The correct answer is B.** The first heart sound ("lub") is the atrioventricular valves (tricuspid and bicuspid) closing in response to the ventricles contracting and increasing intraventricular pressure.

32. **The correct answer is C.** Visual processing occurs within the occipital lobe of the cerebral cortex, which is protected by the occipital bone. The frontal bone (choice A) covers the frontal cortex, which is involved in, among other things, behavioral and motor events. The parietal bone

(choice B) covers the parietal cortex, which is involved in sensory integration processes, while the temporal bone (choice D) protects the temporal lobe, which is involved in audition.

33. **The correct answer is A.** Veins have large lumens and thin, distensible walls; they contain up to 65 percent of the body's total blood supply at any time.

34. **The correct answer is B.** The patella is a sesamoid bone, a special type of short bone.

35. **The correct answer is A.** The automaticity of the heart is normally a function of the sinoatrial (SA) node, which leads to atrial depolarization. The atrioventricular (AV) (choice B) node may become a pacemaker under certain pathological conditions.

36. **The correct answer is A.** Arteries are under the greatest pressure due to the force from the contraction of the heart and the elastic properties of arterial walls.

37. **The correct answer is D.** Ninety-nine percent of the water filtered at the glomerulus is returned by osmosis, most of which occurs within the proximal convoluted tubule.

38. **The correct answer is D.** Type I diabetes mellitus results from inadequate insulin production by the beta cells of the pancreas; high insulin (choice A) levels would reflect just the opposite. Ineffective insulin receptors (choice B) are associated with Type II diabetes. Both Type I and Type II diabetic patients display high blood glucose levels.

39. **The correct answer is A.** The sympathetic division of the autonomic nervous system is involved in dealing with emergencies and stress. Parasympathetic (craniosacral) (choices B and C) activity is primarily involved with energy conservation and "vegetative" functions.

40. **The correct answer is B.** The sympathetic division of the autonomic nervous system is anatomically the thoricolumbar division because of its spinal levels of origin. The parasympathetic division is, anatomically, the craniosacral division.

41. **The correct answer is C.** Cellular respiration, the utilization of oxygen and glucose, occurs within mitochondria. Rough endoplasmic reticulum (choice A) is involved in protein synthesis, and smooth endoplasmic reticulum (choice B) is involved in synthesis of lipid materials. Golgi apparatus (choice D) are involved in cellular packaging and delivery.

42. **The correct answer is B.** Flexion decreases the angle of a joint, bringing the two bones closer together. Extension (choice C) increases the angle of a joint, moving the bones farther apart. Retraction and rotation (choices A and D) are not joint "bending" in nature.

43. **The correct answer is A.** Mitosis leading to the formation of new epidermal cells occurs within the stratum germinativum basale, the deepest layer of the epidermis, which has the advantage of being near the blood supply of the underlying dermis.

44. **The correct answer is C.** Compared to males, females have a larger percentage of fat (and a lower content of water), which is deposited within the subcutaneous layer under the influence of estrogen.

45. **The correct answer is A.** Mucosal membranes line structures such as components of the digestive, respiratory, and reproductive tracts, which access the outside world. Serous membranes (choice B) line cavities that do not access the external environment, such as the pleural cavities. Synovial membranes (choice C) line joint cavities, and cutaneous membranes (choice D) comprise the skin.

46. **The correct answer is B.** The epidermis does not contain blood vessels and depends upon the vascular supply of the underlying dermis for its needs.

47. **The correct answer is B.** Smooth muscle is found within visceral structures (e.g., digestive, reproductive), does not have a striated histological appearance, and is generally under autonomic (involuntary) control. Skeletal muscle (choice A) is striated and voluntary. Cardiac muscle (choice C) is striated but involuntary. Postural muscles (choice D) are skeletal muscles.

48. **The correct answer is B.** Although carried by the circulatory system and influenced by the endocrine systems, blood cell formation is largely a function of spongy bone within the skeletal system.

49. **The correct answer is B.** Parathyroid hormone elevates serum calcium levels by initiating mobilization of calcium from the digestive system. Calcitonin (choice A) lowers blood calcium and leads to deposition of calcium within bone.

50. **The correct answer is A.** Eccrine sweat glands of the face, palms, and soles are active in children. Apocrine sweat glands (choice B) become active at puberty. Sebaceous glands (choice C) produce sebum and are not found on the soles or palms. Ceruminous glands (choice D) are found within the external auditory meatus.

51. **The correct answer is B.** The biceps brachii is a flexor of the elbow, and the triceps femoris is a flexor of the knee.

52. **The correct answer is A.** Apocrine sweat glands become active at puberty under the influence of sex hormones. Eccrine, sebaceous, and ceruminous (choices B, C, and D) glands are active in children.

53. **The correct answer is B.** Calcitonin is responsible for lowering an elevated serum calcium, partially by depositing the excess mineral in bone. Parathormone will elevate serum calcium levels.

54. **The correct answer is B.** Although hormones are produced by endocrine glands, their delivery to target organs is primarily via the cardiovascular system.

55. **The correct answer is D.** Myelin, an insulating substance, is responsible for salutatory conduction in which the impulse "skips" from one Node of Ranvier to the next and is rapidly conducted to the end of the cell. The larger the diameter of an axon, the less resistance present and the faster the axon can conduct. Myelinated, large-diameter axons comprise the axons with the fastest conduction velocities.

56. **The correct answer is B.** The nephron is the basic functional unit of kidneys. Nephrons include Bowman's capsule, the proximal convoluted tubule, the loop of Henle, the distal convoluted tubule, and the collecting duct. The glomerulus (choice A) is part of the circulatory system, the ureters (choice C) convey urine from the kidneys to the bladder, and the urethra (choice D) carries urine out from the bladder.

57. **The correct answer is B.** The esophagus enters the stomach below the fundus at the cardiac region, which contains the cardiac sphincter. The body of the stomach is below, and the pyloric region marks the most distal portion of the stomach adjacent to the duodenum of the small intestine.

58. **The correct answer is C.** Oxytocin, produced by the hypothalamus and released by the posterior pituitary, causes contraction of uterine smooth muscle and plays a role in labor and delivery. ADH (choice A) is also released by the posterior pituitary, but its role is in water conservation within the kidneys.

59. The correct answer is B. ADH, antidiuretic hormone, when released from the posterior pituitary, causes an increased permeability of the collecting duct of the kidneys and leads to water reabsorption and conservation. Inhibition of ADH release, produced for example by the ingestion of alcohol, leads to an increase in urine output.

60. The correct answer is D. FSH (choice A) begins the maturation process of follicles, but it is the elevation of LH levels that leads to the release of mature egg cells (ovulation). ADH and prolactin (choices B and D) do not participate in the process.

61. The correct answer is B. The cardiac sphincter is located at the junction of the esophagus and the stomach and is responsible for preventing gastric reflux. The pyloric sphincter (choice A) is at the junction of the stomach and the small intestine, the ileocecal valve (choice C) is at the junction of the small and large intestines, and the epiglottis (choice D) prevents solids and liquids from entering the trachea.

62. The correct answer is C. Bile, produced in the liver and released from the gallbladder, is involved in fat metabolism in the small intestine. Lipase (choice A) is a pancreatic enzyme that catalyzes the breakdown of fats. Amylase is an enzyme that converts starch and glycogen into simple sugars. HCl is a component of gastric acid.

63. The correct answer is B. Although some digestion takes place within all of the structures listed, the majority of digestive processes take place within the duodenum.

64. The correct answer is C. Visual receptors, rods and cones, are located at the back of the eye on the retina. The lens and cornea (choices A and B) are involved in transmission of light rays from the environment on to the retina; the optic tract (choice D) is part of the optic neural pathway.

65. The correct answer is C. Food absorption takes place primarily within the ileum and jejunum. Functions of the stomach and duodenum (choices A and D) are primarily digestive, while the colon (choice B) is principally involved in water reabsorption, some digestion, and vitamin synthesis.

66. The correct answer is C. The medulla begins at, and is indistinguishable from, the rostral end of the spinal cord, forming the lowest portion of the brain stem, which also includes the pons (choice B) and the midbrain (choice A), both superior. The thalamus (choice D), part of the diencephalon, is yet further rostral.

67. The correct answer is B. Although stored and delivered by the gallbladder (choice C), bile is manufactured within the liver. The duodenum (choice A) is the major site of digestion, where it receives digestive materials from the pancreas (choice D).

68. The correct answer is B. Thyroid hormone contributes to growth and maturation of the nervous system. A hypothyroid infant will show both physical and mental deficits not seen in the adult, since skeletal and brain development have been completed in the adult.

69. The correct answer is C. Rods and cones are located on the retina at the back of the eye. Cones provide color vision, while rods (choice B) provide vision in black and white. Hair cells (choice A) are receptors within the auditory and vestibular systems.

70. The correct answer is A. Lining the inside of the digestive system is the epithelial mucosal layer, which provides an appropriate setting for absorption of materials into the submucosal layer that contains blood vessels, lymphatics, and nerves.

Serosal (choice D) membranes surround the digestive tract to form a protective layer.

71. **The correct answer is B.** The pancreas is classified as an endocrine gland because of its production of insulin and glucagon, which are secreted directly into blood. As an exocrine gland, the pancreas produces a series of enzymes contained in pancreatic juice, carried by the pancreatic duct.

72. **The correct answer is C.** Lacrimation is the activity of the lacrimal glands, which produce lacrimal fluid or tears.

73. **The correct answer is A.** Olfaction, the sense of smell, is the domain of the first cranial nerve, the olfactory nerve. Nerves II, III, and IV (choices B, C, and D) are involved in the sensory and motor functions of the head and face but not the sense of smell.

74. **The correct answer is D.** Immediately distal to the neck of the bladder is the prostate gland. Its enlargement, common in males beginning at about the age of 40, interferes with urine outflow. Benign hyperplasia prostate (BHP) is a nonmalignant enlargement of the gland, which is also a common site for cancer in males. Although located in the same general area, the seminal vesicles (choice B) and bulbourethral (Cowper's) glands (choice C) do not normally hypertrophy with aging.

75. **The correct answer is B.** Linear (vertical and horizontal) acceleration is sensed by receptors within the utricles and saccules; the semicircular canals (choice A) contain receptors activated by rotational movement. Receptors within the cochlea (choice C) detect sound, and the middle ear (choice D) does not contain auditory or vestibular receptor devices.

76. **The correct answer is B.** Although the globulins and fibrin are blood proteins,

albumin is the protein in the highest plasma concentration.

77. **The correct answer is A.** Union of sperm and egg normally occurs within the fallopian (uterine) tubes prior to implantation within the uterus. Implantation at non-uterine sites is termed an ectopic pregnancy.

78. **The correct answer is B.** Depression may result from low levels of serotonin or decreased responsiveness of sertotonergic receptors in the brain, and this is the basis for the use of serotonin reuptake inhibitors in the treatment of clinical depression. High levels of catechol amines may contribute to clinical anxiety.

79. **The correct answer is B.** Lymphatic vessels begin as lymphatic capillaries, blind pouches found in peripheral tissue. Lymph nodes (choice C) are more proximal structures, and lymphocytes (choice D) are forms of white blood cells.

80. **The correct answer is A.** HCG rises to detectable levels following egg fertilization, and its presence in blood and urine forms the basis of pregnancy testing. The function of HCG is to maintain the corpus luteum, which is responsible for maintaining estrogen and progesterone levels, and their effects on the endometrium, during early and middle pregnancy.

81. **The correct answer is C.** Sweet, sour, and salty taste sensations result from activity in the facial nerve, the seventh cranial nerve. The first (choice A) cranial nerve is involved in olfaction; the fifth (choice B) is involved in motor and sensory mechanisms of the head and face. The tenth nerve, the vagus (choice D), is not involved in taste from the tongue.

82. **The correct answer is B.** The parasympathetic division of the autonomic nervous system is primarily involved with energy production and conservation. Its outward

effects can be by the acronym SLUD: salivation, lacrimation, urination, and defecation.

83. **The correct answer is A.** After their formation within the seminiferous tubules, sperm are stored within the epididymis lying alongside the testes. The epididymis leads to the vas deferens (choice B), which ultimately empties into the urethra, which receives material from the seminal vesicles (choice C).

84. **The correct answer is B.** Glucagon elevates blood glucose by (1) promoting the breakdown of glycogen to glucose (glycogenolysis), (2) promoting glucose synthesis (gluconeogenesis), and (3) promoting the release of glucose from liver.

85. **The correct answer is B.** Erythrocytes (red blood cells) are much more numerous than white blood cells (choice A). Globulins and albumin (choices C and D) are proteins, not formed elements.

86. **The correct answer is A.** Although not as powerful as pH-regulating mechanisms in the respiratory or renal systems, buffer systems essentially act at the rate of chemical reactions. The liver (choice D) is not involved in the normal control of blood pH.

87. **The correct answer is B.** Arterial blood pH is critically maintained between 7.35 and 7.45. Either a decline of pH (acidosis) to a level of 7.0 or an increase in pH (alkalosis) to 8.0 is potentially fatal.

88. **The correct answer is B.** While the hematocrit reveals the level of plasma, it is intended to evaluate the percentage of erythrocytes (red blood cells) in whole blood and subsequently the oxygen-carrying capacity of blood. Normal hematocrit values for females are 37–47 percent, 42–54 percent for males. Platelet and white cell enumerations are also useful diagnostics but do not involve the hematocrit.

89. **The correct answer is B.** Although about 5 liters of blood are pumped through the heart per minute, the myocardial muscle is dependent upon the coronary arteries for delivery of oxygen.

90. **The correct answer is B.** The term *hair cell* is applied to receptors within the auditory and vestibular systems. Rods and cones (choices A and C) are visual receptors, and muscle spindles (choice D) are the receptors for stretch reflexes.

91. **The correct answer is A.** Blood typing is based on determining the antigen(s) located on the surfaces of erythrocytes; the "opposite" antibody is located within the individual's plasma. A type A patient therefore has the A antigen and the anti-B antibody. Rh antigens are also located on erythrocyte surfaces leading to an individual being typed as Rh positive (antibody present) or Rh negative (no Rh antigen).

92. **The correct answer is D.** Sickle cell anemia develops when hemoglobin forms long crystalline chains within erythrocytes, forcing the cells into their bizarre shapes. Pernicious anemia (choice A) refers to abnormal destruction of red blood cells; iron deficiency (choice B) and aplastic anemias (choice C) involve abnormal blood cell formation.

93. **The correct answer is D.** Hair cells are the auditory receptors located within the cochlea, part of the inner ear. Auditory ossicles (choice C) are small bones involved in conduction of vibration through the middle ear (choice B).

94. **The correct answer is D.** Female menopause follows aging of the ovaries and is characterized by low estrogen levels, which, in turn, result in high levels of GnRH,

FSH, and LH. The latter two appear to be correlated with the "hot flashes" of menopause.

95. **The correct answer is B.** Hyperventilation can lead to a decreased arterial CO_2 level, which may result in alkalosis of respiratory origin. Extreme alkalosis may lead to convulsions and may produce seizure activity in epileptic patients.

96. **The correct answer is C.** Plasma is approximately 90 percent water, with the rest being comprised of numerous solutes, including proteins, nutrients, gases, hormones, ions, and products of cell activity.

97. **The correct answer is B.** Estrogen is involved in a feedback loop to the hypothalamus such that high levels of estrogen inhibit the release of GnRH, which reduces levels of LH and prevents ovulation.

98. **The correct answer is D.** Heparin is an endogenous anticoagulant produced by basophils. Fibrin, calcium, and thrombin (choices A, B, and C) are all promoters of the coagulation process.

99. **The correct answer is B.** GnRH (choice C) from the hypothalamus controls the release of FSH (choice A) and LH (choice B) from the anterior pituitary. FSH initiates follicle development, and LH leads directly to ovulation, the release of a mature egg.

100. **The correct answer is D.** Testosterone is produced by interstitial (Leydig) cells under the influence of ICSH, interstitial cell stimulating hormone. The epididymis and prostate (choices C and A) gland are not involved in testosterone synthesis.

Test 4: Anatomy, Physiology, and Health Science

1. B	9. B	17. D	25. C	33. D
2. B	10. D	18. C	26. A	34. A
3. D	11. C	19. B	27. C	35. B
4. A	12. B	20. A	28. B	36. A
5. D	13. B	21. B	29. D	37. B
6. A	14. D	22. B	30. A	38. D
7. A	15. C	23. D	31. B	39. C
8. C	16. B	24. B	32. B	40. C

1. **The correct answer is B.** Sphincters are circular muscles that contract when stimulated.

2. **The correct answer is B.** Bile is released into the duodenum and breaks down the undigested fats into small droplets.

3. **The correct answer is D.** Urea is filtered from the blood by the kidneys and excreted in urine.

4. **The correct answer is A.** Group AB blood contains both group A and B antigens and neither A nor B antibodies; therefore, it cannot clump any donor red cells containing A and B antigens.

5. **The correct answer is D.** Caffeine is a stimulant found in coffee.

6. **The correct answer is A.** Dried milk is an inexpensive but valuable source of protein.

7. **The correct answer is A.** Tendons, connective tissue made of dense fibers in the shape of a cord, have great strength.

8. **The correct answer is C.** Testosterone is the hormone that regulates male sex characteristics.

9. **The correct answer is B.** Hinge joints allow movement in only two directions.

10. **The correct answer is D.** Peristalsis is the progressive, wavelike movement that occurs involuntarily to force food forward.

11. **The correct answer is C.** The parotid gland is a large salivary gland that is affected by mumps.

12. **The correct answer is B.** The electron is the unit of negative electricity.

13. **The correct answer is B.** Capillaries connect arterioles with venules and function as exchange vessels.

14. **The correct answer is D.** Erythrocytes (red blood cells) contain hemoglobin.

15. **The correct answer is C.** Proteins are nutrients essential for growth and repair of tissue.

16. **The correct answer is B.** The diffusion of gas occurs across the thin, squamous epithelium lining of the alveoli.

17. **The correct answer is D.** The SA node, located in the right atrium, starts each heartbeat.

18. **The correct answer is C.** The mitral valve, located between the left atrium and left ventricle of the heart, is also called the bicuspid valve.

19. **The correct answer is B.** Viruses are so small that they can be seen only through special electron microscopes.

20. **The correct answer is A.** The pulmonary artery carries deoxygenated blood from the heart.

21. **The correct answer is B.** When water intake is excessive, the kidneys excrete generous amounts of urine; if water intake is lost, they produce less urine. The process is regulated by hormones.

22. **The correct answer is B.** Iodine makes up about 65 percent of thyroxine, a hormone secreted by the thyroid gland.

23. **The correct answer is D.** Scurvy is a disease caused by a deficiency of vitamin C.

24. **The correct answer is B.** Leukocytes (white blood cells) destroy bacteria when there is an infection in the body.

25. **The correct answer is C.** The islets of Langerhans are located in the pancreas and produce insulin.

26. **The correct answer is A.** Gastric and intestinal enzymes gradually break down the protein molecule into its separate amino acids.

27. **The correct answer is C.** Glucose is the end product of carbohydrate digestion.

28. **The correct answer is B.** When one muscle contracts, the opposing muscle must relax; in this way, movements are coordinated and normal functions are carried out.

29. **The correct answer is D.** The medulla oblongata is located between the pons and the spinal cord, and the vital centers are located in it.

30. **The correct answer is A.** Rays pass through a series of transparent, colorless eye parts. On the way, they undergo a process of bending called refraction, which makes it possible for light from a large area to focus on the retina.

31. **The correct answer is B.** The cornea is referred to frequently as the "window" of the eye.

32. **The correct answer is B.** A calorie is the unit of measure of heat—the amount of heat required to raise the temperature of 1 kilogram of water by 1°C.

33. **The correct answer is D.** Vitamin D is referred to as the "sunshine" vitamin because it is formed in the body by the action of the sunshine on the cholesterol products in the skin.

34. **The correct answer is A.** Digestion is the process whereby the enzymes in the body change food into simple substances that can be readily used by the body.

35. **The correct answer is B.** The thyroid gland needs iodine for the formation of thyroxine.

36. **The correct answer is A.** Vitamin K helps the liver to produce substances necessary for the clotting of blood.

37. **The correct answer is B.** Thiamine is another name for vitamin B_1.

38. **The correct answer is D.** Peristalsis is a wave-like progression of muscular contractions that moves food through the alimentary canal.

39. **The correct answer is C.** The thigh bone is the femur. It is the longest and strongest bone in the body.

40. **The correct answer is C.** Plasma is the liquid portion of the blood in which corpuscles are suspended.

Test 5: Anatomy, Physiology, and Health Science

1. C	**7.** C	**13.** D	**19.** B	**25.** B
2. D	**8.** B	**14.** A	**20.** C	**26.** B
3. C	**9.** C	**15.** B	**21.** A	**27.** A
4. B	**10.** B	**16.** D	**22.** C	**28.** C
5. A	**11.** A	**17.** B	**23.** D	**29.** B
6. C	**12.** C	**18.** D	**24.** D	**30.** D

1. **The correct answer is C.** Blood pressure is the force of the blood exerted against the wall of the blood vessel.

2. **The correct answer is D.** Relative humidity refers to the amount of moisture in the air in relation to the temperature.

3. **The correct answer is C.** A specimen is a laboratory sample used to help the physician make a diagnosis.

4. **The correct answer is B.** Defecation is the act of having a bowel movement or removing solid waste materials from the body.

5. **The correct answer is A.** *Sterile* means that an object is completely free of all microorganisms. Steam under pressure (autoclave) will give complete sterilization.

6. **The correct answer is C.** Carbon dioxide stimulates the respiratory center in the brain (medulla oblongata).

7. **The correct answer is C.** The presence of excessive amounts of the protein albumin in the urine is called albuminuria. It results from the failure of the kidneys to filter.

8. **The correct answer is B.** Protein, the body's vital building material, makes up the basic structure of all cells.

9. **The correct answer is C.** The gallbladder stores and concentrates bile, which is used to break down fats into droplets and aids in the absorption of fatty acids and glyceral.

Therefore, fats are restricted when there are diseases of the gallbladder.

10. **The correct answer is B.** Water-soluble vitamins include vitamin C and vitamin B complex.

11. **The correct answer is A.** Iron and calcium are the minerals most often deficient in the American diet.

12. **The correct answer is C.** Tetany, which is due to lack of calcium, may be corrected by increasing the consumption of milk or milk products, which are rich in calcium salts. Drugs containing high amounts of calcium may be given intravenously in emergencies.

13. **The correct answer is D.** Constriction of the blood vessels prevents loss of heat from the blood through the skin.

14. **The correct answer is A.** Milk contains only about 0.1 milligram of iron per cup. The recommended daily amount is 15–18 milligrams.

15. **The correct answer is B.** Food proteins supply our bodies with nitrogen to replace that lost in urine, feces, and perspiration.

16. **The correct answer is D.** The electrical charge results when a neutral atom or group of atoms loses or gains one or more electrons during chemical reactions.

17. **The correct answer is B.** The cell is the unit of structure and function of all living things. The simplest organisms consist of only one cell.

18. **The correct answer is D.** Osmosis is the diffusion of water through a semipermeable membrane from a region of greater concentration to a region of lesser concentration.

19. **The correct answer is B.** *Cardiologist* comes from the word *cardiology*, meaning the study of the heart's physiology and pathology.

20. **The correct answer is C.** Greenstick fractures are incomplete fractures with a longitudinal split of the shaft. They usually occur in long bones of children.

21. **The correct answer is A.** Environmental factors are the relationships of living things to their surroundings.

22. **The correct answer is C.** The fluid-like residue of digestion found in the colon contains valuable water, which is absorbed into the bloodstream.

23. **The correct answer is D.** After ovulation, the egg travels into the fallopian tube. If sperms are present, the union of the sperm and the egg (fertilization) takes place in the fallopian tube.

24. **The correct answer is D.** Photosynthesis is the process by which certain living plant cells combine carbon dioxide and water, in the presence of chlorophyll and light energy, to form carbohydrates and release oxygen as a waste product.

25. **The correct answer is B.** The atmosphere is composed of about 78 percent nitrogen.

26. **The correct answer is B.** Enzymes are protein substances that act as biochemical catalysts. They affect the rate at which a specific reaction occurs.

27. **The correct answer is A.** Essential amino acids are those that cannot be manufactured by the body and, therefore, must be included in the daily diet.

28. **The correct answer is C.** The barometer is an instrument used to measure air pressure and forecast weather.

29. **The correct answer is B.** An elevation of body temperature above normal is referred to as fever or pyrexia.

30. **The correct answer is D.** The otoscope is a lighted instrument used to examine the ear canal, eustachian tube, eardrum, and the middle ear.

Test 6: Body Structure and Function

1. A	7. D	13. C	19. B	25. C
2. D	8. C	14. B	20. B	26. D
3. C	9. C	15. D	21. A	27. B
4. B	10. A	16. C	22. B	28. A
5. C	11. B	17. B	23. C	29. A
6. B	12. D	18. A	24. A	30. B

1. **The correct answer is A.** During homeostasis, the body is constantly stabilizing and equalizing its environment to prevent any sudden or severe changes.

2. **The correct answer is D.** During mitosis, the DNA molecules in the nucleus of a cell duplicate themselves and the cell divides, forming two cells.

3. **The correct answer is C.** In acquiring passive immunity, the body of the recipient plays an active part in response to an antigen.

4. **The correct answer is B.** The nucleus is the functional unit suspended near the center of the cell that has the property of division.

5. **The correct answer is C.** Produced by the thyroid gland, thyroxin controls the rate at which glucose is burned and converts it to heat and energy.

6. **The correct answer is B.** Sweat glands are distributed in the skin and produce perspiration, primarily water.

7. **The correct answer is D.** Melanin, a brown pigment, increases when exposed to sun.

8. **The correct answer is C.** Estrogen and progesterone promote development of female sex characteristics and regulate menstruation.

9. **The correct answer is C.** Epithelial tissue has many forms—flat and irregular, square, long and narrow—that are arranged in single or multiple layers to form a protective covering and lining.

10. **The correct answer is A.** The ball-shaped head of the femur fits into the concave socket of the hipbone and allows for a wide range of motion.

11. **The correct answer is B.** Adrenaline is released from the adrenal medulla to prepare the body for emergency situations.

12. **The correct answer is D.** A small opening into the nose at the inner corner of the eye allows the fluid to drain through.

13. **The correct answer is C.** Many gray-matter areas that form the cranial nerves are located in the medulla oblongota and are involved in the control of vital activities.

14. **The correct answer is B.** As peristalsis moves content along, water is absorbed through the walls into the circulation, and the remaining cellulose passes on to the rectum.

15. **The correct answer is D.** Aldosterone is the hormone released from the adrenal cortex that helps regulate sodium and potassium balance.

16. **The correct answer is C.** The shedding of the lining of the uterus (menstruation) occurs if the egg has not been fertilized by the sperm.

17. **The correct answer is B.** *Dorsal* pertains to the back; the cranial and spinal cavities contain the brain and the spinal cord.

18. **The correct answer is A.** Deoxygenated blood returns from the body tissues via the superior and inferior vena cava into the right atrium.

19. **The correct answer is B.** The left ventricle has the major responsibility for pumping blood into the aorta to be dispersed throughout the body.

20. **The correct answer is B.** The vitreous humor is the jelly-like substance that prevents the eyeball from collapsing inward.

21. **The correct answer is A.** The endocardium is a smooth lining, which helps blood flow smoothly through the heart.

22. **The correct answer is B.** The perineum, which forms the pelvic floor, is the external region between the vulva and anus in the female or between the scrotum and anus in the male.

23. **The correct answer is C.** The greater trochanter is the ball-like head that articulates with the hipbone.

24. **The correct answer is A.** The gluteus maximus is part of the hips and buttocks.

25. **The correct answer is C.** Nephrons are responsible for the processes of filtration, absorption, and secretion.

26. **The correct answer is D.** Normal urine has a low specific gravity.

27. **The correct answer is B.** Aldosterone is released by the adrenal cortex in response to decreased blood volume, decreased blood sodium ions, or increased potassium ions.

28. **The correct answer is A.** Water plus creatinine and urea, which are nitrogenous wastes, are normal substances in urine.

29. **The correct answer is A.** The left motor control center in the brain controls the right side of the body because of the crossing of the nerve tracts within the brain.

30. **The correct answer is B.** When the water intake is excessive, the kidneys excrete generous amounts of urine; if the water intake is lost, they produce less urine. The process is regulated by hormones.

Test 7: Physiology and Health Science

1. B	15. D	29. B	43. B	57. D
2. A	16. C	30. C	44. C	58. A
3. B	17. A	31. B	45. B	59. B
4. C	18. C	32. C	46. A	60. A
5. A	19. C	33. D	47. B	61. B
6. B	20. D	34. A	48. A	62. C
7. A	21. B	35. B	49. D	63. A
8. B	22. A	36. C	50. B	64. D
9. B	23. C	37. C	51. D	65. B
10. A	24. A	38. C	52. B	66. A
11. A	25. C	39. C	53. A	67. D
12. C	26. A	40. B	54. B	68. C
13. C	27. D	41. A	55. C	69. A
14. B	28. B	42. B	56. C	70. B

1. **The correct answer is B.** Insulin increases the permeability of the cell membrane to glucose, thus enhancing the uptake of glucose from the blood by the cells. If insulin is deficient, glucose is not removed from the blood and utilized by the cells, resulting in an excess of glucose in the blood and leading to other symptoms of diabetes.

2. **The correct answer is A.** The amnion is one of the extraembryonic structures formed during embryonic development. It surrounds the embryo and becomes filled with fluid in which the embryo floats. The amniotic fluid probably provides protection from mechanical shock for the embryo.

3. **The correct answer is B.** Sebaceous glands are associated with hair follicles: the cells lining the glands form the secretion, and the entire cellular lining, plus the fatty secretion, form sebum, which is expelled into the hair follicle. Sebum serves to keep the hair and skin pliable.

4. **The correct answer is C.** DNA (deoxyribonucleic acid) is found in the nucleus of each cell and "stores" genetic information, or the genetic code. DNA replicates itself before mitosis or meiosis begins, and genetic information is distributed equally to the daughter nuclei. RNA (ribonucleic acid), transcribed on DNA, translates the genetic or hereditary information.

5. **The correct answer is A.** Melanin is a dark pigment found in the cells of the basal layers of the skin. Skin color varies with the size and density of the melanin particles: the more melanin present, the darker the skin.

6. **The correct answer is B.** Each person has a set of 20 deciduous teeth, as contrasted to 32 permanent or nondeciduous teeth. The set of deciduous teeth contains no bicuspids, and only two molars per quadrant rather than three. A set per quadrant of deciduous teeth includes two incisors, one canine, and two molars; a set per quadrant of nondeciduous teeth includes two incisors, one canine, two premolars (bicuspids), and three molars.

7. **The correct answer is A.** Cementum covers the surface of roots of teeth; enamel (choice C) covers the surface of the crowns of teeth.

8. **The correct answer is B.** The bulk of a hemoglobin molecule consists of four subunits, each one of which is a chain of amino acids. Iron (choice C) is also present in hemoglobin but does not comprise as large a part of the entire molecule as the four chains of amino acids. Ferritin (choice A) is an iron-containing molecule stored in the liver. Myosin (choice D) is a major component of muscle cells.

9. **The correct answer is B.** The XY chromosomes are found in the male, while the female carries XX. As a result of meiosis, a sperm will carry either an X or Y chromosome; all eggs will carry one X. Fertilization of an X-bearing egg by a Y-bearing sperm produces an XY zygote, which develops into a male. Fertilization of an X-bearing egg by an X-bearing sperm produces an XX zygote, which develops into a female.

10. **The correct answer is A.** The fetus and the mother have independent circulatory systems. Fetal blood passing to and from the placenta by way of the umbilical blood vessels is separated from the mother's blood in the placenta by thin tissues; food, gases, and metabolic wastes can diffuse through these tissues between the two bloodstreams. After birth, the placenta's function has ended, and as the baby's systems become "active," there is no longer an exchange of materials between the two bloodstreams.

11. **The correct answer is A.** The major difference between plasma and blood is cellular content. Plasma is the liquid portion of the blood. Whole blood consists of plasma with its dissolved materials and the blood cells.

12. **The correct answer is C.** Thrombocytes disintegrate when blood flows from a blood vessel, releasing a phospholipid, thrombokinase, that acts to convert prothrombin in the plasma to thrombin. Thrombin acts enzymatically on fibrinogen in the plasma, converting it to fibrin, which is insoluble and forms a mesh, trapping blood cells. This mesh is the blood clot.

13. **The correct answer is C.** The femur is the thigh bone of the leg. It is the longest, strongest, and heaviest bone of the body.

14. **The correct answer is B.** Iron is a part of the hemoglobin molecule, the red, oxygen-carrying pigment of red blood cells. If iron is deficient, hemoglobin cannot be produced, and the formation of red blood cells is inhibited.

15. **The correct answer is D.** Peristalsis is the wave of muscular contractions that pushes food through the esophagus into the stomach and through the intestine. Food must reach the digestive sites, the stomach and small intestine, for digestion to occur. Transamination, glucogenolysis, and the Krebs cycle (choices A, B, and C) are involved in metabolic processes, not in digestion.

16. **The correct answer is C.** The liver is the largest glandular organ of vertebrates and has the important function of regulating organic materials such as wastes, glucose, and proteins in the blood. It can also perform other essential functions, such as fat digestion and storage functions, immune responses, protein metabolism, and detoxifying blood by converting toxic substances into harmless wastes. It is essential for life.

17. **The correct answer is A.** The cell walls of gram-negative bacteria are more complex than gram-positives—with less peptidoglycan and more lipopolysaccharides—which renders them more difficult for drugs to cross.

18. **The correct answer is C.** Nerve fibers from the retina of the eye form the optic nerve of the eye; at the crossover point (optic chiasma), fibers from the nasal halves (inner halves) of each retina cross to the opposite side of the brain, while fibers of the temporal halves (outer halves) of each retina remain uncrossed. Thus, each optic nerve, after the chiasma, contains fibers from both retinas. This means that objects in one field of vision (either left or right) produce effects in two eyes that are transmitted to one side of the brain. In other words, the two halves of the retina of each eye are represented on opposite sides of the brain, producing a stereoscopic effect and permitting perception of depth.

19. **The correct answer is C.** Many aquatic animals excrete ammonia as their nitrogenous waste; egg-laying animals excrete uric acid, and intra-uterine animals excrete urea.

20. **The correct answer is D.** Estrogen is a complex of female sex hormones responsible for the appearance of secondary sex characteristics, such as widening of the pelvis, breasts, etc. Estrogen also functions in the menstrual cycle, preparing the uterus for implantation of the embryo.

21. **The correct answer is B.** A polymer is a large, chain-like organic molecule formed by bonding together many smaller organic molecules of the same kind. A protein is a chain of many amino acid molecules joined to one another by peptide bonds. The amino acid molecules present, and the sequence in which they are joined, are considered the primary structure of the protein and determine its physical or chemical properties.

22. **The correct answer is A.** Red blood cells are produced in the bone marrow in the adult. The other statements are incorrect as follows: vitamins typically are consumed with food (two possible exceptions); glucose is a product of digestion, and bile is stored in the gallbladder; water is a part of almost all tissues; and fats are refined by the bile from the liver.

23. **The correct answer is C.** Connective tissues are those whose cells are not contiguous but scattered throughout a noncellular matrix. Connective tissues can bind and support other tissues; therefore, they are widely distributed. Some examples of connective tissues are blood, bone, cartilage, adipose, and tissues composing tendons or ligaments.

24. **The correct answer is A.** The limited amount of ATP stored in muscle tissue supplies immediate energy for contraction when the ATP is converted to ADP. When the ATP is used up, it is recreated by energy from a reserve, creatine phosphate. When the creatine phosphate is consumed, oxidation of glucose to CO_2 and water provides energy for muscle contraction and for the resynthesis of creatine phosphate. Lactic acid can form anaerobically during severe muscle exertion, and its accumulation is partly responsible for the feeling of fatigue. Lactic acid diffuses out of the muscle tissue into the bloodstream and thus to the liver, where some of it is oxidized to produce further energy, and some can be converted to glycogen for carbohydrate storage.

25. **The correct answer is C.** Adrenalin, or epinephrine, secreted by the adrenal medulla, is normally released in small quantities and helps to regulate blood circulation and carbohydrate metabolism. Under stressful conditions, the adrenal medulla is stimulated to release larger amounts of adrenalin, which increases blood pressure, heart rate, carbohydrate metabolism, and conversion

of glycogen to sugar, thus raising the blood sugar level, etc. This prepares the body to cope with the stressful situation—hence, the "flight or fight" response.

26. **The correct answer is A.** Exercise will cause perspiration, which evaporates from the skin. Perspiration is a liquid composed of water, salt, and a small amount of urea and is drawn from the bloodstream (from capillaries in the sweat glands) and released to the body surface through pores. Thus, rigorous exercise will cause the body to lose sodium (salt) and water.

27. **The correct answer is D.** Cholesterol is a lipid that is insoluble in fluids such as blood; therefore, it is bound to proteinaceous carriers for transport. Evidence indicates that cholesterol is involved in the fatty deposits in arteries, even infiltrating cells and the intercellular spaces of arterial walls, if carried by certain carriers. This can lead to plaque and clot formation, blocking off the arteries and interfering with blood circulation. This same plaque and clot formation can occur in the coronary artery supplying heart muscle, causing a heart attack.

28. **The correct answer is B.** The endocrine glands secrete hormones directly into the bloodstream. The hormones are transported throughout the body, but only specific "target" cells or tissues can pick up a specific hormone. Thus, the hormone may regulate cellular activities in tissues some distance from the cells that secreted it. By regulating cellular activities of tissues, hormones regulate bodily activities.

29. **The correct answer is B.** The thyroid hormone controls the rate of cellular metabolism for the release of energy. An overactive gland secretes an excess of hormone, which will increase the metabolic rate. A deficiency of thyroid hormone causes the rate of metabolism to be lowered.

30. **The correct answer is C.** The alveolus is a small, thin-walled sac of the lung; it is the blind end of the smallest bronchioles. Each alveolus (approximately 300 million are present in human lungs) is surrounded by, or adjacent to, small capillaries. It is here that gaseous exchange between the blood and lungs occur. Carbon dioxide passes into the alveolus from the blood, and oxygen passes from the alveolus into the bloodstream through the capillary walls.

31. **The correct answer is B.** A hemorrhoid is a dilation of veins in the anal region. This can lead to an enlargement of tissue, especially the rectal sphincter, which is a ring-shaped muscle controlling the anal opening.

32. **The correct answer is C.** The amino nitrogen must be removed from amino acids in order to give them the basic hydrocarbon skeleton similar to carbohydrates. After the amino group is removed, the resulting compounds may enter the same metabolic pathways used by carbohydrates.

33. **The correct answer is D.** The chemistry of life is closely dependent upon the chemistry of water. Water, in the presence of the proper enzymes, must be added to the bonds that bind monosaccharides in carbohydrates, amino acids in proteins, and fatty acids and glycerol in fats to degrade these polymers to their subunits.

34. **The correct answer is A.** Energy production, in the degradation of foods, is associated with the release of hydrogen (oxidation). The ratio of hydrogen to oxygen is significantly greater in fats than in carbohydrates and proteins.

35. **The correct answer is B.** Oxygenated blood passes from the lungs to the left atrium of the heart by way of the pulmonary veins. From the left atrium, blood

moves to the left ventricle, from which it is pumped through the aorta to the arterial system of the body, and thus throughout the body, where oxygen is diffused into the cells and carbon dioxide is picked up by the blood. The carbon-dioxide-laden blood is returned to the heart, entering the right atrium, and passing to the right ventricle. From the right ventricle, it is pumped to the lungs through the pulmonary arteries, where it becomes oxygenated again.

36. **The correct answer is C.** Studies conducted by Dr. Allan Roses and D. Warren Stuttmatter at the Duke University Medical Center and reported in the Wall Street Journal (October 19, 1995) indicated that the apoliprotein E gene occurs as E-2, E-3, and E-4 subtypes. The potential of gene E for promoting cell maintenance and protection against Alzheimer's, heart disease, and diabetes is in order of potency of E-2 > E-3 > E-4. Therefore, E-2 is the good gene and E-4 is the bad form.

37. **The correct answer is C.** The three basic kinds of muscle tissue are smooth, skeletal, and cardiac. Smooth muscle is characteristic of the digestive tract and arteries, organs not under voluntary control. Cardiac muscle is found in the heart. Skeletal muscle (striated) makes up the muscles associated with voluntary movement. The kidney is nonmuscular.

38. **The correct answer is C.** Gaseous exchange between the respiratory system and the circulatory system occurs by means of the capillaries present in the lungs surrounding alveoli. These are referred to as the pulmonary capillaries.

39. **The correct answer is C.** The hybridoma, formed by fusing lymphocytes with cancer cells, produces a single type of antibody. The hybridoma can be injected into a mouse or cultured, in vitro, to increase production of the single antibody type.

40. **The correct answer is B.** Blood in systemic veins is returning to the right atrium of the heart from the cells of the body. Therefore, it is high in concentrations of carbon dioxide and metabolic wastes that were received from the cells as a result of cellular metabolism. Venous blood of the pulmonary system is returning to the left atrium of the heart from the lungs, where it gave up carbon dioxide to be expelled from the body and acquired oxygen. Therefore, it has a higher concentration of oxygen.

41. **The correct answer is A.** The first division of meiosis results in a reduction of the number of chromosomes, because the members of each pair of chromosomes are separated from one another. Each daughter nucleus resulting from meiosis receives only one chromosome of each pair present in the parent nucleus, or one half the number of chromosomes of the parent nucleus. Nuclei resulting from meiosis are haploid, as contrasted to the diploid condition of the parent nucleus.

42. **The correct answer is B.** Fraternal, or nonidentical, twins result from two fertilized eggs, or zygotes. If two eggs are released during ovulation and both are fertilized (one sperm per egg), fraternal twins result. These twins are like ordinary siblings, whereas identical twins resulting from a single zygote are genetically identical.

43. **The correct answer is B.** Restriction fragment length polymorphisms are differences in the lengths of fragments of DNA produced by exposing DNA from genetically different individuals to a bacterial restriction enzyme that cuts DNA at specific points.

44. **The correct answer is C.** Specialized muscle cells, known as the "pacemaker" of the heart, make up a region of the right atrium. When these cells are excited, the atria are stimulated to contract, emptying the blood into the ventricles. Certain muscle fibers then carry the excitation stimulus, by way of the atrio-ventricular node, to muscles of the ventricles, stimulating them to contract and force blood from the heart.

45. **The correct answer is B.** The XY chromosomes are found in the male, while the female carries XX. As a result of meiosis, a sperm will carry either an X or a Y chromosome; all eggs will carry an X. Fertilization of an X-bearing egg by a Y-bearing sperm produces an XY zygote, which develops into a male. Fertilization of an X-bearing egg by an X-bearing sperm produces an XX zygote, which develops into a female.

46. **The correct answer is A.** Red blood cells contain the pigment hemoglobin, which has as its function the transport of oxygen. If the number of red blood cells is decreased, the ability of the blood to transport oxygen is decreased.

47. **The correct answer is B.** Temperatures greater than 40°C will denature (destroy) the molecular geometry of most proteins. In many plant and animal cells, special proteins (heat shock proteins) are synthesized to prevent denaturation at these temperatures.

48. **The correct answer is A.** The cerebrum is the largest division of the central nervous system of humans. It originates thinking and controls learning, memory, thought, some voluntary movements, and the senses. In the animal kingdom, observations indicate that intelligence increases with cerebrum size. Humans have the largest cerebrum, in proportion to body size, in the animal kingdom.

49. **The correct answer is D.** The stapes, cochlea, and tympanic membrane are all parts of the ear. The stapes is one of the vibrating bones of the middle ear, the cochlea is the receptor portion of the inner ear from which electrical impulses ("messages") are transmitted to the brain through the auditory nerve, and the tympanic membrane is the eardrum. The cornea, on the other hand, is the transparent covering over the front of the lens of the eye.

50. **The correct answer is B.** Human activities (e.g., agricultural and industrial) generally destroy food and alter physical conditions required to complete the life cycle in some species. The overall effect is a reduction in the total number of species that occupy a habitat.

51. **The correct answer is D.** Acidity is determined by the concentration of hydrogen ion H^+s per unit of volume. Strong bases allow fewer H^+s to escape in aqueous solution than weak bases, producing weaker acids (e.g., Cl^- is a weak base, making HCl a strong acid, whereas HCO_3 is a strong base, making H_2CO_3 a weak acid).

52. **The correct answer is B.** The arrows directed to the right in chemical equations represent products generated from the forward reaction, and those directed to the left represent reactants produced by the reverse reaction. The arrow length symbolizes the concentration of the substances on both sides of the equation.

53. **The correct answer is A.** In humans and other animals, it is normal for an individual to have two copies of each type of chromosome in the nucleus of any body cell, except an egg or a sperm. There are 23 different types of chromosomes in humans;

therefore, the normal complement of chromosomes in human cells is 46. Individuals with Down syndrome receive an extra copy of chromosome 21 from one of their parents. They have three copies of chromosome 21 and a total of 47 chromosomes in the nuclei of their cells.

54. **The correct answer is B.** In cellular metabolism, glycolysis is an anaerobic process (requires no O_2), produces reduced nicotinamide adeninedinucleotide ($NADH_2$) and small amounts of ATP, and occurs in all types of cells.

55. **The correct answer is C.** Osmosis is the movement of water across cell membranes from solutions of low solute concentration to solutions with higher concentrations of solute. The salt gives the water a higher solute concentration than the frog's intracellular fluids. Therefore, the water concentration inside the cells would decrease as water flowed to the outside.

56. **The correct answer is C.** The air (atmosphere) around the earth exerts a normal pressure of 760 mmHg (1.0 atmosphere). The pressure in interplanetary space is zero (a vacuum). Since the pressure inside the astronaut's blood vessels is greater than zero, the vessels would push outward.

57. **The correct answer is D.** All of these viruses have been associated with cancer: adenoviruses (respiratory tract tumors), retroviruses (leukemia and AIDS), and papovaviruses (cervical cancer).

58. **The correct answer is A.** Cereals (grains) are rich in certain members of the vitamin B complex; because of the starchy endosperm in seeds, cereals also are high in carbohydrates.

59. **The correct answer is B.** Labels on canned goods may include a variety of information about the product, but the net contents by weight or volume and the quality should always be included. The number of portions may vary per net contents, according to the nature of the product, so knowledge of the number of servings is useful information. Other information may also be included on the label.

60. **The correct answer is A.** Caloric needs vary with age as well as with physiological state, activity, and the size of the individual. Both physical and mental growth and development are more rapid during infancy and early childhood than at any other time in one's life. Therefore, more food is needed in proportion to size to provide the needed calories of energy and to provide the materials for growth. A proper diet is essential for normal development.

61. **The correct answer is B.** Genes shown to cause cancerous growths are called oncogenes.

62. **The correct answer is C.** Many individuals believe that the use of tissues from aborted fetuses is ethically unacceptable.

63. **The correct answer is A.** The AIDS virus uses its surface glycoproteins to bind to membrane receptors of host cells, initiating the infection by infusing viral RNA into the host cell.

64. **The correct answer is D.** The AIDS virus uses an enzyme—reverse transcriptase—as the normal pattern of synthesis (using DNA as a template to produce RNA) to a reverse method (using RNA as a template to form DNA).

65. **The correct answer is B.** The inability to pass Cl– to the outside of cells in cystic fibrosis patients causes water to enter the cells by osmosis, making the intercellular mucus thicker than normal.

66. **The correct answer is A.** Cell membranes maintain their high external Na^+ and high

internal K$^+$ concentrations by using ATP to energize membrane carrier proteins that form the sodium-potassium pump. This is an active transport mechanism, which moves both ions against concentration gradients.

67. **The correct answer is D.** The general procedure for cloning includes: isolating DNA plasmid from a bacterium, isolating the DNA comprising the gene of interest from a different cell type, mixing the gene of interest with the plasmid to form a hybrid type of DNA called recombinant DNA, infecting a vector (bacteria or virus) with the recombinant DNA, and culturing the vector (containing the recombinant DNA) to produce many identical copies of itself (clones).

68. **The correct answer is C.** Plasmids—small, circular self-duplicating DNA molecules isolated from bacteria—are major requirements for recombinant DNA technology.

69. **The correct answer is A.** The restriction enzymes recognize and fragment the DNA (at the proper location) of the genes to be cloned.

70. **The correct answer is B.** The splicing of DNA from two different sources is accomplished by the enzyme, DNA ligase, which catalyzes bonding by the complementarity of base pairing.

Reading Comprehension

OVERVIEW

Unit 16

READING COMPREHENSION ANSWER SHEET

Test 1

1. Ⓐ Ⓑ Ⓒ Ⓓ   2. Ⓐ Ⓑ Ⓒ Ⓓ   3. Ⓐ Ⓑ Ⓒ Ⓓ   4. Ⓐ Ⓑ Ⓒ Ⓓ   5. Ⓐ Ⓑ Ⓒ Ⓓ

Test 2

1. Ⓐ Ⓑ Ⓒ Ⓓ   3. Ⓐ Ⓑ Ⓒ Ⓓ   4. Ⓐ Ⓑ Ⓒ Ⓓ   5. Ⓐ Ⓑ Ⓒ Ⓓ   6. Ⓐ Ⓑ Ⓒ Ⓓ

2. Ⓐ Ⓑ Ⓒ Ⓓ

Test 3

1. Ⓐ Ⓑ Ⓒ Ⓓ   3. Ⓐ Ⓑ Ⓒ Ⓓ   4. Ⓐ Ⓑ Ⓒ Ⓓ   5. Ⓐ Ⓑ Ⓒ Ⓓ   6. Ⓐ Ⓑ Ⓒ Ⓓ

2. Ⓐ Ⓑ Ⓒ Ⓓ

Test 4

1. Ⓐ Ⓑ Ⓒ Ⓓ   2. Ⓐ Ⓑ Ⓒ Ⓓ   3. Ⓐ Ⓑ Ⓒ Ⓓ   4. Ⓐ Ⓑ Ⓒ Ⓓ   5. Ⓐ Ⓑ Ⓒ Ⓓ

Test 5

1. Ⓐ Ⓑ Ⓒ Ⓓ   2. Ⓐ Ⓑ Ⓒ Ⓓ   3. Ⓐ Ⓑ Ⓒ Ⓓ   4. Ⓐ Ⓑ Ⓒ Ⓓ   5. Ⓐ Ⓑ Ⓒ Ⓓ

answer sheet

TEST 1

5 Questions • 8 Minutes

Review Unit 7, Reading Comprehension, before attempting this test.

> **Directions:** Carefully read the following passage and then answer the accompanying questions, basing your answers on what is stated or implied in the passage. When you have decided which choice is best, fill in the corresponding space on your answer sheet. There is only one best answer for each question.

How can we know that the birds we see in the South in the winter are the same ones that come north in the spring? John J. Audubon, a bird lover, wondered about this. Every year, he watched a pair of little phoebes nesting in the same place. He wondered if they were the same birds and so decided to put tiny silver bands on their legs. The next spring, back came the birds with the bands to build their nests on the walls of farm buildings in the neighborhood. The phoebe, it was learned, wintered wherever it was warm enough to find flies. In summer, phoebes could be seen from Georgia to Canada; in winter, anywhere from Georgia to Florida and Mexico. The phoebe was the first kind of bird to be banded, and Mr. Audubon was the first birdbander. Today there are thousands of birdbanders all over America, people who band all kinds of birds.

The government of the United States has a special birdbanding department that makes all the birdbands. The bands do not hurt the birds because they are made of aluminum and are very light. They come in different sizes for different-sized birds. Each band has a special number and the words, "Notify Fish and Wildlife Service, Washington, DC." Anyone who finds a dead bird with a band on one of its legs is asked to send the band to Washington with a note telling where and when the bird was found. In this way naturalists add to their knowledge of the habits and needs of birds.

1. The title below that best expresses the main theme or subject of this selection is
   A. "The Migration of Birds."
   B. "The Work of John Audubon."
   C. "The Habits and Needs of Birds."
   D. "Studying Bird Life Through Birdbanding."

2. According to the selection, Audubon proved his theory that
   A. birds prefer a diet of flies.
   B. birds return to the same nesting place each spring.
   C. silver is the best material for birdbands.
   D. phoebes are the most interesting birds to study.

3. Audubon's purpose in banding the phoebes was to
   A. satisfy his curiosity.
   B. notify the government.
   C. start a birdbanding department.
   D. gain fame as the first birdbander.

4. The migration habits of phoebes depend upon
   A. nesting places.
   B. the help of bird lovers.
   C. the available food supply.
   D. the number of young birds.

5. Which statement is true according to
the selection?

A. Residents of Georgia may expect to
see phoebes all year long.

B. The weight of a band causes a bird
considerable discomfort.

C. The government offers a reward for
information about dead birds.

D. Phoebes are more plentiful in the East
than any other kind of bird.

STOP

IF YOU FINISH BEFORE TIME IS CALLED, YOU MAY
CHECK YOUR WORK ON THIS SECTION ONLY. DO NOT
TURN TO ANY OTHER SECTION IN THE TEST.

TEST 2

6 Questions • 10 Minutes

Review Unit 7, Reading Comprehension, before attempting this test.

Directions: Carefully read the following passage and then answer the accompanying questions, basing your answers on what is stated or implied in the passage. When you have decided which choice is best, fill in the corresponding space on your answer sheet. There is only one best answer for each question.

It is important to understand just what we mean when we talk about stress, and theoretical definitions of stress abound. Probably the best definition was offered by the renowned stress researcher Hans Selye, who summarized stress as "... any bodily change produced as a response to a perceived demand being placed upon the individual." This definition highlights the notion that there are two important facets to stress: the psychological (or mental) and the physiological (or physical).

Stress can be typically negative events, called "distress," as well as the more positive happenings in life that nonetheless demand change and adjustment. After a demand is perceived, bodily or physical changes occur as a reaction. These biological responses typically include increased heart rate, respiration rate, rising blood pressure, and muscular tension, shallow (rather than deep) breathing, and the increased release of certain so-called stress hormones such as adrenaline and cortisol.

Such bodily changes occur for what is commonly known as the "fight-or-flight" response. The fight-or-flight response served a purpose ages ago, when acute, sudden stressors such as animal predators immediately threatened a person's existence. Successfully fighting off or fleeing from the threat greatly increased one's chance of survival. And, as with other creatures, our fight-or-flight stress reaction became "wired in" as a protective mechanism.

Stress continues to serve us today, as mild to moderate levels of stress can sharpen our alertness and motivate positive growth, spur the need to accept challenges, and promote change in our lives. Stress becomes a problem only when you consider the nature of some of our stressors. Unlike the saber-tooth tigers of long age, today's stressors tend to be more chronic in nature. Most people struggle with the demands of health problems, interpersonal difficulties, financial worries, and negative or critical self-imaging, to name just a few. These concerns have a propensity to stick around. When you begin to experience any one of them, your body reacts with predictable changes. However, because these stressors usually stay around and dominate parts of our existence for long stretches of time, the bodily changes that get "turned on," stay "turned on," which can cause or influence numerous undesirable consequences.

Chronic stress can contribute to such physical problems as migraine headaches, lower back pain, ulcers, digestive disorders, TMJ (temporomandibular joint) syndrome, suppressed immunity, and, of particular concern to people with diabetes, difficulty controlling rising blood sugar. There is even some evidence that cardiovascular disease, high blood pressure, and certain types of cancer can be adversely affected by stress. Chronic stress also appears to contribute to many psychological and behavioral disorders such as depression, anxiety disorders, and low self-esteem.

Everyone attempts to cope with the stress in his or her life, whether doing so consciously and deliberately or not. Unfortunately, many of the strategies people use to deal with stress actually produce additional sources of stress. Overeating, excessive alcohol consumption, cigarette smoking, and drug use are examples of stress management attempts gone awry.

Any effective strategy of stress management needs to do more than just distract you from that which is causing the stress. It needs to address both the physical and the psychological aspects of stress.

—"Women and Diabetes: Strategies for Handling Stress" Reprinted with permission from *Diabetes Self-Management*. Copyright © 1997 R.A. Rapaport Publishing, Inc.

1. According to Hans Selye, stress is stimulated by a(n)

   A. environmental change.

   B. bodily change.

   C. perceived demand.

   D. physiological and psychological conflict.

2. The physiological symptoms of stress are a result of

   A. secretion of adrenalin and cortisol.

   B. suppression of adrenaline.

   C. accumulation of cortisol.

   D. absence of adrenaline and cortisol.

3. The main problem presented by stress in diabetics is that the

   A. blood sugar rises.

   B. blood pressure drops.

   C. immune system is suppressed.

   D. stomach develops ulcers.

4. The theoretical basis for the effects of stress is based on the

   A. interaction of the physiological and psychological self.

   B. interaction of the self with the environment.

   C. relationship between change and coping.

   D. relationship between change and growth.

5. An effective method of coping with stress would be

   A. focusing on the pleasure of eating.

   B. inducing relaxation by drinking alcoholic beverages.

   C. delaying stopping smoking.

   D. adapting to change.

6. According to this passage,

   A. stress causes cancer.

   B. stress can be controlled.

   C. all stress is harmful.

   D. all stress is continuous.

STOP

IF YOU FINISH BEFORE TIME IS CALLED, YOU MAY CHECK YOUR WORK ON THIS SECTION ONLY. DO NOT TURN TO ANY OTHER SECTION IN THE TEST.

TEST 3

6 Questions • 10 Minutes

Review Unit 7, Reading Comprehension, before attempting this test.

> **Directions:** Carefully read the following passage and then answer the accompanying questions, basing your answers on what is stated or implied in the passage. When you have decided which choice is best, fill in the corresponding space on your answer sheet. There is only one best answer for each question.

Since 1910, more American women have died of heart disease than of any other cause. But for most of this century, physicians and researchers treated heart disease almost exclusively as a man's problem. When the American Heart Association held its first public conference for women in 1964, it focused on how women could help protect their husbands' hearts.

How could doctors and scientists overlook such a clear threat to women's health for so long?

For many years, heart-disease researchers concerned themselves primarily with premature heart attacks—heart attacks that strike down the young or middle-aged rather than the elderly. When women get heart disease, however, they tend to develop it 10 to 15 years later than men; thus, they are more likely to have heart attacks when they are past middle age.

For much of their lives, the sex hormone estrogen offers women substantial protection from heart disease. Only around age 55 does the rate of heart disease in women start to climb, both because estrogen levels drop after menopause and because other risk factors for heart disease become more common at the same age.

The age difference makes heart disease appear a more dramatic problem in men than in women; it's somehow more shocking when a heart attack hits a 50-year-old than when a 65-year-old is the victim. Indeed, the fact that men develop heart disease earlier than women means the disease may have a greater impact on their lives, and offers some justification for putting a greater emphasis on studying heart disease in men than in women. But until recently, researchers have done much more than that: They have systematically and almost completely excluded women from studies of all aspects of coronary heart disease. One major heart-disease study did include women in virtually equal numbers with men, but the data were misinterpreted in a way that actually added to the confusion over women's risks. The Framingham Heart Study has been following more than 5,000 men and women since 1948 to chart the causes and course of heart disease. Among other factors, the researchers identified people with chest pain, and assumed that they were suffering from angina, a symptom indicating that narrowed coronary arteries are supplying inadequate amounts of oxygen to the heart muscle.

Angina often precedes a heart attack. But in the mid-1950s, the Framingham researchers found that men with chest pain were much more likely than women with chest pain to have a heart attack within five years. They concluded that heart disease was simply not much of a threat to women.

There are two problems with that conclusion. First, many women with chest pain turn out not to have angina at all. A major study published in 1982 revealed that fully half of all women with chest pain who underwent coronary angiography—an X-ray procedure for visualizing the arteries of the heart—did not have blockages. (The same was true of only 17 percent of the men.) And second, in the 1950s most of Framingham's women were still too young to be at high risk for heart attack. A later analysis of the Framingham data showed that heart disease in women develops more gradually than in men. Women are more likely to experience angina for an extended period of time before suffering a heart attack.

Clinical trials—studies that test the effects of different treatments on a disease, rather than simply trying to understand the factors that lead to illness—have also tended to exclude women. Investigators have traditionally steered clear of testing any new treatments on women of child-bearing age to avoid the confounding effects their hormonal cycles might have on test results, and to avoid unwittingly exposing a fetus by giving a drug to a woman who doesn't yet know she is pregnant. Many researchers have also excluded people over age 65, the age when women have the greatest heart-disease risk, out of concern that other illnesses in these older people would muddy the data. In clinical trials conducted over the past 30 years to evaluate treatments for heart attack, fewer than 20 percent of the total 151,000 subjects were women, according to a recent analysis in the Journal of the American Medical Association.

As a result, physicians have proceeded on the assumption that a treatment tested in men will work about equally well in women. Not necessarily. It is now clear, for instance, that the drug propranolol (Inderal), a beta-blocker commonly prescribed for high blood pressure and angina, is broken down far more slowly in women's bodies—an important consideration for dosage. Moreover, the potential of estrogen treatment to prevent heart disease in postmenopausal women is only now being tested in large clinical trials.

In 1985, the U.S. Public Health Service Task Force on Women's Health Issues ordered the National Institutes of Health to include more women in research, particularly research on heart disease. After several years of foot-dragging, the NIH established an office to ensure that women are appropriately represented in NIH-funded studies. Several large-scale clinical trials including women are now in the planning stage or underway. The clinical trial portion of the Women's Health Initiative—a $600 million, 14-year effort—will study the effects of a low-fat diet and hormonal therapy in preventing cardiovascular disease (as well as cancer and osteoporosis). It may be many years, however, before the decades of neglect are overcome.

—"Heart Disease: Women at Risk" Reprinted by permission from *Consumer Reports*, May 1993. Copyright © 1993 by Consumers Union of U.S., Inc., Yonkers, NY 10703-1057

1. The theory that estrogen protects women from heart disease is supported by the fact that

   A. the rate of heart disease in women drops after age 55.

   B. the rate of heart disease in women increases after age 55.

   C. the incidence of heart disease in women is far less than in men.

   D. only post-menopausal women have heart disease.

2. Physicians and researchers have placed emphasis on heart disease in men more than in women because

   A. men develop heart disease earlier than women.

   B. more men die from heart disease than women.

   C. men are more prone to heart disease than women.

   D. men respond to treatment more readily than women.

3. When comparing the occurrence of angina in men and women,

   A. women have angina for a longer period of time before a heart attack.

   B. angina usually precedes a heart attack in both men and women.

   C. the occurrence is more frequent in females.

   D. the occurrence is less frequent in males.

4. The age when women are at greatest risk for heart disease is

   A. 45–49.

   B. 50–59.

   C. 60–65.

   D. over 65.

5. It is important to conduct clinical research on both men and women because

   A. preventive techniques are the same for both men and women.

   B. age differences in occurrence of heart disease indicate differences in causes.

   C. physiological differences lead to differences in responses to treatment.

   D. the impact of heart disease on an individual's life is the same for men and women.

6. The focus of the NIH clinical trials for Women's Health Initiative is to study the

   A. relationship between the aging process and the occurrence of heart disease.

   B. factors that lead to high risk for heart disease.

   C. female responses to drugs used to treat heart disease.

   D. effects of diet and hormonal therapy on prevention of heart disease.

STOP

IF YOU FINISH BEFORE TIME IS CALLED, YOU MAY CHECK YOUR WORK ON THIS SECTION ONLY. DO NOT TURN TO ANY OTHER SECTION IN THE TEST.

TEST 4

5 Questions • 8 Minutes

Review Unit 7, Reading Comprehension, before attempting this test.

> **Directions:** Carefully read the following passage and then answer the accompanying questions, basing your answers on what is stated or implied in the passage. When you have decided which choice is best, fill in the corresponding space on your answer sheet. There is only one best answer for each question.

Can creativity evolve with aging—maybe even flower with aging? If you belong to the "can't teach an old dog new tricks" school of thought, you may think that unless you have been an artist or writer or musician your whole life you are unlikely to be one in midlife—that increased creativity isn't compatible with growing old.

But research into fields as varied as neurology, behavioral science and art history says otherwise. So do the thousands of people who are finding that different types of creativity can accompany aging.

There is the artistic creativity of people like Bill Traylor, a folk art painter who did not pick up a paintbrush until he was 85 years old.

There is the exhilaration of the 81-year-old whose late-life burst of creativity led to her discovery of literature, a discovery she felt changed her life.

Then there is social creativity, a deftness with interpersonal relationships, that older people, the keepers of the culture, have traditionally offered.

The point is not that every older person can or should be a Picasso, but that aging precludes neither productivity nor creative energy. Moreover, creative capacity after age 65 is considerably more common than most people realize.

Creativity at older ages is not just a matter of anecdote; science has shown that the potential for intellectual growth with aging has biological underpinnings. Studies of the brain show that, in response to a more stimulating or challenging environment, brain cells sprout new extensions, improving their communication with other brain cells.

The same studies, along with behavioral research, indicate that brain cells respond to mental exercise just as muscle cells respond to physical exercise. Science, in short, supports the maxim "use it or lose it" when it comes to the aging brain.

There are several ways of categorizing the creative impulses of older persons:

- creativity that continues with aging;
- creativity that commences with aging;
- creativity that changes with aging;
- creativity in response to late-life loss.

There are famous examples of older people exuding creativity throughout their lives—Picasso experimenting with new styles of painting in his 90s, Verdi composing new operas in his 80s, George Bernard Shaw writing new plays in his 90s.

—"Contemplating Creativity"
by Dr. Gene Cohen Reprinted with permission from
AARP Bulletin, April 1997 Copyright © 1997 by AARP

1. According to this passage, the relationship between aging and creativity can be
   A. direct.
   B. indirect.
   C. mutually exclusive.
   D. unpredictable.

2. Bill Traylor is an example of which one of the following types of creativity?
   A. Composing music
   B. Social creativity
   C. Literature discovery
   D. Folk art painting

3. A theoretical basis for creativity at older ages is that
   A. intercommunication among brain cells expands in response to physical exercise.
   B. intercommunication among brain cells expands in response to stimulating environments.
   C. intellectual growth increases in the aging brain.
   D. intellectual growth decreases in the aging brain.

4. The point of this article is to explain
   A. different types of creativity.
   B. the scientific and behavioral research studies about creativity and aging.
   C. that aging and creativity are compatible.
   D. the different stages related to creativity and aging.

5. Which one of the following statements is true?
   A. All aged people are creative.
   B. Only people who have been creative in younger life can be creative in older life.
   C. The first sign of creativity may occur in older life.
   D. Only one type of creativity is seen in aged people.

STOP

IF YOU FINISH BEFORE TIME IS CALLED, YOU MAY CHECK YOUR WORK ON THIS SECTION ONLY. DO NOT TURN TO ANY OTHER SECTION IN THE TEST.

TEST 5

5 Questions • 9 Minutes

Review Unit 7, Reading Comprehension, before attempting this test.

> **Directions:** Carefully read the following passage and then answer the accompanying questions, basing your answers on what is stated or implied in the passage. When you have decided which choice is best, fill in the corresponding space on your answer sheet. There is only one best answer for each question.

A nearby flow of water is a very convenient place to dispose of waste materials, and people have been doing this for many years. If the right chemicals are dumped into the water, it can be beneficial. Lakes tend to follow a course from being deep, clear, nutrient-poor lakes to becoming shallow and more productive nutrient-rich lakes. This is the natural course of most lakes, and the addition of chemicals such as phosphates and nitrates can actually accelerate this process. To a certain extent, this is beneficial, and it has been done intentionally in some cases. But when carried to extremes, it can lead to a human-caused natural disaster. The water produces so much algae that most other forms of life cannot exist, and the lake chokes to death. In most cases, factories and sewage drains have carried this addition of chemicals too far.

Another consequence of dumping waste material into waterways, especially lakes, occurs when the waste contains metals, such as copper. Some metals literally cover the lake bottom and kill off all the bottom-dwelling organisms. Since many of these organisms are responsible for the decomposition of organic material on the bottom, the removal of these animals results in a great deal of the organic material remaining undecomposed, decreasing the nutrient content of the environment.

The dumping of waste materials from combustion into the air is quite obvious every time you look at the skyline of any major industrial area. Dumping poisonous materials into the environment has resulted in the destruction of many of our oxygen-producing plants and has driven many animals from our immediate environment. Another result that strikes perhaps closer to home is the increase in lung disease attributed to air pollution. Moreover, the propellants from aerosol cans cause problems by deteriorating the ozone layer of the atmosphere. This depletion allows greater amounts of ultraviolet radiation to reach the surface of the Earth. This higher level of radiation reputedly causes an increase in skin cancer.

Both air and water pollution are a retaliation by nature to human abuse. We assume that the dumping of wastes into the environment is a one-way process, and we do not count on any repercussions. But the cost of dumping garbage into the environment is slowly coming back to haunt us. Whether it be by the return of mercury and DDT to us in our food, or the destruction of shields in the atmosphere that protect us from being burned by the sun's radiation, we will pay for our assaults on the environment.

1. What title would best express the main idea of this section?
   A. "Save Our Lakes"
   B. "Humans' Responsibility Toward Nature"
   C. "Air Pollution"
   D. "How Pollution Causes Cancer"

2. According to this passage, one of the negative results of dumping waste chemicals into lakes is the
   A. increased growth of algae, which kills other organisms.
   B. discoloration of water.
   C. limitation of recreational activities.
   D. increased temperature in the water.

3. Two causes of air pollution are
   A. smoke and copper.
   B. aerosol cans and recycling of waste materials.
   C. decomposition of organisms and deoxygenation of plants.
   D. dumping of waste materials and use of aerosol cans.

4. The author's attitude toward environmental protection is
   A. complacency.
   B. pro-conservation.
   C. indifference.
   D. apathy

5. The author's reference to the driving of animals from our immediate environment implies
   A. migration.
   B. extinction.
   C. destruction.
   D. poaching.

STOP

IF YOU FINISH BEFORE TIME IS CALLED, YOU MAY CHECK YOUR WORK ON THIS SECTION ONLY. DO NOT TURN TO ANY OTHER SECTION IN THE TEST.

ANSWER KEYS AND EXPLANATIONS

Test 1

1. D	2. B	3. A	4. C	5. A

1. **The correct answer is D.** The title of a piece typically reflects the main idea of that piece. Only choice D is broad enough to cover the range of information in the passage. Choices A, B, and C focus on just one detail in the passage.

2. **The correct answer is B.** The answer is found in sentence 5 of paragraph 1.

3. **The correct answer is A.** The answer is found in sentence 4 of paragraph 1.

4. **The correct answer is C.** The answer is found in sentence 6 of paragraph 1.

5. **The correct answer is A.** The answer can be inferred by putting together the information in the two clauses in sentence 7 of paragraph 1.

Test 2

1. C 2. A	3. A	4. A	5. D	6. B

1. **The correct answer is C.** The answer is stated in sentence 2 of paragraph 1.

2. **The correct answer is A.** The answer is stated in the last sentence in paragraph 2.

3. **The correct answer is A.** The answer is stated in sentence 1 in paragraph 5.

4. **The correct answer is A.** The answer can be found by integrating information in sentence 1 and sentence 3 in paragraph 1.

5. **The correct answer is D.** The answer can be inferred from information in paragraphs 6 and 7.

6. **The correct answer is B.** The answer can be inferred from information in paragraphs 6 and 7.

answers

Test 3

1. B 2. A	3. A	4. D	5. C	6. D

1. **The correct answer is B.** The answer is stated in sentence 2 of paragraph 4.

2. **The correct answer is A.** The answer is stated in sentence 1 of paragraph 3.

3. **The correct answer is A.** The answer is stated in the last sentence in paragraph 7.

4. **The correct answer is D.** The answer is stated in sentence 3 in paragraph 8.

5. **The correct answer is C.** The answer can be inferred from information in paragraph 9.

6. **The correct answer is D.** The answer is stated in sentence 4 in the last paragraph.

Test 4

1. A	2. D	3. B	4. C	5. C

1. **The correct answer is A.** That there is a direct relationship between aging and creativity is the main idea of the entire passage.

2. **The correct answer is D.** The answer is stated in paragraph 3.

3. **The correct answer is B.** The answer is stated in sentence 2 in paragraph 7.

4. **The correct answer is C.** When a question asks about the point of a passage, it's asking for the main idea of the passage. Look for the broadest, that is, the most general answer. In this case, it's choice C. The other answer choices give just one detail of the passage, not the general idea of what the passage is about.

5. **The correct answer is C.** The answer is found in the second bullet point in paragraph 9.

Test 5

1. B	2. A	3. D	4. B	5. A

1. **The correct answer is B.** Any question that asks you to choose the best title for a passage is really asking you to identify the main idea of the piece. Look for the title that is the broadest, the most general. In this set of answers, it's choice B. The other choices focus on just one detail in the passage.

2. **The correct answer is A.** The answer is stated in sentence 6 in paragraph 1.

3. **The correct answer is D.** The answer is stated in sentences 1 and 4 in paragraph 3.

4. **The correct answer is B.** All the information in the passage suggests that the author supports conservation, so his or her attitude, or tone, is *pro-conservation*.

Choice A is incorrect because *complacency* means "a feeling of self-satisfaction," which doesn't fit the information chosen by the author to include in the passage. *Indifference* (choice C) is also incorrect because the word means "lacking concern or care for something." Choice D is incorrect because *apathy* means "a lack of interest, being indifferent."

5. **The correct answer is A.** The answer can be inferred from sentence 2 in paragraph 3. If the sentence didn't have the phrase "our immediate environment," then either choice B or choice C could be correct. Choice D is incorrect because there is no indication that illegal shooting of animals is involved.

Judgment and Comprehension in Practical Nursing

OVERVIEW

- **Using Professional Judgment in Practical Nursing**
- **Judgment and Comprehension in Practical Nursing Answer Sheet**
- **Judgment and Comprehension in Practical Nursing Test**
- **Answer Key and Explanations**

USING PROFESSIONAL JUDGMENT IN PRACTICAL NURSING

The Psychological Services Bureau (PSB) Aptitude for Practical Nursing Examination includes a section titled "Judgment and Comprehension in Practical Nursing Situations." According to PSB, "This test is concerned with the measurement of the exercise of judgment and comprehension in the working relationships experienced by the practical and vocational nurse as a student and as a practitioner" (http://psbtests.com/available-tests/). This section consists of 50 multiple-choice questions (A–D) to be answered in 30 minutes.

The questions in this section each provide a clinical scenario that requires a response from the practical or vocational nurse. To answer these questions, you must apply your intuition and knowledge of the responsibilities of practical and vocational nurses in clinical practice and in their working relationships by selecting the answer that provides the most appropriate action or response by the nurse.

Below is a practice test to help familiarize you with this type of question and evaluate your ability to apply your intuition, judgment, and knowledge to practical nursing situations.

JUDGMENT AND COMPREHENSION IN PRACTICAL NURSING ANSWER SHEET

1. Ⓐ Ⓑ Ⓒ Ⓓ   5. Ⓐ Ⓑ Ⓒ Ⓓ   9. Ⓐ Ⓑ Ⓒ Ⓓ   13. Ⓐ Ⓑ Ⓒ Ⓓ   17. Ⓐ Ⓑ Ⓒ Ⓓ
2. Ⓐ Ⓑ Ⓒ Ⓓ   6. Ⓐ Ⓑ Ⓒ Ⓓ   10. Ⓐ Ⓑ Ⓒ Ⓓ   14. Ⓐ Ⓑ Ⓒ Ⓓ   18. Ⓐ Ⓑ Ⓒ Ⓓ
3. Ⓐ Ⓑ Ⓒ Ⓓ   7. Ⓐ Ⓑ Ⓒ Ⓓ   11. Ⓐ Ⓑ Ⓒ Ⓓ   15. Ⓐ Ⓑ Ⓒ Ⓓ   19. Ⓐ Ⓑ Ⓒ Ⓓ
4. Ⓐ Ⓑ Ⓒ Ⓓ   8. Ⓐ Ⓑ Ⓒ Ⓓ   12. Ⓐ Ⓑ Ⓒ Ⓓ   16. Ⓐ Ⓑ Ⓒ Ⓓ   20. Ⓐ Ⓑ Ⓒ Ⓓ

answer sheet

JUDGMENT AND COMPREHENSION IN PRACTICAL NURSING TEST

20 Questions • 10 Minutes

1. As you begin your shift, a coworker approaches you and says, "Did you hear what Linda did at the party last night?" Linda is another coworker. Your best response would be to

   A. encourage the coworker to share the story so you can better bond with her.

   B. listen politely and then report the coworker's behavior to your supervisor.

   C. threaten to report the coworker for spreading gossip if she continues this behavior.

   D. change the subject to something more appropriate.

2. In an interview for a practical nurse position at a hospital, the interviewer asks whether you attend religious services in your community. The most appropriate response would be to say:

   A. "I don't see how my religious beliefs are relevant to this position, so I'd prefer to move on to another question."

   B. "It's illegal for you to ask me that question; expect to hear from my lawyer soon."

   C. "I'd be happy to discuss my religious beliefs; what would you like to know?"

   D. "Organized religion is for haters."

3. A patient reports her pain level as 8 out of 10. You ask her whether she would like more of her pain medication, which her provider has prescribed to be used as needed. The patient shakes her head "no" and smiles, but you notice that she is grimacing as she does so. The most appropriate response would be to

   A. urge the patient to take the medication.

   B. respect her wishes and move on to your next task.

   C. ask if there is a reason she doesn't want to take it.

   D. hide the medicine in her food.

4. You enter a patient's room and greet him. You would like to learn about how he did overnight. The best thing to say would be:

   A. "Did you sleep well last night?"

   B. "Tell me about how you did last night."

   C. "Did the pain medication help last night?"

   D. "Are you feeling well-rested this morning?"

5. When you ask a patient whether she needs to get up to use the bathroom, she replies, "I went a few hours ago." Your best response would be to

   A. begin to raise the head of her bed so you can assist her to the bathroom.

   B. move on to your next task, as it seems she is fine.

   C. say, "Would you like some water?"

   D. say, "Are you telling me that you do not need to go to the bathroom now?"

6. You have arrived at a patient's room to take him to imaging services to have some x-rays taken. Your next action should be to

   A. begin raising the head of his bed to make it easier for him to transfer to a wheelchair.

   B. explain to the patient where you are taking him and why.

   C. ask him whether he has any metal plates in his body.

   D. ask him whether he has fasted for at least 12 hours.

7. Practical and vocational nurses often access a patient's personal health information. The quality most important for this task is

   A. confidentiality.

   B. empathy.

   C. creativity.

   D. flexibility.

8. You are wheeling a patient into the imaging services department to have some x-rays taken when the radiology technician informs you that there's been some mistake and that the patient is not due for imaging now. Your best response is to

   A. confirm the patient's identity with the technician and then report the mix-up to your supervisor.

   B. demand that the technician apologize to you and the patient for the error.

   C. take the patient back to his room and then file a complaint through your supervisor.

   D. give the technician a stern look and then take the patient back to his room.

9. A nurse's main responsibility is

   A. diagnosing disease.

   B. treating disease.

   C. collecting health data.

   D. caring for patients.

10. You are about to enter the room of a patient to give him his daily bed bath when you notice that several of his family members who just arrived from out of town are visiting him. Your best response is to

    A. knock on the door and politely ask the family members to step out while you bathe the patient.

    B. enter the room, ignoring the visitors, and begin setting up to administer the bath.

    C. plan to return later in your shift to give the patient his bed bath.

    D. skip the patient's bath and move on to your next task.

11. In working with a patient, you are following the steps of the nursing process. Your first action would be

    A. planning nursing care.

    B. implementing nursing care.

    C. assessing the patient.

    D. evaluating nursing care.

12. You enter the room of a patient who is wearing a hijab, or Muslim head covering. You notice that her food which includes pork is untouched. When you ask about why she is not eating, she replies, "I am Muslim. I cannot eat this." The most appropriate response is:

    A. "I'm sorry for the mix-up. Would you like me to see what other food options we have?"

    B. "There's nothing in your health record about special dietary needs. I'll need to check with my supervisor about this."

    C. "Oh, it won't kill you to eat it just this once. Go ahead and try it."

    D. "Sorry about that. Your next meal will be breakfast, and it should be safe."

13. You are meeting a newly admitted patient for the first time, who appears to be a woman in her 90s. She is accompanied by several family members. When asking about her health history, you should address

    A. the patient's daughter.

    B. the patient directly using your normal tone of voice.

    C. the patient directly with a loud voice.

    D. the whole family, speaking very slowly and clearly.

14. The 7-year-old sister of an infant recently admitted to the hospital for a serious birth defect appears frightened by the situation, and her mother is occupied with speaking to the surgeon in the patient's room. The most appropriate nursing action would be to say:

    A. "Your brother has spina bifida, which is a serious condition and requires immediate surgical repair."

    B. "Don't worry, sweetie; the doctors will fix your brother and everything will be fine."

    C. "I understand your being scared, but we will do everything we can to take care of your little brother."

    D. "This is no place for a little girl; your mother needs to take you home."

15. A patient in the ER complains of severe abdominal pain and asks for some pain medication. The patient has not yet been examined by a physician. Your best response would be to

    A. locate some appropriate pain medications and administer them immediately.

    B. tell the patient he must be examined first and that only the physician can prescribe him pain medication.

    C. ignore the patient and go on about your business.

    D. ask the patient whether he has an addiction to prescription pain relievers.

16. While observing you administer an injection to a patient, your supervisor criticizes your technique. Your best response is to

    A. accept the criticism and ask for direction on how to improve.

    B. explain that you are doing the best you can and that it's not reasonable to expect you to do it perfectly.

    C. explain that this is the way you learned in school, so it must be right.

    D. apologize and say that you think you're not cut out to be a nurse.

17. You are early in your first interview at a hospital for a practical nurse position, and the interviewer asks you whether you have any questions. The best response at this point would be:

    A. "No, I can't think of any off the top of my head."

    B. "What is the staff-to-patient ratio like in this unit?"

    C. "What is the pay for this position?"

    D. "How many vacation days would I get in this position?"

18. Practical and vocational nurses often must change their approach to patient care as the patient's condition and other key factors can change unexpectedly. The quality most important in these situations is

    A. compassion.

    B. dependability.

    C. adaptability.

    D. effective communication skills.

19. One of your coworkers has an approach to bathing patients that is different from the way you learned in school and that annoys you. The appropriate response is for you to

    A. educate your coworker on the approach you learned and explain why it is better.

    B. report the coworker's behavior to your mutual supervisor.

    C. apologize later to the patient for your coworker providing inferior care.

    D. ignore the differences in your approaches and mind your own business.

20. A patient who is under the care of one of your coworkers loses control of her bladder while ambulating in the hall with a nursing assistant and leaves a trail of urine behind her. Your coworker is providing wound care to another patient currently and is unavailable. Your best response would be to

    A. set up caution signs in the hall and ask your coworker to clean it up later.

    B. clean up the urine yourself immediately to prevent any falls.

    C. report the mess to your supervisor.

    D. ignore the mess, knowing that someone else will clean it up at some point.

ANSWER KEY AND EXPLANATIONS

1. D	5. D	9. D	13. B	17. B
2. A	6. B	10. C	14. C	18. C
3. C	7. A	11. C	15. B	19. D
4. B	8. A	12. A	16. A	20. B

1. **The correct answer is D.** Spreading gossip about coworkers is not appropriate or professional, nor is encouraging such behavior. The response in this situation would probably be to change the subject to something more appropriate, to diffuse the gossip. Choice A is incorrect because this would promote rather than discourage the gossip, and there are healthier ways to bond with coworkers than through sharing gossip. Choice B is incorrect because listening politely also encourages the gossip, and reporting the behavior to your supervisor, unless it is a chronic problem with this coworker, is not warranted. Choice C is incorrect because threatening to report a coworker is inappropriate in this context as a simpler, less antagonistic option is available.

2. **The correct answer is A.** It is, indeed, illegal for an employer to ask questions in an interview about an applicant's age, gender, race, ethnicity, nationality, religion, or sexual orientation. Religious beliefs are not an appropriate topic in an interview for a nursing position as they are not relevant. In this case, the best response would be to point out the lack of relevance of the question and to ask to move on to another question. Choice B is incorrect because, although it is true that such questions are illegal, threatening to bring a lawsuit is unnecessarily provocative and would likely end any chances of getting the position, which might still be desirable despite the interviewer's improper question. Choice C is incorrect because, even if you are comfortable talking about your religious beliefs, they are not an appropriate topic for an interview. Choice D is incorrect because, like answer B, it is unnecessarily provocative.

3. **The correct answer is C.** The patient in this scenario is clearly in pain and would likely benefit from taking the medication but for some reason is refusing to take it. The best response would be to find out the reason she does not want to take it; then, the nurse may be able to help resolve whatever objection the patient has so that she can take the medication. Choice A is incorrect because the nurse should never coerce the patient to take medication against her will. Choice B is incorrect because it misses the opportunity to learn more about the patient's refusal of the medication and to potentially help overcome it. Choice D is incorrect because the nurse should not deceive the patient or force her to take the medication against her will.

4. **The correct answer is B.** When communicating with patients, it is usually better to ask open-ended questions or requests rather than yes-or-no questions, as open-ended questions usually elicit more information from the patient. This allows us to rule out choices A, C, and D, which are all yes-or-no questions.

5. **The correct answer is D.** The patient does not directly answer the nurse's question and may have even misunderstood it. The nurse's best response would be to clarify the patient's response by asking a follow-up

question. Choice A is incorrect because the patient has not clearly indicated that she needs to go to the bathroom. Choice B is incorrect because the nurse has not confirmed that the patient does not need to use the bathroom. Choice C is incorrect because it does not address whether, in fact, the patient needs to use the bathroom.

6. **The correct answer is B.** You should always explain to the patient what action you are about to take and why before performing the action. Choice A is incorrect because this should be done after explaining where you are taking him and why. Choice C is incorrect because metal plates are a concern when a patient is undergoing magnetic resonance imaging, not an x-ray. Choice D is incorrect because patients are not required to fast before x-rays.

7. **The correct answer is A.** When dealing with a patient's personal health information, the privacy of which is protected by law, confidentiality is a key quality for the nurse to possess. Empathy, creativity, and flexibility, although important qualities to have when performing other tasks, are not as important as confidentiality when it comes to working with a patient's personal health information.

8. **The correct answer is A.** Honest mistakes happen all the time in the hospital, and there is no need to demand an apology, file a complaint, or even give the radiology technician a stern look, which allows us to rule out choices B, C, and D. However, it would be prudent to double-check the patient's identity with the radiology technician just to make sure you are referring to the same patient and then to report the mix-up to your supervisor in case further action or follow-up is necessary.

9. **The correct answer is D.** The nurse's primary responsibility is caring for patients.

Diagnosing and treating disease are the primary responsibilities of physicians, nurse practitioners, and other healthcare providers, although nurses assist in carrying out these responsibilities. This allows us to rule out choices A and B. Nurses also collect health data, but that is not their main responsibility, so we can rule out choice C.

10. **The correct answer is C.** When a task is not urgent and a patient is visiting with family, it would be appropriate to return later in your shift to perform it, so as to not unnecessarily interrupt their visit. Choice A is incorrect because it is an interruption to the family's visit. Choice B is incorrect because it interrupts the visit and also because the patient may not be comfortable being bathed with others present in the room. Choice D is incorrect because the patient should receive a bath and this can be performed later in your shift.

11. **The correct answer is C.** The steps in the nursing process are (1) assess the patient, (2) make the nursing diagnosis, (3) plan the nursing care, (4) implement the nursing care, and (5) evaluate the nursing care.

12. **The correct answer is A.** It is important for nurses to be sensitive to their patients' unique needs related to their culture and make every effort to provide culturally appropriate food options. Choice B is incorrect because if the food restriction is not noted in the patient's record, it does not mean that the nurse shouldn't offer other food options. Choice C is culturally insensitive, and choice D is negligent.

13. **The correct answer is B.** When working with an older patient, you should directly address them just as you would any other patient. Do not assume that just because a person is older that they are mentally incompetent or deaf.

14. **The correct answer is C.** The best nursing response in this situation is to comfort the child without giving her false reassurance. Choice A is incorrect because, although true, it is not comforting and not at the appropriate level for a 7-year-old. Choice B is incorrect because it is providing false reassurance to the child. Choice D is incorrect because the girl has the right to be in her brother's room in the hospital and because there may not be anyone else available to keep her other than her mother.

15. **The correct answer is B.** Not only is it beyond the scope of a practical nurse to prescribe medications to a patient or administer a medication for which a patient has no prescription, it is a serious ethical and legal breach. This rules out choice A. Choice C is incorrect because ignoring the patient's request is inappropriate as it does not address his concern. Choice D is incorrect because it is an unfounded assumption and unnecessarily provocative and rude.

16. **The correct answer is A.** When your supervisor gives a correction related to your performance, you should graciously accept the criticism without complaining or making excuses, and ask for direction on how to improve. Choices B and C are incorrect because they are defensive and seek to shift the blame to someone else. Choice D is incorrect because making a mistake is normal and not an indication that you are not suited to be a nurse.

17. **The correct answer is B.** Generally, it is best to wait to discuss wages and benefits until the interviewer brings up this topic, which typically occurs later in the interview or series of interviews. This allows us to rule out choices C and D. Choice A is incorrect because not taking the opportunity to ask a question of the interviewer when offered may give the appearance of a lack of interest or preparation on the part of the applicant.

18. **The correct answer is C.** Changing one's approach unexpectedly requires much adaptability. Compassion, dependability, and effective communication skills are all important for other tasks but not as important as adaptability in this situation.

19. **The correct answer is D.** There are often many acceptable ways to perform various nursing tasks, such as bathing a patient, and you should not assume that the way you learned is necessarily superior to anyone else's way. So, in this case, it would be best to ignore the differences in approaches and mind your own business. Choice A is incorrect because it is arrogant to assume your way is better and also inappropriate for you to correct a coworker who does not report to you. Choice B is incorrect because your coworker has done nothing wrong and so you should not report the coworker's behavior to your supervisor. Choice C is incorrect because your coworker has not provided inferior care and because it is unprofessional to criticize your coworker's performance in front of a patient.

20. **The correct answer is B.** The best response would be for the nurse to take the initiative and clean up the mess. Choice A is incorrect because setting up caution signs, although better than doing nothing, still exposes others to the risk of slipping and falling and only postpones the inevitable job of cleaning up the mess. Choice C is incorrect because cleaning up the mess is a simple task that you can perform without informing your supervisor. Choice D is incorrect because ignoring the mess is negligent and dangerous.

NOTES

NOTES